Diseases of the Veins

Pathology, Diagnosis and Treatment

Diseases of the Veins

Pathology, Diagnosis and Treatment

Norman L Browse MD, FRCS

Professor of Surgery, United Medical and Dental Schools of Guy's and St Thomas's Hospitals.
Consultant Surgeon, St Thomas' Hospital, London

Kevin G Burnand MS, FRCS

Reader in Surgery, United Medical and Dental Schools of Guy's and St Thomas's Hospitals.
Consultant Surgeon, St Thomas' Hospital, London

Michael Lea Thomas MA, PhD, FRCP, FRCR

Senior Physician in Radiology, St Thomas' Hospital. Honorary Lecturer, United Medical and Dental
Schools of Guy's and St Thomas's Hospitals, London

Edward Arnold

A division of Hodder & Stoughton

LONDON   BALTIMORE   MELBOURNE   AUCKLAND

© Norman L Browse, Kevin G Burnand and Michael Lea Thomas, 1988

First published in Great Britain 1988

British Library Cataloguing in Publication Data

Browse, Norman
    Diseases of the veins: pathology, diagnosis and treatment.
    1. Veins——Diseases
    I. Title   II. Burnand, Kevin G.   III. Lea Thomas, M.
    616.1′4   RC695

    ISBN 0-7131-4523-4

Typeset in 10/11 pt Times by Colset Private Ltd, Singapore
Printed and bound in Great Britain for Edward Arnold, the educational academic and medical publishing division of Hodder and Stoughton Limited, 41 Bedford Square, London WC1B 3DQ by Butler & Tanner Ltd, Frome and London

Preface

Interest in the physiology and pathology of the veins has waxed and waned over the centuries. The development of methods of measuring blood pressure and blood flow gave an enormous impetus to the study of the circulation but the new methods were mainly applied to the heart and arteries. For the first forty years of this century the veins could truly be thought of as the Cinderella of the circulation, neglected, and almost forgotten.

The past forty years has seen a steady change in this attitude brought about by the efforts of a relatively small number of physiologists, surgeons and radiologists such as Kenneth Franklin, Edwin Wood, John Shepherd, John Ludbrook, Robert Linton, Harold Dodd, Frank Cockett, Robert May, Carl Arnoldi, JC dos Santos, Gunnar Bauer, T Greitz, A Gullmo and Orsten Almen.

The scientific study of venous disease began when JC dos Santos introduced phlebography. By chance the beginning of our own interest in venous thrombosis, pulmonary embolism, venous ulceration, the post-thrombotic syndrome and varicose veins coincided with the invention and acceptance of the X-ray contrast media that made phlebography safe – a technical 'breakthrough' that enabled our inquisitiveness to flourish, produce over 300 publications and to write this book.

A book describing and criticizing every publication about the veins would extend into many volumes. We therefore chose to write a book which analyses and discusses what we consider to be the important publications on venous disease but which also presents our own views and attitudes to venous problems, with ample references for the reader who wishes to seek out the sources on which our opinions are based.

We hope that the result is a practical, readable book containing something for medical students, residents and consultants, which quotes facts but which questions current views and stimulates the reader to begin his own enquiries.

We are particularly indebted to Dr Graham Miller for his excellent chapter on Pulmonary Embolism. All the other chapters have been written by ourselves.

Two areas have been intentionally omitted, the intracerebral veins and the portal venous system, because disorders of these veins are usually fully discussed in textbooks of neurosurgery and gastroenterology as they tend to present to specialists in these fields rather than to generalists or phlebologists.

Many of the views presented in this book have developed from our association with the physiologists, radiologists and surgeons already mentioned, our former research associates and residents, J Ackroyd, MR Andress, P Baskerville, R Beard, JN Bowles, GM Briggs, A Chilvers, EW Fletcher, L Gray, P Jarrett, G Layer, R Leach, D Negus, T O'Donnell, A Pimm, J Waters, S Whitehead, and our excellent Technical Staff, D Rutt, D Sizeland, Marian Morland and Gill Clemenson. This book is the fruit of all our labours. We hope it is a worthwhile contribution to the dissemination of knowledge about diseases of the veins.

London, 1988

NLB
KGB
MLT

Acknowledgements

All three of us owe much to the stimulation of our colleagues and teachers. Many have been mentioned in the preface but three deserve special mention, John Shepherd, John Kinmonth and Frank Cockett. Our interest in the veins and the peripheral circulation would never have begun if we had not met and worked with these men.

Our research has depended upon the devoted support of the technical staff of the Department of Surgery and Radiology of St Thomas' Hospital, London, guided by Mr DL Rutt, Senior Chief Medical Laboratory Scientific Officer and Miss DA Hannigan, Senior Radiographer.

The illustrations have been produced by Mr TW Brandon and his colleagues in the Department of Photography.

We are most grateful to Sterling Research Laboratories for defraying the cost of the coloured illustrations.

The burden of typing the manuscript has fallen on our secretaries, Julia Hague, Solveig Joannides, Barbara Neal and Linda Lewis. In addition to working on the manuscript, Vivienne Beckett and David Sizeland have catalogued and checked all the references.

We are greatly indebted to all those mentioned and many others for their support and encouragement and particularly to our Publishers, Edward Arnold, who encouraged us to write the book yet accepted the delays that are inevitable when busy clinicians try to write.

Contents

1

Milestones, pebbles and grains of sand

Time, and the judgement of our successors, will decide which of the papers on venous disease published in this century have made a major contribution to the advancement of our knowledge and understanding. Even the smallest paper helps to expand our knowledge. The greatest house needs grains of sand in its cement to hold the bricks and the keystones in place.

This chapter presents the publications, in chronological order, which we think have advanced contemporary understanding. They show that man has had a considerable empirical understanding of the treatment of venous problems for at least 2000 years but that a real appreciation of the physiological and pathological processes involved had to await the greatest advance of all, William Harvey's description of the circulation of the blood.

The story begins in Ancient Egypt.

1550 BC
The first 'venous' publication?

The Ebers papyrus was written in 1550 BC. One section contains a description of three types of lump, together with the advice that two types can be treated surgically but 'certain *serpentine windings* are not to be operated upon because that would be head on the ground'.

Majno and others[13,17,20] have suggested that the term 'serpentine windings' means varicose veins which should not be incised lest a fatal ('head on the ground') haemorrhage occur. If this interpretation is correct, this is the first known, 'venous' publication.

Ebers papyrus, 1550 BC.

4th century BC
The first illustration of a varicose vein?

Figure 1.1 is a votive tablet found at the foot of the Acropolis in Athens. It shows the medial side of a massive leg with a long serpentine swelling which has all the characteristics of a varicose vein. Is the small mortal performing a Trendelenberg test on his God, or does the God have gross hypertrophy of the limb with congenitally abnormal veins? This is the oldest known illustration of a varicose vein. Perhaps Doctor Amynos, to whom the tablet is dedicated, was one of the first phlebologists.

6th century BC
The first description of a function for the veins?

In his description of the life and works of Alcmaeon of Croton, Codellas states that Alcmaeon believed that 'sleep was the retreat of blood to the veins and awakening its forth pouring' and that death was caused by 'the total retreat of blood to the veins'.[7]

The works of Alcmaeon of Croton, 6th century BC.

460–377 BC
Hippocrates and the veins

There are many references to the vascular system and to ulcers in the works of Hippocrates.[1,6,15]

In *De carnibus* he states that 'two vessels arise from the heart, the one called an artery the other called a vein.' When discussing wounds he describes the fact that a loose tourniquet will cause

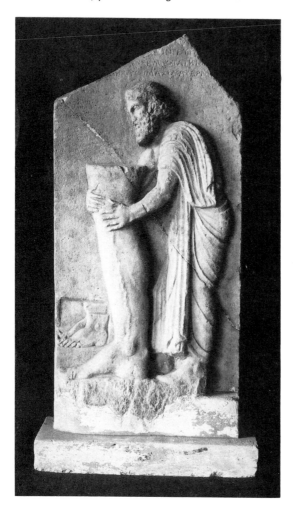

Fig. 1.1 This votive tablet was found on the site of the sanctuary (temple) of the hero, Doctor Amynos, at the base of the west side of the Acropolis in Athens. According to the inscription it was offered and dedicated to Doctor Amynos by Lysimachidis of Acharnes, son of Lysimachos. It is estimated to date from the end of the 4th century. It is the earliest known depiction of varicose veins.

(We are grateful to the National Archeological Museum of Greece for permission to reproduce this illustration and for the historical information.)

excessive bleeding whereas a tight tourniquet may cause gangrene.

In *De ulceribus* he states that 'in the case of an ulcer it is not expedient to stand, more especially if the ulcer be situated in the leg' and then describes the causes of ulcers including, possibly, venous thrombosis.

He also says, 'We must avoid wetting all ulcers except with wine, unless the ulcer be situated near a joint, for the dry is nearer to the sound and the wet to the unsound.'

A little later he warns, 'When a varix is on the fore part of the leg and is superficial, or below the flesh, and the leg is black and seems to stand in need of having the blood evacuated from it, such swellings are not by any means to be cut open, for generally large ulcers are the consequences of the incisions'. Is this a warning against the treatment of superficial thrombophlebitis in the gaiter area of the leg by incision and evacuation of the thrombosis?

Majno[18] has compiled a description of how Hippocrates would have treated a fat woman with varicose veins and a venous ulcer based on the many references to ulcers found throughout the Hippocratic texts. He suggests that Hippocrates would have given the following advice.

- Wash the ulcer, only puncture it once in a while lest a large sore follow.
- If necessary, cut out the ulcer and then compress it to squeeze out the blood and humours.

Perhaps this is the first reference to compression dressings for venous ulceration even though the main objective was to keep the ulcer open to let out the 'evil humours'.

Hippocrates. *De ulceribus* and *De carnibus*, 460–377 BC.

479–300 BC
Did the Chinese recognize venous ulceration?

The Yellow Emperor's Classic of Internal Medicine was written by Huang Ti Nei Ching Su Wen. Although the Yellow Emperor lived in 2600 BC, the book was probably written between 479 and 300 BC making it contemporary with Hippocrates. It certainly describes the treatment of ulcers but whether it refers to varicose veins depends entirely upon the translator's interpretation of the ancient text.[27] This interpretation varies considerably in different translations making it difficult to decide whether the Chinese physicians recognized a connection between venous abnormalities and ulceration.

Huang Ti Nei Ching Su Wen. *The Yellow Emperor's Classic of Internal Medicine.* 400 BC.

335 BC
Veins are different from arteries

Praxagoras of Cos was probably the first physician to differentiate between arteries and veins when he stated that the veins contained blood whereas the arteries contained air.[14,24]

The Writings of Praxagoras, 335 BC.

270 BC
The ligation of blood vessels. The beginning of vascular surgery

The foundation of the Alexandrian School of Medicine in Egypt and the innovations of its two greatest physicians, Herophilos and Erasistratos were the progenitors of vascular surgery. These physicians invented artery forceps and were the first to ligate blood vessels, thus controlling bleeding and making surgery possible.[19] They noticed that the valves of the heart stopped retrograde blood flow[16]and, although they thought that the arteries contained air, Erasistratos knew that a tourniquet caused congestion of the venous blood in a limb but did not know how this occurred because he did not appreciate that the blood circulated.[4,21]

Burggraeve states that Herophilos discovered the lacteals.[3]

The works of these remarkable men were lost when the great library at Alexandria was destroyed in AD 391, a tragic event that delayed the advance of medicine for 1000 years.

200 BC
Indian ulcers

The practice of medicine developed in India at the same time and just as swiftly as in the Mediterranean. The main textbook of Indian surgery was the *Sushruta Samhita* which describes the treatment of ulcers with maggots to clear away necrotic material, curettage, and dressings using leaves. It also describes the use of Chinese cloth bandage for the treatment of ulcers. This inelastic material would have acted in the same way as a modern impregnated bandage.

The Sushruta Samhita. 200 BC. Translated by K.L. Bhishogratna. Chowkhamba Sanskrit Series Office. India, Varanasi 1907-1911.

AD 14-37
Roman ulcers

Celsus was the great Roman physician. He lived during the Emperorship of Tiberius. In many of the Hippocratic texts it is not clear whether the term ulcer is used in its modern sense or as a collective noun that includes all forms of wounds. Celsus distinguished between wounds and ulcers[5] and advised the use of plasters and linen bandages to pull ulcers together. He described the ligation of veins that were bleeding, the double clamping and division of veins between ligatures, and treated varicose veins by avulsion and cauterization. He used antiseptics on wounds and described the four cardinal physical signs of inflammation.

Celsus AC. *De medicina* AD 25.

AD 130-200
Galen – the beginning of varicose vein surgery

Galen of Pergamum described the treatment of ulcers and varicose veins by venesection. He noticed that the walls of the veins were always much thinner than the walls of arteries and that veins contained dark blood. He described the use of silk ligatures and advised that varicose veins should be treated by incision and tearing out with a blunt hook.[12,28]

The works of Claudius Galen. AD 130-200.

AD 502-575

According to Anning, Aetius of Amida re-described the ligation of varicose veins in the 6th century AD.[2]

AD 900
Keep the ulcer open!

In AD 900 Avicenna was still supporting the Hippocratic view that ulcers should not be allowed to heal because they were a site from which 'evil humours' could escape. If an ulcer did heal, he advised that it should be deliberately broken down again.[26]

Avicenna. *De ulceribus*. Lib IV. 10th century.

1306
Wrong reasons, right result

Although Maitre Henri de Mondeville described the use of bandages on the limbs to drive out the 'evil humours' from ulcers, he correctly realized that compression bandaging helped the ulcer to heal.[22] He would probably have explained ulcer healing by claiming that it was no longer needed once the bandages had expelled all the bad humours.

Chirurgie de Maitre Henri de Moneville. 1302–1320.

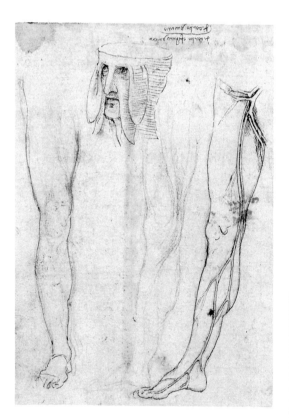

Fig. 1.2 Leonardo's drawing of the superficial veins of the lower limb. This leg did not have a posterior arch vein, often called Leonardo's Vein, nor are any communicating veins visible.

1452
The anatomy of the veins as seen by a great artist

The masterly anatomical drawings of Leonardo da Vinci (Figs. 1.2, 1.3 and 1.4) show how clearly he observed the venous system. Interestingly, the leg in Fig. 1.2 does not have a posterior arch vein, which is often called Leonardo's vein, and no communicating veins are shown.

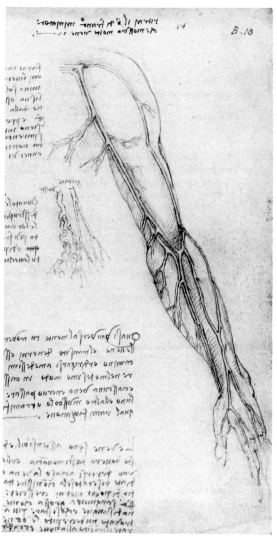

Fig. 1.3 Leonardo's drawing of the superficial veins of the arm.

1510–1590
A local compression dressing

Ambroise Paré described the ligation of varicose veins and the long saphenous vein in the thigh[23]. While he was employed as a surgeon to Henri II in 1553, he cured the ulcer of his captor, Lord Vandeville, by regular bandaging. His method was to 'roule the leg beginning at the foote and finishing at the knee, not forgetting a little bolster upon the varicose veine'.

The works of Ambroise Paré. c. 1560–1580.

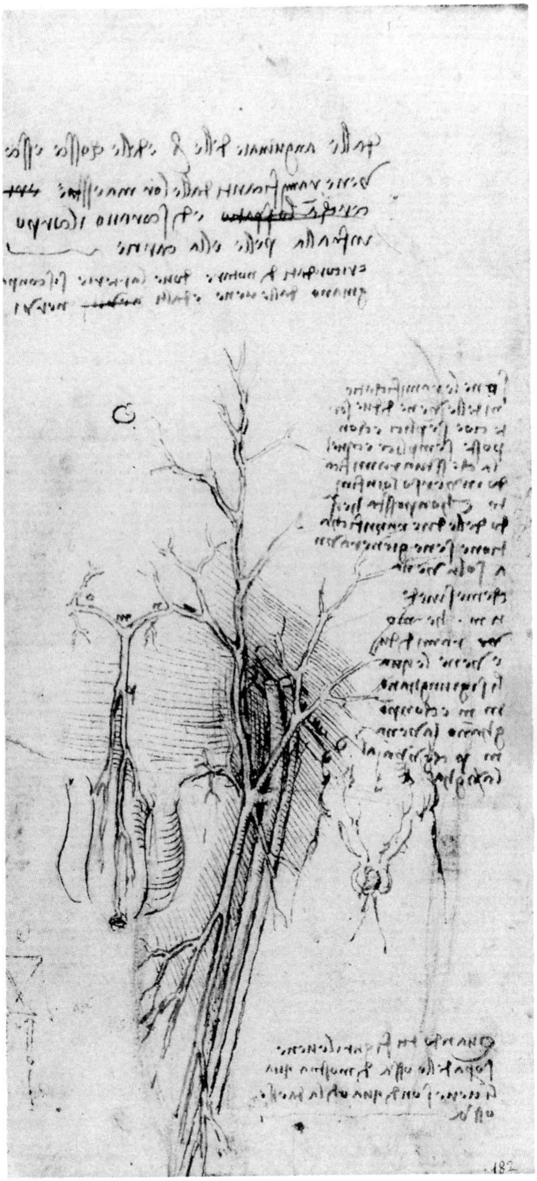

1547–1580
Venous valves

In 1562 Fallopius stated that Amatus Lusitanus testified to him that JB Canano had described the valvular fold in the azygos vein to him (Amatus) in 1547. It is possible that this was the first description of a venous valve. In 1551 Amatus stated that the veins contained valves and that it was he that had given proof of this a thousand times since 1547. Whether Canano or Amatus was the first to demonstrate the valves will never be known. Franklin[9] and Friedenwald[10] have reviewed the arguments over the historical precedence. Withington[29] and Friedenwald[10] concluded that Amatus showed the valves to Canano, Friedenwald believing that Fallopius misunderstood the description of the dissections in Ferrara in 1547, conducted by Canano and Amatus together.

Lusitanus A. *Centuriae I*, Curat. 52, 1551; *Centuriae V*, Curat. 70, 1560.

1514–1564
The first complete anatomical description of the veins (but no valves!)

Vesalius described the venous system in detail. It seems certain that he was told about the valves by Canano in 1546, when visiting Ratisborn. He then looked for them himself, could not find them and subsequently denied their existence.[11]

Vesalius *Fabrica*. 1555.

1585
A drawing of a valve, at last

Figure 1.5 is believed to be the first recorded drawing of a valve in a vein. It was published by Saloman Alberti in 1585.

Alberti, S. *De valvutis membraneis quorundam vasorum*. Tres orations. Norimb. 1585.

Fig. 1.4 Leonardo's detailed drawing of the tributaries of the long saphenous vein in the groin. (Royal Library, Windsor Castle. R.L. 19113R [QIV8r] Copyright reserved. Reproduced by gracious permission of Her Majesty The Queen.)

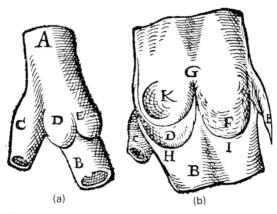

(a)   (b)

Fig. 1.5 (a and b)   These illustrations, published by Saloman Alberti in 1585, are the first known drawings of a venous valve.

(a) This shows the outside of a leg vein (AB) with a muscle tributary (C). D and E are the bulging valve sinuses.

(b) This shows the opened veins with the mouth of the tributary (K), the valve cusp (E) cut away to reveal the sinus (F), the agger of each cusp (H and I) and the cornua of the cusps (G).

1593–1603
A full description of the valves

Hieronymus Fabricius of Aquapendente re-described the valves in his work entitled *De venarum ostiolis* after he had demonstrated them at public dissections in 1579. He noticed that they stopped retrograde flow but thought that they participated in the control of the ebb and flow of blood described by Galen.

Fabricius may have described the relationship between gangrene and venous thrombosis in his book *Gangraena et Sphacelo*, and he definitely described the double ligature and division between the ligatures of varicose veins in his book *Opera Chirurgica*.

It is significant that William Harvey worked with Fabricius between 1599 and 1603 and that Fabricius was a pupil of Fallopius who was in turn a pupil of Vesalius.

Fabricius H. *De venarum ostiolis*. 1603.
Fabricius H. *De gangraena et sphacelo*. Cologne 1593.
Fabricius H. *Opera chirurgica*. 1593.

1620
A connection between varicose veins and ulcers

In 1620 Fallopio stated that 'varices carry faeculent humours which cause ulceration'.[8]

Fallopio G. *La chirurgica*. Venice. 1620.

1628
The great revolution: the blood circulates

William Harvey published *De Motu Cordis* in 1628. This work produced the greatest revolution of physiological thought since medicine began and was the foundation of our present understanding of the circulation. Figure 1.6 illustrates the fundamental observation made by Harvey that the valves in the veins are there to ensure unidirectional blood flow.

Harvey W. *Exercitatio anatomica de motu cordis et sanguini in animalibus* Frankfurt. W. Fitzer. 1628.

1644
Venous occlusion observed

Schenck described an occlusion of the inferior vena cava.

Schenck. *Observationum Medicum Rariorum* 1644 Lugduni. Lib 3; 339.

1669
The first use of the term 'venous tone' and the first description of the calf muscle pump

Richard Lower used the words 'relaxato venarum tono' in his book *De Corde*. This is the first description of 'venous tone'. In his next book, *Tractatus de corde item de motu et colore sanguinis et chyli in eum transitu*, Lower clearly appreciated the effect of the limb muscles on blood flow, so giving the first description of the peripheral muscle venous pump.

Lower R. *De Corde*. 1669.
Lower R. *Tractatus de corde item de motu et colore sanguinis et chyli in eum transitu*. London. Allestry 1670.

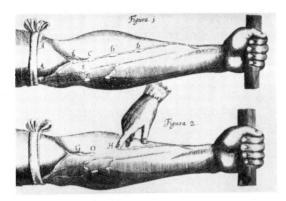

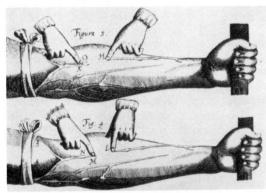

Fig. 1.6 The illustration from *De Motu Cordis* that depicts the simple but incontrovertible experiment that convinced William Harvey that the blood circulates.

Fig. 1. The text states: 'Let an arm be ligated above the elbow in a living human subject as if for blood letting. [AA] At intervals there will appear, especially in country folk and those with varicosis, certain so to speak nodes and swellings [BCDEF] not only where there is a point of division [EF] but even

where none exists [CD] and those nodes are produced by valves, which show up in this way in the outer part of the hand or of the elbow. If by milking the vein downwards with the thumb or a finger [*Fig. 2*, O to H] you try to draw blood away from the node or valve [*Fig. 2*, O], you will see that none can follow your lead because of the complete obstacle provided by the valve; you will also see that the portion of vein [*Fig. 2*, O H] between the swelling and the drawn-back finger has been blotted out, though the portion above the swelling or valve is fairly distended [*Fig. 2*, O G]. If you keep the blood thus withdrawn [back to H] and the vein thus emptied, and with your other hand exert a pressure downward towards the distended upper part of the valves [*Fig. 3*, K], you will see the blood completely resistant to being forcibly driven beyond the valve [*Fig. 3*, O]. And the greater the effort you put into your performance, the greater will be the swelling and distension of the vein which you will see at the valve or swelling [*Fig. 3*, O], though below that the vessel is empty [*Fig. 3*, H O].

Moreover, if, with the arm ligated as before [AA] and the veins swelling up, you press on one of them some distance [*Fig. 4*, L] below a selected swelling or valve, and thereafter with a finger [M] stroke the blood upwards to the region above the valve [N], you will see that part of the vein remaining empty and the blood to pass back through the valve [as in *Fig. 2*, H O]. When, however, you take your finger [*Fig. 2*, H] away, you will see the stretch of vein fill up again from the parts below, and become as in *Fig. 1*, D C. *Whence it is clearly established that the blood moves in the veins from parts below to those above and to the heart, and not in the opposite way.'* (Authors' italics.)

Based on K.J. Franklin's translation of *De Motu Cordis*. Springfield. Ill. C.C. Thomas, 1957.

1676
'Varicose' ulcers and a compression stocking

Richard Wiseman, Sergeant Surgeon to Charles II and a neighbour of Richard Lower, redescribed the association between varicose veins and ulceration. He appreciated the effect that venous dilatation had on the valves and used the term 'varicose ulcer'. He invented a leather lace-up stocking for the treatment of venous disease of the lower limb which was the forerunner of the modern elastic stocking (see Fig. 15.2) and also described a case of postpartum white leg.

In 1652 Wiseman was an assistant to Edward Molins, Surgeon to St Thomas's Hospital, and so would have worked at St Thomas's, a privilege enjoyed by the authors who have often considered re-introducing his lace-up stocking to their own practice.

Figure 1.7a–d shows four abstracts from Wiseman's book which describes the treatment of varicose veins and varicose ulcers and reveals his deep understanding of the problems.

Wiseman R. *Severall Chirurgicall Treatises*. London. Royston and Took 1676.

(a)

and fuffers the reft of the ftream to pafs by it. This moft commonly happens in cutaneous Veffels, where the Veins have no affiftance from mufcular Flefh which by frequent preffure would otherwife be apt to fqueeze it forwards. To which it may be added, that the Valves of the Vein fo fwelled, whether naturally or accidentally, are weakened, and do not fufficiently fupport the Blood in its afcent; fo that, falling down upon the fides of the Veffel, the weight of it is too great to be driven forward by the venal motion of the Blood.

(b)

The *Varices* ought not to be cured, unlefs they be painful, or that they be extended into a large Tumour, or ulcerate and bleed much: for, as I have faid, they preferve Health. But if there be a neceffity of curing them, it ought to begin with Purging and Bleeding, not once or twice, but often repeated; and if the *Vifcera* be in fault, they ought to be ftrengthned and amended; after which the Cure may be endeavoured by aftringent and exficcant Medicaments, and thofe to be applied with convenient Bandage, to prefs back the Blood coagulating in the Veffel, and moderately refift the Current. If thefe fuffice not, then, according to the ancient practice, you are to proceed by Section, dividing the Skin, and feparating the Teguments; and having raifed the varicous Vein, you are to pafs a Ligature above and another beneath it, making a deligation of them; then flit the Vein, caft out the grofs Blood, and afterwards digeft and heal it, as is after faid in an *Aneurifma*. With what fuccefs this hath been done, you may read in the Works of *Fabricius Hildanus*: and whether the Pain be

(c)

Such another was commended to my hands by Doctor *Weatherly*. The Ulcer was in the Leg, and had been very vexatious to the Patient: it was accompanied with fome little Fluxion, enough to relax the Parts, and keep the Ulcer from digefting, and confequently from healing. I dreffed it as in the former Obfervation hath been faid; only inftead of a Rowler I put on a laced Stocking: by the wearing of which the Humours were reftrained, and the Patient cured himfelf in a few days by the Unguents fore-mentioned.

(d)

which it fwelled, and became more humid. After fome while, when I faw the temper of the Member alter, I ordered a laced Stocking to be put on, for that I could not with a Rowler make fuch a Compreffion fo near the Ancle as I would, without caufing a fwelling in his Foot. I dreffed it with Pled-

Fig. 1.7 Excerpts from Richard Wiseman's book *Severall Chirurgicall Treatises*. Fourth Edition. London. Benjamin Tooke 1705.

(a) Book I Chapter XIV 'of a Varix' Page 64 lines 10–16.
This refers to superficial thrombophlebitis which Wiseman considered occurred in cutaneous vessels because there is no 'assistance to blood flow from the muscles', a clear reference to the calf muscle pump, and also states that 'the valves of dilated veins are weakened and cannot support the blood'.

(b) Book I Chapter XIV 'of a Varix', Page 65 lines 12–15.
A description by Wiseman of the surgical method for curing varicose veins. After describing the surgical cure he says 'I have never met one patient that cared to hear of the Cure by ligature nor indeed have I seen any great reason for it. For if the unsightliness and pain be in the legs it may be helped by the wearing of a laced stocking'.

(c) Book II Chapter II 'Of a simple ulcer' page 166 lines 25–31.
This describes the use of the laced stocking instead of a bandage (Rowler) followed by ulcer healing in a few days.

(d) Book II Chapter III 'Of Ulcers with Intemperies' page 171 lines 14–17. This describes the application of local compression with the laced stocking. Wiseman observes that tight compression with a bandage caused swelling of the foot.

1733
Measurement of venous pressure

The Reverend Stephen Hale measured arterial and venous pressures in conscious animals.

Hale S. *Statistical Essays Containing Haemastatics or an Account of Some Hydraulic and Hydrostatical Experiments made on the Blood and Blood-vessels of Animals* Vol 2. London. W Innys and R Manby 1733.

1758
Gravity

Sharp, in his book *A Treatise on the Operations of Surgery*, stated that 'the indisposition of these sores (leg ulcers) is in some measure owing to the gravitation of the humours downward', thus showing an appreciation that gravity affects the blood and interstitial fluid within the lower limb. Newton described his Laws of Gravity 71 years earlier in 1687.

Sharp. *A Treatise on the Operations of Surgery*. London. Touson 1758.

1688
Tumours spread inside veins

Blancardus observed the intraluminal venous spread of a tumour when he described an inferior vena cava 'filled with neoplastic "steatomatous" matter'.

Blancardus. *Anatomica Practica Rationalis*. 1688 Obs. XVI; 38.

1759–1768
Milk oedema

Pusoz, Levret and Astruc all thought that postpuerperal white leg was due to excess milk in the legs.

Pusoz N. *Traite des Accouchemens*. Paris. Deslandes 1759.
Levret. *L'art des Accouchmens* 3rd edition. Paris. Didot 1766.
Astrud J. *Traite de Maladies des Femmes*. Paris. Cavelier 1761–1765.

1769
A system opposed to coagulation

Morgagni noticed that the blood failed to clot after a sudden death.

Morgagni GB. *De sedibus et causis morborum per Anatomen Indigatis*. Venice. 1769.

1784
Lymphoedema

White suggested that the postpuerperal white leg was caused by rupture of the lymphatics.

White C. *An Enquiry into the Nature and Cause of the Swelling in One or Both Legs which Sometimes Happens to Lying Women*. Warrington. 1784.

1786
Venous oedema

Haller described the oedema that follows the ligation or obstruction of a major vein.

Haller A. *First Lines of Physiology*. 1786.

1793
Stasis causes thrombosis

Baillie gave the first British description of inferior vena caval obstruction and stated that a reduction in the rate of blood flow leads to thrombosis. This was perhaps the first reference to 'stasis' as a cause of thrombosis.

Baillie M. *Transactions of a Society for the Improvement of Medical and Chirurgical Knowledge* I, 1793; 119.

1794
Fright keeps the blood liquid

John Hunter noticed that the blood of a stag hunted to death had not coagulated.

Hunter J. *A Treatise on the Blood, Inflammation and Gunshot Wounds*. London. 1794; 26.

1797
Hydrostatic forces matter

Home stated that the patient's height and weight affected the pressure in the veins and the development of ulcers. He also said that the symptoms of venous disease varied with the weather.

Home E. *Practical Observations on the Treatment of Ulcers on the Legs Considered as a Branch of Military Surgery*. London. Nichol 1797.

1799
A paste bandage

In a book on the management of all forms of leg ulcer, Baynton reported that ulcers were situated on the distal part of the limb because they were remote from 'the foundation of life and heat' and were at a disadvantage for the return of blood and lymph from the legs. He introduced a primitive form of paste bandage.

Baynton T. *A New Method of Treating Old Ulcers of the Legs*. Bristol. Emery and Adams 1799.

1810
White leg is not exclusively a complication of pregnancy

Ferriar described a case of phlegmasia alba dolens associated with typhus and, though he still thought this was caused by a lymphatic abnormality, this is probably the first description of deep vein thrombosis other than in childbirth.

Ferriar J. An affectation of the lymphatic vessels hitherto misunderstood. *Medical Histories and Reflections* 1810; Vol 3: 129.

1822
The relationship between phlegmasia alba and thrombosis finally established

Davis described how deep vein thrombosis caused phlegmasia alba dolens and re-emphasized its relationship to childbirth.

Davis DD. The proximate cause of Phlegmasia Dolens. *Med Chir Trans* 1822; 12: 419.

1824
A thesis on venous disease

In 1824 Briquet wrote a detailed thesis on venous disease. He pointed out that phlebectasy was most pronounced in the superficial veins near large communications with deep veins. He understood that the calf muscles acted as a pump but thought that all the blood flowed out of the lower limb through the superficial veins, having passed from the deep to the superficial veins through the communicating veins.

Briquet. *These de Paris.* 1824.

1824
Physiological explanations of therapy

Astley Cooper stated that compression of varicose veins restored the competence of the valves. He also reiterated the importance of varicose veins in the genesis of leg ulcers.

Cooper A. *The Lectures of Sir Astley Cooper Bart. on the Principles and Practice of Surgery* London. Thomas 1824.

1845
An invention that revolutionized medical science

Francis Rynd invented the hypodermic needle in 1845. This led to the development of sclerotherapy, the measurement of intravascular pressures and the analysis of blood samples.

1846
A clinical test of incompetence

Brodie described reflux down the long saphenous vein and its prevention by direct digital pressure. This was the first description of a clinical test of venous incompetence. He used plaster and bandages to heal ulcers and recognized that some dressings caused skin sensitivity reactions.

Brodie B. *Lectures on Pathology and Surgery.* 1846.

1852
Initial injury causes thrombosis

Rokitansky reported that venous thrombosis occurred in a vein at the site of an injury or where the vein was adjacent to an area of inflammation. He came very close to describing Virchow's well-known triad, which was published 8 years later.

Rokitansky C. Venous thrombosis due to vein injury, neighbouring inflammation, or blood changes. In: *Pathological Anatomy.* 4 London. Sydenham Society 1852; 336.

1854
The medicated compressing bandage

Unna described the use of a non-compliant plaster dressing for the treatment of ulcers, which became known as the 'Unna Boot'.

Unna PG. Veber Paraplaste eine neue form medikaneutoser Pflaster. 1854 *Wien Med Wochenschr* 1896; **46**: 1854.

1855
A connection between deep and superficial vein incompetence

Verneuil, in his book on varicose veins, described the anatomy of the veins of the leg in detail and stated that varicose veins were caused by incompetence of the deep veins.

He observed that the valves in the communicating veins, which he also described, stopped blood flowing from the deep to the superficial system.

Verneuil A. Du Siege reel et primitif des varices des membres inférieurs. *Gazette Medicale Paris* 1855; **10**: 524.

1859
The source of pulmonary emboli, the causes of thrombosis, and a hint of fibrinolysis

Virchow described the association between thrombosis in the legs and emboli in the lung in 1846 and, later in other publications, and his seminal book *De Cellular Pathologie* he described the three predisposing causes of thrombosis – changes in the vessel wall, the blood flow and the blood. He also recorded that blood remained fluid in the capillaries after death.

Propagating thrombus and pulmonary emboli were clearly depicted in Virchow's great book (Figs. 1.8, 1.9 and 1.10).

Virchow R. Die Verstopfung den Lungenarteries und ihre Folgen. *Beitr z exper Path u Physiol* 1846; **21**.
Virchow R. Neuer Fall von todlicher Emboli der Lungerarteries. *Arch path Anat* 1856; **10**: 225.

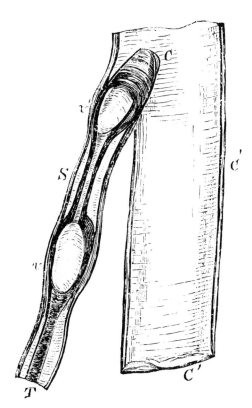

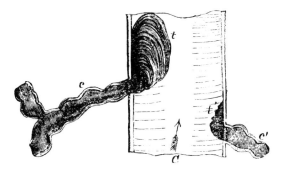

Fig. 1.10 This is Figure 71 of the English translation of Virchow's *Cellular Pathology* (1860). It shows 'two small varicose circumflex veins of the thigh filled with autochthonous (original) thrombus projecting beyond the orifices into the trunk of the femoral vein. The prolonged thrombus (t) is produced by concentrically opposed deposits from the blood. The prolonged thrombus (t¹) is irregular because fragments (emboli) have become detached from it'. This figure clearly shows that Virchow had seen and recorded how thrombus is formed by successive layers of thrombus deposition producing what are now called the 'Lines of Zahn', 15 years before the mechanism was described by Zahn.[30]

Fig. 1.8 This is Figure 69 of the English translation of Virchow's *Cellular Pathology* (1860). It shows 'thrombosis of the saphenous vein(s), thrombi seated on the valves (v,v¹) in process of softening and connected by more recent and thinner portions of coagulum: Prolongation of the plug (C) projecting beyond the mouth of the saphenous vein into the femoral vein'.

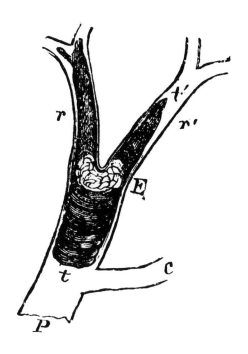

Fig. 1.9 This is Figure 72 from the English translation of Virchow's *Cellular Pathology* (1860). It illustrates the features of a pulmonary embolus. 'The embolus (E) is astride the angle formed by the division of the pulmonary artery (P). The capsulating (secondary) thrombus (t and t¹) reaches in front of the embolus (t) to the next highest collateral vessel, behind the embolus (t¹) it fills in great measure the diverging branches (r and r¹) ultimately terminating in the form of a cone'.

Virchow R. *Die Cellular Pathologie*. Berlin. Verlag von August Hirschwald 1859.

1863
Bed-rest and elevation

In his book *Rest and Pain* Hilton observed that venous ulcers were frequently above the medial malleolus, that ulcers can be healed by rest and that incompetent communicating veins are probably ulcerogenic.

Hilton J. *Rest and Pain* London. Bell and Daldy Lecture IX 1863.

1864
The beginning of sclerotherapy

In his book on varicose veins Chapman reported that a Frenchman, Monsieur Pravaz 'has tried to sclerose varicose veins by injecting perchloride of iron'.

Chapman HT. *Varicose Veins, their Nature, Consequence and Treatment* London. Churchill 1864.

1866
Thrombosis damages the valves – a classic example of clinical and autopsy observation

In 1866 John Gay published a book based on a series of Lettsomian lectures. The illustrations in this book are obviously hand-drawn by Gay from autospy dissections and are rather crude but they clearly show the communicating veins and the posterior arch vein. (Figs. 1.11, 1.12, 1.13 and 1.14).

Gay appreciated that leg ulcers were more difficult to heal if varicose veins were present, commenting that 'when the varicose veins are relieved the ulcers are as readily cured as ulcers in general'. His drawings clearly show post-thrombotic deep vein damage and even old thrombi in the deep veins, the significance of which he fully appreciated and recognized.

Gay J. *On Varicose Disease of the Lower Extremities*. Lettsomian Lecture. London. Churchill 1866.

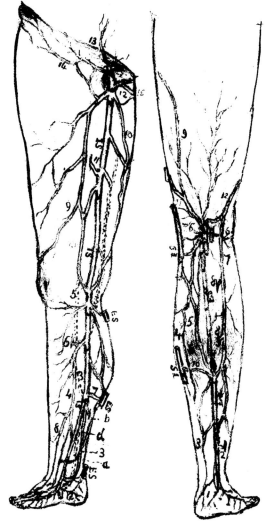

Fig. 1.11 This drawing from John Gay's lecture on 'Varicose Disease of the Lower Extremities' shows the anatomy of the long and short saphenous vein. It depicts and labels the posterior arch vein (which he calls the loop vein) (3) and the medial communicating veins (b, d and 6).

1868
Venous not varicose ulcers

Spender published his book on ulcers and venous disease 2 years after Gay's book, and similarly recorded the fact that ulcers could occur in the absence of varicose veins if there had been post-thrombotic damage to the deep veins, the first

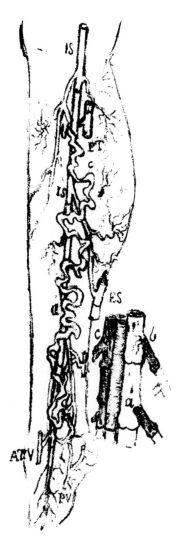

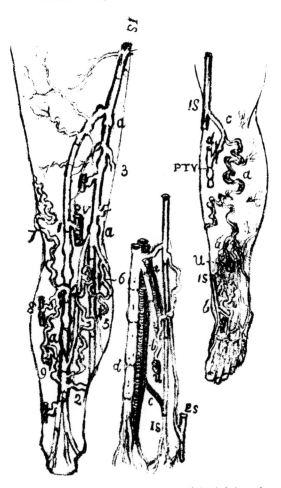

Fig. 1.12 John Gay's illustration of the varicose veins in the right leg of a 56-year old woman who died of erysipelas of the left leg. The inset shows the tributaries of the posterior tibial veins filled with old thrombus (6). The text states that 'the posterior tibial artery was so encrusted that its cavity was almost entirely obliterated'. An example of combined venous and arterial insufficiency.

Fig. 1.13 John Gay's dissection of the left leg of a 55-year old man with ulcers on both legs. The anterior view shows the long saphenous vein connecting with the posterior tibial vein (PTV), and in the inset a vein from beneath the ulcer (u) connecting with the saphenous vein and a deep vein (b). The text states: 'The peroneal and the outer posterior tibial venae comitantes were narrowed throughout, and their channels obstructed by old blood clot which pervaded their tributaries to the first valves as well as a large branch (Inset, c) by which the latter of these veins was connected with the internal saphena.'

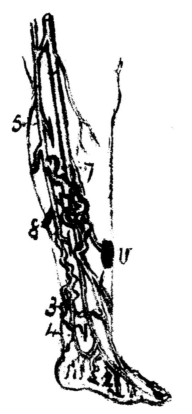

Fig. 1.14   John Gay's drawing of the veins on the medial side of the leg of a 56-year old man with a venous ulcer. It clearly shows the posterior arch vein and the text describes three communicating veins (3, 8 and 5).

indication that the term varicose ulcer was misleading. Both Gay and Spender referred to venous rather than varicose ulcers.

Spender JK. *A Manual of the Pathology and Treatment of Ulcers and Subcutaneous Diseases of the Lower Limbs.* London. Churchill 1866.

1870
The long saphenous vein is often normal when its tributaries are varicose

In Holmes *Surgery* Callender pointed out that superficial varices mainly occur in the tributaries of the long saphenous vein, not in the long saphenous vein itself.

Callender in Holmes *Surgery* 1870.

1871
Primary venous tumours

Perl described a primary vein wall tumour.

Perl L. Ein Fall von Sarkom der Vena Cava Inferior. *Virchows Arch Pathol Anat* 1871; **53**: 378.

1878
Elastic compression bandages

In 1878 Martin wrote a long letter to the *British Medical Journal* describing the use of india-rubber bandages for the treatment of leg ulcers. He gave a detailed description of their method of application and the way in which they produced compression.

Martin HA. The india-rubber bandage for ulcers and other diseases of the legs. *Brit Med J* 1878; **2**: 624.

1891
The logical surgical treatment of long saphenous incompetence

Trendelenberg described the ligation of the long saphenous vein in the upper third of the thigh to prevent long saphenous vein reflux. He did not advocate a flush ligation of the long saphenous vein at the sapheno-femoral junction.

Trendelenberg F. Uber die Unterbindung der Vena Saphena magna bie unterschenkel varicen. *Beitrag Z clin Chir* 1891; **7**: 195.

1894
The first operation for deep venous insufficiency

Parona (cited by Turner Warwick)[25] described ligation of the popliteal vein for venous problems because he believed that superficial varicose veins were secondary to deep varicose veins.

Parona. Poloclinico. *Chirurgie* 1894; **8**: 9.

1894
The connection between surgery and deep vein thrombosis

Von Strauch observed and recorded the occurrence of deep vein thrombosis after a surgical operation.

Von Strauch M. Uber venen thrombose der unteren extremitaten nach koliotomien bei bechenhock largering und athernarkose. *Zentrac f Gynak* 1894; **18**: 304.

1895
A test of deep vein obstruction

Perthes described his walking test for detecting obstruction of the communicating veins.

Perthes G. Uber die Operation der Unterschenkel-varicen nach Trendelenburg. *Dtsch med Wechr* 1895; **21**: 253.

1899
Silent and symptomatic thrombosis

Welch described 'bland' and 'infective' thrombus. He noticed that pulmonary emboli could come from latent as well as from overt deep vein thrombosis. This was the beginning of the notion that there were two types of thrombosis – thrombophlebitis and phlebothrombosis, a concept which has now been abandoned.

Welch WH. *A System of Medicine 6*: 155 C. Albutt. London. Macmillan 1899.

1905 and 1906
Stripping

Keller and Mayo described techniques for stripping out the long saphenous vein.

Keller. A new method of extirpating the internal saphenous and similar veins in varicose conditions. *New York Med J.* 1905; **82**: 385.
Mayo CH. Treatment of varicose veins. *Surg Gynec Obstet* 1906; **2**: 385.

1906
The advent of reconstructive venous surgery

Carrel and Guthrie, in their Nobel Prize winning work on vascular anastomosis, made the first attempts at vein transplantation.

Carrel A, Guthrie CC. Uniterminal and bi-terminal venous transplantation. *Surg Gynec Obstet* 1906; **2**: 266.

1911
The beginning of physiological measurements on peripheral veins

Hooker noticed that exercise affected the pressure in the veins of the lower limb but he did not measure it precisely.

Hooker DR. The effect of exercise upon the venous blood pressure. *Am J Physiol* 1911; **28**: 235.

1916 and 17
Primary and secondary varicose veins

Homans described the treatment of varicose veins and classified them as primary if the deep veins were normal, and as secondary if the deep veins showed evidence of post-thrombotic damage. He suggested that leg ulcers were caused by post-thrombotic deep vein damage and introduced the concept that venous stasis was the ultimate cause of venous ulceration.

Homans J. The operative treatment of varicose veins and ulcers, based upon a classification of these lesions. *Surg Gynec Obstet* 1916; **22**: 143.
Homans J. The aetiology and treatment of varicose ulcers of the leg. *Surg Gynec Obstet* 1917; **24**: 300.

1923
Phlebography

Berberich and Hirsch described their first attempt at venography using strontium bromide.

Berberich J, Hirsch S. Die roentgenographische Dorstellung der Arterien und Venen am lebenden Menschen. *Klin Wschr* 1923; **2**: 2226.

1924
The pathology of the thrombus

Aschoff, in his lectures on pathology, argued that iliofemoral thrombus began at the groin and propagated downwards. He also described the pathological feature of thrombus formation and growth, which Virchow had drawn 65 years earlier (see Fig. 1.10).

Aschoff L. *Lecture Notes on Pathology*. New York. Hoeber 1924.

1926
Venous thrombectomy

Basy described a case of thrombosis of the right axillary vein treated by phlebotomy, removal of the thrombus and suture of the vein. This is probably the first description of venous thrombectomy.

Basy L. Thrombose de la veine axillaire droite (thrombo-phlebite par effort). Phlebotomie, ablation de caillots, suture de la veine. *Mem Acad Chir* 1926; **52**: 529.

1928
Anatomy of venous valves

Franklin's historical survey of the discovery of the valves of the veins signalled a resurgence of interest in venous physiology and pathology.

Franklin KJ. Valves in veins. An historical survey *Proc R Soc Med Section of History of Medicine.* 1928; **21**: 1.

1930
'Gravitational' ulcers and safer phlebography

Dickson Wright described the use of local dressings and adhesive bandages (Elastoplast) for the treatment of venous ulcers and introduced the term 'gravitational' ulcer.

Ratschow introduced the first water-soluble X-ray contrast material, a di-iodinated pyridine derivative, for phlebography.

Ratschow M. Uroselektan in der Vasographie unter spezieller Berucksichtigung der Varikographie. *Forschr Rontgenstr* 1930; **42**: 37.
Wright D. Treatment of varicose ulcers *Brit Med J* 1930; **2**: 996.

1931
An early 'gold standard'

In 1931 Turner Warwick published an important monograph on varicose veins which stimulated interest in the surgical treatment of venous disease. Much of his thoughts were based on the work of Gay, Spender, Briquet and Verneuil. In this book he described the 'bleed-back' test which is still used at operation to test the competence of the valves in the communicating veins.

Turner Warwick W. *The Rational Treatment of Varicose Veins and Varicocele.* London. Faber 1931.

1933
Fibrinolysis

Tillett and Garner observed that the haemolytic streptococcus produced a substance which broke down fibrin.

Tillett WS, Garner RL. The fibrinolytic activity of haemolytic streptococci. *J Exper Med* 1933; **58**: 485.

1936
Plasmin

Schmitz described the nature of plasmin.

Schmitz A. Uber die Proteinase des fibrins. *Zeitschrift fur Physiologische Chemie* 1936; **244**: 89.

1937
The destructive effect of thrombosis

Edwards and Edwards showed that a venous thrombosis destroyed the valves but was frequently followed by recanalization.

Edwards FA, Edwards JE. The effect of thrombophlebitis on the venous valve. *Surg Gynec Obstet* 1937; **65**: 320.

This year also saw the publication of Franklin's important monograph on the physiology of the veins, the first book of our era solely concerned with this topic.

Franklin KJ. *A Monograph on Veins.* Springfield. Thomas 1937.

1937
Heparin

After many years of basic research Murray and his co-workers described the use of heparin in animals as a form of preventing thrombosis after vascular injury.

This was followed by Crafoord's description of the use of heparin in man.

Murray DWG, Jaques LB, Perrett TS, Best CH. Heparin and the thrombosis of veins following injury. *Surgery* 1937; **2**: 163.

Crafoord C. Preliminary report on post-operative treatment with heparin as a preventative of thrombosis. *Acta Chir Scand* 1937; **79**: 407.

Natural fibrinolysis

In 1937 MacFarlane described postoperative hyperfibrinolysis.

MacFarlane RG. Fibrinolysis following operation. *Lancet* 1937; **1**: 10.

1938
Thrombectomy and the mechanism of venous gangrene

Gregoire established that gangrene can be caused by deep vein thrombosis, and Lawen described the removal of a thrombus from a leg vein.

Gregorie M. La phlebite bleu (Phlegmatia Caerulea Dolens) *Presse Med* 1938; **46**: 1313.
Lawen A. Weitere erfahrungen uber operative Thrombanentfernung bei venethrombose. *Arch Klin Chir* 1938; **193**: 723.

1938
Clinical phlebography

Dos Santos described a clinically applicable technique of phlebography.

Dos Santos JC. La phlebographie directe. Conception, technique, premier resultats. *J Int Chir* 1938; **3**: 625.

Communicating vein ligation

In 1938 Linton described the operation of subfascial ligation of the medial lower leg communicating veins.

Linton RR. The communicating veins of the lower leg and the operative technique for their ligation. *Ann Surg* 1938; **107**: 582.

1939
Heparin and deep vein thrombosis

Crafoord described the use of heparin for the treatment of postoperative deep vein thrombosis.

Crafoord C. Heparin and post-operative thrombosis *Acta Chir Scand* 1939; **82**: 319.

1939
Thrombectomy accepted

Leriche described a technique of thrombectomy for deep vein thrombosis.

Leriche R, Geisendorf W. Resultats d'une thrombectomie precoce avec resection veineuse dans une phlebite grave des deux membres inférieurs. *Presse Med* 1939; **47**: 1239.

1939
'osis or 'itis

Oschner and DeBakey established (temporarily) the use of the terms 'phlebothrombosis' and 'thrombophlebitis' in an extensive review of the current knowledge of venous thrombosis.

Oschner A, DeBakey M. Therapy of phlebothrombosis and thrombophlebitis. *Southern Surgeon* 1939; **8**: 269.

1940
The clinical application of phlebography

Bauer applied phlebography to define the state of the deep veins in patients with deep vein thrombosis. This important publication set the scene for our present understanding of the post-thrombotic syndrome and the value of anticoagulant therapy.

Bauer G. A venographic study of thromboembolic patients. *Acta Chir Scand* 1940; **84**: Suppl. 61.

1941
The prevention of postoperative thrombosis with heparin

Crafoord and Jorpes attempted to prevent postoperative deep vein thrombosis by fully anticoagulating their patients with heparin. These patients had no pulmonary emboli, and surprisingly few bleeding complications in spite of the fact that they were given doses of 30–40 000 units daily.

Crafoord C, Jorpes E. Heparin as a prophylactic against thrombosis. *JAMA* 1941; **116**: 2831.

The effect of heparin on established deep vein thrombosis

Bauer continued his studies with phlebography and showed that the exhibition of anticoagulants early in the course of a deep vein thrombosis stopped its progression.

Bauer G. Venous thrombosis. Early diagnosis with aid of phlebography and abortive treatment with heparin. *Arch Surg* 1941; **43**: 463.

1942
The post-thrombotic syndrome

By performing further phlebograms on the patients he had studied 5 or more years earlier Bauer was able to describe the sequelae of deep vein thrombosis. He showed that a large proportion of patients who had had a major deep vein thrombosis developed post-thrombotic sequelae.

Bauer G. A roentgenological and clinical study of the sequels of thrombosis. *Acta Chir Scand* 1942; **86**: Suppl 74.

1946
Physiological fibrinolysis

MacFarlane and Biggs having observed that blood, taken after an operation, which had clotted later dissolved spontaneously, developed the concept that trauma, fear and anaesthesia stimulate fibrinolytic activity.

MacFarlane also developed the concept of the coagulation cascade.

MacFarlane RG, Biggs R. Observations on fibrinolysis, spontaneous activity associated with surgical operations and trauma. *Lancet* 1946; **2**: 862.

1947
Tissue plasminogen activator

In 1947 Astrup and Permin described tissue plasminogen activator, the initiator of fibrinolysis.

Astrup T, Permin PM. Fibrinolysis in the animal organism. *Nature* 1947; **159**: 681.

1948
The Bisgaard regimen

Bisgaard described his method of massage and bandaging for the treatment of venous ulceration.

Bisgaard H. *Ulcers and Eczema of the Leg. Sequels of Phlebjtis*. Copenhagen. Munksgaard 1948.

1948
Fibrinolysis balances coagulation

MacFarlane and Biggs described the presence of intrinsic fibrinolysis within the blood and postulated that it acted as a counterbalance to the coagulation system.

MacFarlane RG, Biggs R. Fibrinolysis: its mechanism and significance. *Blood* 1948; **3**: 1167.

1949
A test of venous function

Pollack and Wood measured the pressure in the saphenous vein at the ankle while the subject was standing and lying down and observed that the venous pressure fell during exercise.

Pollack AA, Taylor BE, Myers TT, Wood EH. The effect of exercise and body position on the venous pressure at the ankle in patients having venous valvular defects. *J Clin Invest* 1949; **28**: 559.
Pollack AA, Wood EH. Venous pressure in the saphenous vein at the ankle in man during exercise and changes in posture. *J Appl Physiol* 1949; **1**: 649.

1950
Low-dose heparin for the prevention of deep vein thrombosis

De Takats suggested that the injection of a low dose of heparin would prevent deep vein thrombosis after operation.

De Takats G. Anticoagulant therapy in surgery. *JAMA* 1950; **142**: 527.

1951–54
Therapeutic thrombolysis

Astrup described the isolation of a substance derived from tissues which was capable of activating the proteolytic enzymes in the blood. This was the beginning of the era of thrombolysis.

Innerfield, Schwarz and Angrist showed that trypsin dissolved thrombi; and Johnson and Tillett showed that intravascular thrombi could be dissolved by streptokinase.

Clifton and Sherry showed that plasmin could dissolve artificially induced femoral vein thrombi and arterial thrombi.

Mullertz showed that there is always a degree of fibrinolytic activity in human blood.

Astrup T. The activation of a proteolytic enzyme in the blood by animal tissue. *Biochem J* 1951; **50**: 5.
Astrup T, Stage A. Isolation of a soluble fibrinolytic activator from animal tissue. *Nature* 1952; **170**: 929.
Clifton EE, Grossi CE, Connamela DA. Lysis of thrombi produced by sodium morrhuate in the femoral vein of dogs by human plasmin (fibrinolysin). *Ann Surg* 1954; **139**: 52.

Innerfield I, Schwarz A, Angrist A. Intravenous trypsin. The anticoagulant fibrinolytic and thrombolytic effects. *J Clin Invest* 1952; **31**: 1049.

Johnson AJ, Tillett WS. The lysis in rabbits of intravascular blood clots by streptococcal fibrinolytic system (streptokinase). *J Exp Med* 1952; **95**: 449.
Mullertz S. A plasminogen activator in spontaneously active human blood. *Proc Soc Exper Biol Med* 1953; **82**: 291.
Sherry S, Titchner A, Gottesman L, Wasserman P, Troll W. The enzymatic dissolution of experimental arterial thrombi in the dog by trypsin, chromotrypsin and plasminogen activators. *J Clin Invest* 1954; **33**: 1303.

1953
'Blow-out veins'

In 1953 Cockett described the 'Ankle blow out syndrome' and its treatment by the extrafascial ligation of incompetent communicating veins. This paper revived European interest in the surgical treatment of venous ulceration.

Cockett FB, Jones DE. The ankle blow-out syndrome. A new approach of the varicose ulcer problem. *Lancet* 1953; **1**: 17.

1954
Phlebography for all

In 1954 sodium diatrozoate (a tri-iodinated con-

trast material) was introduced, heralding the widespread use of contrast phlebography. These agents are still in use but are being replaced by the much safer, virtually non-thrombogenic, low osmolality, non-ionic media.

Almen T. Contrast agent design: some aspects of the synthesis of water soluble contrast agents of low osmolality. *J Theo Biol* 1969; **24**: 216.

A deep vein bypass operation

Warren and Thayer published the first description of the use of the saphenous vein for bypassing a post-thrombotic occlusion of the superficial femoral vein.

Warren R, Thayer T. Transplantation of the saphenous vein for postphlebitic stasis. *Surgery* 1954; **35**: 867.

1956
Education

In 1956 Dodd and Cockett published their book on the treatment of venous disease of the lower limb. This book became the standard textbook on the treatment of venous disease and stimulated many surgeons throughout the world to develop an interest in this field of surgery.

Dodd H, Cockett FB. *The Pathology and Surgery of the Veins of the Lower Limb*. Edinburgh. Livingstone 1956.

1957
Bed-rest and thrombosis

Gibbs published a detailed description, based on autopsy studies, of the site of venous thrombosis and its relation to rest in bed.

Fontaine discussed the value of venous thrombectomy and reported that Leriche had performed a venous thrombectomy in the 1920s.

Gibbs NM. Venous thrombosis of the lower limb with particular reference to bed rest. *Br J Surg* 1957; **45**; 209.
Fontaine R. Remarks concerning venous thrombosis and its sequelae. *Surgery* 1957; **41**: 6.

1958
A source of fibrinolytic activator

Todd described the production of a fibrinolytic

activator from the wall of the veins. This was the beginning of our understanding of the role the endothelium and other cells in the production of fibrinolytic activator.

Todd AS. Fibrinolysis autographs. *Nature* 1958; **181**: 495.

Femoro-femoral vein bypass

In 1958 Palma described his femoro-femoral bypass operation for the relief of iliac vein obstruction.

Palma EC, Risi F, De Campo F. Tratamiento de los trastornos postflebiticos mediante anastomosis venosa safeno-femoral contro-lateral. *Bull Soc Surg Uruguay* 1958; **29**: 135.

1959
The first proof that pulmonary embolism can be prevented

In 1959 Sevitt and Gallagher published a study which showed that oral anticoagulants significantly reduced the mortality and the incidence of fatal pulmonary embolism following hip fractures.

Sevitt, S, Gallagher NG. Prevention of venous thrombosis and pulmonary embolism in injured patients. A trial of anticoagulant prophylaxis with phenindione in middle aged and elderly patients with fractured necks of femur. *Lancet* 1959; **2**: 981.

1959
Streptokinase will lyse venous thrombi

In 1955 Tillett, Johnson and McCarty demonstrated that streptokinase can be given safely to humans, and then showed that it could lyse artificially induced human venous thrombi *in vivo*.

Tillet WS, Johnson AJ, McCarty WR. The intravenous infusion of the streptococcal fibrinolytic principle (streptokinase) into patients. *J Clin Invest* 1955; **34**: 169.
Johnson AJ, McCarty WR. The lysis of artificially induced intravascular clots in man by intravenous infusion of streptokinase. *J Clin Invest* 1959; **38**: 1627.

1960
The detection of venous thrombi with radiosotopes

Hobbs and Davies described a series of animal experiments which showed that labelled fibrinogen could be used to detect the presence of venous thrombosis. This study led to the development of the Fibrinogen Uptake Test, a method of diagnosis which has greatly enlarged our understanding of the aetiology and natural history of venous thrombosis in all types of patient.

Hobbs JT, Davies JWL. Detection of venous thrombosis with[131] I labelled fibrinogen in the rabbit. *Lancet* 1960; **2**: 134.

1960–1987

From the 1960s onwards there has been a vast expansion in the number of publications concerning venous disease. It would be invidious to pick out the contributions of any of our many friends and colleagues from around the world for special mention because only time will tell whether contemporary contributions will be considered to be significant by our successors. The rest of this book refers to many hundreds of publications, the contents of which indicate how much thought and development has gone into investigation and treatment of venous disease.

References

1. Adams EF. *The Genuine Works of Hippocrates*. London. Sydenham Press 1949.
2. Anning ST. Historical aspects. In: Dodd H, Cockett FB (Eds) *The Pathology and Surgery of Veins of the Lower Limb* Edinburgh. Livingstone 1956.
3. Burggraeve A. *Etudes sur Andre Vésale Gaud*. Annott-Braeckman 1841.
4. Caelius Aurelianus. *De Morbis Chronicis*. II 186/Amman; 416.
5. Celsus AC. *Of Medicine in Eight Books*. Trans by Grieve J. London. Wilson & Durham 1756.
6. Chadwick J, Mann WN. *The Medical Works of Hippocrates*. Blackwell. Oxford 1950.
7. Codellas PS. Alcmaeon of Groton, his life, work and fragments. *Proc R Soc Med* 1932; **25**: 1041.
8. Fallopio G. *La Chirurgica di Gabriel Fallopio*. Trans by Cio Petro Maffei. Venice 1620.
9. Franklin KJ. Valves in veins, an historical review. *Proc R Soc Med* 1927; **21**: Sec His Med 1.

10. Friedenwald H. Amatus Lusitanus. *Bull Inst Hist Med* 1937; **5**: 603.
11. Friedenwald H. Amatus Lusitanus. *Bull Inst His Med* 1937; **5**: 644.
12. Galen C. *Claudi Galeni Opera Omnia*. CG Kühn, ed Lipsiae. Off Libr C Cnobochii 1821–1833 22 vols.
13. Ghalioungni P. *The House of Life (Per Ankh)*. Amsterdam. Israel 1973; 81 and 83.
14. Harris CRS. *The Heart and Vascular System in Ancient Greek Medicine from Alcmaeon to Galen*. Oxford. Clarendon 1973; 108.
15. Littré E. *Oeuvres Completes d'Hippocrate: Traduction Nouvelle avec le Texte* Grec en Regard. Paris. Bailliére. 1839–1861 (10 vols).
16. Lonie IM. The paradoxical text "On the Heart". *Medical History* 1973; **17**: Part II p137.
17. Majno G. *The Healing Hand*. Cambridge. Harvard University Press 1975; 90.
18. Majno G. *The Healing Hand*. Cambridge. Harvard University Press 1975; 153.
19. Majno G. *The Healing Hand*. Cambridge. Harvard University Press 1975; 328.
20. Major RH. *A History of Medicine*. Oxford. Blackwell 1954 Vol 1.
21. Michler M. *Die Alexandrinischen Chirurugen. Eine Sammlung und Answertung ihre Fragmente*. Wiesbaden. Steiner 1968; 13.
22. Mondeville H de. *Chirurgie de Maitre Henri Mondeville composée de 1306 á 1320*. Trans by Nicaise E. Paris. Alcan 1893.
23. Paré A. *The works of that famous surgeon Ambrose Paré*. Trans by Johnson T. London. Cotes and du Gard 1649.
24. Soury J. *Le systéme nerveux central. Structure et fonctions. Histoire critique de théories et des doctrines*. Paris. Carré et Naud 1899.
25. Turner Warwick W. *The Rational Treatment of Varicose Veins and Varicocele*. London. Faber & Faber 1931.
26. Underwood M. *A Treatise upon Ulcers of the Legs*. London. Mathews 1783.
27. Veith I. *Huang Ti Nei Ching Su Wen. The Yellow Emperor's Classic of Internal Medicine*. Berkeley. University of California Press 1966.
28. Walsh J. Galen's writings and influences inspiring them. *Ann Med Hist* 1934; Part **I**: 14.
29. Withington. *Medical History from the Earliest Times*. London 1894; 276.
30. Zahn W. Untersuchungen über Thrombose. Bildung der Thromben. *Virchows Arch Path Anat* 1875; **62**: 81.

2

Embryology and radiographic anatomy

A knowledge of the normal anatomy of the venous system and its many variations is essential for a full understanding of venous disease. As much of living anatomical knowledge is derived from contrast phlebography, this chapter is deliberately presented as radiological anatomy with surgically important features emphasized where appropriate.

Development and congenital anomalies

Initially, the cardinal veins form the main venous drainage system of the embryo. They consist of the anterior cardinal veins, which drain the cephalic part of the embryo, and the posterior cardinal veins, which drain the remaining part of the body of the embryo. The anterior and posterior cardinal veins join before entering the sinus horn to form the short common cardinal veins. During the fourth week the cardinal veins form a symmetrical system.

During the fifth to the seventh week of embryonic life a number of additional veins is formed: the subcardinal veins, which mainly drain the kidneys; the sacrocardinal veins which drain the lower extremities; and the supracardinal veins which drain the body wall by way of the intercostal veins thereby taking over the function of the posterior cardinal veins (Fig. 2.1a).

Characteristic of the formation of the vena caval system is the appearance of anastomoses between left and right so that blood from the left is channelled to the right side.

The anastomosis between the anterior cardinal veins develops into the left brachio-cephalic (innominate) vein. Most of the blood from the left side of the head and the upper extremities is then channelled to the right. The terminal portion of the left posterior cardinal vein entering the left brachio-cephalic vein is retained as a small vessel, the left superior intercostal vein. This vessel receives blood from the second and third intercostal spaces. The superior vena cava is formed by the right common cardinal vein and the proximal portion of the right anterior cardinal vein.

The anastomosis between the subcardinal veins is formed by the left renal vein. When this communication has been established the left subcardinal vein disappears and only its distal portion remains as the left gonadal vein. Hence the right subcardinal vein becomes the main drainage channel and develops into the renal segment of the inferior vena cava.

The anastomosis between the sacrocardinal veins is formed by the left common iliac vein. The right sacrocardinal vein finally becomes the sacrocardinal segment of the inferior vena cava. When the renal segment of the inferior vena cava connects with the hepatic segment, which is derived from the right vitelline vein, the inferior vena cava is complete. It consists then of a hepatic segment, a renal segment and a sacrocardinal segment.

With the obliteration of the major portion of the posterior cardinal veins, the supracardinal veins gain in importance. The fourth to eleventh right intercostal veins empty into the right subcardinal vein, which, together with a portion of the posterior cardinal vein, form the azygos vein. On the left the fourth to seventh intercostal veins enter the left supracardinal vein. After development of a communicating vessel between the two supracardinal veins the left supracardinal vein enters into the azygos vein and this is then known as the hemi-azygos vein (Fig. 2.1b).[25]

This complex development, coupled with the persistence of parts of the embryological trunks, gives rise to a number of anomalies.[29] It has been

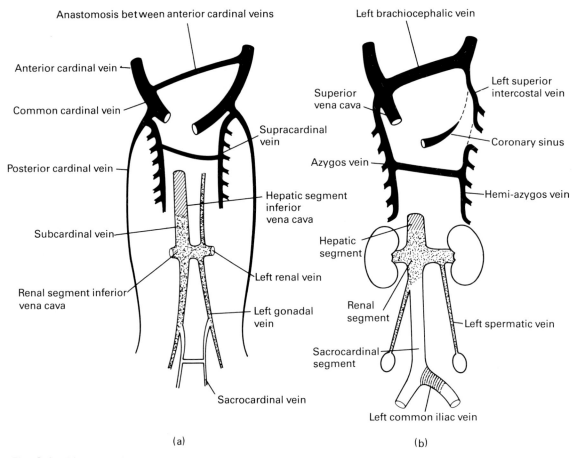

Fig. 2.1 Diagrams showing the development of the inferior vena cava, the azygos veins and the superior vena cava.

(a) In the seventh week. Note the anastomoses which have formed between the subcardinal, the supracardinal, the sacrocardinal and the anterior cardinal veins.

(b) The venous system at birth. Note the three components of the inferior vena cava. (After Langman.)[25]

estimated that one per cent of otherwise normal subjects have anomalies of the inferior vena cava or its tributaries.[36]

Two anomalies of the inferior vena cava are of particular clinical interest, a double inferior vena cava below the renal veins, and hypoplasia or complete absence of the inferior vena cava.

A double inferior vena cava exists if the left sacrocardinal vein fails to lose its connection with the left subcardinal vein. The incidence of this anomaly is between 0.2 and 3 per cent.[21] The two cavae may be of equal size but the right cava is usually larger. The left inferior vena cava drains into the right inferior vena cava via the left renal vein (Fig. 2.2a and b).

Absence of the inferior vena cava occurs when the right subcardinal vein fails to connect with the liver. Blood from the lower half of the body returns to the heart by the azygos vein and the superior vena cava. The hepatic veins enter the right atrium directly from below. This anomaly is usually associated with other cardiac malformations (Fig. 2.3a and b).[25]

A persistent left sacrocardinal vein resulting in a left-sided inferior vena cava has an incidence of 0.2–0.5 per cent.[14,20,42] The left inferior vena cava drains into the left renal vein, crosses the spine and continues cranially as a normal right-sided inferior vena cava (Fig. 2.4).

Persistence of the right posterior cardinal vein

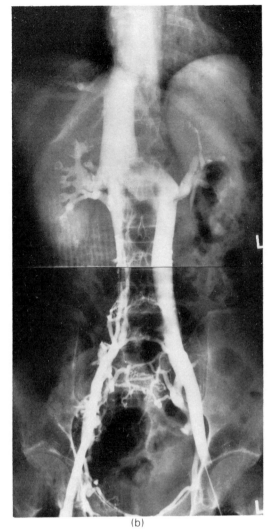

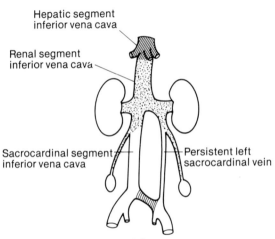

Hepatic segment
inferior vena cava

Renal segment
inferior vena cava

Sacrocardinal segment
inferior vena cava

Persistent left
sacrocardinal vein

(a)

(b)

Fig. 2.2 (a) Diagram of a double inferior vena cava at lumbar level caused by persistence of the left sacrocardinal vein. (After Langman.)[25]

(b) Duplication of the inferior vena cava shown by phlebography. The plexus of vessels to the right of the spine are remnants of a full sized right-sided vessel which has become thrombosed following plication for pulmonary embolism. A phlebogram was not carried out pre-operatively and the patient had a pulmonary embolus through the left vena cava.

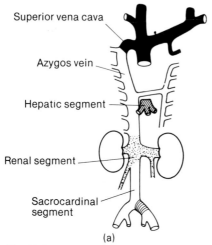

Superior vena cava

Azygos vein

Hepatic segment

Renal segment

Sacrocardinal segment

(a)

Fig. 2.3 (a) Diagram of an absent inferior vena cava. The lower half of the body is drained by the azygos vein which enters the superior vena cava. The hepatic vein enters the heart at the site of the inferior vena cava. (After Langman.)[25]

results in a retrocaval or retroiliac ureter. The distal ureter lies dorsal to the inferior vena cava. This anomaly is recognized on an excretion urogram or retrograde ureterogram by the medial displacement of the ureter. When a ureter is obstructed by this abnormality of the inferior vena cava the pelvi-calyceal system and proximal third of the ureter is dilated (Fig. 2.5). Failure of the anastomosis between the two sacrocardinal veins leads to agenesis of the left common iliac vein (see Chapter 23).[26]

The most common congenital anomaly of the superior vena cava is a persistent left superior vena cava. This occurs in 0.3 per cent of the population but more frequently (4.3 per cent) in patients with congenital heart disease.[8,9] Although a left superior vena cava may occur in isolation, it is more often found in association with a separate right superior vena cava. The left superior vena cava drains into the coronary sinus (Fig. 2.6a). Another anomaly is a double superior vena cava caused by persistence of the left anterior cardinal vein and failure of the left brachiocephalic (innominate) vein to develop (Fig. 2.6b).

Development of the limb veins

The primitive capillary plexus of the flattened

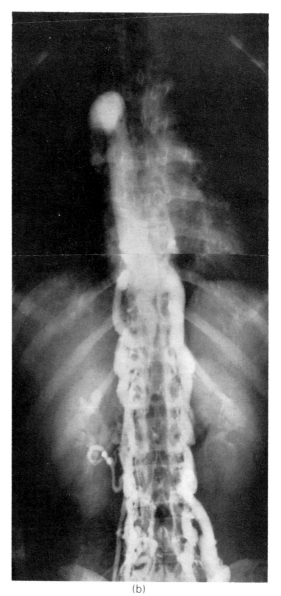

(b)

Fig. 2.3 (b) A phlebogram showing absence of the inferior vena cava. The venous return is through both ascending lumbar veins and the azygos and hemiazygos veins. This was thought to be congenital in origin because it was noted early in life and there was no history to suggest venous thrombosis.

limb buds organizes to form a peripheral border vein which serves as the primitive outflow tract for blood brought in by the axial arteries. Along the cranial border of the limb bud this vein is small and largely disappears, but on the caudal margin

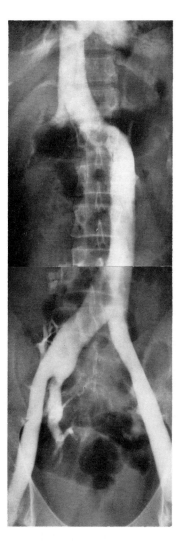

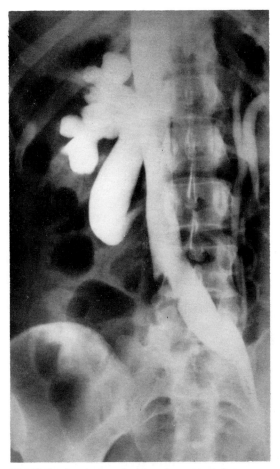

Fig. 2.5 A retrocaval ureter shown by inferior vena cavography. The calyces and upper ureter on the right are dilated due to obstruction by the abnormal inferior vena cava. Below the obstruction the ureter is displaced towards the mid-line. The excretion urogram resulted from the contrast injection for the phlebogram. The vena cava is not distorted by the position of the ureter.

Fig. 2.4 A pure left-sided inferior vena cava. The vein crosses to the right to continue cranially as an otherwise normal inferior vena cava.

it transforms into a permanent vessel. The border vein appears in the arm and leg between the sixth and eighth weeks, the adult venous anatomy being outlined during the next 2 weeks.

In the arm the radial extension of the border vein atrophies, the ulnar portion of the vein persists to form, at different levels, the subclavian, axillary and basilic veins. The border vein originally opens into the posterior cardinal vein but as the heart descends, the subclavian vein ultimately opens into the precardinal (internal jugular) vein. The cephalic vein develops secondarily in associa-tion with the radial border vein. At first the cephalic vein anastomoses with the external jugular vein but finally it opens into the axillary vein. The external jugular veins and the subclavian veins develop independently and attach later.

In the leg the tibial continuation of the primi-tive border vein disappears while the fibular segment largely persists. The long saphenous vein arises seperately from the posterior cardinal vein, gives off the femoral and posterior tibial veins, and then incorporates the tibial border vein at the level of the knee. Distally, the border vein deve-

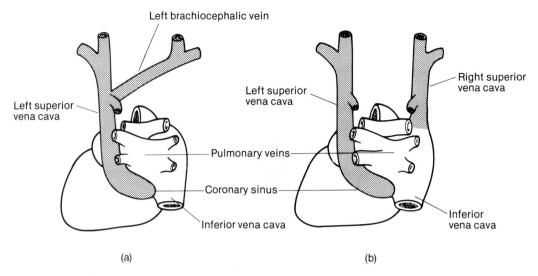

Fig. 2.6 (a) Diagram of a left superior vena cava draining into the right atrium by way of the coronary sinus (dorsal view).

(b) A double superior vena cava. The communicating (brachio-cephalic) vein between the two anterior cardinal veins has failed to develop. (After Langman.)[25]

lops into the anterior tibial and short saphenous veins.[2]

Abnormal development of these systems gives rise to some of the congenital venous anomalies which are discussed in Chapter 23.

Structure of veins

The walls

The walls of the veins, like those of the arteries, are composed of three coats, the tunica intima, the tunica media and the tunica adventitia. The main difference between the walls of the arteries and those of the veins is that, in the latter, there is a comparative weakness of the muscular layer and a much smaller proportion of elastic tissue. In small veins these coats are difficult to distinguish.

The media varies considerably between veins of different calibre. In the venules it is thin and composed almost exclusively of muscle. In the medium sized veins it consists of a thick layer of connective tissue with elastic fibres and some smooth muscle fibres, usually arranged circumferentially. The larger veins such as the femoral, iliac, axillary, subclavian and innominate veins have much less smooth muscle in the tunica media, and in the inferior and superior venae

cavae smooth muscle is almost entirely absent. The saphenous veins contain large amounts of smooth muscle in their walls.

Valves

Unlike arteries, veins possess valves which direct the blood flow towards the heart. The valves have two leaflets consisting of folds of intima reinforced with an intervening layer of connective tissue.

There are no valves in the superior and inferior venae cavae but there are valves in the tributaries from both the upper and lower limbs, the number of valves increasing towards the periphery of each limb. Valves do not appear to play an important part in controlling the circulation within the upper limbs and there is no equivalent of the calf and thigh muscle pumps in the arm. Venous return is largely the result of 'vis-a-tergo' in the upper limbs.[38] Consequently, although thrombosis in upper limb veins damages the valves as severely as it does in the lower limb, it rarely produces serious late sequelae.

The valves in the lower limb play an important role in controlling the direction of blood flow (see Chapter 3).

There are no valves in the sinusoidal veins of the

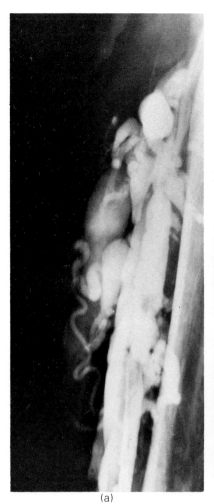

(a)

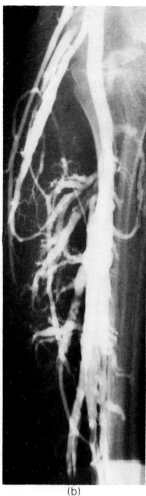

(b)

Fig. 2.7 (a) Soleal muscle veins which are baggy and valvelèss.
(b) Normal calf veins. There are numerous valves in the gastrocnemius veins, and in the paired stem veins.

soleal muscles (Fig. 2.7a) but the venous arcades which drain the soleal and gastrocnemius muscles have numerous valves (Fig. 2.7b). All the deep veins of the calf are densely valved with valves occurring at approximately 2 cm intervals (Fig. 2.8a). The popliteal vein usually has two valves in the region of the knee joint; damage to these valves may have serious consequences on the calf muscle pump.[3] There is a valve in the femoral vein just distal to its junction with the deep femoral vein in 90 per cent of all legs and a valve in the upper third of the popliteal vein just distal to the adductor canal in 96 per cent of legs. The other valves in the deep veins of the thigh are inconstant in number and position and not only vary from person to person but also vary between the right

and left legs (Fig. 2.8b).[13,40] There are eight to ten valves in the long and short saphenous veins. There is invariably a valve at the proximal end of the long saphenous vein which is thought to be important in preventing reflux down the long saphenous vein (Fig. 2.9).

The valves in the communicating veins between the superficial and deep venous systems of the leg are arranged so that blood flows from the superficial to the deep veins, and the high pressure in the deep venous system is prevented from reaching the superficial veins. The valves in the communicating veins are both superficial and deep to the deep fascia (Fig. 2.10).

There is some doubt about the significance of the valves in the communicating veins of the feet;

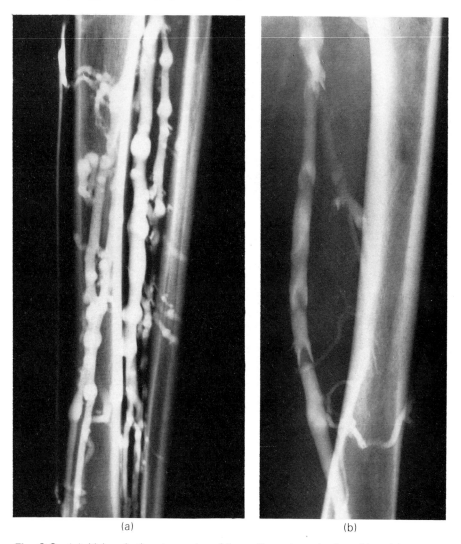

(a)   (b)

Fig. 2.8   (a) Valves in the stem veins of the calf causing a 'string of beads' appearance.
   (b) Valves in the superficial and deep femoral veins and the popliteal vein. There are fewer valves in these more proximal veins. In this phlebogram the clearly defined bicuspid valves are clearly shown because a Valsalva manoeuvre is being performed.

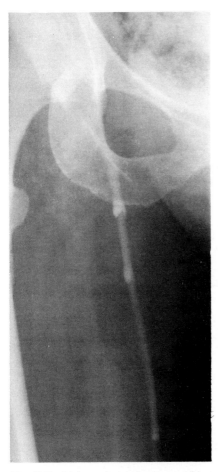

Fig. 2.9 Valves shown in a normal long saphenous vein by a Valsalva manoeuvre.

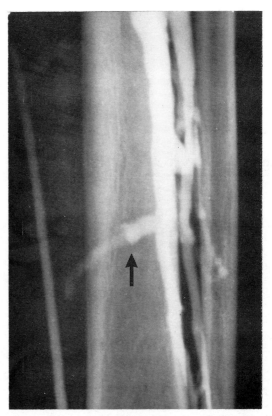

Fig. 2.10 A phlebogram showing a valve in a normal communicating vein 10 cm above the ankle joint (arrowed). Venous valves are frequently shown to be slightly incompetent on phlebography.

it seems likely that these veins are only partly valved so that blood can flow from the feet into both the deep and superficial venous systems.[19,23] As a consequence of this bi-directional flow in the foot, in contrast to the situation in the rest of the leg, the foot veins have no major haemodynamic importance.

Anatomy of the lower limb veins

The foot veins

The venous drainage of the foot consists of the following systems.

The superficial dorsal venous arch (i.e. the long and short saphenous vein, joined together by the arch and its tributaries)

The plantar cutaneous arch joining the medial and lateral marginal veins

The deep venous system of the sole (i.e. the lateral and medial plantar veins, which become the posterior tibial veins)

The communicating veins, which connect the deep and superficial networks (Fig. 2.11a and b)[37]

The deep veins of the leg

The deep veins of the lower leg consist of three paired stem veins which are venae commitantes accompanying the arteries: the anterior tibial veins, the posterior tibial veins and the peroneal veins. Each vein may divide into several trunks which surround the artery and anastomose freely with each other. The anterior tibial veins drain the

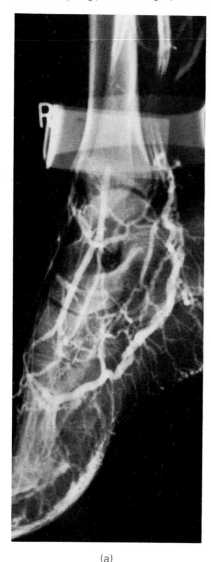

(a)

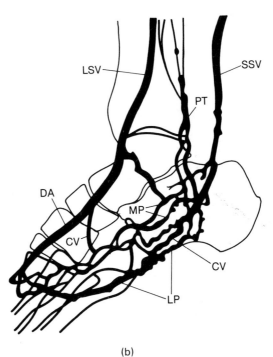

(b)

Fig. 2.11   (a) A normal foot phlebogram.
   (b) Schematic drawing of the foot veins.
LSV – long saphenous vein; SSV – short saphenous
vein; PT – posterior tibial veins; DA – dorsal venous
arch (medial limb); MP – medial plantar vein;
LP – lateral plantar vein; CV – communicating veins
connecting the medial plantar veins with the medial
limb of the dorsal venous arch and the lateral plantar
veins with the lateral marginal vein. (After Pegum
and Fegan.)[37]

blood from the dorsum of the foot and run in the deep part of the anterior (extensor) compartment close to the interosseous membrane. The posterior tibial veins are formed by the confluence of the superficial and deep plantar veins behind the ankle joint beneath the flexor retinaculum. The peroneal veins lie directly behind and medial to the fibula.

In a phlebogram taken in an antero-posterior or postero-anterior projection with the foot internally rotated, the peroneal veins lie between the images of the tibia and fibula, the anterior tibial veins lie more laterally often overlying the fibula,

and the posterior tibial veins lie medially running obliquely upwards to cross the lower third of the shaft of the tibia. Individual veins are easier to identify in a lateral projection (Fig. 2.12a and b). Collectively, these veins are referred to as the stem veins of the calf. The main deep veins of the lower limb are shown diagramatically in Fig. 2.13.

The veins of the calf muscles are either large, baggy and valveless, the so-called sinusoidal veins which are dilated segments of the venous arcades joining the posterior tibial and peroneal veins (see Fig. 2.7), or thin and straight with valves (Fig. 2.14). The former predominate in the soleal

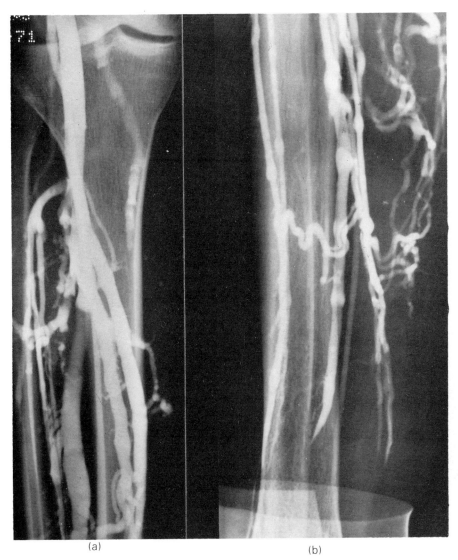

(a)   (b)

Fig. 2.12   The three paired stem veins of the calf: the anterior tibial, peroneal and posterior tibial veins. In the upper part of the calf the veins merge into single trunks and then unite to form the popliteal vein.

(a) Anterior projection with the foot internally rotated.

(b) Lateral projection. The lateral phlebogram gives a better demonstration of the individual stem and muscle veins of the calf. The veins which lie behind the tibia and pass upwards towards it are always the posterior tibial veins. Interconnections between the deep veins are common.

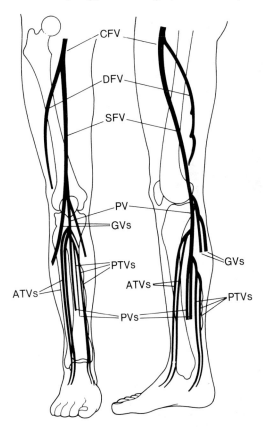

Fig. 2.13 Diagram of the main deep veins of the leg.

PVs – peroneal veins; ATVs – anterior tibial veins; PTVs – posterior tibial veins; GVs – gastrocnemius veins; PV – popliteal vein; CFV – common femoral vein; SFV – superficial femoral vein; DFV – deep femoral vein. (After May and Nissl.)[30]

The terms common femoral, superficial femoral and deep femoral vein are frequently used clinically and throughout this book even though they are not absolutely accurate anatomical terms.

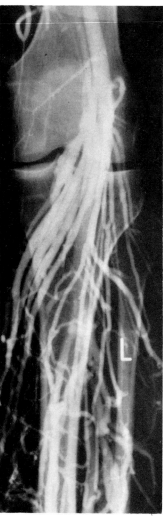

Fig. 2.14 The gastrocnemius veins. These veins which drain the gastrocnemius muscles are straight and valved and join the upper popliteal vein. They tend to be multiple with up to seven medial and lateral tributaries.

muscle and the latter in the gastrocnemius muscles.

In the upper part of the calf the paired stem veins merge to form single trunks and then unite at different levels to form the popliteal vein. If they unite above the knee joint they produce an apparently duplicated popliteal vein (Fig. 2.15). The veins from the soleal muscle drain into the stem veins or the lower part of the popliteal vein. The veins from the gastrocnemius muscles drain into the lower and upper parts of the popliteal vein (see Fig. 2.14).

The deep veins of the thigh

The superficial femoral vein is the continuation of the popliteal vein and on a phlebogram passes obliquely upwards and medially across the lower third of the femur. Approximately 9 cm below the inguinal ligament it receives the deep femoral vein which is only demonstrated fully in about a third of phlebograms when there is a direct connection between the lower part of the superficial femoral vein and a tributary of the deep femoral vein

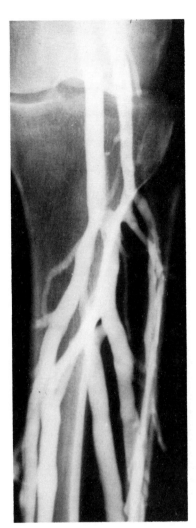

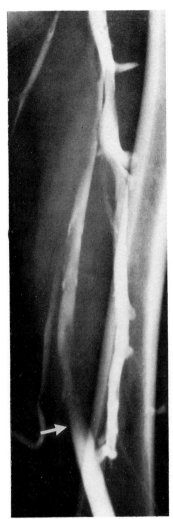

Fig. 2.15 A phlebogram of a double popliteal vein caused by a high termination of the stem veins of the calf.

Fig. 2.16 A phlebogram showing a direct connection between the superficial (white arrow) and deep femoral veins so that both fill completely.

This direct communication occurs in about one-third of all legs and has surgical implications for ligation to prevent propagation of popliteal vein thrombosis.

(Fig. 2.16). Mavor and Galloway[31] found the deep femoral vein connecting directly to the popliteal vein in 38 per cent of limbs and with a tributary to the popliteal vein in 48 per cent. These findings suggest that ligation of the femoral vein below the entrance of the deep femoral vein may often be ineffective in preventing thrombus from propagating down into the popliteal vein.[31]

There are frequent and considerable variations in the anatomy of the popliteal vein, the superficial femoral vein and the deep femoral vein. Duplication occurs in 2 per cent of legs. It has been suggested that the classical anatomical pattern is present in only 16 per cent of legs.[6]

The common femoral and external iliac veins

The common femoral vein is formed by the confluence of the superficial femoral and deep femoral veins and becomes the external iliac vein as its

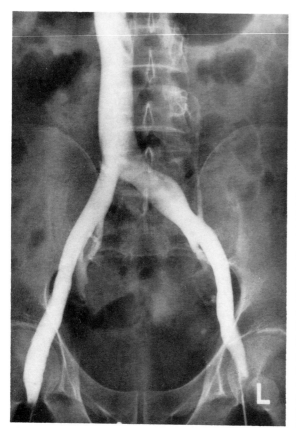

Fig. 2.17 A normal pelvic phlebogram showing the external iliac veins, the common iliac veins and the lower inferior vena cava. The internal iliac veins are shown with a Valsalva manoeuvre as far as competent valves permit.

There is a slight translucency at the termination of the left common iliac vein due to compression by the right common iliac artery. This is a normal appearance found in about half of all iliac phlebograms.

passes beneath the inguinal ligament. As the inguinal ligament is not visible on a radiograph, its level must be inferred from a knowledge of its anatomical position. The distinction between the common femoral vein and external iliac vein is somewhat artificial, and tributaries commonly ascribed to one often drain into the other. The external iliac vein is the continuation of the common femoral vein. It runs from the inguinal ligament to the sacro-iliac joint where it is joined infero-medially by the internal iliac vein emerging from the true pelvis (Fig. 2.17). The main tributaries of the external iliac vein anastomose with

each other across the floor of the pelvis to form important collaterals in iliac vein obstruction (Fig. 2.18a and b).[32]

The common iliac veins

The common iliac veins are short wide vessels which ascend from the level of the sacro-iliac joints to unite on the right side of the fifth lumbar vertebra to form the inferior vena cava. The right common iliac vein and the inferior vena cava run upwards in an almost straight line whereas the left common iliac vein runs transversely to join the left common iliac vein at a right angle. At this level the left common iliac vein is pushed forwards by the convexity of the lumbo-sacral spine and crossed by the right common iliac artery. This causes a variable degree of antero-posterior compression at the termination of the left common iliac vein which appears as a radiological filling defect in approximately 50 per cent of pelvic phlebograms (see Fig. 2.17). Excessive compression at this site may predispose to thrombosis and is discussed in detail in Chapter 9. The only tributary of the common iliac vein is the ascending lumbar vein which is larger on the left side than on the right side. The vein forms one of the main collateral pathways around a common iliac vein or lower inferior vena caval obstruction. Its iliac tributaries, draining the muscles of the false pelvis, form collaterals in external iliac vein obstruction (Fig. 2.19).

The internal iliac veins

The internal iliac veins are formed on the floor of the true pelvis by the gluteal, internal pudendal and obturator veins together with the veins of the sacral and visceral pelvic plexuses. These plexuses may form valuable collaterals across the pelvis in unilateral common iliac vein obstruction (Fig. 2.18a and b). The internal iliac veins can only be fully demonstrated radiologically by the intraosseous technique (Fig. 2.20).

The inferior vena cava

The inferior vena cava is formed by the confluence of the common iliac veins at the level of the fifth lumbar vertebra and terminates at the right atrium (Fig. 2.21a and b). It lies to the right of the vertebral bodies and it receives a variable

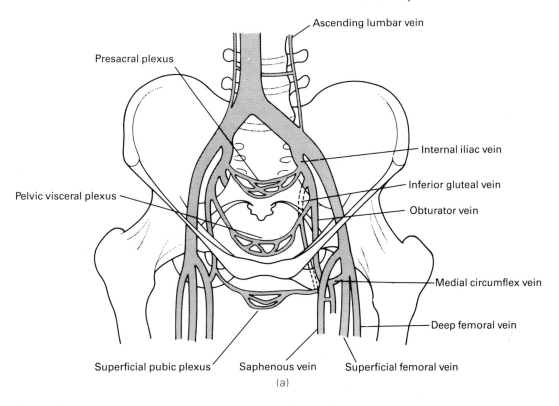

Ascending lumbar vein

Presacral plexus

Internal iliac vein

Inferior gluteal vein

Obturator vein

Pelvic visceral plexus

Medial circumflex vein

Deep femoral vein

Superficial pubic plexus   Saphenous vein   Superficial femoral vein

(a)

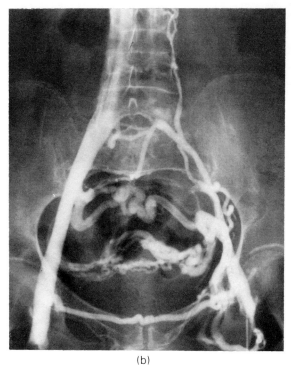

(b)

Fig. 2.18 (a) Diagram of the potential collateral pathways in pelvic vein obstruction. (After Mavor and Galloway).[32]

(b) A pelvic phlebogram with left common iliac vein occlusion and replacement of the left external iliac vein by a collateral representing a vena commitans of the adjacent artery. Note the extensive collateral circulation from left to right through the pubic veins and the visceral and pre-sacral plexuses.

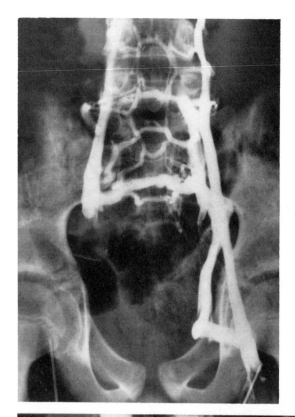

Fig. 2.19 A left femoral vein injection phlebogram showing localized occlusion of the left common iliac vein probably congenital in origin. There are collaterals from the pre-sacral plexus, both ascending lumbar veins, and the vertebral plexuses. An enlarged obturator vein joining the left internal iliac vein is also a collateral.

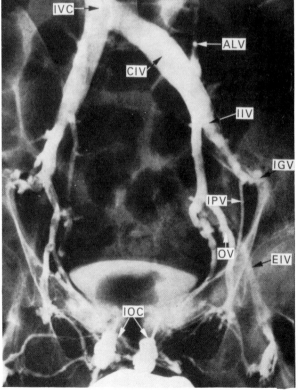

Fig. 2.20 The internal iliac veins shown by bilateral intraosseous injections into the pubic bones in the supine position. This technique allows complete visualization of all the tributaries but is rarely required. (IOC – intraosseous cannulae; IIV – internal iliac vein; EIV – external iliac vein; CIV – common iliac vein; IVC – inferior vena cava; ALV – ascending lumbar vein; OV – obturator vein; IPV – internal pudendal vein; IGV – inferior gluteal vein).

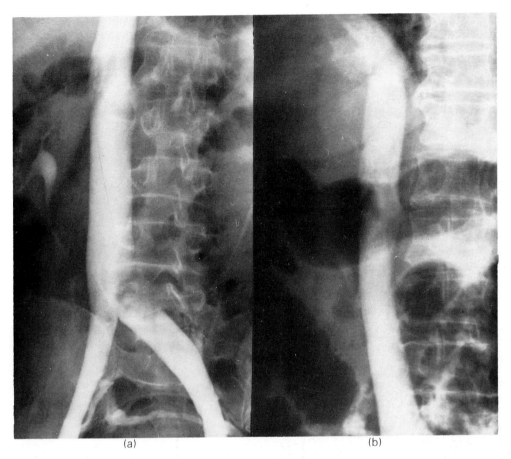

Fig. 2.21 A normal inferior vena cavagram.
 (a) Antero-posterior projection.
 (b) 20 degree left anterior oblique projection. The cava lies to the right of the vertebral column. Non-opacified blood can be seen entering from the renal veins and hepatic veins.

number of short, wide lumbar veins which connect with the vertebral venous plexuses, the left gonadal vein, the right renal vein, the right adrenal vein, the phrenic veins and the hepatic veins. Many of these tributaries can only be shown by selective phlebography.

Potential routes for collaterals in inferior vena caval obstruction are almost limitless and the most complete analysis of these is that of Pleasants[39] but this was before the advent of vena cavography.[12] Ferris *et al.* have described the channels most often demonstrated by phlebography,[14,15] and even these may require special techniques such as balloon occlusion cavography, selective catheterization or intraosseous studies to show them fully. Ferris and his colleagues, for convenience, divided the collaterals into central,

intermediate, portal and superficial groups. The central channels comprise the lumbo-azygos system, the vertebral plexuses and the cava above the occlusion; the intermediate channels comprise the gonadal veins, the ureteric veins and the left renal-azygos system; the portal collaterals are via the rectal plexus; and the extensive superficial routes include the superficial epigastric, the circumflex iliac veins, the thoraco-abdominal, the lateral thoracic and the axillary veins together with the superior vena cava (Fig. 2.22a, b and c).[16,27]

The superficial veins of the lower limb

The superficial venous system of the leg consists of two main veins, the long and short saphenous

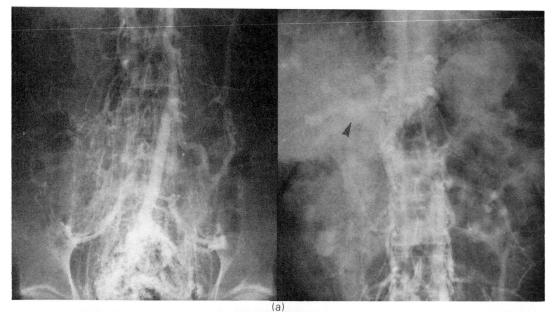

(a)

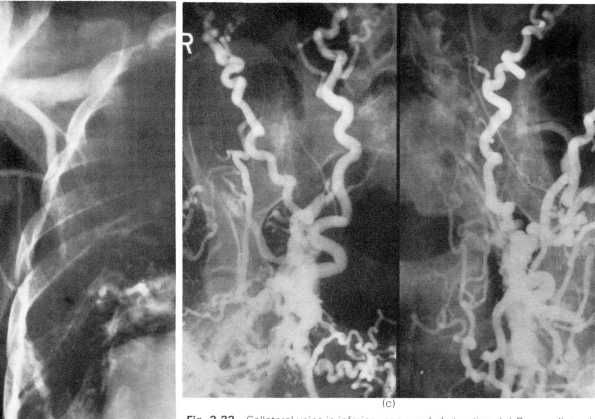

(b)

R

(c)

Fig. 2.22 Collateral veins in inferior vena caval obstruction. (a) Deep collaterals from the rectal venous plexus joining the portal vein (arrow) via the inferior mesenteric vein. (b) Lateral thoracic veins joining the axillary vein demonstrated by intraosseous pertrochanteric phlebography. (c) The lower inferior vena cava and the external and common iliac veins are occluded. The superficial collateral veins bypassing the obstruction are the superficial epigastric veins medially and the superficial circumflex iliac veins laterally. These collaterals should be clinically obvious.

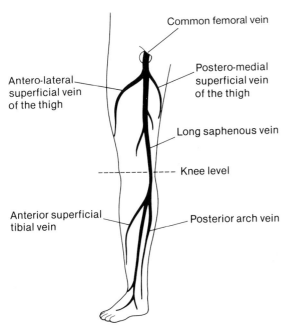

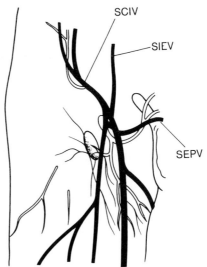

Fig. 2.23 The anatomy of the superficial venous system of the lower extremity. (After Haeger).[17]

Fig. 2.24 The most constant tributaries of the saphenous vein in the fossa ovalis. SIEV – superficial inferior epigastric vein; SEPV – superficial external pudendal vein; SCIV – superficial circumflex iliac vein.

veins (both of which are valved) and their tributaries (Fig. 2.23).

The long saphenous vein

The long saphenous vein is formed by the union of the veins from the medial side of the sole of the foot with the medial dorsal veins. It runs upwards in front of the medial malleolus along the length of the antero-medial aspect of the limb, gradually inclining posteriorly to pass behind the medial condyles of the tibia and femur. It is accompanied by the saphenous branch of the femoral nerve which may be avulsed if the vein is stripped below the knee. In the thigh the long saphenous vein runs in a slight curve towards its junction with the femoral vein, the breadth of two fingers (3 cm) below and lateral to the pubic tubercle, at the fossa ovalis. Just before it enters the fossa, it is joined by the superficial circumflex iliac, the superficial inferior epigastric and the superficial external pudendal veins (and occasionally by the deep internal pudendal vein, although this usually drains directly into the common femoral vein) together with as many as seven other superficial unnamed veins (Fig. 2.24).[17] The long saphenous

vein receives several tributaries in its course along the lower leg. The medial superficial veins from the sole join it near its anatomical origin and the posterior arch vein joints its posterior aspect in the upper leg. The posterior arch vein is important because it is connected to the deep venous system by at least two or three major medial ankle communicating veins. It should be noted that stripping the long saphenous vein from the ankle upwards does not avulse these communicating veins. The anterior superficial tibial vein joins the long saphenous vein at about the same level as the posterior arch vein (see Fig. 2.23).

Two large tributaries join the long saphenous vein in the thigh. They are probably best referred to as the postero-medial and antero-lateral superficial veins of the thigh. The postero-medial vein usually originates from a confluence of veins on the postero-medial border and the posterior aspect of the thigh. It often connects with the upper part of the short saphenous vein just before that vein pierces the deep fascia. It runs around the medial aspect of the thigh as it ascends and ends by joining the upper part of the long saphenous vein. The antero-lateral superficial vein of the thigh runs from the lateral aspect of the knee obliquely across the anterior aspect of the thigh to join the long saphenous vein usually just below its termination but sometimes as low as 15 cm below the fossa ovalis. Both medial and lateral superficial thigh veins may be quite large and can be mistaken at operation for the main long saphenous vein (Fig. 2.23, Fig. 2.25).

There are many variations of anatomy in the region of the fossa ovalis where the long saphenous vein joins the common femoral vein, mainly consisting of the direct entry of one or more of the tributaries of the long saphenous vein into the common femoral vein.[10] These variations will be recognized at the time of surgery if the sapheno-femoral junction is adequately displayed. Varicography or saphenography can give pre-operative information about these anatomical variations (see Chapters 4 and 6).

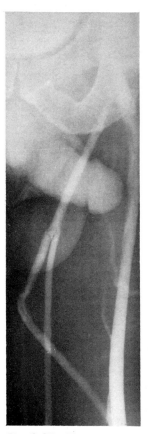

Fig. 2.25 The postero-medial superficial vein of the thigh shown by saphenography. This vein and the antero-lateral superficial vein of the thigh may be quite large and mistaken for the main long saphenous vein at surgery.

In approximated 15–20 per cent of legs the superficial external pudendal artery crosses in front of the long saphenous vein. This can be safely divided to expose the deep structures of the sapheno-femoral junction. The reported frequency of duplication or reduplication of the long saphenous vein varies between 1 per cent and 27 per cent.[18,33] In the authors' experience, based on saphenography in patients without previous surgery for varicose veins, the frequency of duplication is approximately 5 per cent. There are two rare, but clinically important, variations of the termination of the long saphenous vein; a low termination in which the saphenous vein joins the femoral vein 3–5 cm below the inguinal ligament with the external pudendal and superficial epigastric veins joining at the usual higher site,[4] and a high termination in which the long saphenous vein terminates in a vein in the subcutaneous tissues of the abdominal wall.[43]

The short saphenous vein

The short saphenous vein begins at the outer border of the foot behind the lateral malleolus as a continuation of the dorsal venous arch.[22] It is joined above the malleolus by a communicating vein which may be important when ulcers are present in this area. It enters the popliteal vein between the heads of the gastrocnemius muscle. The short saphenous vein is best seen in the lateral projection of a phlebogram where it can be seen lying superficially and following the curve of the calf muscles (Fig. 2.26). There are a number of variable connections between the long and short saphenous vein in the region of the knee and these may cause confusion when trying to decide whether varices are connected to dorsal tributaries of the long saphenous vein or to tributaries of the short saphenous vein. The short saphenous vein usually joins the posterior aspect of the popliteal vein lateral to the tibial nerve producing a characteristic 'S'-shaped loop on a saphenogram. Duplication of the short saphenous vein, in contrast to that of the long saphenous vein, is extremely rare – 0.25 per cent.[24] The close proximity of a lateral gastrocnemius vein which may be indistinguishable from the short saphenous vein is often mistaken for duplication (Fig. 2.27). Approximately 60 per cent of all short saphenous veins join the popliteal vein in the popliteal fossa within 8 cm of the knee joint; 20 per cent join the

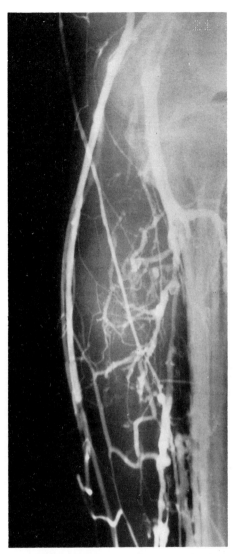

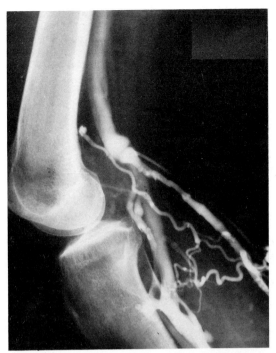

Fig. 2.27   A saphenogram showing a small but entirely normal short saphenous vein joining the popliteal vein in the popliteal fossa. Deep to this is a lateral gastrocnemius vein which is often mistaken for a duplication.

Fig. 2.26   The short saphenous vein shown by short saphenography. The vein can be recognized in a lateral projection lying superficially in the subcutaneous tissues following the curve of the calf muscles.

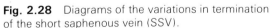

Fig. 2.28   Diagrams of the variations in termination of the short saphenous vein (SSV).

(a)   A small tributary extending superficially onto the back of the thigh.

(b)   The short saphenous vein joining the superficial postero-medial vein of the thigh which drains into the long saphenous vein.

(c)   The short saphenous vein passing deeply to join a gluteal vein draining into the internal iliac vein. (After Kosinski.)[24]

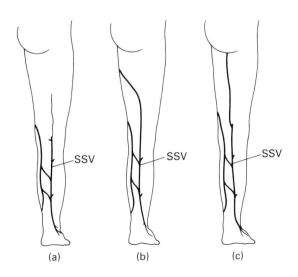

(a)   (b)   (c)

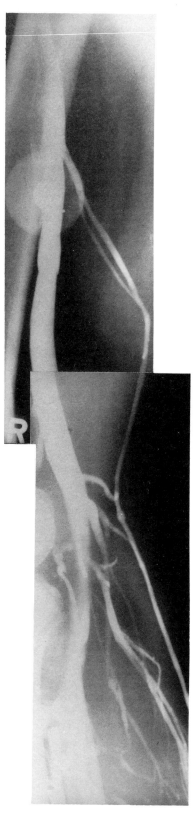

long saphenous vein via the postero-medial or antero-lateral superficial thigh veins at varying levels in the thigh; and the remainder join the superficial femoral vein, the deep femoral vein, or even tributaries of the internal iliac veins (Fig. 2.28a, b and c).[25,35] Wherever the principal termination, and however high, there is usually a small vestigal connection with the popliteal vein. As the precise termination of the short saphenous vein is difficult to find by clinical examination, the site of its termination by saphenography or varicography can be very useful as a pre-operative investigation (Fig. 2.29).

The communicating veins

The deep and superficial venous system of the lower extremity are separated by fascia and joined by communicating veins with valves which direct the blood from the superficial to the deep venous system. These communicating veins are sometimes called perforating veins because they pierce the deep fascia (see Chapter 3). The communicating veins have been further divided into direct (i.e. connecting a superficial vein directly with a deep vein) or indirect, when the connection is through one or more sinusoids in the muscles.[28] This distinction is somewhat artificial but the direct communicating veins are generally more constant in position, larger and haemodynamically more important than the indirect veins.

The largest communicating veins are the terminations of the long and short saphenous veins where they join the deep venous system but they are only part of a system of more than 100 veins in each leg which connect the superficial to the deep veins. The communicating veins of the foot allow the blood to pass in either direction and are of little physiological importance.

In the lower leg there are medial and lateral communicating veins. On the medial side there is one perforating vein just below the medial malleo-

Fig. 2.29 A montage showing a short saphenous vein with a high termination into the superficial femoral vein in the thigh. Note that there is a tributary joining the popliteal vein at the usual site in the popliteal fossa.

The ball-bearings are of known size and enable correction for magnification to be made when assessing the diameter of the vein for use for bypass surgery.

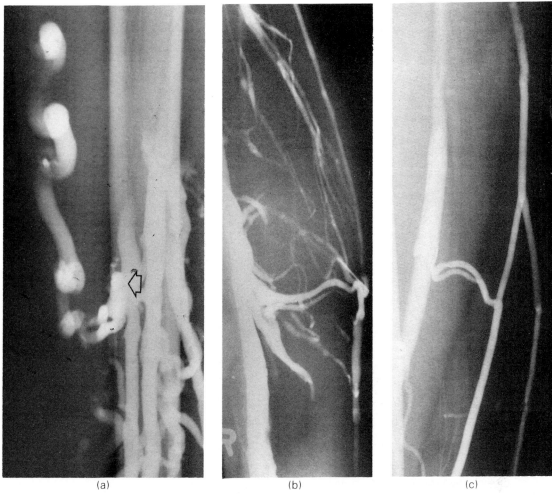

| (a) | (b) | (c) |

Fig. 2.30 Examples of communicating veins shown by ascending phlebography.

(a) A medial ankle communicating vein of Cockett. The vein demonstrated here is incompetent because it fills from the posterior tibial (i.e. a deep vein), it is dilated and joins a varicose vein.

(b) The soleus 'point'. This communicating vein connects veins in the soleal muscle with the short saphenous vein or its tributaries. The gastrocnemius point (not illustrated, see Fig. 2.31) connects veins in the gastrocnemius muscle with the superficial veins.

(c) Mid thigh communicating veins (Dodd's group). These veins in Hunter's canal are frequently multiple. The two veins shown here are almost certainly competent being less than 3 mm in diameter.

lus and three or four above the malleolus behind the tibia. The medial lower leg communicating veins, often called Cockett's veins, connect the posterior arch vein with the posterior tibial veins but do not drain directly into the long saphenous vein, (Fig. 2.30a).[7] The lowest medial communicating vein is usually found at approximately 7 cm, the middle vein at 12 cm and the upper vein 18 cm above the tip of the medial malleolus. A further communicating vein may be present above these.[34] Another communicating vein which may become incompetent is situated on the medial aspect of the calf 10 cm below the knee joint. It joins the main trunk of the long saphenous vein to the posterior tibial veins and is sometimes called Boyd's vein.[5]

The most important communicating vein on the lateral side of the lower leg is not constant in posi-

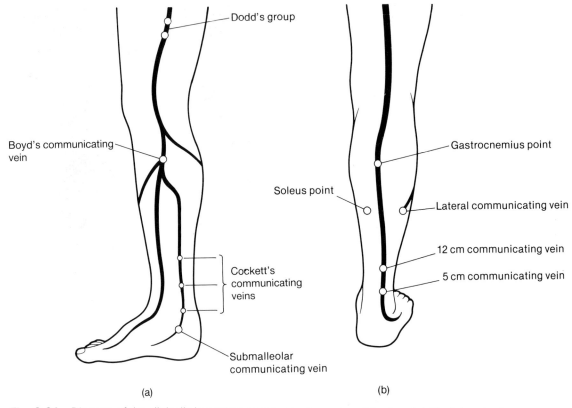

Fig. 2.31   Diagram of the clinically important communicating veins of the leg. (a) Medial projection. (b) Postero-lateral view. (After May and Nissl.)[34]

tion. It connects the short saphenous vein with the peroneal veins anywhere from just above the lateral malleolus to the junction of the lower and middle thirds of the calf. Two more constant communicating veins also joining the short saphenous vein with the peroneal veins are situated posteriorly approximately 5 cm and 12 cm above the os calcis. These are the two posterior mid calf communicating veins which sometimes cause recurrent varicose veins. They join the short saphenous vein or its tributaries to the soleal or gastrocnemius muscle veins near the mid line (Fig. 2.30b) and are referred to as the soleal and gastrocnemius points.

In the thigh there are several connections between the long saphenous vein and the femoral vein. The most important group, sometimes called Dodd's veins[11] consist of one or more veins which pass through the subsartorial (Hunter's) canal to join the long saphenous vein with the superficial femoral vein (Fig. 2.30c). These veins are usually, but not invariably, destroyed when the long saphenous vein is stripped out and so are an important cause of recurrent varicose veins. After saphenous ligation, without stripping, an incompetent mid-thigh communicating vein may be responsible for an early recurrence of varicose veins on the medial aspect of the leg in the region of the knee.

The most important communicating veins of the legs are shown diagrammatically in Fig. 2.31.

Whilst the communicating veins which have been described are relatively constant and surgically important, other communicating veins may be the cause of primary or secondary varicose veins or ulceration at unusual sites. For this reason their accurate localization by ascending phlebography or varicography is often required as discussed in Chapter 4.

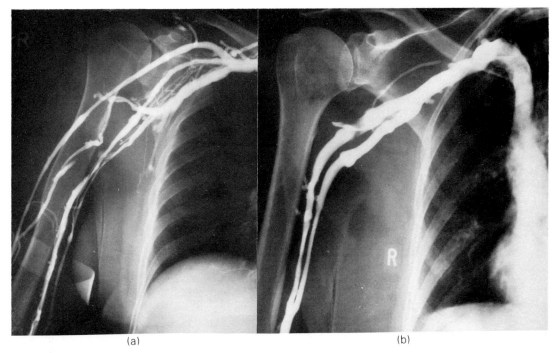

(a)   (b)

Fig. 2.32 (a) A phlebogram showing the superficial veins of the arm. The cephalic vein is often paired, as in this example. Both cephalic veins can be seen on the lateral aspect of the upper arm entering the axillary vein just below the medial part of the clavicle. The basilic vein can be seen on the medial aspect of the arm. It passes deeply to join the usually paired brachial veins to become the axillary vein at the outer border of the scapula. The phlebogram is not taken in the true anatomical position of the arm which is why the cephalic and basilic veins are not as clearly separated as they are in life or when shown diagrammatically.

(b) The deep veins of the arm. The paired brachial veins become the axillary vein at the outer border of the scapula. At the outer border of the first rib the axillary vein continues as the subclavian vein. The brachio-cephalic (innominate) vein is formed behind the sternoclavicular joint by the junction of the subclavian and the internal jugular vein. The innominate vein can be seen in this phlebogram passing downwards to enter the superior vena cava. Before doing so it is joined by the right innominate vein and both veins drain into the right atrium.

Anatomy of the upper limb veins

The upper limb has a superficial and a deep system of veins, both of which drain into a single outflow tract, the axillary vein. The superficial veins drain the dorsal aspect of the hand laterally through the cephalic vein, and medially through the basilic vein. At the elbow these veins are joined by the median cubital vein and the blood is carried proximally by both the cephalic and basilic veins which join the deep veins at different levels near the shoulder. The basilic vein pierces the fascia of the upper arm to join the deep brachial vein and become the axillary vein. The cephalic vein pierces the clavi-pectoral fascia to join the axillary vein (Fig. 2.32a). The deep veins draining the palmar surface of the hand continue as paired venae commitantes of the radial and ulnar arteries. A third group of veins, the interosseous veins, join with the radial and ulnar veins to form a pair of brachial veins which become in turn the axillary, subclavian and brachio-cephalic (innominate) veins.

The right and left brachio-cephalic veins unite to form the superior vena cava which descends on the right of the ascending aorta to enter the right atrium at the level of the third costal cartilage (Fig. 2.33). In its upper half the superior vena cava is covered on its anterior, posterior and right side by the pleura. In its lower half it lies within

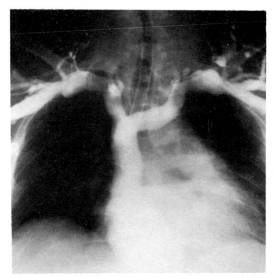

Fig. 2.33 A normal superior vena cava, formed by the confluence of the brachio-cephalic (innominate) veins, entering the right atrium.

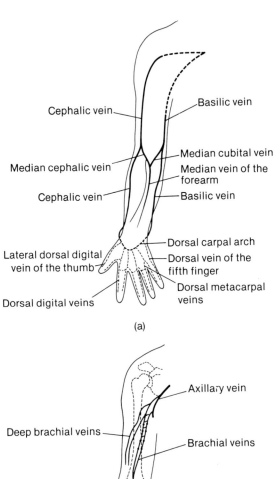

Cephalic vein

Basilic vein

Median cephalic vein

Median cubital vein

Median vein of the forearm

Cephalic vein

Basilic vein

Dorsal carpal arch

Lateral dorsal digital vein of the thumb

Dorsal vein of the fifth finger

Dorsal digital veins

Dorsal metacarpal veins

(a)

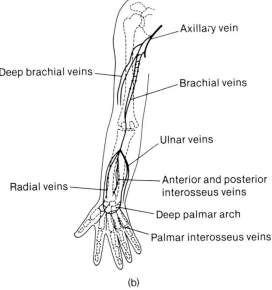

Axillary vein

Deep brachial veins

Brachial veins

Ulnar veins

Radial veins

Anterior and posterior interosseus veins

Deep palmar arch

Palmar interosseus veins

(b)

Fig. 2.34 (a) Diagram of the superficial veins of the upper limb. (b) Diagram of the deep veins of the upper limb.

the pericardium. Before it enters the pericardium it is joined posteriorly by the azygos vein.

The axillary vein begins, by definition, at the lower border of the subscapularis muscle but as this cannot be seen on radiographs it is usually considered to begin at the outer border of the scapula. It ends at the outer border of the first rib where it becomes the subclavian vein which in turn ends just medial to the mid-point of the clavicle. The brachio-cephalic veins are formed by the junction of the subclavian and internal jugular veins behind the sterno-clavicular joints and end where they unite to form the superior vena cava behind the lower border of the fifth right costal cartilage (see Fig. 2.32b).

The usual arrangement of the superficial and deep veins of the upper limb are shown diagrammatically in Fig. 2.34a and b.

Variations in the anatomy of the veins of the upper limb occur frequently but as primary varicose veins are absent in the upper limb, venous surgery is rarely required and the variations are therefore much less significant than those of the lower limb. Sometimes the median cubital vein is large and carries all or most of the blood from the cephalic into the basilic vein, the proximal part of the cephalic vein being either absent or proportionally diminished. The accessory cephalic vein arises from small tributaries on the back of the forearm and from the ulnar side of the dorsal venous network and joins the cephalic vein below the elbow. In some arms it arises from the cephalic vein above the wrist and joins it higher up. A large oblique tributary frequently joins the cephalic vein on the back of the forearm. Sometimes the brachio-cephalic veins open independently into the right atrium, the right vein taking the course of the normal superior vena cava and the left vein becoming a persistent left superior vena cava (see Fig. 2.6a).

The superficial and deep veins of the arm are linked by a few valved communicating veins, one of the largest being in the cubital fossa. The venous drainage of the upper limb is largely the result of cardiac function, and as there is no muscle pump the valves have little physiological importance. These differences between the upper and lower limbs, which presumably evolved in parallel with man's erect posture, may explain why pathological conditions of the upper limb of venous origin are so uncommon. Only a few patent veins are required for adequate venous drainage and most venous occlusions are rapidly compensated by collaterals. Few, if any, symptoms occur if thrombosis in the upper limb veins damages the valves.[38] Valvular incompetence does not produce symptoms in the upper limb.

The azygos and vertebral venous systems

Venous blood enters the heart via the superior and inferior vena cavae. If either or both of these veins is obstructed drainage is maintained by collaterals formed mainly by the azygos and vertebral venous systems.[44]

The origin of the azygos vein is inconstant but it can generally be regarded as the continuation of the ascending lumbar vein into the thorax. Similarly, the hemi-azygos vein is the continuation of the left ascending lumbar vein. In approximately 60 per cent of people the left renal vein communicates with the hemi-azygos system. The hemi-azygos vein crosses the vertebral column at the level of the nineth lumbar vertebra to join the azygos vein. The azygos vein ascends into the thorax to the level of the fourth thoracic vertebra where it passes anteriorly to join the superior vena cava (Fig. 2.35).

In approximately 0.5 per cent of the population the azygos vein continues upwards in a more lateral position before entering the superior vena

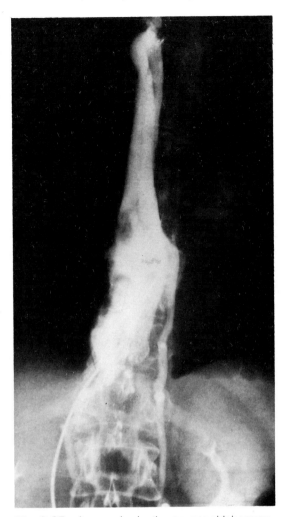

Fig. 2.35 A normal selective azygos phlebogram. The right ascending lumbar vein becomes the azygos vein as it enters the thorax. On the left of this phlebogram the ascending lumbar vein can be seen passing upwards becoming the hemi-azygos vein and crossing the mid-line at D9 to enter the azygos vein.

cava at a higher level giving rise to an azygos lobe of the right lung.[20] The azygos and hemi-azygos veins have a few imperfect valves but their tributaries have functioning venous valves. The veins of the vertebral column form an intricate plexus extending along its entire length, divisible into the external and internal plexuses, outside and inside the vertebral canal. These veins are devoid of valves, anastomose freely with each other, and

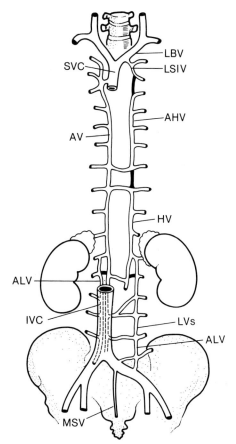

Fig. 2.36 Diagram of the azygos, hemi-azygos and ascending lumbar veins. Shaded segments indicate variable communications. (IVC – inferior vena cava; ALV – ascending lumbar veins; SVC – superior vena cava; LBV – left brachio-cephalic vein; LSIV – left superior intercostal vein; AHV – accessory hemi-azygos vein; HV – hemi-azygos vein; AV – azygos vein; LVs – lumbar veins; MSV – median sacral vein.) All these veins, together with the vertebral plexuses are potential collaterals in superior vena cava obstruction. (After Hemingway).[20]

drain into the intercostal veins, and into the ascending lumbar veins through the intervertebral veins.

In aplasia or hypoplasia or obstruction to either the superior or inferior vena cava the azygos systems and the vertebral plexuses provide the main channels for venous drainage (Fig. 2.36).[11,20] Apart from these circumstances the detailed anatomy of this complex and incon-stant venous network is of little practical importance.

References

1. Abrams HL. The vertebral and azygos veins. In: Abrams HL (Ed) *Angiography* 3rd edition. Boston. Little Brown 1983; 895.
2. Arey LB. *Development Anatomy*. Philadelphia and London. WB Saunders 1974.
3. Basmajian JV. The distribution of valves in the femoral, external, iliac and common iliac veins and their relationship to varicose veins. *Surg Gynec Obstet* 1952; **95**; 537.
4. Bevan PE, Green SH, Stammers FAR. Low ter-mination of the internal saphenous vein. *Br Med J* 1956; **1**: 610.
5. Boyd AM. Discussion on primary treatment of varicose veins. *Proc R Soc Med* 1948; **41**: 633.
6. Cockett FB. Abnormalities of the deep veins of the leg. *Postgrad Med J* 1954; **30**: 512.
7. Cockett FB. The pathology and treatment of venous ulcers of the leg. *Br J Surg* 1955; **43**: 260.
8. Campbell M, Deuchar DC. Left sided superior vena cava. *Br Heart J* 1954; **16**: 423.
9. Cha ME, Khoury GH. Persistent left superior vena cava: Radiologic and clinical significance. *Radiology* 1972; **103**: 375.
10. Daseler EH, Anson BJ, Reimann AF, Beaton LE. The saphenous venous tributaries and related structures in relation to the technique of high ligation. *Surg Gynec Obstet* 1946; **82**: 53.
11. Dodd H. The varicose tributaries of the superficial femoral vein passing into Hunter's canal. *Postgrad Med J* 1959; **35**: 18.
12. dos Santos R. Phlébographie d' une veine cave inférieure suture. *J Urol Med Chir* 1935; **39**: 586.
13. Eger SA, Casper SL. Etiology of varicose veins from the anatomic aspect based on dissections of 38 adult cadavers. *JAMA* 1943; **123**: 148.
14. Ferris EJ, Hipona FA, Kahn PC, Phillips E, Shapiro JH. *Venography of the Inferior Vena Cava and its Branches*. Baltimore. Williams and Wilkins 1969.
15. Ferris EJ. The inferior vena cava. In: Abrams HL (Ed) *Angiography* 3rd edition. Boston, Little Brown 1983.
16. Fletcher EWL, Lea Thomas M. Chronic post-thrombotic obstruction of the inferior vena cava investigation by cavography. A report of two cases. *Am J Roentgenol* 1968; **102**: 363.
17. Haeger K. Practical anatomy. In: Haeger K (Ed) *Venous and Lymphatic Disorders of the Leg*. Lund. Scandanavian University Books 1966.

18. Haeger K. The anatomy of the veins of the leg. In: Hobbs JT (Ed). *The Treatment of Venous Disorders*. Lancaster. MTP Press 1977.

19. Hach W. *Phlebographie der Bein – und Beckenvenen*. Konstantz. Schnetztor Verlag 1976.

20. Hemingway AP. Venography. In: Grainger RG Allison DJ (Eds). *Diagnostic Radiology*. Edinburgh. Churchill Livingstone, 1986.

21. Hirsch DM, Chan K. Bilateral inferior vena cava. *JAMA* 1963; **185**: 729.

22. Holinshead WH. *Anatomy for Surgeons*. Volume 3. Philadelphia. Harper and Row 1982; 603.

23. Jacobsen B. The venous drainage of the foot. *Surg Gynec Obstet* 1970; **131**: 22.

24. Kosinski G. Observations on the superficial venous system of the lower extremity. *J Anat* 1926; **60**: 131.

25. Langman J. *Medical Embryology* 4th edition. Baltimore/London. Williams and Wilkins 1981: 191.

26. Lea Thomas M, Posniak HV. Agenesis of the iliac veins. *J Cardiovasc Surg* 1984; **25**: 64.

27. Lea Thomas M, Fletcher EWL, Cockett FB, Negus D. Venous collaterals in external and common iliac vein obstruction. *Clin Radiol* 1967; **18**: 403.

28. Le Deutu A. *Recherches Anatomiques et Consideratiuns Physiologiques sur la Circulation Vein use du Pied et de la Jambe*. Thesis, Paris. 1967.

29. McClure EF, Butler EG. The development of the vena cava inferior in man. *Am J Anat* 1925; **35**: 331.

30. May R, Nissl R. *Die Phlebographie der Unteren Extremitat*. Stuttgart, Thieme 1959.

31. Mavor GE, Galloway JMD. The iliofemoral venous segment as a source of pulmonary emboli. *Lancet* 1967; **1**: 871.

32. Mavor GE, Galloway JMD. Collaterals of the deep venous circulation of the lower limb. *Surg Gynec Obstet* 1967; **125**: 561.

33. May R, Nissl R. Surgery of the veins of the leg and pelvis. In: May R (Ed) *Anatomy*. Stuttgart, Georg Thieme 1979.

34. May R, Nissl R. Nomenclature of the surgically most important connecting veins. In: May R, Patsch H, Staubesand J (Eds) *Perforating veins*. Munchen. Urban and Schwarzenberg 1981.

35. Mullarky RE. *The Anatomy of Varicose Veins*. Springfield, Ill. Thomas 1965.

36. Negus D. The surgical anatomy of the veins of the lower limb. In: Dodd H, Cockett FB (Eds) *The Pathology and Surgery of the Veins of the Lower Limb*. Edinburgh. Churchill Livingstone 1976.

37. Pegum JM, Fegan WG. Physiology of venous return from the foot. *Cardiovasc Res* 1967; **1**: 249.

38. Picard JD. *La Phlebographie des Membres Inferieurs et Superieurs*. Expansion scientifique Francaise. Paris 1975.

39. Pleasants JH. Obstruction of inferior vena cava with a report of 18 cases. *John Hopkins Hospital Report* 1911; **16**: 363.

40. Powell T, Lynn RB. The valves of the external, iliac, femoral and upper third of the popliteal veins. *Surg Gynec Obstet* 1951; **92**: 453.

41. Raivio E. Untersuchungen uber die Venen der unteren Extremitaten mit besonderer Berucksichtigung der gegenseitigen Verbindungen zwischen den oberflachigen und tiefen Venen. *Ann Med exp Fenn* 1948; **26**: 1.

42. Seib GA. The azygos system of veins in American whites and American negroes, including observations on the inferior caval venous system. *Am J Phys Anthropol* 1934; **19**: 39.

43. Sieglbauer F. *Lehrbuch der Normalen. Anatomie des Menschen*. Wien. Urban & Schwarzenberg 1944.

44. Yao JST, Neiman HL. Upper extremity venography. In: Neiman HL, Yao ST (Eds) *Angiography of Vascular Disease*. New York, Churchill Livingstone 1985.

3

Physiology and functional anatomy

Although the veins form almost one-half of the circulatory system and contain two-thirds of the blood, our understanding of venous physiology has lagged behind our understanding of arterial physiology.

There are two reasons why the physiology of the veins has been neglected. Firstly, there are no obvious fatal venous diseases. Consequently, there has not been the stimulus from the physician to the physiologist to explore venous physiology in the way that there has been the stimulus from physicians to investigate the kidney, bowel, heart and arteries. Secondly, veins are extremely difficult to study. Their variable anatomy, ever changing pressure and flow characteristics and susceptibility to so many local external influences makes measurement of their physiological properties difficult to achieve and interpret. Fortunately, the last 40 years have witnessed a tremendous improvement in measurement techniques and many of these methods have been applied to the veins. There are now numerous books on venous physiology, the subject is vast.[4,33,75] The purpose of this chapter is to introduce some of the important aspects of venous physiology which are relevant to the study of abnormalities of the peripheral veins, and in particular the function of the calf muscle pump.

Physiology

Venous pressure

The pressure in a foot vein which is measured *when the subject is supine* represents the increment of pressure that remains after the dissipation of the kinetic energy generated from the heart by the resistance of the arterioles and capillaries. It is approximately 15 mmHg (20 000 dynes/cm²).

The right atrial pressure is normally between 0 and 2 mmHg so the venous return to the heart when the subject is supine is generated by a pressure gradient of 13–15 mmHg.

When the body is erect the column of blood between the heart and the foot exerts a gravitational force – the hydrostatic pressure. The foot vein pressure is then 15 mmHg plus the pressure exerted by the column of blood between the foot and the point used as the zero reference for the pressure measurement – usually the level of the manubrium sterni. This hydrostatic pressure is exerted equally by the blood in the arteries and the veins, so the perfusion pressure, the pressure difference between the arteries and veins, is unchanged. In a man who is 180 cm (6 ft) tall the hydrostatic pressure (the gravitational potential energy) is approximately 100 mmHg. This means that the measured foot vein pressure will be 100 + 15 mmHg and the mean foot arterial pressure will be 100 + 90 mmHg, the pressure gradient across the capillaries remaining unchanged (Fig. 3.1).

If only the pressure measurements are considered, it may seem that arterial blood is flowing from the heart to the foot against the pressure gradient. It is, but the gravitational *energy* (not the pressure) is 0 mmHg at the foot and 100 mmHg at heart level because the energy resides at the top of the column of blood. Thus the total energy at heart level is 200 mmHg (the 100 mmHg of kinetic pressure energy generated by the heart plus the gravitational energy of 100 mmHg) whereas the total energy at the ankle is 90 mmHg (the 90 mmHg kinetic pressure energy produced by the heart plus *no* gravitational energy). The blood is flowing down to the foot against the pressure gradient but with the energy gradient.

The vein wall contains the same mixture of muscle fibres, elastin and collagen arranged in the

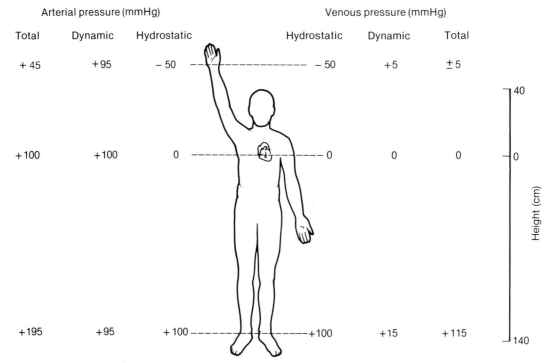

Arterial pressure (mmHg)				Venous pressure (mmHg)		
Total	Dynamic	Hydrostatic		Hydrostatic	Dynamic	Total
+ 45	+95	− 50		− 50	+5	± 5
+100	+100	0		0	0	0
+195	+95	+ 100		+100	+15	+ 115

Fig. 3.1   The arterial and venous blood pressure when standing.

If the heart is used as the zero reference point for pressure measurements, the pressure at any point in the circulation is the sum of the dynamic pressure generated by the heart and the hydrostatic pressure exerted by the column of blood between the site of measurement and the zero reference point.

tunica adventitia, media and interna as other blood vessels. The collagen and muscle fibres are arranged in a spiral. The smooth muscle supplies the active tone, and the elastin and collagen supply the passive elasticity.

When a vein relaxes it collapses flat. As it distends it passes through an eliptical form to become circular (Fig. 3.2). The resistance to blood flow becomes less as the cross-section changes

Cross-section of vein lumen

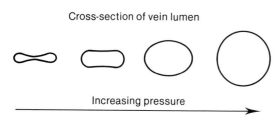

Increasing pressure

Fig. 3.2   When a vein is collapsed its transverse section is 'dumbell'-shaped. As it distends it becomes elliptical before becoming circular. The resistance to flow becomes slightly less as it changes from an elipse to a circle.

from an elipse to a circle. Until the cross-section becomes circular, the vein can accommodate an increasing volume of blood without a significant increase in distending pressure. The distending pressure is the transmural pressure (i.e. the intraluminal pressure minus the extraluminal [tissue] pressure). Once the cross-section is circular, further increases in volume are associated with a disproportionate increase in pressure (i.e. the pressure–volume curve has reached its plateau). (Fig. 3.3).

The shape of the pressure–volume curve is particularly relevant to venous disease in the lower limb. The erect posture or venous obstruction caused by thrombosis both fill and distend the distal superficial limb veins so that when the body is upright they are always full and circular in cross-section. In these circumstances the addition of even a small volume of blood by a disordered pump leaking through incompetent communicating veins will cause a significant increase in superficial venous pressure. This is illustrated in the pressure–volume curve in Fig. 3.3. A 0.5 ml/100

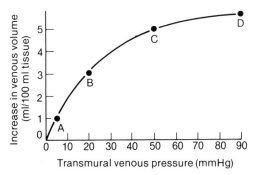

Fig. 3.3 The pressure–volume curve of the veins of the lower limb.

Between points A and B an increase in volume of 0.5 ml/100 ml tissue causes an increase in pressure of 4 mmHg. Between points C and D the same volume change increases the pressure by 50 mmHg.

ml change of volume anywhere between A and B causes only a small (4 mmHg) change in pressure whereas the same change in volume between C and D increases the pressure by 50 mmHg.

The veins contain two-thirds of the total blood volume. Blood volume is generally controlled by the kidney responding to alterations of its blood flow and through hormonal control of tubular function. Rapid changes in the volume of blood in different parts of the circulation are usually controlled by reflex changes of venous tone in response to changes in central venous pressure which is in turn regulated by arteriolar and venular resistance.

The valves

The direction of venous blood flow is controlled by the valves.[39]

Vein valves are bicuspid. The cusps of the valves of the superficial veins lie with their free edges parallel to the skin surface.[27]

The distribution of the valves in the veins of the lower limb is shown in Fig. 5.2, page 153.[51,67] The inferior vena cava and common iliac veins have no valves and 75 per cent of external iliac veins have no valves, but only 25 per cent of common femoral veins are valveless. It has been suggested that the lack of valves in the iliac and common femoral veins is the starting point for the development of a progressive descending valvular incompetence that causes varicose veins (see Chapter 5).[50] Below the inguinal ligament the number of valves in each

segment steadily increases so that the calf veins have valves which are 5 cm apart. Valves are present in veins of 1 mm diameter, but not in smaller veins or the venules.[78]

The terms given to each part of a valve are shown in Fig. 3.4. The valve sinus is always wider than the vein above and below the cusps,[22] and so it has been postulated that the valve cusps do not lie flat against the wall of the vein when the valve is open but float in the longitudinal axis of the vein. There are four reasons for believing that this is correct.

1. The valves are often seen in this position on phlebograms.
2. Valve cusps have been seen in this position during B mode ultrasound imaging.
3. This is the ideal position to ensure that the cusps close when retrograde flow occurs because if they lie flat against the vein wall, they will not fill and balloon out into the bloodstream as reflux begins, whereas if they lie in the bloodstream away from the vein wall, some refluxing blood must flow into the sinus and push the valve towards the mid-line.
4. Thrombosis frequently starts in a valve sinus which suggests that they always contain some blood.[35]

The valves in the axial veins prevent blood flow

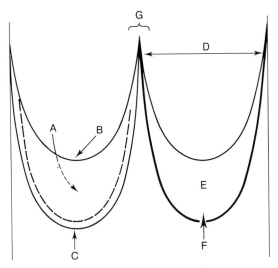

Fig. 3.4 The nomenclature of the valve.
A = sinus; B = free border of cusp; C = attached border of cusp; D = cornua; E = cusp; F = agger; G = commissure. Redrawn after Franklin.[33]

away from the heart. The valves in the communicating veins of the calf stop blood flowing from the deep to the superficial veins but most of the valves in the communicating veins of the foot point in the opposite direction and tend to prevent blood flowing from the superficial veins on the dorsum to the deep veins in the muscles of the sole of the foot.[34,63]

Valves are extremely strong even though they are just a thin layer of collagen fibres covered with endothelium.[3]

The mechanical properties of strips of normal human femoral vein valve cusp cut parallel to the free edge of the cusp, and longitudinal and circumferential strips of the vein wall are shown in Fig. 3.5. The valve cusps are stronger and more elastic than the vein wall. Although calculations of tensile strength have to be related to the thickness of the tissue being studied, this only partly explains the difference in tensiometer measured tensile strength and breaking strain between the valves and the vein wall. There is no doubt that the valves are extremely strong structures.

Circumferential strips of vein are slightly less elastic than longitudinal strips (possibly because of the disposition of the spiral fibres) but circumferential strips from the sinus are more elastic – a property which may help the sinus to 'balloon-out' more easily and turn the combined cavities of the two valve sinuses into a sphere.

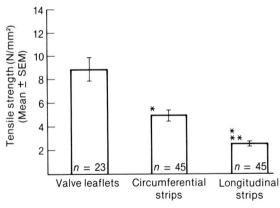

Fig. 3.5 The tensile strength of valve cusps and circumferential and longitudinal strips of human femoral vein.
* = strength significantly different from valve leaflet. $P < 0.001$
** = strength significantly different from circumferential strip. $P < 0.001$

It is customary to think of valve function as solely the result of cusp movement. In fact it is a complex change involving cusp movement and valve sinus distention which tightens the edges of the cusps by separating the commissures. If this does not happen and the valve edge remains loose, because of lack of vein distensibility or because the free edges of the cusps elongate, the edge of the cusp may evert (prolapse) and the valve become incompetent (see Fig. 8.9, page 260).

Venous blood flow

Venous blood flow in the lower limb is produced by the 'vis a tergo', the calf pump and the changes of intra-abdominal and intrathoracic pressure. These factors are discussed later in the section describing the physiology of the calf pump (page 60). Venous tone has an effect on the rate of blood flow but is more involved in the distribution of the blood throughout the body.

Venous tone

Active and variable tone is provided by the smooth muscle in the tunica media. The passive tone is provided by the elastic properties of the vein wall; this cannot be changed and, in the resting state, is probably the major source of tone. Most veins have little active tone when the body is at rest, especially the large collecting deep veins of the limbs and trunk.

Changes in tone are mediated through the sympathetic nerves and by circulating smooth muscle stimulants. Changes of venous tone are part of a number of cardiovascular reflexes.

The smooth muscle of the vein wall constricts when stimulated by noradrenaline.[38,56,95] Acetylcholine can cause both constriction and relaxation.[2,45,68,86] Most prostaglandins dilate the veins but some cause venoconstriction.[36,54]

All veins have an adrenergic innervation,[24,42] through nerve endings which terminate in the tunica media.[21] The density of the nerve endings varies from vein to vein.[10] The splanchnic and cutaneous veins have a rich innervation whereas the veins of skeletal muscles have few endings and so show a minimal response to sympathetic nerve stimulation.[48]

Sympathetic adrenergic stimulation causes venoconstriction.[16] Some parasympathetic nerves (e.g. the vagus) have an acetylcholine mediated constrictor effect.[19] Venodilatation is normally achieved through a reduction in adrenergic tone, provided this is present. Active neurogenic vaso-dilatation mediated through the autonomic nervous system remains unproven.

Sympathetic venous tone is controlled from the brain stem[8] in which there are pressor and depressor areas which cause venoconstriction and venodilatation respectively, by modifying the sympathetic discharge. A few venous reflexes are spinal,[15] but the majority pass through the brain stem. There is also an important thermoregulatory area in the brain stem which controls the tone of the subcutaneous veins.[89]

Tone in the subcutaneous veins is affected by the following.

- Emotion and pain, which cause venoconstriction[25,55]
- Sleep, which causes venorelaxation[88]
- An increased body-core temperature (pyrexia), which causes venorelaxation[69]
- A deep breath, which causes venoconstriction[15,23,71]
- Exercise, which causes venoconstriction[11,12]
- Standing upright, which causes a transient venoconstriction[70]

Overall, the most important reflex role of the subcutaneous veins is in thermoregulation. The only other potent causes of reflex venoconstriction are emotional stress and changes in ventilation (Fig 3.6).

The apparent venoconstriction and dilatation seen in response to local cooling and heating is mainly a passive effect secondary to changes in arteriolar resistance and blood flow. Local temperature changes have only a small direct effect on the vein wall but do modify the response of the veins to thermoregulatory reflexes.[1,89] Thus the veins of a hand placed in hot water are dilated by two mechanisms, a small direct reflex reduction in the tone of the veins and an increased blood flow and consequently an increased venous filling secondary to reflex arteriolar dilatation.

Changes in blood pressure have little or no effect on the subcutaneous veins.[28] Orthostatic hypotension is an arteriolar not a venous failure.

A reduced partial pressure of oxygen in the inhaled air causes venoconstriction, probably via a chemoreceptor reflex.[41]

The veins also respond to local stimuli. A direct injury usually causes venospasm but conversely

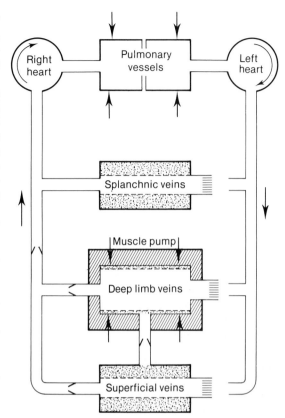

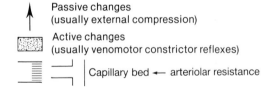

Fig. 3.6 A schematic representation of the sites of passive (usually external compression) and active (usually venomotor constrictor reflexes) changes of venous volume. Adapted from Shepherd.[75]

venospasm can be overcome by repeated gentle blunt trauma (e.g. tapping with the finger).[32]

There are myelinated nerve fibres in the vein wall[94] some of which are involved in the perception of pain, some in detecting changes of temperature and some in the pressure/stretch reflexes.[80]

The endothelium

The endothelium of the blood vessels not only

provides an anti-thrombotic lining but manufactures and secretes a number of substances which affect the condition of the blood and the interstitial fluid. Vascular endothelium is a secretory organ.

Endothelial cells produce coagulation Factor VIII, prostacyclins and activators of fibrinolysis. The precise role of the endothelium in Factor VIII production is not clear.[44] Insufficient Factor VIII causes a bleeding diathesis – haemophilia – but the endothelium is not the sole source of this factor and haemophilia is mainly caused by a loss of hepatic production of Factor VIII. Nevertheless, vascular endothelium does participate in the control of the levels of circulating coagulation factors.

Endothelial cells produce prostacyclins which have antiplatelet aggregating properties.[90] Whether they play a role in preventing the adherence of platelets to the endothelium itself or to any uncovered collagen is uncertain but it is believed that the antithrombotic effect of endothelium is related to the balance between platelet thromboxane and endothelium prostacyclin production.

The endothelial cells of the veins are a major source of fibrinolytic activator. Whereas coagulation factors and prostacyclin are produced by all vascular endothelium, much more fibrinolytic activator is produced by the endothelium of the major veins and their vasa venora than by the endothelium of arteries.

The existence of a system opposed to coagulation has been known for many years.[53,57] Its site of production was established when Todd showed that slices of veins incubated on fibrin plates produced areas of fibrinolysis (see Fig. 16.3, page 450).[83,84,85] The effect of this endothelial activity on the blood can be demonstrated by measuring the increased fibrinolytic activity which follows venous congestion.[46,61,74,82]

The presence of a small but natural and varying blood fibrinolytic activity derived from the venous endothelium led Fearnley to propose the concept of 'natural fibrinolysis'.[30,31,72]

Many workers have since sought a connection between thrombotic disease and reduced fibrinolytic activity.[20,29,43] Nilsson[60] and the authors[14] have shown such a relationship between recurrent thrombosis and vein wall fibrinolytic activity; we have also found a reduced fibrinolytic activity in patients with severe chronic venous insufficiency.[18]

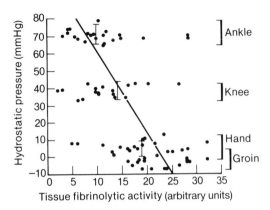

Fig. 3.7 The relationship between vein wall fibrinolytic activity and resting (hydrostatic) venous pressure in 20 patients. The lower the hydrostatic pressure the greater the activator activity.[47]

The inability of normal lower leg veins to produce as much fibrinolytic activator as arm veins and the relationship between venous pressure and activator release[47,62,93] (Fig. 3.7) mean that venous pressure changes and venomotor reflexes cannot be considered to have only a haemodynamic effect. Changes in vein wall configuration, tension and pressure will all affect the productive capacity of the endothelium, adding another dimension to our difficulties in understanding the effects of calf pump malfunction on the microcirculation.

The functional anatomy of the calf pump

The deep and superficial veins of the lower limb occupy two distinct compartments, separated by the deep fascia. Although there are many different types of vein in each compartment, they can, for physiological purposes, be regarded collectively as two entities, a deep chamber and a superficial chamber (Fig. 3.8).[17]

The deep compartment (the pump chamber)

The deep compartment below the knee forms the chamber of the calf pump. The soleal sinuses and gastrocnemius veins actually lie within the muscles. The posterior, anterior tibial, and peroneal veins lie between the muscles. The intermuscular veins are not compressed by muscular contraction as forcefully as the intramuscular

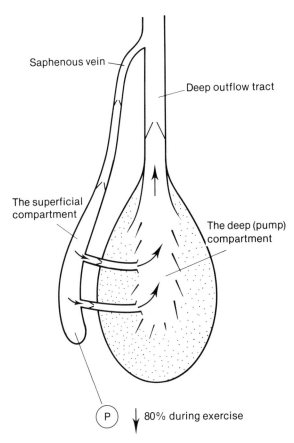

Saphenous vein

Deep outflow tract

The superficial compartment

The deep (pump) compartment

P ↓ 80% during exercise

Fig. 3.8 The functional anatomy of the veins of the lower limb.
The arrows indicate the normal direction of blood flow. During exercise the superficial vein pressure falls by 80 per cent.

veins, and they also act as the outflow tract for the foot. All the deep veins of the calf join to form the popliteal vein which is the calf pump outflow tract. As this vein continues up the limb it passes through the 'thigh' pump but in a position, the subsartorial canal, that protects it from much of the compressive forces generated by thigh muscle contraction. The outflow tract continues through the abdomen and the thorax where it is subject to the intermittent positive and negative pressures associated with respiration. The influence of these extramural pressures is discussed later. .

The superficial compartment

The superficial compartment comprises a net-work of venules and veins in the skin and subcutaneous tissues that empty into both the deep (pump) chamber and the pump outflow tract. The two main superficial veins, the long and short saphenous veins, drain directly into the outflow tract, but there are many other connections between the superficial veins and the veins of the deep compartment.

The superficial tributaries of the saphenous systems collect blood from the skin and subpapillary dermal plexus and then progressively unite to form the two main veins. The saphenous veins themselves lie in a deeper layer of the subcutaneous tissues underneath a thin but quite strong layer of connective tissue. The veins in the dermal plexus and the subcutaneous fat are well situated for their role in thermoregulation but are poorly supported against distending forces.

The valves ensure that blood flows into the pump and towards the heart. Blood leaves the superficial compartment by flowing up the saphenous veins into the femoral or popliteal veins or directly into the pump through the many communicating veins.[13,81]

Communications between the superficial and deep compartments

The superficial compartment has two large constant connections with the outflow tract, the sapheno-femoral and the sapheno-popliteal junctions (see Figs. 2.23 and 2.28, pp. 41, 43). They are protected by valves which normally prevent reflux from the deep to the superficial compartments. The common femoral and popliteal veins are not inside the muscle pumps. They lie relatively unsupported in the loose fatty connective tissue which surrounds the femoral and popliteal neurovascular bundles.

In addition to these two main communications between the deep outflow tract and the superficial compartment there are many other veins which drain into veins beneath the deep fascia which are within the pump, though not always actually within the muscles.

The named communicating veins on the medial aspect of the lower leg (see Figs. 2.30 and 2.31a, pp. 45, 46) connect the superficial veins with the posterior tibial veins. These veins do not connect the long saphenous vein directly to the deep compartment but drain the whole superficial system including the long saphenous vein into the pump indirectly through their connections with the posterior arch vein.

There are also a number of communicating veins on the lateral and posterior aspects of the limb that connect the superficial veins with the peroneal vein and veins within the soleus and gastrocnemius muscles (see Fig. 2.31b, p. 46).

In addition to the named communicating veins there are between 50 and 100 small *unnamed veins* which connect the deep and superficial system. Anatomically, they are similar in muscle and collagen content to superficial veins. They are usually accompanied by a small artery and are primarily venae comitantes of the artery. They do not play a significant part in the normal physiology of the calf pump.

The valves in the communicating veins are arranged so that they prevent flow from the deep to the superficial compartments. There may be one, two or three valves depending upon the length and course of the vein. The valves are invariably in that part of the vein beneath the deep fascia (Fig. 3.9).[47,48]

The course of the communicating veins beneath the deep fascia varies according to their destina-tion. Some are short and direct, others run between or into muscles before connecting with the intermuscular veins.[79] It is not known whether these variations have any pathophysiological significance (Fig. 3.10).

Phlebologists argue about the generic name of these veins. Many like to call them *perforating* veins because they pierce the deep fascia, and some anatomists think the term 'communicating vein' should be reserved for veins that connect vessels within the same compartment.

The important physiological role of these veins is, however, the *connection* that they make between the deep and superficial compartments. We therefore prefer the term *communicating* vein on physiological grounds and do not call them 'perforators' or 'blow outs'. Others have also expressed a preference for this term.[49,51,79]

The physiology of the calf pump

The action of the calf pump is best understood if the many superficial and deep veins are considered as two compartments with a few interconnections and a single outflow tract. It is, how-

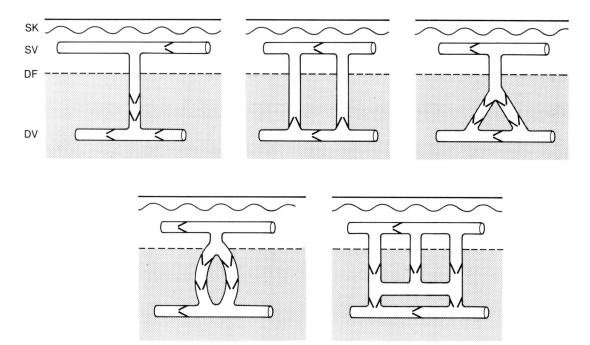

Fig. 3.9 The position of the valves and some common variations of the communicating veins. Redrawn after Pirner.[64]

SK = skin; SV = superficial vein; DF = deep fascia; DV = deep vein. Hatched area = muscle pump.

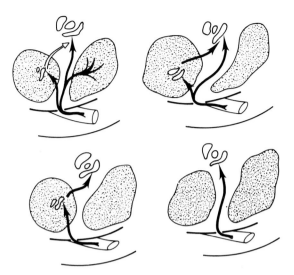

Fig. 3.10 Variations in the pathways taken by veins connecting the superficial to the deep veins. Adapted from Stolic.[79]

ever, important to remember that the superficial compartment communicates with both parts of the deep compartment, the pump chamber and the outflow tract.

The calf pump has been called the peripheral heart. We have found it helpful to develop this comparison because the left side of the heart is also a two chamber system. Figure 3.11 compares our compartmentalized concept of the calf pump with that of the left side of the heart. The calf pump is the equivalent of the left ventricle. The venous outflow tract is the equivalent of the aorta and its valve. The superficial compartment is the equivalent of the left atrium, and the communicating veins are comparable to the mitral valve. The difference between the leg and the heart is that there is a direct connection between the superficial compartment and the pump outflow tract which, if it was present in the heart and not protected by a valve, would be equivalent to a large arteriovenous fistula and add a considerable load to the heart. This is exactly what happens when saphenous vein incompetence refills the superficial chamber with regurgitating blood and subsequently overloads the pump.

The pump

Systole When the calf muscles and the muscles in the deep posterior compartment of the lower leg contract they raise the pressure in and around all the structures contained within the deep fascia. All the intramuscular veins are completely compressed because the muscles generate pressures of 200–300 mmHg.[7,51,91] The pressure which is deep to the fascia but outside the muscles does not rise as high but reaches levels of 100–150mmHg.[37,52,77]

These pressures squeeze the blood out of the veins, the valves ensuring that the blood flows only towards the heart. Flow from the deep to the superficial compartment is prevented by the valves in the communicating veins.[5]

The large veins within the gastrocnemius and soleus muscles form the main chamber of the pump but all the other deep veins participate.

The average volume of the calf is 1500–2000 ml, and the calf blood volume is 60–70 ml.[92] Continuous exercise reduces the calf blood volume by 1.5–2.0 ml/100 ml. Most of this reduction is from compression of the veins in the pump chamber, and the average expelled volume is approximately 30–40 ml, only 50 per cent of all the blood within the pump. The pump will normally expel this volume in four to five contractions, though one single sustained contraction can expel almost as

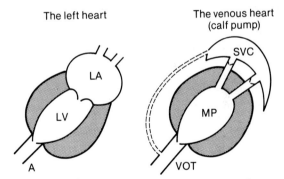

Fig. 3.11 A comparison between the left side of the heart and the calf pump.
LA = left atrium; LV = left ventricle; A = aorta; SVC = superficial venous compartment; MP = deep venous compartment (the muscle pump); VOT = venous outflow tract.
Continuing the analogy:
   Mitral incompetence = Communicating vein incompetence.
   Myocardial failure = Calf muscle weakness.
   Aortic incompetence = Deep vein valve incompetence in the outflow tract.
   Aortic stenosis = Deep vein obstruction in the outflow tract.

much. When the rate of exercise increases, the muscle blood flow may increase to 20–30 ml/100 ml/min. This places an additional load of 600 ml/min on the calf pump. The calf must contract at least 20 times every minute to expel this increased blood flow. Normal walking at 80 steps/min contracts each calf 40 times/min so the pump can easily deal with the high blood flow of exercise hyperaemia.

The outflow tract from the pump is a very large bore vein which offers virtually no resistance to flow. As the gradient of 10–15 mmHg between the small veins and the heart is sufficient to ensure venous blood flow when the subject is supine, the increase in gradient of 100–200 mmHg produced by the pump[6] is more than enough to ensure an adequate rapid venous return to the heart during vigorous erect muscle exercise.

Diastole The pump chamber is refilled by the arterial inflow and the flow from the superficial compartment during diastole. Just as blood flows from the left atrium to the left ventricle during ventricular diastole, so blood flows from the superficial to the deep compartment when the calf muscles relax.[13]

At the moment when the calf muscles relax their contained veins are empty, at zero pressure and as yet unfilled by arterial inflow. As the veins are collapsed they are also unaffected by hydrostatic pressure. Conversely, the superficial veins are full and subjected to hydrostatic pressure plus the remnant of cardiac generated pressure, the 'vis a tergo'. The pressure gradient between the two compartments is therefore 100–110 mmHg. Blood immediately flows from the superficial to the deep compartment through the many communicating veins.[13] This empties the superficial compartment *and reduces its pressure.*[9,37,40,66,73,76,87] Measurements of foot vein pressure during exercise show it to fall by 60–80 per cent (Fig. 3.12). This reduction in pressure is essential for the preservation of healthy skin and subcutaneous tissues. The exposure of the subcutaneous veins to a persistent high pressure may eventually cause cell death (see Chapter 11).

Thus calf pump activity performs two vital functions.

1. It ensures venous return from the lower limbs during exercise.
2. It reduces superficial vein pressure thus removing the damaging effect of the hydrosta-

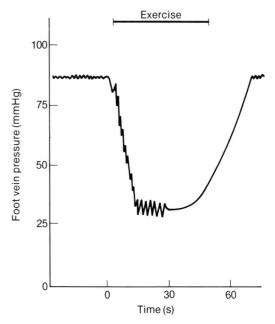

Fig. 3.12 The changes in foot vein pressure during heel raising exercise (Ex).

In a normal limb the pressure drops by 60–80 per cent and, after exercise, takes 15–25 seconds to return to resting levels.

tic pressure that is inseparable from man's upright posture.

It is therefore normal to have a low pressure in the subcutaneous veins during exercise and when supine. Superficial vein pressure only rises when standing still and when the calf pump fails. *The absence of venous hypotension during exercise is the ultimate cause of almost all 'venous' pathology.*

Respiration

The movements of the diaphragm affect the resistance of the outflow tract because they change intra-abdominal and intrathoracic pressure. During inspiration the abdominal pressure increases and obstructs venous return. At the same time the intrathoracic pressure falls so that the pressure gradient between the abdomen and thorax increases, encouraging venous blood flow from the abdominal to the thoracic veins.[58,59] Thus during inspiration blood flow from the limbs to the abdomen is impeded but blood flow from the abdomen to the thorax is accelerated.[26]

As soon as each inspiration stops the abdominal pressure falls and venous blood flow recommences from the lower limbs to the abdomen. There is still a positive but smaller gradient between the abdomen and the chest so blood flow from the abdomen to the chest continues.

Flow from the upper limbs into the chest is directly related to the positive and negative intrathoracic pressures of respiration.

The causes of calf pump failure

The pump

Four abnormalities may reduce the efficiency of the pump itself.

(a) *Muscle weakness* Weakness of the calf pump is the equivalent of heart failure. The calf muscles rapidly waste and weaken with disuse. Disuse accompanies major injuries, neurological disease, vascular insufficiency, debilitating diseases, myositis, and bone and joint pain. If the veins and their valves are normal, a weak calf muscle alone rarely causes symptoms of venous insufficiency but, if there is a pre-existing venous abnormality and the muscle becomes weak, symptoms are exacerbated.

Sometimes venous disease itself causes calf muscle wasting. A painful venous ulcer or fibrous ankylosis of the ankle joint caused by chronic venous insufficiency may cause the patient to limp to avoid painful ankle movements. The absence of calf contractions exacerbates the venous hypertension and its complications and causes calf muscle disuse atrophy. A vicious circle develops as valve damage causes skin complications, which cause pain and walking difficulties, which diminish pump function, which causes further deterioration of the skin.

(b) *Pump chamber contraction* (reduced end-diastolic volume) Extensive deep vein thrombosis may leave many of the deep veins of the calf, within and between the muscles, permanently occluded. They cannot hold all the blood delivered to them during pump diastole, pump vein pressure consequently rises rapidly, the veins that are patent dilate, their valves become incompetent and the pump begins to fail.

The volume of blood that can be squeezed from the calf by external compression is reduced in patients with old deep vein damage.[92]

(c) *Pump chamber dilatation* (Increased end-diastolic volume) (Fig. 3.13) Obstruction to the outflow of blood from the pump caused by occlusion of veins within the pump or in the main outflow tract causes the veins within the pump to dilate and their valves to become secondarily incompetent. Valvular incompetence of the intramuscular veins alone may not be particularly important but, if the communicating veins become incompetent, calf pump efficiency is seriously reduced. A major degree of outflow obstruction is usually caused by axial vein thrombosis.

(d) *Pump vein valve incompetence* All veins lying along the axis of the limb need valves to prevent retrograde flow. Not all the veins within the calf muscles have valves (e.g. the soleal sinuses), but these particular vessels are U-shaped with both ends emptying towards the heart.

An absence of valves in the deep veins puts additional strain on the valves in the communicating veins.

Isolated segments of deep veins with damaged valves rarely cause symptoms presumably because the potential volume of reflux into them is small. Extensive destruction of the valves can, however, cause venous claudication as well as communicating vein incompetence.

Outflow tract obstruction (Fig. 3.14)

Anything that blocks the outflow of blood from the pump will cause secondary dilatation of the veins within the pump and the communicating veins.

Collateral vessels are rarely adequate and therefore obstruction usually causes a slow but progressive deterioration of calf pump efficiency, just as aortic stenosis affects cardiac function.

Once the communicating veins dilate and become incompetent they become collateral vessels by carrying blood out into the superficial system during calf pump systole to bypass the deep obstruction.

Outflow tract incompetence (Fig. 3.15)

Pure deep vein incompetence without obstruction is rare. The pump refills rapidly during diastole and has to eject more blood during systole. The pump develops a high end-diastolic volume. Provided the muscle is strong and the communicating veins remain competent this abnormality rarely

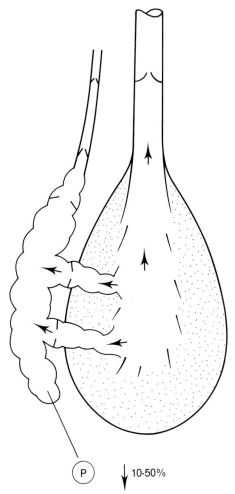

P   ↓ 10-50%

Fig. 3.13 Communicating vein incompetence.
   Dilatation of the veins within the pump leads to dilatation and incompetence of the communicating veins with reflux of blood into the superficial compartment during calf muscle contraction. Communicating vein dilatation may also occur as part of the varicose vein diathesis.
   The arrows indicate the direction of blood flow.
   During exercise the foot vein pressure falls by 10–50 per cent.

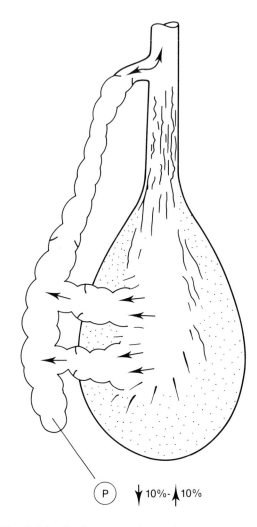

P   ↓ 10%- ↑ 10%

Fig. 3.14 Outflow tract obstruction.
   Deep vein obstruction causes dilatation of the pump chamber and secondary incompetence of the communicating veins because these veins become part of the collateral outflow tract.
   During exercise the foot vein pressure will fall slightly or even rise.

causes symptoms. Ultimately, the veins within the pump and the communicating veins dilate and become incompetent and the symptoms of venous insufficiency begin to appear.

Communicating vein incompetence (Fig. 3.13)

Communicating veins have been mentioned

repeatedly throughout this discussion on calf pump insufficiency. Their valves form an essential protection between the high pressures that develop within the pump and the low pressures produced by the pump in the subcutaneous compartment. If their valves fail, the pump pushes blood into the superficial veins as well as into the outflow tract during systole. The situation is

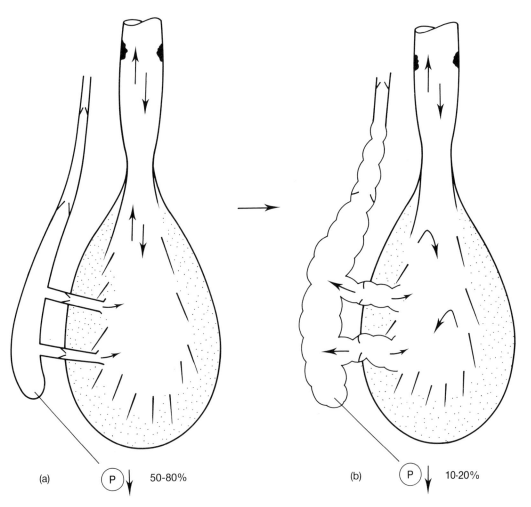

Fig. 3.15 The calf pump can compensate for pure deep vein (outflow tract) incompetence by increasing its output (a). If the dilatation of the veins within the pump affects the communicating veins (b) the pump begins to fail and foot vein pressure is only reduced by 10–20 per cent during exercise.

analogous to mitral valve incompetence. The clinical effect depends upon the balance between forward normal outflow tract blood flow, retrograde communicating vein flow and superficial compartment distention, the latter determines the effect of the retrograde flow on superficial pressure.

The two causes of communicating vein valve incompetence are valve cusp destruction by thrombosis and valve ring dilatation secondary to downstream post-thrombotic venous obstruction or as part of the progressive vein dilatation of the primary varicose vein diathesis.

Superficial vein incompetence (Fig. 3.16)

A segment of a superficial vein with incompetent valves may become dilated and tortuous but will not damage the local tissues provided there is a competent valve between it and the deep veins. Superficial vein incompetence is mainly a cosmetic problem. Its only effect on calf pump function is to increase the volume of blood that has to be pumped out of the lower leg. Incompetent superficial veins (varicose veins) only contain 5–10 per cent of the total blood in the lower limb, but the volume of blood refluxing through them

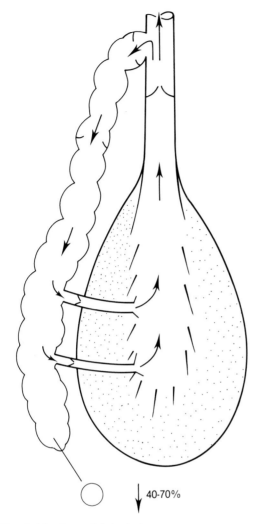

40–70%

Fig. 3.16 Superficial vein incompetence allows reflux of blood down the superficial veins but, providing the communicating veins are competent, the calf pump can usually cope with the additional load and reduce the foot vein pressure during exercise by 40–70 per cent.

may be considerable. Eventually, usually after very many years, this added load can jeopardize calf pump function and cause skin damage. Long-standing primary varicose veins can, though rarely, cause venous ulceration.

The arm veins

The anatomy of the arm veins is described in Chapter 2. The arm muscles exert a pumping effect which is similar to that of the calf muscles but the superficial veins form a greater part of the outflow tract than the superficial veins in the leg and the valves in the communicating veins point in the opposite direction. As the hydrostatic pressure in the arms is so low, venous malfunction never causes the skin changes and ulceration which are seen in the lower limb.

References

1. Abdel-Sayed WA, Abboud FM, Calvelo MG. Effect of local cooling on responsiveness of muscular cutaneous arteries and veins. *Am J Physiol* 1970; **219**: 1772.
2. Ablad B, Mellander S. Comparative effects of hydralazine, sodium nitrate and acetylcholine on resistance and capacitance vessels and capillary filtration in skeletal muscle in the cat. *Acta Physiol Scand* 1963; **58**: 319.
3. Ackroyd JS, Pattison M, Browse NL. A study of the mechanical properties of fresh and preserved human femoral vein wall and valve cusps. *Br J Surg* 1985; **72**: 117.
4. Alexander RS. The peripheral venous system In: Hamilton WF, Dow P (Eds) *Handbook of Physiology*. Section 2. Circulation. Bethesda, Maryland. American Physiological Society 1963; 1075.
5. Almen T, Nylander G. Serial phlebography of the normal lower limb during muscular contraction and relaxation. *Acta Radiol Scand* 1962; **57**: 264.
6. Barcroft H, Dornhorst AC. Demonstration of the muscle pump in the human leg. *J Physiol (Lond)* 1949; **108**: 39.
7. Barcroft H, Dornhorst AC. The blood flow through the human calf during rhythmic exercise. *J Physiol (Lond)* 1949; **109**: 402.
8. Baum T, Hosko MJ. Response of resistance and capacitance vessels to central nervous stimulation. *Am J Physiol* 1965; **209**: 236.
9. Beecher HK, Field ME, Krogh A. The effect of walking on the venous pressure at the ankle. *Scand Arch Physiol* 1936; **73**: 133.
10. Bevan JA, Hosmer DW, Ljung B, Pegram BL, Su C. Innervation pattern and neurogenic response of rabbit veins. *Blood Vessels* 1974; **11**: 172.
11. Bevegard BS, Shepherd JT. Changes in tone of limb veins during supine exercise. *J Appl Physiol* 1965; **20**: 1.
12. Bevegard BS, Shepherd JT. Effect of local exercise of forearm muscles on forearm capacitance vessels. *J Appl Physiol* 1965; **20**: 968.
13. Bjordal R. Simultaneous pressure and flow recordings in varicose veins of the lower extremity. *Acta Chir Scand* 1970; **136**: 309.

14. Browse NL, Gray L, Jarrett PEM, Morland M. Blood and vein wall fibrinolytic activity in health and vascular disease. *Br Med J* 1977; **1**: 478.

15. Browse NL, Hardwick PJ. The deep breath venoconstriction reflex. *Clin Science* 1969; **37**: 125.

16. Browse NL, Lorenz RR, Shepherd J. Response of capacity and resistance vessels of dog's limb to sympathetic nerve stimulation. *Am J Physiol* 1966; **210**: 95.

17. Browse NL. The treatment of venous insufficiency of the lower limb.*Vasc Diag Th* 1982; **3**: 27.

18. Burnand KG, Browse NL. The postphlebitic leg and venous ulceration In: Russell RCG (Ed) *Recent Advances in Surgery II*. Edinburgh. Churchill Livingstone 1982; 225.

19. Burnstock G. Evolution of the autonomic innervation of visceral and cardiovascular systems in vertebrates. *Pharmacol Rev* 1969; **21**: 247.

20. Chakrabarti R, Birks PM, Fearnley GR. Origin of blood fibrinolytic activity from veins and its bearing on the fate of venous thrombi. *Lancet* 1963; **1**: 1288.

21. Coimbra A, Ribeiro-Silva A, Osswald W. Fine structural and autoradiographic study of the adrenergic innervation of the dog lateral saphenous vein. *Blood Vessels* 1974; **11**: 128.

22. Cotton LT. Varicose veins. Gross anatomy and development. *Br J Surg* 1961; **48**: 589.

23. Deluis W, Kellerova E. Reaction of arterial and venous vessels in the human forearm and hand to deep breath or mental strain. *Clin Sci* 1971; **40**: 271.

24. Donegan JF. The physiology of the veins. *J Physiol (Lond)* 1921; **55**: 226.

25. Duggan JJ, Love VL, Lyons RH. A study of reflex venomotor reactions in man. *Circulation* 1953; **7**: 869.

26. Duomarco JL, Rimini R, Energy and hydraulic gradients along systemic veins. *Am J Physiol* 1954; **178**: 215.

27. Edwards EA. The orientation of venous valves in relation to body surfaces. *Anat Rec* 1936; **64**: 369.

28. Epstein SE, Beiser GD, Stampfer M, Braunwald E. Role of the venous system in baroreceptor mediated reflexes in man. *J Clin Invest* 1968; **47**: 139

29. Fearnley GR, Banfort GU, Fearnley E. Evidence of diurnal fibrinolytic rhythm with a simple method of measuring natural fibrinolysis. *Clin Sci* 1957; **16**: 645.

30. Fearnley GR. A concept of natural fibrinolysis. *Lancet* 1961; **1**: 992.

31. Fearnley GR. *Fibrinolysis*. Baltimore. Williams and Wilkins 1965.

32. Franklin KJ, McLachlin AD. Dilatation of veins in response to tapping in man and in certain other mammals. *J Physiol* 1936; **88**: 257.

33. Franklin KJ. A Monograph on Veins. Illinois. Thomas 1937.

34. Gardner AMN, Fox RH. The venous pump of the human foot. *Bristol Med Chir J* 1983; **109**: 112.

35. Gibbs NM. Venous thrombosis of the lower limbs with particular reference to bedrest. *Br J Surg* 1957; **45**: 209.

36. Greenberg RA, Sparks HV. Prostaglandins and consecutive vascular segments of the canine hind limb. *Am J Physiol* 1969; **216**: 567.

37. Höjensgard IC, Stürup H. Static and dynamic pressures in superficial and deep veins of the lower extremity in man. *Acta Physiol Scand* 1953; **27**: 49.

38. Haddy FJ, Fleishman M, Emanuel D. Effect of epinephrine, norepinephrine and serotonin upon systemic small and large vessel resistances. *Circ Res* 1957; **5**: 247.

39. Harvey W. *Exercitatio Anatomica de Motu Cordis et Sanguinis in Animalibus*. Francofurti. Sumptibus Gulielusi Fizeri 1628.

40. Henry JP. The influence of temperature and exercise on venous pressure in the foot when in the erect posture. *Am J Med* 1948; **4**: 619.

41. Hintze A, Throh HL. Das ferhalten der menschlichen handvenen bei akuter arterieller hypoxie. *Pflügers Arch Ges Physiol* 1961; **274**: 227.

42. Hooker DR. The veno-pressor mechanism. *Am J Physiol* 1918; **46**: 591.

43. Isacson S. Low fibrinolytic activity of blood and vein walls in venous thrombosis. *Scand J Haematol* 1971; Suppl **16**.

44. Jaff EA, Hoyer LW, Nachman RL. Synthesis of antihaemophilic factor antigen by cultured human endothelial cells. *J Clin Invest* 1973; **52**: 2757.

45. Kjellmer I, Odelråm M. The effect of some physiological vasodilators on the vascular bed of skeletal muscle. *Acta Physiol Scand* 1965: **63**: 94.

46. Kwaan HC, Lo R, McFadzean AJS. Production of plasma fibrinolytic activity within veins. *Clin Sci* 1957; **16**: 241.

47. Leach RD, Clemenson G, Morland M, Browse NL. The relationship between venous pressure and vein wall fibrinolytic activity. *J Cardiovasc Surg* 1982; **23**: 505.

48. Lesh TA, Rothe CF. Sympathetic and haemodynamic effects on capacitance vessels in dog skeletal muscles.*Am J Physiol* 1969; **217**: 819.

49. Linton RR. John Homan's impact on diseases of the veins of the lower extremity with special reference to deep thrombophlebitis and the post-thrombotic syndrome with ulceration. *Surgery* 1977; **81**: 1.

50. Ludbrook J, Beales G, Femoral venous valves in relation to varicose veins. *Lancet* 1962; **1**: 79.

51. Ludbrook J. *Aspects of Venous Function in the Lower Limbs*. Illinois. Thomas 1966.

52. Ludbrook J. The musculo-venous pumps of tne human lower limb.*Am Heart J* 1966; **71**: 635.

53. Macfarlane RK. Fibrinolysis following operation. *Lancet* 1937; **1**: 10.

54. Mark AL, Schmid PG, Eckstein JW, Wendling MG. Venous responses to prostaglandin F2α. *Am J Physiol* 1971; **220**: 222.

55. Marshall RJ, Shepherd JT. *Cardiac Function in Health and Disease*. Philadelphia. WB Saunders 1966.

56. Mellander S. Comparative studies on the adrenergic neuro-hormonal control of resistance and capacitance blood vessels in the cat. *Acta Physiol Scand* 1960; **50**: Suppl 176.

57. Mole RH. Fibrinolysis and the fluidity of the blood postmortem. *J Pathol Bacteriol* 1948; **60**: 413.

58. Moreno AH, Burchell AR, Vanderwonde R, Burke JH. Respiratory regulation of splanchnic and systemic venous return. *Am J Physiol* 1967; **213**: 455.

59. Moreno AH, Katz AI, Gold LD. An integrated approach to the study of the venous system with steps toward a detailed model of the dynamics of venous return to the right heart. *IEEE Trans Biomed Eng* 1969; **16**: 308.

60. Nilsson IM, Isacson S. New aspects of the pathogenesis of thromboembolism. In: Allgower M (Ed) *Progress in Surgery 11*. Basel. Karger 1973; 46.

61. Nilsson IM, Robertson B. Effect of venous occlusion on coagulation and fibrinolytic components in normal subjects. *Thromb Diath Haemorrh* 1968; **20**: 397.

62. Pandolfi M, Nilsson IM, Robertson B, Isacson S. Fibrinolytic activity of human veins. *Lancet* 1967; **2**: 127.

63 Pegum JM, Fegan WG. Physiology of venous return from the foot. *Cardiovasc Res* 1967; **1**: 249.

64. Pirner F. Über die Bedentung Form und Art der Klappen in den V communicates der unteren Extremitat. *Anat Anz* 1956; **103**: 450.

65. Pirner F. Die Bedentung der insuff V.perforans fur die Kramfaderoperation. *Chir Praxis* 1963; **7**: 112.

66. Pollack AA, Wood EH. Venous pressure in the saphenous vein at the ankle in man during exercise and changes in posture. *J Appl Physiol* 1949; **1**: 649.

67. Powell T, Lynn RB. The valves of the external iliac, femoral and upper third of the popliteal vein. *Surg Gynec Obstet* 1951; **92**: 453.

68. Rice AJ, Long JP. An unusual venoconstriction induced by acetylcholine. *J Pharmacol Exp Ther* 1966; **151**: 423.

69. Rowell LB. Human cardiovascular adjustments to exercise and thermal stress. *Physiol Rev* 1974; **54**: 75.

70. Sammueloff SL, Browse NL, Shepherd JT. Response of capacity vessels in human limbs to head-up tilt and suction on the lower body. *J Appl Physiol* 1966; **21**: 47.

71. Samueloff SL, Bevegard BS, Shepherd JT. Temporary arrest of circulation to a limb for the study of venomotor reactions in man.*J Appl Physiol* 1966; **21**: 341.

72. Samuels PB, Webster DR. The role of venous endothelium in the inception of thrombosis. *Ann Surg* 1962; **136**: 422.

73. Seiro V. Über blutdruck und blulkreislauf in den krampfadern der unteren extremitaten. *Acta Chir Scand* 1938; **80**: 41.

74. Shaper AG, Marsh NA, Patel I, Kater F. Response of fibrinolytic activity to venous occlusion. *Br Med J* 1975; **3**: 571.

75. Shepherd JT, Vanhoutte PM. *Veins and their Control* . Philadelphia. Saunders 1975.

76. Smirk RH. Observations on the causes of oedema in congestive heart failure. *Clin Science* 1936; **2**: 317.

77. Stürup H, Höjensgard IC. Venous pressure in the deep veins of the lower extremity of patients with primary and post thrombotic varicose veins. *Acta Chir Scand* 1950; **99**: 526.

78. Stanbesand J, Rulffs W. Die klappen kleiner venen. *Z Anat Entwickl Gesch* 1958; **120**: 392.

79. Stolic E. Terminology, division and systematic anatomy of the communicating veins of the lower limb. In: May R, Partsch H, Straubesand J (Eds) *Perforating Veins*. Wien. Urban & Schwarzenberg 1981; 19.

80. Thompson FJ, Barnes CD. Evidence for thermosensitive elements in the femoral vein. *Life Sci, I*. 1970; **90**: 309.

81. Tibbs DJ, Fletcher EWL. Direction of flow in superficial veins as a guide to venous disorders in lower limbs. *Surgery* 1983; **93**: 758.

82. Tighe JR, Swan UT. Fibrinolysis in venous obstruction. *Clin Sci* 1963; **25**: 219.

83. Todd AS. Fibrinolysis autographs. *Nature* 1958;**181**: 495.

84. Todd AS. Histological localization of fibrinolysis activator. *J Path Bact* 1959; **78**: 281.

85. Todd AS. Localisation of fibrinolytic activity in tissues. *Br Med Bull* 1964; **20**: 200.

86. Vanhoutte PM, Shepherd JT. Venous relaxation caused by acetylcholine acting on the sympathetic nerves. *Circ Res* 1973; **32**: 259.

87. Walker AJ, Longland CJ. Venous pressure measurement in the foot in exercise as an aid to investigation of venous disease in the leg. *Clin Sci* 1950; **9**: 101.

88. Watson WE. Distensibility of the capacity blood

vessels of the human hand during sleep. *J Physiol (Lond)* 1962; **161**: 392.

89. Webb Peploe MM, Shepherd JT. Response of superficial limb veins of the dog to changes in temperature. *Circ Res* 1968; **22**: 737.

90. Weksler BB, Marcus AJ, Jaff EA. Synthesis of prostaglandin I_2 by cultured human and bovine endothelial cells. *Proc Natl Acad Sci USA* 1977; **74**: 3922.

91. Wells HS, Youmans JB, Miller DG. Tissue pressure, intracutaneous, subcutaneous and intramuscular, as related to venous pressure, capillary filtration and other factors. *J Clin Invest* 1938; **17**: 489.

92. Whitehead S, Clemenson G, Browse NL. The assessment of calf pump function by isotope plethysmography. *Br J surg* 1983; **70**: 675.

93. Wolfe JHN, Morland M, Browse NL. The fibrinolytic activity of varicose veins. *Br J Surg* 1979; **66**: 185.

94. Woollard HH. The innervation of blood vessels. *Heart* 1926; **13**: 319.

95. Zsoter T, Tom H. Adrenoreceptive sites in the veins. *Br J Pharmacol Chemother* 1967; **31**: 407.

4

Techniques of investigation

There are many different methods available for the investigation of the venous system. All these techniques provide incomplete information on either the anatomy or function of the veins, or both. They vary from simple clinical examination to methods using modern sophisticated electronic apparatus. Each method has its own particular advantages, and disadvantages, and sometimes three or four different methods actually measure the same thing. There are, for example, four methods of calf plethysmography all of which measure the change in blood volume within the calf, and these, together with foot volumetry and photoplethysmography, make six techniques which measure calf pump function.

It is essential to understand which aspect of venous anatomy or function a test measures and how accurately it does this. Knowledge of the methodology of the tests, though secondary to this understanding, is also very important when interpreting the results. This chapter describes all the tests in common use. It concentrates upon the principle of each test, the method and the reasons for inaccuracies. The place of each test in the investigation of chronic venous insufficiency and venous thrombosis is discussed in the relevant chapter.

It has become customary to express the value of a test, not only in terms of accuracy, but in terms of sensitivity, specificity and predictive value. These are mathematical forms of assessment which are undoubtedly useful when evaluating a new test but they should also be used to evaluate any test, however old, when you introduce it into your own regimen of investigation as a way of comparing your own ability to perform the test against the published results of other workers.

These mathematical expressions of validity depend upon a comparison between the test being evaluated and an established test of the same function whose accuracy is known. The key word in the preceding sentence is 'accurate'. The most accurate test available is commonly referred to as *the gold standard*. Unfortunately, there are few gold standards in venous investigation. Phlebography almost comes up to the 100 per cent accuracy level required of a gold standard for anatomical delineation but there are no perfect tests of venous physiological function. When talking about the specificity or sensitivity of a test therefore, always remember to specify or enquire about the gold standard against which the new test is being compared. More often than not you will find that the gold standard is not totally reliable (a base metal, often gold lacquer covering lead). After such a discovery you will properly appreciate the value of the calculated expressions of sensitivity and specificity.

Accuracy Accuracy is a word we all understand. It is the simple expression of the number of correct diagnoses obtained by the test, whether they be positive or negative, as a proportion of the total number of tests performed ($\times$ 100 to make it a percentage).

$$\text{Accuracy} = \frac{\text{Number of correct tests}}{\text{Total number of tests}} \times 100$$

(The numerator which is the total number of correct tests, both positive and negative, is based upon a comparison with the gold standard.)

Sensitivity The sensitivity of a test tells you how often a positive test actually indicates real disease. It is therefore the ratio between the number of correctly positive tests and the true incidence of the disease.

$$\text{Sensitivity} = \frac{\text{Number of correct positive tests}}{\text{Number with disease}} \times 100$$

(The numerator is determined by the gold standard, the denominator is the sum of the correct positive tests and the incorrect negative tests (true-positives plus false-negatives) again determined by comparison against the gold standard.)

Specificity The specificity of a test tells you how often a negative test actually indicates no disease.

$$\text{Specificity} = \frac{\text{Number of correct negative tests}}{\text{Number without disease}} \times 100$$

(The denominator is the sum of the correct negative tests and the incorrect positive tests [true-negative plus false-positive].)

We find the terms sensitivity and specificity confusing. They are words whose meanings bear no relation to what they are trying to tell us – the ability to detect disease and the ability to identify the absence of disease respectively. Unfortunately, they have become firmly established amongst those workers who have developed and who perform many of these non-invasive vascular laboratory tests and therefore all of us have to remember their definitions.

The question that the clinician is more likely to ask, apart from overall accuracy, is 'How often is a positive (or a negative) test likely to be correct?' This question implies that a test may be better at detecting disease than detecting normality, or *vice versa*. This question can be easily answered by calculating what has become known as the positive (or negative) predictive value – another cumbersome expression which would be much simpler and easier to comprehend if it was changed to positive (or negative) test accuracy.

Positive test accuracy

$$\underset{\text{(positive predictive value)}}{\text{Positive test accuracy}} = \frac{\text{Number of correct positive tests}}{\text{Number of positive tests}} \times 100$$

(The numerator is derived from a comparison against the gold standard. The denominator is all the positive tests, that is the sum of the correct [true] and the incorrect [false] positive tests.)

Negative test accuracy

This is similar to positive test accuracy.

$$\underset{\text{(negative predictive value)}}{\text{Negative test accuracy}} = \frac{\text{Number of correct negative tests}}{\text{Number of negative tests}} \times 100$$

(The denominator is the sum of the correct and the incorrect negative tests [true-negatives and false-negatives].)

Example Suppose you have developed a new test of venous thrombosis which you have performed on 300 limbs and compared against phlebograms performed on the same limbs, the phlebogram being accepted as the gold standard, even though we know that it is not quite 100 per cent accurate.

Two hundred of the new tests are positive, 100 tests are negative. When, however, the tests are compared against the phlebograms:

- 180 of the new test's positive results are correct (true positives)
- 20 of the new test's positive results are incorrect (false-positives)
- 70 of the new test's negative results are correct (true-negatives)
- 30 of the new test's negative results are incorrect (false-negatives)

Overall accuracy of the test is $\dfrac{180 + 70}{300} \times 100 = 83\%$

Positive test accuracy of the test is (positive predictive value) $\dfrac{180}{200} \times 100 = 90\%$

Negative test accuracy of the test is (negative predictive value) $\dfrac{70}{100} \times 100 = 70\%$

Sensitivity of the test is $\dfrac{180}{180 + 30} \times 100 = 86\%$

Specificity of the test is $\dfrac{70}{70 + 20} \times 100 = 77\%$

These calculations suggest that our new test is moderately good. Overall it gets the answer right in 4 out of 5 cases (accuracy 83 per cent). It is, however, better when a thrombosis is present (9 out of 10 positive test accuracy) than when the leg is normal (7 out of 10 negative test accuracy). Overall its ability to detect disease is 86 per cent (sensitivity) and its ability to exclude disease is almost as good – 77 per cent (specificity).

Think about these ways of expressing the value of a test and decide which you most readily understand and prefer.

Clinical examination

The many and varied symptoms and signs of venous disease are described and discussed in those chapters dealing with specific venous abnormalities. The majority of symptoms and signs are non-specific.[78,134]

History

Venous disease affects all age groups, though varicose veins in children are likely to be associated with a congenital rather than an acquired abnormality, and deep vein thrombosis is rare in children.

Pain, swelling and unsightliness are the dominant symptoms.

Superficial venous insufficiency causes a dull aching pain which is relieved by rest; deep vein thrombosis causes a persistent more severe pain. Venous outflow obstruction, whether acute (following a deep vein thrombosis) or chronic, causes a bursting pain during muscle exercise. A patient with an acute thrombosis is unlikely to try to walk because the muscles are also painful at rest.

Night cramps are common.

Swelling of the leg may be localized, or general. General swelling may vary from a little oedema around the ankle to gross swelling of the whole limb. There is no difference between the swelling of deep vein thrombosis and that of chronic venous insufficiency; it is a low protein oedema caused by the venous obstruction.

Unsightliness is related to the size and extent of the varicose veins, intradermal venules, pigmentation, scarring and swelling.

A carefully taken clinical history is an essential part of the investigation of venous disease and often helps exclude or pinpoint other differential diagnoses. Chest symptoms in a patient with deep vein thrombosis should always be assumed to be caused by pulmonary embolism until proved otherwise.

Examination

Always examine the legs twice, first when the patient is standing and then when the patient is lying down, except when muscle pain and discomfort are severe.

Inspection Three abnormalities may be visible on inspection, dilated superficial veins, changes in the skin and swelling.

Dilated veins may be large incompetent tortuous subcutaneous veins (i.e. varicose veins) or fine intradermal venules ('venous stars'). The position of the dilated veins may indicate their anatomical origin and connections. Veins on the medial side of the thigh are most likely to be connected to the long saphenous system but below the knee the position of a varicose vein does not allow its attribution to any particular system. A varicose vein on the medial side of the calf may be connected to the long saphenous system but it could be connected to the short saphenous system or it could be independent of both.

Skin changes range from mild eczema and pigmentation through thickening and hardening of the skin and fat (lipodermatosclerosis) to weeping eczema and frank ulceration. Although the majority of these skin changes are found on the lower medial third of the lower leg, they can occur anywhere. Conversely, other forms of ulceration more common on other parts of the leg can occur in the 'gaiter' area and so never assume that skin changes are venous in origin just because of their site. The clinical features of venous ulcers are discussed in Chapter 14. The presence of skin changes indicates a severe disturbance of calf pump function, whereas quite large varicose veins may exist with little or no functional abnormality.

The extent of diffuse swelling caused by venous disease usually correlates with the site and severity of the venous outflow obstruction. Localized swelling is usually caused by local inflammatory changes (e.g. superficial thrombophlebitis).

Palpation The size and tension of the veins can easily be assessed with the finger tips. The presence of an *expansile cough impulse* indicates the absence of functioning valves between the palpating finger and the thorax. Always examine for this impulse at the sapheno-femoral junction, whether there be a palpable vein or not, and over any other visible veins. Veins that cannot be seen can often be felt, especially in the thigh.

A calf that is the site of a deep vein thrombosis will be warmer than the normal calf. Recently thrombosed veins are firm, incompressible and tender. The tenderness fades with the inflammation but the vein gets harder and the overlying skin often becomes pigmented.

Skin changes are not usually tender to palpation except when there is acute lipodermatosclerosis when the skin, which is red–brown, and the fat, which is thickened with a palpable edge between it and the normal tissues, are both tender.

The surface of an ulcer is painful if it is infected or necrotic. Clean, healing chronic venous ulcers are usually neither painful nor very tender.

The oedema of venous obstruction is soft and 'pits' easily with firm pressure.

The thickening of lipodermatosclerosis sometimes looks like oedema but is hard and incompressible and can even become calcified. Veins amongst thickened hard tissues feel like hollow pits when the patient is lying flat and the venous pressure is low. It is easy to be misguided by this appearance into thinking that these pits are fascial defects corresponding to the site of superficial-to-deep communicating veins.[25]

Deep tenderness within the muscles, particularly the calf, is a physical sign of deep vein thrombosis but also of a multitude of other abnormalities within the muscle such as local trauma, myositis, arteritis, ischaemia and malignant change. Varicose veins rarely cause muscle tenderness. Even in conditions where deep vein thrombosis is the most likely diagnosis (e.g. postoperation) calf tenderness has a positive test accuracy of only 50 per cent (using the fibrinogen uptake test as the gold standard).[102] Nevertheless, it is important to palpate the deep tissues of the leg as well as the skin, subcutaneous tissues and veins. Attempts to quantify tenderness by applying known pressures with a pneumatic cuff have not been helpful.[16,125,127]

Careful palpation may reveal tender defects in the deep fascia on the medial side of the lower leg which sometimes correspond to the site of dilated communicating veins.[25]

Percussion A dilated blood-filled vein will conduct a percussion impulse in the direction of normal blood flow and retrogradely if the valves are incompetent. Thus tapping on a vein and feeling downstream can be used as a method for detecting the course and connections of a dilated vein, and tapping and feeling upstream can be used as a way of testing for incompetent valves in the segment of vein between the two hands.[44]

Auscultation Do not forget to place a stethoscope over large bunches of varicosities, especially if they are in an abnormal position. On rare occasions there will be a 'machinery murmur' indicating the presence of an arteriovenous fistula.

Elevation If the veins in a limb are distended when the patient is lying down, slowly raise the limb until the veins collapse. The height to which the limb has to be raised corresponds to the pressure in the veins and indicates the severity of the venous obstruction.

General examination

No patient with venous disease should have just their veins examined. It is essential to examine all the systems of the limb, particularly the arteries and nerves, and the *whole patient*. Varicose veins can be caused by abdominal tumours. Deep vein thrombosis and superficial thrombophlebitis can be secondary to occult carcinoma, especially of the lung, stomach, pancreas and kidney. Failure to examine the whole patient even though they present with only a few varicose veins is negligent.

The tourniquet tests

The tourniquet tests are simple bed-side tests which help to assess the direction of blood flow and the source of refilling of the superficial veins.[33,34,63,192] They are tests whose accuracy very much depends on the operator (i.e. they get more accurate as the experience and understanding of the clinician performing the test grows).

If the subcutaneous veins of the lower limb are occluded by a narrow tourniquet placed around the limb when the patient is lying down, filling of the veins below the tourniquet when the patient stands up indicates that there is an incompetent connection between the deep and superficial veins below the tourniquet (Fig. 4.1).

The level of this incompetent connection can be determined by repeating the test with the tourniquet at different levels or by using multiple tourniquets. Venous filling can be accelerated by mild exercise, such as repeated heel raising.

If the tourniquet is placed around the limb when the patient is standing and the superficial veins are distended, exercise should reduce the pressure and volume of blood in the veins below the tourniquet if the deep veins are functioning normally, and increase their pressure and volume if the deep veins are obstructed. This test, usually called Perthes test,[163] is more difficult to perform than the simpler reflux test, which is loosely called Trendelenburg's test.[33]

Tourniquet tests are useful in patients with chronic venous insufficiency and especially in those with superficial varicosities (see Chapter 6). In conjunction with clinical examination they provide a sufficient understanding of the venous

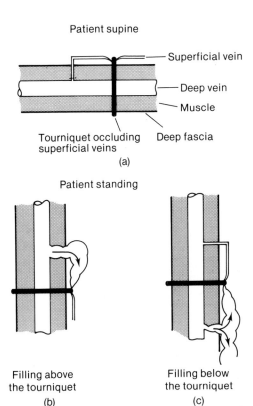

Patient supine

— Superficial vein

— Deep vein

— Muscle

Tourniquet occluding   Deep fascia
superficial veins

(a)

Patient standing

Filling above   Filling below
the tourniquet   the tourniquet
(b)   (c)

Fig. 4.1 The principle of the tourniquet test.
(a) A tourniquet is placed around the leg to occlude the superficial veins when the patient is supine and the superficial veins empty. The patient is then asked to stand.
(b) Filling of the veins above the tourniquet indicates an incompetent deep-to-superficial communication above the tourniquet.
(c) Filling of the veins below the tourniquet indicates an incompetent connection below the tourniquet.

abnormality for management decisions in 80–90 per cent of patients (see Chapter 7).

Photography

Colour photographs can be used to record the size and extent of superficial varicosities and ulcers (see colour plate section).

Photographs are the only way in which changes in the appearance of the skin may be recorded over a period of time but they are only useful if the photographic technique is carefully controlled and kept constant between photographs. Widmer used photography effectively as part of his prevalence study of venous disease in Basle.[204] The important aspects of his technique are given below.

Position

The patient must stand in a standardized reproducible position with legs apart and feet externally rotated as much as possible to ensure that the whole of the inner side of both legs is visible on the anterior view, and the lateral sides are visible on the posterior view. Oedema is best shown in an anterior view with the long axis of the foot in the sagittal plane.

Views

Anterior, posterior and oblique views (at a standard angle) should be taken.

Lighting

Although oblique lighting gives shadows which reveal large varicosities it does not illuminate the skin sufficiently to reveal fine intradermal veins. A direct light does not give many shadows but demonstrates minor colour differences in the skin much more clearly. The intensity and colour of the light used must be kept constant between photographs. A flash is not necessary if optimum lighting and a good camera are used.

Colour

Colour film reveals minor variations of skin pigmentation but intradermal venules show up better on black and white film. The type and make of film must not be altered as different brands have different colour sensitivities.

Camera

Any good camera will suffice provided the focal distance, aperture and exposure are kept constant.

The changes in ulcers may also be recorded with serial photographs provided the same constraints about constant position, lighting, film and camera are applied. Serial close-up views are most informative provided a centimetre scale is placed on the skin to enable measurements from the photograph to be calibrated.

Infra-red photography

The blood in the superficial veins heats the overlying skin. This temperature difference can be detected by infra-red photography, a method which is less sensitive but similar to thermography. Large veins appear as dark areas, even intradermal venules show up but the technique is not very valuable except when the clinician suspects that there are many varices that he cannot see or feel (Fig. 4.2).

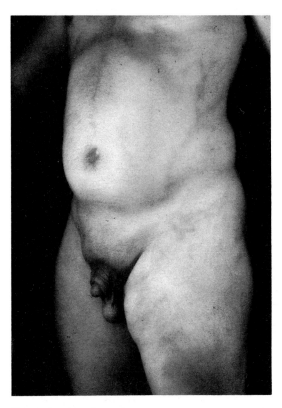

Fig. 4.2 An infra-red photograph of a patient with an occlusion of the inferior vena cava. There were no visible veins on the abdominal wall but the infra-red photograph revealed dilated subcutaneous collateral veins on the lateral side of the abdomen.

The fluorescein test

The use of fluorescein to reveal the site of incompetent communicating veins was described by us in 1970.[45] When fluorescein is injected into a foot vein below a tourniquet at the ankle (which occludes the superficial veins), it ascends into the calf through the deep veins and then into the superficial veins if the communicating veins are incompetent. The point where it appears beneath the skin can be seen as a yellow fluorescent area if the leg is illuminated in a darkened room with ultraviolet light. When compared against phlebography, however, this method has a positive test accuracy of only 47 per cent[67,156] and is no better than many other simpler and less invasive tests; it has never been adopted as a routine investigation.

Thermography

A thermographic system detects differences in skin temperature by measuring the infra-red emissions from the skin with an infra-red detector – usually indium–antimonide or cadmium–mercury–telluride cooled with liquid nitrogen. The object under study is scanned by a scanning camera which focuses the infra-red emissions onto the detector. The electrical impulses from the detector are converted into a video signal so that a visual television image is produced which can be examined directly or photographed with a polaroid camera.[50]

If the patient is lying in bed, the legs can be scanned from the foot of the bed by viewing them through a mirror held over them at an angle of 45°. To examine the deep veins, the legs must be elevated to eliminate superficial venous pooling.[49]

It is important for the limbs to be exposed for 10 minutes in an ambient temperature of 18–20°C and in a room without any draughts. Any movement of air will affect the thermogram. The common convention is to display the hot areas as white and the cold areas as black. It is, however, best to focus the image so that there is the maximum number of grey tones. Some systems have a colour coded presentation.

The normal image of the leg reveals an even temperature throughout with a slightly colder area over the tibia and patella anteriorly and a warmer area over the popliteal fossa posteriorly (Fig. 4.3 a and b). Sometimes the image has a mottled appearance caused by irregular warm and cool spots. The mechanism and reason for these local variations in skin blood flow is not known.

Deep vein thrombosis This causes an increase in the temperature of the overlying skin. This was first recorded as a clinical observation in 1939[164] and was confirmed with thermography in the early 1970s.[49] Examples of positive thermograms

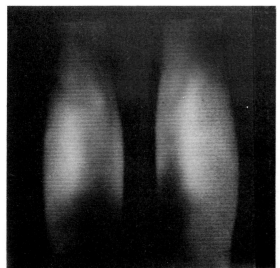

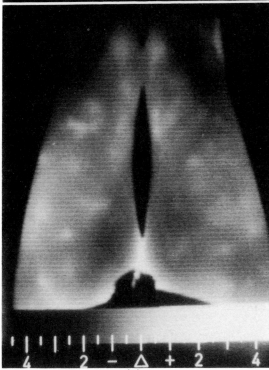

(a)

are shown in Fig. 4.4 a and b. Other conditions which may cause a temperature increase and be confused with deep vein thrombosis are: superficial thrombophlebitis, acute infection, acute arthritis, trauma, ruptured Baker's cysts, Paget's disease of bone, osteomyelitis and bone tumours. The first four also give false-positive results with the fibrinogen uptake test.

Cooke compared thermography against phlebography for the diagnosis of deep vein thrombosis in 164 patients.[50] Thermography had a positive test accuracy of 92 per cent, and a negative test accuracy of 93 per cent. The overall accuracy being 93 per cent. Other investigators[170] have obtained similar results but it must be remembered that the clinicians managing these patients had excluded patients with clinical evidence of conditions expected to cause false-positives before proceeding to thermography. The published studies of thermography show that it is accurate but it has not been widely adopted because the equipment is expensive and the setting up of the test and the control of the environment is cumbersome and time consuming. Simpler and cheaper temperature detectors are now being

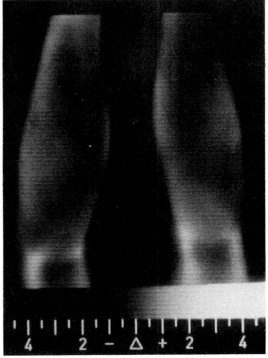

(b)

Fig. 4.3 Normal thermograms.

(a) The anterior view of the thighs and lower legs. White areas are hot; black areas are cold. The legs are symmetrical; the skin over the patellae and subcutaneous borders of the tibiae is cooler (blacker) than the skin over the muscles in the adjacent anterior compartment.

(b) The posterior view of the calves.

We are indebted to Dr ED Cooke for providing these thermograms.

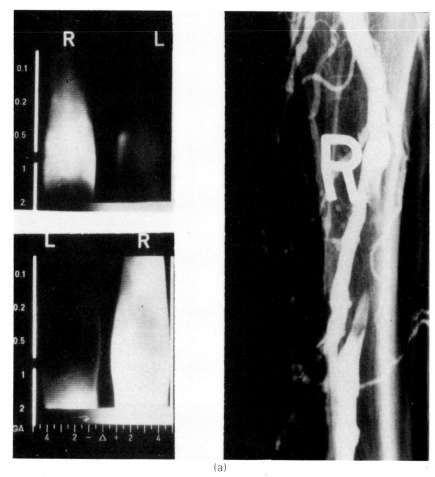

(a)

Fig. 4.4   (a) The thermogram and phlebogram of a patient with calf vein thrombosis.
The anterior and posterior thermographic views of the right leg show a warm skin corresponding to the thrombus visible on the X-ray. The left calf was normal. As the legs are examined through a mirror, their image is upside down.

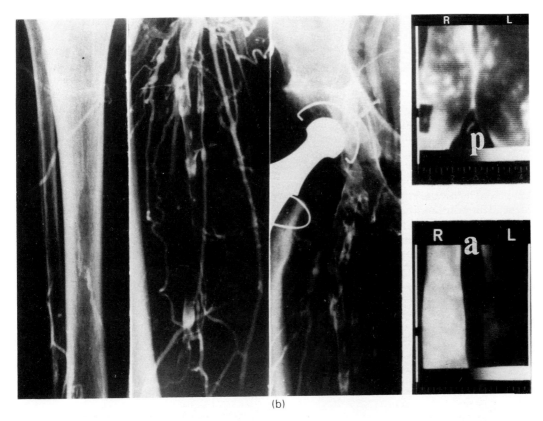

(b)

Fig. 4.4 (b) A thermogram and phlebogram of a patient with a complete right calf, femoral and iliac vein thrombosis following a hip replacement operation.

The right calf and thigh show an increased temperature with loss of the normal cool area over the patella and tibia. These images are obtained through a mirror and are therefore reversed and upside down.

p = pubis; a = ankle.

We are indebted to Dr ED Cooke for providing these illustrations.

introduced.[165,173] Their accuracy compares well with conventional thermography but the effects of air movement, ambient temperature and other conditions causing an increase of skin temperature are just the same.

Varicose veins Varicose veins do not show up on the thermogram if the patient is supine. If the patient stands, the veins appear as irregular lines over the leg; these lines are similar to those seen on an infra-red photograph (Fig. 4.5).

Incompetent communicating veins If the leg is emptied of blood, a superficial vein occluding tourniquet placed below the knee, and the leg then put in a dependent position, the sites at which any blood flows from the deep to the superficial system, through incompetent communicating veins, become hot and can be seen on a thermogram (see

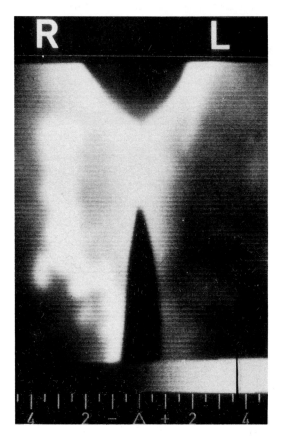

Fig. 4.5 The thermogram of a patient with a large right saphena varix and a dilated long saphenous vein.

We are indebted to Dr ED Cooke for providing this thermogram.

Fig. 6.21). This effect has been used to detect and pinpoint the position of incompetent communicating veins. The accuracy of the method can be increased by cooling the skin of the leg with cold towels before performing the test. This technique has been compared with phlebography and the Turner–Warwick 'bleed back test' at operation.[161,172,206] Compared with operation, thermography has a positive test accuracy of 87 per cent and a negative test accuracy of 84 per cent.

Chronic deep vein insufficiency It has been claimed that in 20 per cent of all patients with chronic venous insufficiency the calf is warmer than a normal calf; this abnormality is detectable by thermography.[48] The increased temperature is patchy and uneven and can therefore be distinguished from the uniform temperature rise of deep vein thrombosis. It is increased by exercise.[82] The significance of this observation and its mechanism needs further investigation but it has been suggested that patients with this abnormality have a nine-fold increase in the incidence of post-operative deep vein thrombosis.

Ultrasound flow detection

The application of ultrasound techniques to the investigation of peripheral vascular disease has produced a significant improvement in our understanding of peripheral vascular physiology. The arteries have yielded some of their secrets more readily than the veins. This is because arterial blood flow is regular and phasic and more susceptible to mathematical analysis than venous blood flow which is irregular and, though ultimately controlled by the heart, is profoundly affected by many other factors (e.g. respiration, abdominal pressure and skeletal muscle contraction).

Doppler flow detection depends upon the principle that the frequency of a sound-wave reflected from a moving object is changed in proportion to the speed of movement of the reflecting object.[180] An object moving away from the source of a sound reflects the sound at a lower frequency; an object moving towards the source of a sound increases the frequency of the sound. The frequency change can be used to detect movement and to measure the velocity of the movement.

The simplest ultrasound probe consists of two piezoelectric crystals; one crystal is excited to

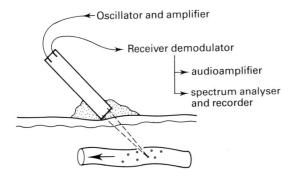

Fig. 4.6 The principle of the Doppler ultrasonic flow detector. Ultrasound is generated by exciting a piezoelectric crystal to vibrate at its resonant frequency. The ultrasound is focused into a beam and directed towards a blood vessel through a coupling jelly. The frequency of the reflected ultrasound is altered, according to the Doppler principle, if the reflecting agent (e.g. a red blood cell) is moving. The reflected ultrasound is received by a second crystal in the transducer and the change in frequency is converted into an audible signal.

transmit ultrasound, the other crystal becomes excited on receipt of the reflected ultrasound (Fig. 4.6). The ultrasound is directed towards a blood vessel by coupling the probe to the tissues with a coupling jelly to stop all the sound being reflected at the air–skin interface. Although other tissue interfaces of different density will reflect some of the sound-waves, the majority are reflected from the red cells because they have a much higher density than their surrounding plasma. Any change in reflected frequency indicates movement of the red cells.

As Doppler ultrasound instrumentation has improved, it has become possible to focus the ultrasound to a precise depth, examine a known volume of blood (the sample volume), use pulsed as well as continuous wave sound, use a zerocrossing frequency-proportional-to-voltage converter to give a signal to drive a strip recorder, make the signal bidirectional and apply Fourier waveform analysis to the signal.

The application of these sophisticated techniques to the arteries is well advanced. Investigators are only beginning to use these techniques on the veins but they will undoubtedly be applied increasingly as the quality of the instrumentation and analysis improves.

Flow detection (vein patency)

Most authorities use a simple handheld 5 MHz pencil probe with stethoscope ear-pieces without a chart recorder for day-to-day use in the ward or office.[23,185] Better tissue penetration is obtained with 5 MHz than with the 8 MHz, commonly used for arterial studies; 5 MHz is the best frequency to use when examining the deep veins. Superficial veins can be studied using an 8 MHz probe, which gives better spatial discrimination but the 5 MHz probe is the most practical frequency, applicable to all veins in the limbs and to the iliac veins in the lower abdomen.

Position The patient must lie *supine* with the head and shoulders above the level of the legs to ensure that the veins are full.

The leg should be slightly abducted and externally rotated with the hip and knee slightly flexed. The popliteal vein can usually be examined with the leg in this position but if the signal is poor, the patient must be turned to a prone position.

When the arm is examined, it should be placed at the patient's side, below the level of the right atrium.

The probe The probe should be placed on the skin within a pool of coupling jelly. When superficial veins are examined the probe should not be pressed hard against the skin otherwise the veins will be compressed.

The probe should be held at 45° to the long axis of the veins (Fig. 4.6). This is usually 45° to the skin surface, except when studying the upper part of the popliteal vein which runs obliquely into the depths of the leg towards the adductor canal. When insonating the upper popliteal vein the probe may have to be held at 90° to the skin.

Finding the vein The deep veins all run alongside arteries; the simplest way to find a vein is therefore to insonate the artery's pulsatile flow, after feeling the pulse with the fingers, and then move or just angle the probe to that side of the artery where the vein should be found. The sound produced by venous flow has a lower pitch than that of the arterial flow, and it is generated by the gentle fluctuations of blood flow caused by respiration. Quick confirmation that the sound is coming from the vein can be obtained by asking the patient to stop breathing. The sounds of venous blood flow should stop immediately and should resume with a rush when breathing recommences. This technique is applicable to the common femoral, superficial femoral, popliteal and posterior tibial veins.

The flow signal   The sound heard through the stethoscope is the amplified combination of the transmitted and reflected ultrasound, the beat frequency. Although ultrasound is inaudible, the beat frequency is audible. You are not actually hearing the blood flow but a noise whose amplitude is proportional to it. It is therefore acceptable to display the sound graphically and call it blood flow, provided the graph is not calibrated.

The effect of respiration   Femoral vein blood flow at rest varies with respiration (Fig. 4.7). As the patient inspires, the flow falls; this is caused by the contraction of the diaphragm and the increased abdominal pressure. A few patients breathe without increasing abdominal pressure during inspiration. In these patients the venous flow may increase during inspiration because of the sucking effect of the negative intrathoracic pressure.

A deep breath or a Valsalva manoeuvre (a deep breath followed by a forced expiration against a closed glottis to raise both intrathoracic and intra-abdominal pressure) stops the blood flow in the femoral vein (Fig. 4.7). When the Valsalva manoeuvre is released, there is a sudden increase in blood flow.

If the blood flow stops in response to a deep breath or a Valsalva manoeuvre, the veins between the heart and the point of examination are patent. The respiratory responses should always be present in the femoral and popliteal veins and can be heard in the posterior tibial veins at the ankle in 80 per cent of patients. The absence of these responses indicates an obstruction

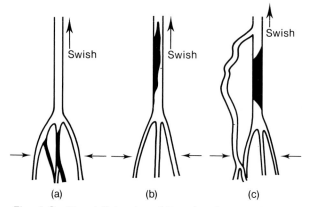

Fig. 4.8   The deficiencies of Doppler ultrasound detection of deep vein thrombosis. This figure shows the three situations in which calf compression will augment femoral vein blood flow in the presence of a deep vein thrombosis thus producing a false-negative test result.

(a)   A small amount of calf thrombus will not prevent the augmentation of flow produced by squeezing the calf.

(b)   A non-occluding femoral vein thrombus will not prevent the augmentation of flow produced by squeezing the calf.

(c)   A large collateral may carry the extra blood flow caused by squeezing the calf into the femoral vein and so mask the presence of a superficial femoral vein occlusion.

between the probe and the chest. The signal just above an obstruction may also have a reduced respiratory fluctuation because the blood flow is reduced by the obstruction.

The effect of venous compression   The blood flow through a vein can be increased by squeezing the vein or the tissues containing the blood that drains into the vein.

If manual compression of the calf augments the flow signal in the common femoral vein, it is reasonable to assume that the veins between the compressing hand and the probe are patent;[68,177,179,184] this is not, however, always true (Fig. 4.8). Large collateral vessels may conduct sufficient blood around an occluded main vein to augment the flow signal above the block, but the augmentation will be dampened, and the audible signal is often recognizably different from the rapid normal response. Before accepting that there is no augmentation in response to compression, it is important to check the position of the probe and make sure that the upstream veins are full of blood before they are squeezed.

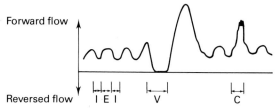

Fig. 4.7   The effect of respiration, a Valsalva manoeuvre and upstream compression on femoral vein blood flow detected by ultrasound.

Blood flow slows with inspiration (I) and increases during expiration (E). A Valsalva manoeuvre (V) stops femoral vein blood flow. Compression of the vein upstream to the flow detector augments flow (C).

It has been suggested that squeezing a calf containing non-adherent thrombus might cause a pulmonary embolus[36,76] but the experience of many thousands of clinicians worldwide who have used this test on countless occasions does not support this view. Squeezing or plantar flexing the foot is an acceptable alternative.[32]

Detection of valvular incompetence

When the clinician tests for valvular incompetence, the patient should be standing upright. If it can be shown that blood can flow downwards (retrogradely) in a vein, its valves cannot be functioning.[133,207]

The two forces commonly used to produce retrograde blood flow are a raised intra-abdominal/intrathoracic pressure (the Valsalva manoeuvre) and venous compression downstream to the probe.

The position of the probe This test can be applied to superficial veins as well as to deep veins. The long saphenous vein at the groin is detected by finding the common femoral vein and then edging the probe downwards and medially to a point where the vein is visible, or palpable, or where the respiratory fluctuations diminish. Unless the long saphenous vein can be seen or felt, it is difficult to be sure that the probe is insonating the saphenous vein and not a deep vein. This problem can be overcome by using an imaging probe. The source of the signal can then be accurately identified. Unfortunately, such equipment cannot be carried in the pocket for immediate use at the bed-side or in the office.

The short saphenous vein is easier to find, as it is in the mid-line below the centre of the popliteal fossa but it is not always possible to be certain whether the superficial vein or the popliteal vein is being insonated (Fig. 4.9).

Other superficial veins can only be studied if they are clearly visible or palpable.

The Valsalva manoeuvre The production of a positive pressure in the chest or abdomen will stop venous blood flow in normal veins but will cause retrograde flow if the valves are incompetent, followed by a sharp increase in flow as the Valsalva manoeuvre is released.

The simple Doppler flow detector does not indicate the direction of blood flow but the examiner hears a continuous flow-sound during the Valsalva manoeuvre in contrast to the silence (no

flow) of a normal limb. A directional flow recording will show that the flow is retrograde (Fig. 4.9).

This method may be used over the femoral and the popliteal vein. It is less reliable on the posterior tibial vein at the ankle.

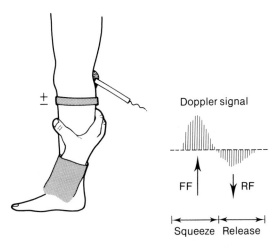

Fig. 4.9 The technique for testing for popliteal vein reflux. The vein is insonated with the probe at an angle of 45° to the skin in a pool of coupling jelly.

Forward flow (FF) is augmented by squeezing the calf. When the compression is released, flow will stop or, if the popliteal vein is incompetent, flow will occur in the opposite direction (RF). To confirm that the retrograde flow is not in the short saphenous vein, the test is repeated with the short saphenous vein occluded with an assistant's finger or a narrow tourniquet.

Downstream (cephalad) compression A similar effect to that caused by the Valsalva manoeuvre can be obtained by compressing the vein downstream (cephalad) to the probe. If the valves are incompetent, there will be retrograde flow; if the valves are competent, the flow will stop – the examiner therefore hears either a louder flow-sound during compression or silence respectively. A directional flow recording will show the retrograde nature of the flow.

The advantage of this method over the Valsalva technique is that much shorter segments of vein in many parts of the leg can be tested and in both the superficial and the deep systems. It is, however, essential to know which vein is being insonated and to know if the same vein is being compressed downstream.

Upstream (caudad) compression When the patient is standing up it is possible to detect retrograde blood flow by compressing the tissues upstream (caudad) to the probe. For example, if the probe is over the popliteal vein and the calf is squeezed, blood will flow forwards during the compression but run backwards when the compression is released (Fig. 4.9). This is the simplest way to detect popliteal vein reflux when the patient is standing.

This test can be confused by the blood running into the top half of a competent popliteal vein and then down and out through an incompetent short saphenous vein. This cause of false-positive results can be abolished by performing the test with the short saphenous vein occluded by manual compression. We have found this test difficult to perform and unreliable (see Chapter 8, page 255).

Communicating vein incompetence

If flow can be detected in a communicating vein or its immediate tributaries during compression of the deep veins, it is probably incompetent. To detect retrograde flow the examiner must squeeze the leg on one side of a tourniquet which occludes the superficial veins and listen for a flow signal with a Doppler probe over the site of a communicating vein on the other side of the tourniquet (Fig. 4.10).[75,141] The tourniquet stops the pressure of the calf squeeze causing blood flow in the superficial veins so any blood flow in the communicating veins must have come via the deep veins and out through an incompetent communicator. The method has two problems – the identification of the site of the communicating vein for the insonation and the uncertainty that the tourniquet

has stopped all blood flow in the superficial compartment. In our hands this technique has not proved to be accurate.

Accuracy

The accuracy of the Doppler technique for detecting venous occlusion depends upon the anatomical complexity of the vein under study. The iliac, femoral and popliteal veins are major axial veins with few collaterals. Occlusion of these vessels by thrombus can be detected with an overall accuracy of 90 per cent, a positive test accuracy of 85 per cent and a negative test accuracy of 95 per cent. Sensitivity (overall ability to detect obstruction) is 95 per cent. Specificity (overall ability to detect normality) is 90 per cent.[185]

The test is less reliable when an occluded vein is part of a plexus of vessels (e.g. in the calf). For detecting deep vein occlusions below the knee the overall accuracy in expert hands is claimed to be 80 per cent, the positive test accuracy is 65 per cent, the negative test accuracy is 95 per cent, the sensitivity is 95 per cent and the specificity is 85 per cent,[185] but the published results are very variable, ranging from those quoted above to false-positive rates of 20–50 per cent.[177,142] We find that Doppler techniques are unreliable for the detection of venous thrombosis below the level of the knee joint. Accuracy can be improved by combining Doppler ultrasound with other techniques such as pulse volumetry.[88]

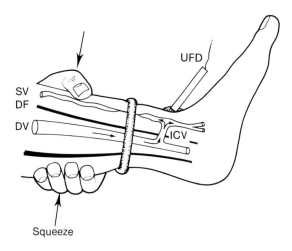

Fig. 4.10 The detection of incompetent communicating veins with the ultrasound flow detector.

The calf is squeezed on one side of a superficial vein occluding tourniquet and the sites of the communicating veins are insonated with an ultrasound flow detector (UFD) on the other. If blood flow is detected in response to the squeeze, the communicating vein must be incompetent.

This test will only work well when performed in this way if the deep vein valves are also incompetent. The effect of the squeeze can be augmented by placing another tourniquet above the knee.

If the position of the probe and squeezing hand are reversed, the test will work even when the deep axial veins are competent but the tissues just above the ankle are difficult to squeeze effectively.

SV = superficial vein; DV = deep vein; ICV = incompetent communicating vein; DF = deep fascia.

UFD

SV
DF

DV

ICV

Squeeze

The accuracy of the Doppler flow detector technique for detecting deep vein reflux has not been studied extensively because many investigators are not prepared to perform descending phlebograms on these patients. Studies using foot vein pressure measurements as the gold standard suggest that this technique has a high accuracy[152] but we do not believe that the ability to reduce foot vein pressure during exercise with and without a superficial vein occluding tourniquet is an acceptable gold standard for measuring deep or superficial vein reflux.

Our unpublished experience comparing descending venography with Doppler flow detection has revealed a low accuracy rate. The inaccuracies of these techniques stem from our inability to define the precise site of insonation. This problem will be solved when the combination of B-mode imaging and directional flow detection is universally available.

Ultrasound imaging

In contrast to the technique of flow detection which solely analyses the frequency changes in ultrasound reflected from a small volume of flowing blood, B-mode images are derived from the amplitude of the reflected ultrasound and the time it has taken to travel from the transmitting to the receiving crystal. This provides a measure of tissue density at known depths and so builds up a picture of the tissues which can be presented in tones of grey; the whiteness is inversely proportional to the density. This is known as greyscale or B-mode imaging.

If a pulsed signal is used in conjunction with a B-mode image, the source of the sample volume giving a Doppler shift can be accurately identified on the image.

The application of B-mode imaging to the veins has lagged behind its application to the arteries. Scanning of the arteries is now highly sophisticated; the operator is able to measure the degree of stenosis and distinguish different forms of atheromatous plaques and ulcers. Although the first report of venous imaging was in the 1970s,[59,197] it was only applied seriously to the veins in the early 1980s.[46,171,182,188]

Method The probes are usually linear arrays of 4 MHz or 8 MHz crystals arranged to give a large image and good penetration. The patient lies supine on a table tipped foot down to 20° to ensure good filling of the leg veins.

The deep veins are scanned by finding the common femoral vein at the groin and following it down the leg to the adductor canal. Placing the probe along the length of the vein gives a longitudinal image of the vessels in which valve cusps can often be seen (Fig. 4.11). Turning the probe through 90° gives a cross-sectional image of the vein. It is easier to scan the popliteal vein when the patient is lying in a lateral or prone position.

The long saphenous vein can be followed from the ankle to the groin. Tributaries joining the posterior arch vein may be visualized, and sometimes the communicating veins between this arcade and the deep veins can be seen (Fig. 4.12).

In general an 8 MHz probe is used to examine the deep veins above the knee and a 4 MHz probe is used for all the deep and superficial veins below the knee. The velocity characteristics of the blood flow in any of these veins may be studied from the Doppler shift, the effect of respiration and distal tissue compression.

Thrombus is recognizable because it prevents the vein from collapsing under pressure and has an echogenicity slightly different from that of blood. As thrombus ages it becomes more dense. It is sometimes possible to determine whether thrombus is adherent or 'floating' (Fig. 4.13).

Results Normal veins and valves are thin-walled and easy to compress. A Valsalva manoeuvre makes the limb veins dilate.

The iliac vein may be obscured by gas shadows. The main thigh veins, except the deep femoral vein, can usually be seen. The calf veins can be seen during 80–90 per cent of examinations, but valves in the calf veins are difficult to see.

Flanagan *et al.*,[73] have studied 511 patients using this technique. Fifty patients with suspected thrombosis had phlebograms and B-mode scans. The overall accuracy was 94 per cent, the positive test accuracy was 92 per cent and the negative test accuracy was 96 per cent.

Although this method of examining the veins is highly 'technician-dependent' it may develop over the next few years into a valuable and perhaps 'first line' method of investigating deep vein thrombosis.

Photoplethysmography (PPG)

The density of the skin and its ability to reflect

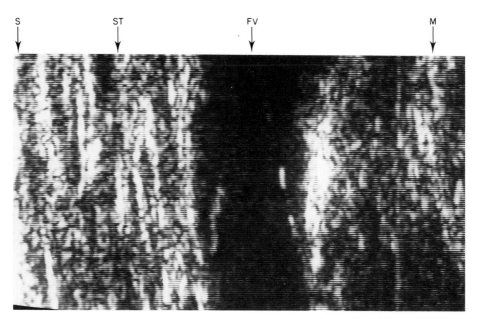

Fig. 4.11 An ultrasound image of the superficial femoral vein showing two valve cusps floating in the stream of blood. S = skin; ST = subcutaneous tissue; FV = femoral vein; M = muscle.
We are indebted to Dr JJ Cranley for providing this illustration.

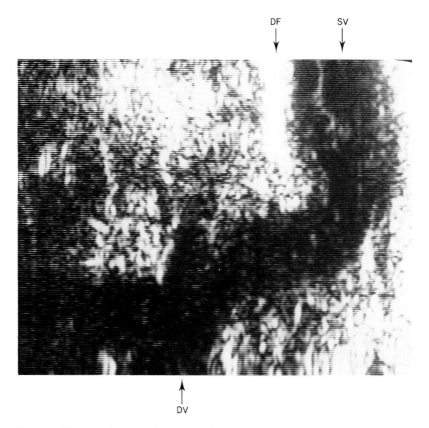

Fig. 4.12 An ultrasound image of a superficial vein (SV) passing through the deep fascia (DF) to unite with a deep vein (DV). We are indebted to Dr JJ Cranley for this illustration.

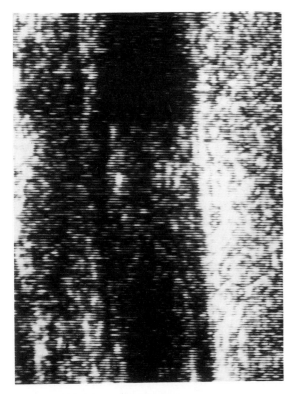

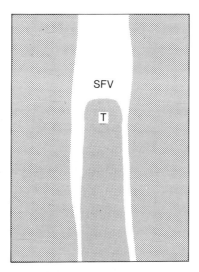

Fig. 4.13 Fresh non-adherent thrombus (T) in the superficial femoral vein (SFV). We are indebted to Dr JJ Cranley for this illustration.

light partly depends upon the volume of blood in the capillaries within the skin.[83,143] The photo-plethysmograph (PPG) contains an infra-red light source (805 nm) and a photoelectric cell which measures the reflectivity of the skin.[43] Many workers have shown that this indirect method of assessing skin blood volume correlates closely with the superficial venous pressure, and in many laboratories PPG has therefore replaced the invasive direct method of pressure measurement for assessing calf pump function.[17,145] PPG cannot be used for measuring blood flow. Rapid changes in skin blood volume can be detected if the photoelectric cell is recorded in the AC mode because the upslope of each pulse is related to blood flow, but it is extremely difficult to calibrate this in absolute terms. The DC mode gives a dampened mean measure of skin reflectivity over a longer course of time and so indicates overall changes of skin blood volume, 70 per cent of which is within the venules and veins.

Method[139,140] The probe must be placed parallel to and in complete contact with the skin surface so that it can only receive reflected light from the skin (Fig. 4.14). The probe is designed so that its outer part masks the sensor from any back-scattered outside direct light.

The probe is fixed to the skin with transparent double-sided adhesive tape.

Any area of skin may be studied but for routine testing the probe is fixed on the medial side of the leg, 4–5 inches (10–12.5 cm) above the medial malleolus. It should not be placed over a visible or palpable large subcutaneous varix.

The normal test procedure is to ask the patient to sit with the feet resting on the floor and then to perform regular heel raises, without weight bearing, in time to a metronome. The sitting position prevents the reduction of calf blood volume produced by the calf muscle contractions which are unavoidable when standing.

Alternatively, the patient is asked to stand with

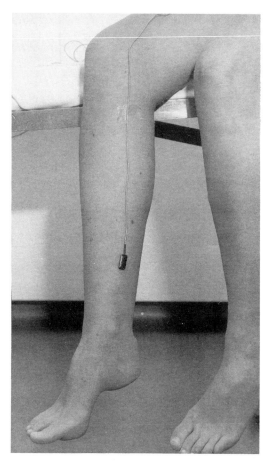

Fig. 4.14 A photoplethysmograph attached with double-sided adhesive tape to the skin of the medial side of the leg, 5 in (12.5 cm) above the medial malleolus.

tion have been shown to correlate moderately well with simultaneous measurements of foot vein pressure.[70,71,98,158]

The shape of the PPG tracing (Fig. 4.15) is similar to that of the foot vein pressure trace on exercise.[1,162] It is therefore possible to measure the *percentage emptying* (provided some attempt has been made at calibration), the *refilling time* (in seconds) or the 50 per cent refilling time (T½).

Refilling is non-linear, and sophisticated analyses of the refilling curve are not justified.

Application Venous refilling after exercise normally comes from the arterial circulation. If the superficial or deep veins are incompetent, blood will reflux down the limb and venous refilling will be accelerated. The PPG can therefore be used to assess the degree of venous reflux.

Reflux through superficial veins can be prevented with a superficial vein occluding tourniquet. If the application of such a tourniquet restores an abnormally short refilling time to normal, the abnormality must be pure superficial vein incompetence.

If the tourniquet is positioned at various levels on the leg, the site of any superficial-to-deep incompetent connections can be determined in a way similar to the clinical tourniquet test.

Accuracy The PPG recovery time correlates well with the foot vein pressure recovery time.[162] When a single superficial vein occluding cuff restores an abnormal trace to normal there is little doubt that the superficial veins are incompetent but when there is only a partial improvement the significance is far less clear. Attempts to define normal ranges of refilling and relate them to disease groups have not been very helpful because of the inherent inaccuracies of PPG and the more

all their weight on one leg whilst performing the heel raising with the non-weight bearing leg. The greater hydrostatic pressure when standing gives the maximum initial venous filling.

Most laboratories use PPG solely for measuring refilling time after exercise because it is not possible to calibrate the PPG tracing in terms of blood volume. A crude calibration can be obtained by adjusting the gain so that the output is zero when the patient is supine and maximal (100 per cent) when standing. The 100 per cent can be equated to the calculated hydrostatic pressure at the site of the probe. The change in reflectivity during exercise can then be expressed as a percentage of the maximum calf volume or as an absolute pressure. Both these methods of calibra-

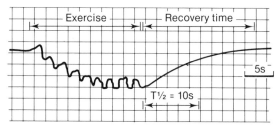

Fig. 4.15 A tracing of a normal photoplethysmograph showing a rapid emptying of venous blood from the calf during exercise (Ex) and a half refilling time (T1/2) of 10 s.

fundamental problem – our lack of gold standards for comparison.

PPG is therefore most useful as a test for *excluding* venous disease. It can identify pure long and/or short saphenous vein incompetence but gives little information about communicating or deep vein disease apart from indicating its presence. The most sensible way to use this apparatus is to establish your own definition of normal refilling and, when a patient's test is in the abnormal range, measure the effect of superficial vein occluding tourniquets above and then below the knee. This will provide an immediate assessment of the contribution of long and short saphenous vein reflux to the rate of refilling and indicate the possibility of deep vein disease. Any attempt to make the PPG tracing provide a more specific and accurate analysis is not worthwhile.

Phleborheography (PRG)

Phleborheography is a sophisticated form of whole leg plethysmography using multiple air-filled cuffs to detect the volume changes.

Plethysmography was first described in 1905[35] and has been used extensively for the measurement of limb blood volume for many years. In the early years water was used as the coupling medium because of its accuracy in transmitting volume and pressure changes but the development of low pressure transducers has permitted the replacement of the water-filled chamber with an air-filled cuff without significant loss of sensitivity.[94] An air-filled cuff[54,55] has another advantage (in addition to convenience) – it can be instantly turned into a pressure-applying cuff when required.

It is obviously not practical to place the whole leg in a single chamber. Multiple air-filled chambers are not only more practical but also allow the study of separate segments of the limb.

Changes in limb volume may be caused by respiration and external compression. The fluctuations of limb volume with respiration, coincident with the flow variations detectable with the Doppler flow meter (see page 82) indicate patent veins. The orthograde transmission of a pulse of blood flow following a foot or calf squeeze also depends upon venous patency. Retrograde flow is prevented by competent valves. The changes of limb volume in response to these stimuli provide much more information about the state of the deep veins.

Method[54]   The patient lies supine on a couch

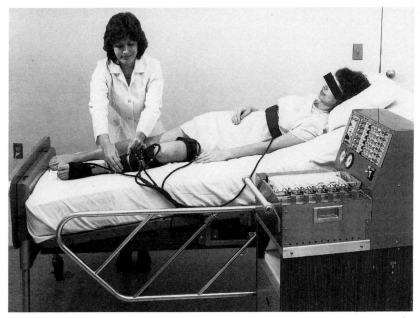

Fig. 4.16   The six cuffs of the phleborheograph and the recorder. Note that the patient lies 10° foot-down to ensure that all the veins of the lower limb are full.
We are indebted to Dr JJ Cranley for this illustration.

with the legs below the level of the heart (approximately 10°). This ensures that the limb veins are full of blood.

Pneumatic cuffs are placed around the chest and the lower third of the thigh. Three cuffs are then placed side-by-side around the upper half of the lower leg and another is placed around the foot – a total of six cuffs (Fig. 4.16).

The cuffs are then inflated to 10 mmHg to ensure that they fit snugly in and around the contours of the limb.

The cuffs are calibrated by the removal of 0.2 ml air from each cuff, the amplification being adjusted so that this change causes a 2 cm deflection of the pen recorder. This is done to ensure

that all six cuffs have the same sensitivity, and to allow comparisons between the traces of one patient obtained at different times and between different patients.

After the wave-forms from all the cuffs have been recorded, the foot cuff is rapidly inflated three times to 50 mmHg to compress the foot and squeeze blood up the leg.

A similar compression stimulus is then applied to the lower of the calf cuffs or the thigh cuff. A similar technique may be used on the arm.[183]

Application PRG detects occlusion of the major axial deep veins. It is therefore valuable for the diagnosis of major deep vein thrombosis. An occluded femoral vein will prevent the respiratory

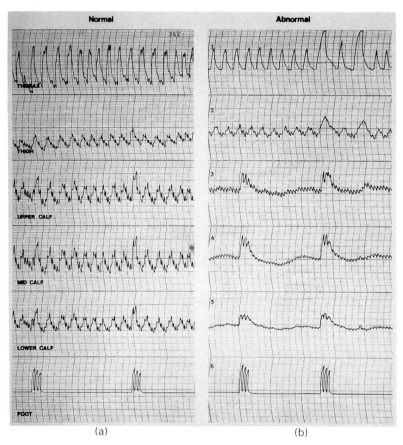

Fig. 4.17 A phleborheograph trace. The upper five traces record the pressures in the chest, thigh and three calf cuffs. The lowest trace indicates that the compression is being applied to the foot cuffs (a) In a normal limb, the foot compression causes a transient rise of calf cuff pressure, and respiratory fluctuations are seen in all five traces.
(b) In a limb with a popliteal vein thrombosis, the respiratory fluctuations are absent in the three calf traces, and foot compression causes an increase in pressure which is slow to return to baseline.
  We are grateful to Dr JJ Cranley for providing this illustration.

waves reaching the calf and will cause the calf volume to rise when the foot is squeezed (Fig. 4.17 and 4.18).

By inflating the thigh cuff to 80 mmHg, the limb can be filled with blood and the time and rate of venous emptying and the maximum venous outflow can be calculated. This can indicate the degree of both acute and chronic venous occlusion, though a chronic occlusion only causes a positive test result when it is causing severe outflow obstruction.

PRG is not suitable for the assessment of superficial venous incompetence but can show retrograde flow in the deep veins if the lower calf expands in response to calf or thigh compression.

Accuracy   There have been many assessments of PRG as a diagnostic tool for deep vein throm-

bosis. When there is occlusive thrombus in a main axial vein the positive test accuracy is 95 per cent and the negative test accuracy is 90 per cent. A mathematical compilation of eight large studies by Cranley gave an overall accuracy of 92 per cent, a sensitivity of 91 per cent and a specificity of 93 per cent.[47,53] In making this last analysis, however, Cranley, the originator of the method, excluded some of the data of one paper[42] because 56 per cent of the patients studied had thrombus in small veins below the knee, justifying this with the statement 'PRG cannot detect thrombus not in the mainstream i.e. veins in the soleus muscle, the deep femoral, internal iliac and saphenous veins'. Many workers consider that this inability to detect thrombosis in small peripheral veins is a serious disadvantage of all forms of

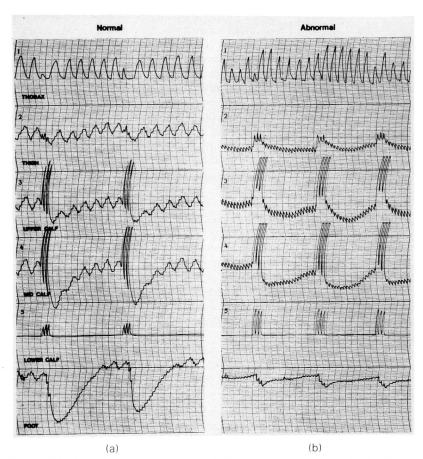

(a)   (b)

Fig. 4.18   A phleborheograph trace with the compression applied to the lower calf cuff.
(a) is from a normal limb. (b) shows a loss of respiratory fluctuation in the thigh cuff and an increase in thigh cuff pressure during calf compression indicating the presence of an ilio-femoral vein occlusion.
   We are grateful to Dr JJ Cranley for providing this illustration.

plethysmography not just of PRG and Doppler flow detection.

The accuracy of all these methods in detecting thrombus in the calf is 50 per cent or less. Non-occlusive non-obstructing thrombus in major veins may also be missed. The claims for a 90 per cent accuracy must therefore be considered in the context of these exclusions. As a means of diagnosing all forms of venous thrombosis (80 per cent of which is confined to the small calf veins) PRG is only approximately 60 per cent accurate and it has a negative test accuracy of 60–70 per cent.

False-positive readings are usually caused by muscle tension compressing veins in nervous patients – sedation or a change in posture usually corrects this abnormality.[56] Pregnancy also causes false-positive recordings.[150]

Strain-gauge plethysmography (SGP)

If a cross-section of the calf is assumed to be circular, it is possible to calculate its area from a measurement of its circumference and hence calculate its volume.[186] The development of electronics in the 1940s led to the invention of the mercury-in-rubber strain gauge, the resistance of which is directly proportional to its length. When placed around the calf any change in the length of the gauge caused by a change in calf volume alters its resistance. If the length–resistance relationship has been determined by precalibration, the volume change of a 1 cm slice of calf can be calculated. Strain gauges have now been refined and have become more reliable; silastic is better than rubber, and indium–gallium alloy is better than mercury. Calibration can be carried out electrically, a 1 per cent change in resistance being equivalent to a 1 per cent change in volume.

A strain gauge can only measure the volume change in the plane of the gauge but many studies have shown a close correlation between the volume changes measured with a strain gauge and direct volume measurements obtained with a water-filled plethysmograph. Provided the tube of tissue being studied is horizontal and almost cylindrical, problems caused by uneven filling and irregularities of shape are therefore insignificant. Strain gauges require a temperature compensation circuit and must fit the limb properly. The ideal gauge length should be 90 per cent of the limb circumference, and the gauge should be stretched by 10 per cent when it is applied so that it completely encircles the limb.

Method[41,58,151] The patient lies supine with the limb elevated above heart level, preferably to 20–30°. This ensures that the veins are as empty as possible before venous congestion is applied.

A gauge, 90 per cent of the circumference to be studied, is stretched around the limb. It should lie comfortably without compressing the skin or any underlying veins (Fig. 4.19).

A large pneumatic tourniquet, at least 20 cm wide, is placed around the thigh. Narrow cuffs and cuffs with bladders that do not encircle the limb will not occlude all the veins in the tissues beneath them. Theoretically, the width of the cuff should be 1 or 2 times the diameter of the limb.

The cuff is inflated to 50 mmHg. After 2 minutes, when the volume curve is almost stable, the cuff is released. (The volume will not become absolutely constant as the venous congestion slowly reduces the venous tone and causes tissue oedema.) This procedure provides a measurement of the total calf volume and the venous outflow.

A second narrow cuff in then placed at the top of the thigh and inflated to 300 mmHg. The large thigh cuff is then rapidly inflated to 50 mmHg. This test can be repeated with a superficial vein occluding tourniquet below the knee. These manoeuvres test deep venous reflux.

The cuffs are removed and the patient then stands and performs a series of heel raises in time to a metronome so that the volume changes during and after exercise can be recorded. This test may be repeated with superficial vein occluding tourniquets.

The test may also be performed while the patient walks on a treadmill[69,87] and similar results can be obtained when a strain gauge is placed around the foot.[175]

Application This method of plethysmography is not as easy to perform as air or impedance plethysmography; it is therefore rarely used in the acute clinical situation presented by venous thrombosis. It is a vascular laboratory investigation most often used to elicit the state of the venous outflow tract and venous reflux.

Calf volume expansion After 2 minutes of congestion at 50 mmHg calf volume expansion is usually 2–3 per cent.[20,79] The presence of acute venous thrombosis reduces this to 1–2 per cent because the veins are already full of thrombus and

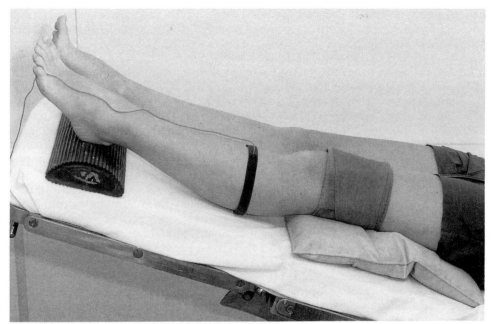

Fig. 4.19 A photograph showing a strain gauge around the calf. The limb is elevated to 20°.

the inflamed vein walls are less distendable. This test is rarely used for the diagnosis of venous thrombosis.

Some patients with chronic venous insufficiency also have a decreased calf volume expansion but measurement of this volume is of no special clinical value.

Maximum venous outflow The rate at which blood flows out of the calf following venous congestion depends upon the outflow resistance and the pressure gradient, which in turn depends upon the venous tone and the venous distention.[18,95] Some authors have used the maximum rate of outflow, derived from the rate of outflow in the first few seconds after congestion, as a measure of obstructive axial vein damage (Fig. 4.20).[21] An outflow less than 20 ml/100 ml/min probably signifies a significant outflow obstruction. Formulae have been devised which incorporate corrections for the degree of venous filling, the volume of the veins under the cuff and the rate of cuff deflation; with the hope that these formulae will make this measurement more discriminatory.[41,95] They have, however, failed. This test only reveals the type of gross obstruction, acute thrombotic or chronic, that is usually obvious on clinical examination.[80] Moderate and mild obstruction are not detected because the stimulus to outflow – a pressure gradient of 50 mmHg – is

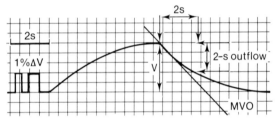

Fig. 4.20 The calculations that can be derived from a strain gauge measurement of calf volume. Calf volume expansion (V), maximum venous outflow (MVO), and 2-s outflow. In this patient V = 2.5 ml/100 ml, the 2-s outflow = 48 ml/ 100 ml/min and the MVO = 56 ml/100 ml/min.

too low. This test has a specificity of 90 per cent for femoral and iliac vein occlusion but its specificity for obstruction caused by calf vein thrombosis is only 60 per cent.[21] If the test could be performed with a constant and greater pressure gradient which was reproducible, it might detect lesser degrees of obstruction.

Venous reflux The inflation of a wide cuff below an arterial occluding cuff will push blood down the leg into the calf if the deep vein valves are incompetent. In a normal limb thigh cuff inflation expands the calf by 3 per cent whereas in a grossly incompetent venous system the expansion may exceed 10 per cent.[19]

This is an uncomfortable test for the patient,

and the scatter of results is so wide that it only detects those patients who have gross abnormalities. It is simpler to measure refilling after erect exercise.[22,87]

The same test can be performed with and without a superficial vein occluding tourniquet to assess superficial vein reflux.

Venous refilling after erect exercise This measurement is identical in concept to the refilling time measured with PPG, foot volumetry or foot vein pressure. In all these tests it is more informative to look at the recording and see the effect of tourniquets rather than to calculate precise refilling times. We find it difficult to measure venous refilling after erect exercise because of the artefacts caused by movement during exercise. One way of avoiding these artefacts is to squeeze the blood out of the calf manually and then record and measure the rate of reflux, provided you can apply a calf compression of reproducible pressure and rate and release it instantaneously.

Impedance plethysmography (IPG)

Impedance plethysmography can measure a change in the volume of blood within a limb from the associated change in tissue electrical resistance (impedance).[57,141] A current of low strength (1 mA) and high frequency (22 KHz) is passed through the limb between two circumferential electrodes. This current cannot be felt by the patient and is too high to stimulate the nerves or muscles. Changes in voltage are recorded from two other electrodes (approximately 10 cm apart) placed inside the first two electrodes. The four electrodes are contained within two Velcro-covered bands. The tissue resistance is principally related to the volume of blood within it so that changes of venous filling and venous emptying can be easily assessed. Other factors which affect tissue impedance are relatively unimportant, and many studies using water, air and strain-gauge plethysmography (SGP) have confirmed the close relationship between tissue impedance and blood volume.

Method[199,200,201] The patient lies supine with the hip and knee slightly flexed and the whole limb raised above heart level by elevating the foot of the bed or couch until it is tilted by 20°.

A wide (8 inch, 20 cm) pneumatic tourniquet is placed around the thigh taking care not to compress the veins and cause distal venous disten-

tion. The electrodes are placed around the calf over a conductive jelly, the inner electrodes being approximately 10 cm apart (Fig. 4.21). The chart recorder is adjusted so that an electrically induced 2 per cent change in impedance produces a 5 mm deflection of the recorder.

The cuff is then inflated to 50 mmHg for 2 or 3 minutes, until the venous volume becomes constant. The cuff is then rapidly deflated.

This procedure is repeated four or five times because the ratio between filling and emptying may change as venous congestion alters the venous tone and as the patient relaxes. Ten per cent of normal tests become abnormal and 20 per cent of abnormal tests become normal between the first and fifth inflations.[92,174,190]

False-positive readings are often caused by leg contractions. These subside with repeated testing. It has been suggested that muscle tone should be monitored with an electromyograph during testing.[30] The maximum venous capacitance and the maximum venous outflow in 3 seconds are then measured directly from the tracing in millimetres (Fig. 4.22).

The results can be plotted on a prepared nomogram which indicates whether the ratio of venous volume to the rate of emptying is normal or abnormal.[201] An alternative nomogram gives the ratios for normal legs and legs with venous thrombosis, including the 95 per cent confidence limits.[92]

Venous obstruction slows the rate of emptying disproportionately to the venous filling. Wheeler has recently related the venous outflow measurements to the actual diameter of the proximal veins measured with ultrasound.[12,199] This has enabled him to indicate the percentage change in vein diameter that must have caused the observed increase of venous outflow obstruction. These studies suggest that an abnormal test indicates a lumen reduction greater than 50 per cent.

Application and accuracy Impedance plethysmography has become widely used for diagnosing main axial vein thrombosis.[13,51,93] Like all forms of plethysmography it cannot detect thrombus in the calf muscle veins, deep femoral or internal iliac veins and will also miss non-obstructing non-adherent thrombi in large axial veins (Fig. 4.23). IPG can claim the same degree of accuracy as phleborheography for major vein occlusion but is not as good at detecting calf vein thrombosis, though it becomes more

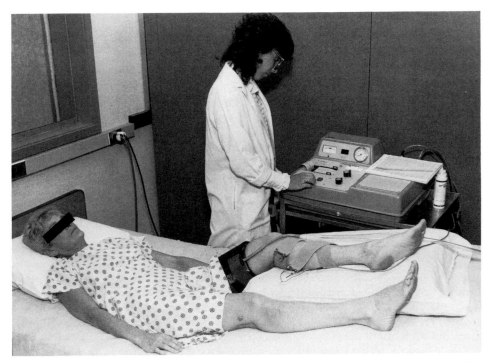

Fig. 4.21   The impedance plethysmograph. Each Velcro band contains two electrodes. The limb is raised above heart level and the venous occluding cuff is around the middle of the thigh.
   We are indebted to Dr H Brownell Wheeler for providing this illustration.

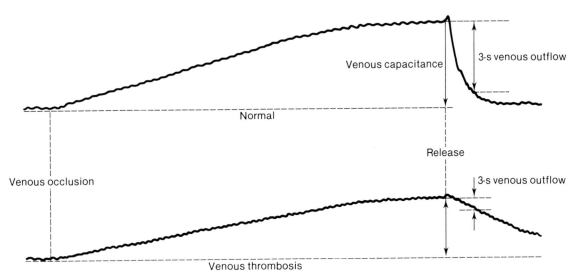

Fig. 4.22   A normal impedance plethysmograph trace and a trace from a patient with femoral vein thrombosis. In the abnormal leg the venous capacitance and the venous outflow in 3 s are both reduced.
   Redrawn from Wheeler.[199]

accurate if repeated daily.[89] For proximal major vein thrombi the sensitivity and specificity are 95 per cent and 90 per cent respectively but for calf vein thrombi the figures are 40 per cent and 85 per cent respectively.

IPG has not yet found a place in the investigation of chronic venous insufficiency,[124] but may do so if measurement of outflow tract resistance (the venous diameter index) becomes simple and accurate.[199]

Isotope plethysmography

Isotope plethysmography is a technique which we have developed and which measures the volume of blood within the calf by counting the radioactivity of the calf after labelling the red blood cells with technetium.[202,203]

If stannous pyrophosphate is injected into the bloodstream, it will adhere to the red cells and absorb any radioactive technetium that is subsequently injected. The label remains fixed to the red cells for 2 hours but does not damage them. Calf radioactivity then directly reflects the calf blood volume.

The advantage of this method is that calf blood volume can be measured during calf muscle exercise or passive compression, while the patient is standing, without causing the type of artefacts seen with photoplethysmography and strain-gauge plethysmography.

Method Stannous pyrophosphate, 3 ml, is injected intravenously followed, 20 minutes later, by 15 mCi technetium-99 m (pertechnate). The patient then stands on an exercise platform and a scintillation counter is loosely fixed to the back of the calf (Fig. 4.24). Exercise is performed by depressing a foot pedal to raise a known weight to a fixed height at a specified rate; thus the work of the exercise is controlled and reproducible. The calf can also be squeezed passively by placing a large pneumatic tourniquet around the whole calf and inflating it to 90 mmHg. Superficial vein occluding tourniquets can be used to eliminate superficial reflux.

Application This technique can measure the calf blood volume, the percentage expelled volume with exercise and passive compression, the rate of emptying during exercise and passive compression, and the rate of refilling following exercise or passive compression. All these measurements can be made with and without superficial vein occlusion and all can be expressed as a percentage of the total calf volume (Fig. 4.25). These are measurements of calf pump efficiency, outflow obstruction and deep and

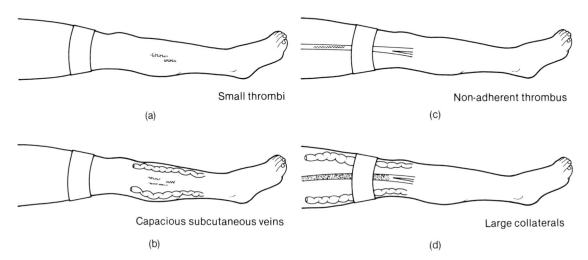

Small thrombi

(a)

Non-adherent thrombus

(c)

Capacious subcutaneous veins

(b)

Large collaterals

(d)

Fig. 4.23 The reasons why all forms of plethysmography are unable to detect minor calf vein thrombosis.
(a) Small thrombi affect neither capacitance nor outflow.
(b) Large subcutaneous veins may mask a reduction of venous capacitance.
(c) Non-adherent thrombus may not affect the rate of outflow.
(d) Large subcutaneous collateral veins may compensate for a deep vein obstruction.

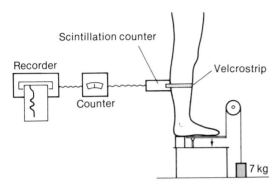

Fig. 4.24   The technique of isotope plethysmography.
   Plantar flexion of the foot moves a 7 kg weight a fixed distance. The radioactivity of the calf is measured with a scintillation counter held in a horizontal mobile rig behind the calf.

superficial reflux respectively. The method therefore measures more aspects of calf pump function than any other technique.

   Isotope plethysmography has been tested against clinical assessment, phlebography and

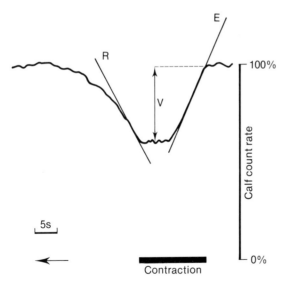

Fig. 4.25   The measurements that can be made from an isotope plethysmograph trace.
   V = volume ejected; E = rate of emptying (%/s); R = rate of re-filling (%/s)
   Each measurement can be made following continuous exercise, a sustained calf contraction or passive compression.

foot volumetry. There is general agreement between these tests when the diagnosis is simple but less correlation when there is a combination of abnormalities. Like many other methods, isotope plethysmography needs to be tested against the surgical correction of the abnormalities it detects by performing the test before and after curative operations.

Foot volumetry

This method is foot plethysmography using an open water-filled plethysmograph.[191] The patient stands in a temperature-controlled water bath, the water reaching up to the narrow part of the ankle, and exercises by performing knee bends in time to a metronome. As the blood is pumped out of the foot so the water level falls. This can be measured precisely with a pressure manometer or an electrical sensor. The method gives an overall indication of calf pump function.

   Method[157]   The foot is placed in the plethysmograph. Water at 32°C is added to a marked level on the tank; this volume subtracted from the known volume of the tank gives the volume of the foot (Fig. 4.26). The plethysmograph is calibrated by withdrawing 10 ml aliquots of water. The patient holds onto a rail and performs 20 knee bends at 1 s intervals. The test is then repeated with superficial vein occluding tourniquets. The tracing should show a reduction of volume during exercise followed by refilling.

   The measurements made from the trace are as follows (Fig. 4.27).

- Absolute expelled volume, ml (EV)
- Expelled volume relative to resting foot volume, ml/100 ml (EVr)
- Refilling or half refilling time (t or tv½)
- Maximum rate of refilling, ml/100 ml/min (Q)
- Ratio of maximum rate of refilling to relative expelled volume (Q/EVr)

   Application   The advantage of this technique is its simplicity. The water bath and baffles can be homemade of perspex, it is therefore very cheap, and water put into such a tank at 32°C remains at this temperature ±2°C for 30 minutes so that a heater and thermostat are not necessary.

   The measurements indicate overall calf pump function (expelled volume – absolute and relative) and the degree of venous reflux, superficial

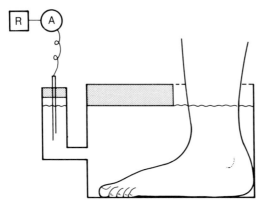

Fig. 4.26 The foot volumeter. In this illustration the water level is sensed by the change in resistance between two electrodes in the side-arm.
A = amplifier; R = recorder.

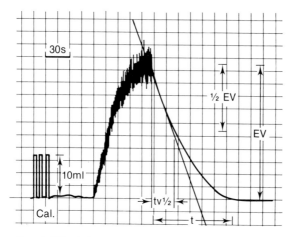

Fig. 4.27 A foot volumetry trace showing the calculation of the expelled volume (EV), the half volume refilling time (tv 1/2), and the refilling time (t).

reflux being separated from deep reflux by the tourniquet test.

Foot volume changes correlate closely with venous pressure changes,[103,160] both of which have been assessed against other forms of diagnosis such as clinical examination and phlebography, though neither are gold standards of peripheral venous physiology.[66] It is easier to use the technique in a qualitative manner by taking note of the shape of the tracing and the effect of the tourniquets rather than the mathematical calculations of expelled volume and refilling time.

Foot vein pressure measurements

When the patient stands upright the calf pump plays an important role in assisting the return of blood to the heart by accelerating the flow of blood to the heart from the veins. The effect of calf pump action is to empty and reduce the pressure in the superficial veins. The absence of venous hypotension during exercise damages the microcirculation of the skin and may lead to skin necrosis (ulceration) (see Chapters 11 and 13). The measurement of the effect of calf muscle exercise on superficial vein pressure is an important test of calf pump function and an indication of the severity of the physiological abnormality.[167]

Three of the techniques already described in this chapter, photoplethysmography, strain-gauge plethysmography and foot volumetry assess the same aspect of calf pump function by measuring the volume of blood in the superficial veins but none correlates perfectly with foot vein pressure which is generally accepted as the gold standard assessment for calf pump function.

A number of studies have shown that the superficial veins constitute a single superficial compartment so that pressure measured in one vein is representative of the pressure throughout the compartment.[14,31,86,126]

Method A suitable (large and straight) vein on the dorsum of the foot is cannulated. Many modern workers use a 21 gauge butterfly needle. We prefer to use a large cannula to ensure a faster frequency response and avoid the damage that the tip of a needle sometimes causes to the inside of the vein during exercise. Always insert the needle when the patient is lying down because a proportion of patients faint if it is done while they are standing.

The needle is connected to a strain gauge which is sensitive enough to detect changes of 2–5 mmHg without excessive amplification and which gives a rapid response (95 per cent +) to changes of at least 10 MHz.

The centre of the transducer is fixed level with the tip of the catheter with the connecting tube as short as is practical to allow exercise.

The system should be checked to ensure that there are no air bubbles. The transducer is connected to a pen recorder and patency and pressure transmission are checked by asking the patient to perform a Valsalva manoeuvre and by putting rapid, brief, high pressure flushes into the system.

The Valsalva manoeuvre should cause a steady rise in foot vein pressure; the flush should produce a vertical rise and fall of pressure. If the fall is not instantaneous and vertical, the system is either damped by bubbles in the system, or the catheter or vein is too narrow, or the catheter is occluded by the vein wall. Repeated flushes are essential throughout the study to check the patency of the system.

Clotting may be prevented by adding a slow constant infusion of heparinized saline to the system.

The patient exercises by raising both heels off the ground every second in time to a metronome, for 10–20 s or until the pressure becomes stable. The patient should hold onto a support throughout the study so that he/she can fully relax between periods of exercise. An alternative exercise is knee bending but this dorsiflexes the ankle whereas heel raising plantar flexes the ankle and is less likely to disturb or occlude the cannula.

If other tests of calf pump function are being performed, one form of exercise should be used which is suitable for all tests.

The test should be repeated with superficial vein occluding cuffs at different levels on the leg. The resting pressure (the hydrostatic pressure) depends upon the height of the patient, provided

there is no cardiac failure, constrictive pericarditis, ascites, abdominal masses, or any other abnormality that will impede venous return.

The fall in pressure during exercise, which is highly reproducible, indicates the efficiency of calf pump function (Figs. 4.28 and 4.29). The rise of pressure after exercise which is produced by the arterial inflow and venous reflux can be expressed as the time taken to refill completely, the time taken for 90 per cent refilling, the time for 50 per cent refilling or the maximum rate of refilling.

Provided a laboratory keeps to a standard exercise and standard method of measuring refilling, the way in which the results are expressed is not particularly important. We find that the T½ is the easiest to measure and, as it includes the period of maximum refilling, it is probably the best simple measure of reflux. The maximum refilling rate is frequently difficult to measure as refilling is often not linear.

Application Foot vein pressures are used to assess calf pump function and detect abnormalities such as chronic deep vein incompetence or obstruction and superficial vein incompetence.[166,193] The use of superficial vein occluding tourniquets can clearly demonstrate the contribution of superficial reflux to pump insufficiency, and the site of incompetent deep-to-superficial

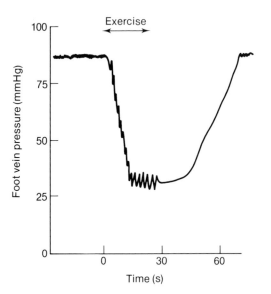

Fig. 4.28 A normal foot vein pressure trace. Exercise causes a fall in pressure of 60–80% which takes 25–30 s to return to normal.

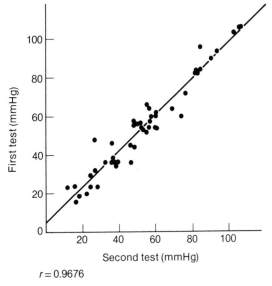

$r = 0.9676$

Fig. 4.29 A comparison between repeated tests of the fall in foot vein pressure in 48 limbs.
The measurement was highly reproducible.

vein connections can be detected by moving the tourniquet up and down the leg in the same way as in the simple clinical tourniquet test.[154,181]

Deep vein obstruction is difficult to measure, except when it is so gross that the foot vein pressure *rises* during exercise.[196]

Foot vein pressure measurements have not been used for detecting deep vein thrombosis, though they would detect a major outflow obstruction, but they have been used to follow changes of calf pump efficiency in the years following thrombosis or operation.[40]

Accuracy It is assumed that the essential function of the calf pump is to lower foot vein pressure during exercise on the basis of finding a close correlation between symptoms and signs and the inability to reduce pressure (see Fig. 11.12, page 315). Pressure has therefore been accepted as the gold standard of calf pump function assessment and other methods have been compared with it. Provided the technique of measurement is meticulous, the tracing should represent the intravenous pressures without any inaccuracies. The meaning of the changes depends upon our understanding of calf pump physiology. The fact that the surgical correction of pump abnormalities changes the pressure profile in the expected direction suggests that our hypotheses of the causes of pressure profile abnormalities are probably correct. The improvement of the pressure profile is, however, always less than expected which means that either our operations do not fully correct the abnormality or that the abnormalities corrected are not the only cause of the pump inefficiency and the abnormal pressure. Many more studies testing the significance of the abnormal features of foot vein pressure profiles need to be performed.

Femoral vein pressure measurements

If there is a gross obstruction to the venous outflow from the leg, the venous pressure will rise during muscle exercise.[147] This abnormality can sometimes be observed in the foot vein pressure profile. Lesser degrees of obstruction only limit the reduction of the foot vein pressure during exercise, a change which is not diagnostic as it can also be caused by axial and communicating vein incompetence.

Consequently, lesser degrees of iliac vein obstruction can only be detected by measuring the pressure during exercise in the femoral vein immediately upstream to the obstruction. This is an essential test before considering any type of iliac vein bypass operation (see Chapter 9).[130]

Method The patient lies supine on a couch, and a fine cannula is inserted into the femoral vein under local anaesthesia. It is helpful to have a previous ascending phlebogram available to confirm the patency and position of the femoral vein. The opposite femoral vein is also cannulated. The precautions required to ensure accurate pressure recordings described in the previous section on foot vein pressure measurement must be observed.

The patient is asked to plantar flex both feet vigorously. Although it is possible to fix the cannulae in place so that the patient can exercise on a bicycle ergometer, this degree of exercise is seldom necessary to reveal a significant obstruction.

If the limbs are normal, the femoral vein pressures will be equal and rise by 2–4 mmHg during calf muscle exercise. If the pressure rises by 10 mmHg or more, there is a significant obstruction to outflow.[147,149] The rate at which the pressure returns to normal will be delayed in the presence of an iliac vein obstruction.

Application and accuracy This technique is the only satisfactory method of diagnosing iliac vein obstruction. Phlebography may arouse suspicions but pressure measurements provide physiological proof of obstruction. We combine pressure measurement with bilateral percutaneous common femoral/iliac vein phlebography as a routine part of the phlebography (see Fig. 9.11, page 280).

In our opinion no iliac vein bypass procedure should be performed without physiological preoperative confirmation of an abnormal femoral vein pressure rise during exercise. It would be a step forward if surgeons were to confirm the adequacy of their bypass operations by showing that the bypass had abolished the pressure rise of exercise by repeating this investigation 3 months and 12 months after the operation; as well as showing that it was patent.

The fibrinogen uptake test (FUT)

The possibility that venous thrombi would incorporate radioactive fibrinogen as they formed was first tested in the rabbit by Hobbs and Davies in

1960,[84] but studies with different isotopes were necessary before the test used today became fully validated.[15,24,77,146,159]

All thrombi are metabolically active, they are not 'silent backwaters' of the circulation. Fibrinogen is not only taken from the circulation and converted into fibrin as a thrombus forms but fibrinogen diffuses in and out of the thrombus throughout its early life. As the fibrin in the thrombus polymerizes and the thrombus ages, the exchange of molecules between it and the blood become less.

The fibrinogen uptake test (FUT) depends upon the incorporation of injected radioactive fibrinogen by thrombus and the detection of the localized radioactivity by external scintillation counting.[74,148] Fibrinogen cannot be autoclaved but since the introduction of small pools of donors and testing for hepatitis B antigen (Australia antigen) and HIV (human immunodeficiency viruses) the risk of giving a patient a serum-transmitted disease has almost been abolished.

Method The patient is given 100 mg of potassium iodide on the day before the labelled fibrinogen is given and daily thereafter for 14 days to block the uptake of radioactive iodine by the thyroid gland. In emergency situations the potassium iodide and the fibrinogen can be given together because the quantity of free iodine released during the first 24 hours is extremely small and most unlikely to damage the cells of the thyroid gland.

The patient should lie comfortably on a bed or couch with the legs elevated (30°) above the heart, to eliminate pooling of blood in the legs.

The legs are examined with a handheld scintillation counter or ratemeter[96] along the line of the femoral vein in the thigh, over the popliteal fossa, and down the centre or either side of each calf.

A standard sodium iodide crystal and 3 in (7.5 cm) collimator will view an area of tissue 4 in (10 cm) in diameter to a depth of 2 in (5 cm). With such a counter the points for counting should be 4 in (10 cm) apart. The smaller crystal and collimator of the common portable ratemeter views an area 2 in (5 cm) in diameter to a depth of 4 in (10 cm) so counting points should be 2 in (5 cm) apart.

In the early days of the test the radioactivity was measured in counts/min using a scaler and a timer; the development of small portable ratemeters has replaced this rather cumbersome apparatus.

The counts emitted from the precordium (the fourth left interspace adjacent to the sternum) are adjusted on the ratemeter to read 100 per cent. The counts from each point along both legs are then recorded as percentages of the precordial count (Figs. 4.30 and 4.31).

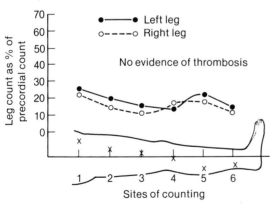

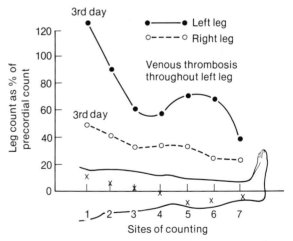

Fig. 4.30 The fibrinogen uptake test of two normal legs. The count rates over the points marked 1–6 are recorded as a percentage of the precordial count. The slight variations in radioactivity are caused by the varying quantities of blood in the tissues beneath the scintillation counter. This study was performed with a 4 inch collimator.

Fig. 4.31 A patient with a raised fibrinogen uptake test (4 in collimator) throughout the left leg 3 days after an abdominal operation. The difference between the legs at points 1, 2, 5 and 6 were greater than 15 percentage points and persisted for 24 hours. This patient had a calf and femoral vein thrombosis.

The initial studies comparing[125]I-fibrinogen uptake with phlebography used a scaler and timer and showed that a difference of 15 percentage points developing between adjacent sites on the same leg or between identical sites on the opposite leg was diagnostic of a thrombosis. Comparisons between the scaler/timer system and the portable ratemeter showed that a difference of 20 percentage points was necessary to make a positive diagnosis with the ratemeter. The increased count rate must persist for more than 24 hours to be significant. Daily investigations are performed to detect changes in the configuration of the thrombus.

The information is kept on a sheet or displayed graphically (Fig. 4.31). A graph makes comparisons easier and shows the day-to-day changes occurring in the thrombus.

Application   This test is best used for the detection of thrombus in circumstances when it is expected that thrombosis will occur (e.g. after operation or during a severe medical illness) so that the radioactive fibrinogen is given *before* the event.

The FUT has been the main research tool used for the study of the prevalance of venous thrombosis and for testing methods of prophylaxis.

It could be used to screen all hospital patients but would be too expensive, though it is used in some centres for screening high risk patients.

It can be used to confirm the diagnosis of established thrombosis but as the thrombus ages so its accuracy diminishes and different diagnostic criteria are required.[37]

Accuracy   Any condition that causes a deposition of fibrin, intravascular or extravascular, will give a positive test.[38,97] Inflammation, bruises, haematomata, arthritis and fresh wounds will all give false-positive results (Fig. 4.32); it must be remembered that in all the studies comparing this test with phlebography, most of these conditions have been diagnosed clinically and excluded from the study. The FUT is only accurate when limbs with disorders that would cause false-positive scans are excluded.

False-negatives occur when ageing thrombus does not take up fibrinogen[37] and when there are fresh thrombi in the upper half of the thigh or pelvic veins[74,148] where the background radioactivity from blood and urine masks the relatively small increase of radioactivity present in a thrombus. These are serious disadvantages and mean

that the FUT can only be used to study or detect calf and lower thigh thrombosis.

The positive and negative test accuracy for thrombi developing after the injection of the radioactive fibrinogen, below the mid-thigh, having excluded obvious causes of false-positives by clinical examination and confirmed that the abnormality is persistant (24 hours), is over 95 per cent, when compared to phlebography. Some investigators consider that this test should be used as the gold standard of calf thrombosis, and it has been suggested that it could replace phlebography for the diagnosis of deep vein thrombosis if it was combined with impedance plethysmography.[90,91]

The positive test accuracy for established thrombus when compared against phlebography is 75 per cent for thrombi less than 7 days old and 65 per cent for thrombi more than 14 days old. These tests may take 48 hours to become positive. Thus, the FUT is not of practical value in the diagnosis of established thrombosis, except when combined with other screening tests which exclude major vein thrombi and indicate that a 48-hour delay in waiting for the test result is safe.

The radioactive plasmin uptake test

The slow entry of fibrinogen into established

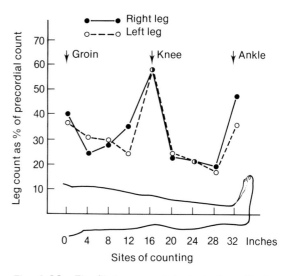

Fig. 4.32   The fibrinogen uptake test of a patient with acute rheumatoid arthritis of the knees and ankles. This was initially interpreted as a positive test until the joints were examined. A phlebogram was normal.

thrombus stimulated a search for a substance that would enter thrombi faster and more easily and so be suitable for the diagnosis of established thrombi. Labelled porcine plasmin was found to do this and it has been used as a clinical test.[4,24,61,153]

This test can detect established unilateral thrombi within 30 minutes of the injection of the labelled plasmin but because of the method of expressing the radioactivity, bilateral symmetrical thrombi are often missed. The advantage of this technique is the rapidity of the result and the absence of radiation of the thyroid gland. Its disadvantage, apart from its failure to detect bilateral disease, is the short half-life of the isotope (6 hours) which means that the plasmin must be labelled for each test and cannot be stored on the shelf.

This test has not been generally adopted because of the difficulties mentioned above together with a low specificity of 40 per cent (i.e. a poor ability to detect the absence of disease).

This test is mentioned to illustrate the continuing search for better and faster ways of detecting deep vein thrombosis – one of which may be ultrasonic imaging.

Phlebography

The term phlebography when used alone refers, by convention, to X-ray contrast phlebography which, until recently, was the only method available for imaging the venous system. The derivation of the word does not preclude its use for other venous imaging techniques but to avoid confusion it is usual to add an adjective to indicate the method being employed (e.g. isotope phlebography).

Berberisch and Hirsch[26] published the first description of phlebography in 1923. They used strontium bromide but it was not until less toxic contrast media became available, diodone in the 1930s, and tri-iodinated benzoic acid compounds (e.g. sodium or meglumine diatrizoate, iothalamate, or metrizoate) in the 1950s, that phlebography became widely employed. As these ionic media are hyperosmolar compared with blood and tissue fluids, side-effects are quite common but they do not outweigh, in most cases, the diagnostic benefits of the investigation.

The next major advance in phlebography was the introduction of low osmolality contrast media, either non-ionic or dimeric in composition, after it was pointed out by Almen[11] that it was the hyperosmolality rather than the chemotoxicity which caused the complications of contrast injections.

Phlebography of the lower limbs

Ascending phlebography

The term ascending phlebography indicates that the contrast medium is injected peripherally and passes centrally towards the heart in the venous bloodstream. Ascending phlebography of the arm entails injecting contrast medium into a hand or elbow vein to outline the arm veins and the superior vena cava. The term is, however, most often used to describe phlebography of the legs when contrast medium is injected into a foot vein. This is the most commonly employed phlebographic technique.

Contrast medium The introduction of low osmolality contrast media has significantly improved patient comfort and safety in all forms of vascular imaging, particularly phlebography. Hyperosmolar agents are painful on injection[111] and can cause thrombosis[137,169] and tissue necrosis when extravasated.[27]

We recommend that low osmolality contrast media should always be used for phlebography[106] but if, because of financial contraints or because the newer agents have not received official approval, hyperosmolar media are used, they should be diluted to bring their osmolality closer to that of plasma.[28] We suggest iopamidol 300 (Niopam) or iohexol 300 (Omnipaque) or sodium/meglumine ioxaglate 200 (Hexabrix) should be used for routine peripheral phlebography. A higher iodine concentration (e.g. iopamidol 300, iohexol 350 or sodium/meglumine ioxaglate 320) may be needed for larger veins such as the vena cava. Iopamidol 300 has a low viscosity (4.5 cP) which allows it to be injected through small needles. Hexabrix is less expensive but has more minor side-effects (e.g. nausea, vomiting and urticaria). All contrast media should be warmed to reduce their viscosity. The amount of contrast medium needed for a particular examination varies considerably according to the type of examination. As an approximate guide, about 50 ml of contrast medium are usually sufficient for ascending phlebography of one leg but four times this volume may be required for the examination of both legs and the proximal veins, or when repeat studies are necessary to display areas about which there is doubt. The poor quality of phlebograms in the past was usually caused by our inability to inject large volumes of contrast media because of their toxicity; this restraint does not apply to low osmolality media.

Equipment Special radiographic apparatus is not required for phlebography. A tilting table is essential and image intensification with television monitoring and an automatic exposure device is highly desirable. The use of television monitoring has improved the diagnostic accuracy of phlebography because it enables the phlebographer to see the direction of flow of the contrast medium and also enables radiographs to be taken when the veins are optimally filled, thus avoiding artefacts. In addition to a fluoroscopy table, a serial film changer allows sequential exposures which, in some circumstances, are necessary to obtain maximum information. Cine radiography has a limited place in dynamic studies of the venous system.

Small 'butterfly' needles are useful for peripheral injections, and larger intravenous plastic cannulae are useful for bolus injections which may require a pressure injection pump. Potts–Cournand needles (Becton–Dickinson, Rutherford, New Jersey, USA) are useful because they have a blunt obturator which allows the needle to be threaded into the vein a short distance thus preventing extravasation. A sphygmomanometer for a controlled Valsalva manoeuvre should also be available.

Position of the patient Ideally, ascending phlebography of the lower limbs should be carried out with the patient in the vertical position. In this position the deep venous system always fills with contrast medium if it is patent, and there is maximum mixing of the contrast medium with the blood thus minimizing artefacts. This position is, however, often not possible for ill patients, and vaso-vagal attacks are quite common, even in healthy patients. To avoid these problems the maximum tilt we use is 60° foot-down but a tilt of 30° is often sufficient when combined with the use of tourniquets. When filling the calf veins with contrast medium it is important to instruct the patient not to bear weight on the leg being examined because calf muscle contraction prevents adequate filling of the calf muscle veins.

Venepuncture Contrast medium can be injected into any vein on the dorsum of the foot. A constant vein is the medial digital vein of the great toe which can often be punctured even in the oedematous foot. Another advantage of this vein is that extravasation can easily be detected. Oedema, however, makes venepuncture difficult. Prolonged local pressure may displace the oedema overlying a vein, and veno-dilatation can be encouraged by applying warm packs or by sitting the patient with the legs dependent and the feet in a bowl of warm water. If the examination is not urgent, bedrest for 24 hours with elevation of the legs will usually disperse enough oedema to make a percutaneous injection feasible. If a vein cannot be found on the foot or ankle, any suitable vein in the lower leg will suffice, provided the tourniquet is applied above the puncture site to direct the contrast medium into the deep veins and a steeper foot-down table tilt is used to encourage the hyperbaric medium to fill the veins below the level of puncture. The degree of filling of veins below a high puncture site is not as good as that from a distal foot injection but is often adequate for the clinical management of deep vein thrombosis. When percutaneous venepuncture is impossible a cut-down can be performed on the long saphenous vein at its known site 2 cm above and anterior to the medial malleolus. Alternatively, an intraosseous injection into the os calcis or medial malleolus can be used (Fig. 4.33). We usually use a 21 gauge 'butterfly' needle but for very small veins a 23 gauge needle may be required. Injection through small needles may require the assistance of an injection pump. A plastic cannula may be used instead of needles to reduce the risk of extravasation but cannulae are not as sharp as needles and the discomfort they cause, if multiple venepunctures are needed, outweighs their advantage.

Tourniquets If a steep foot-down table tilt is used, an ankle tourniquet is not essential to fill the deep veins because there are numerous communicating veins in the foot that connect the superficial veins to the deep veins. If, however, the superficial veins are not occluded by a tourniquet, the superficial and the deep veins are opacified simultaneously, producing a confusing phlebogram with overlap of the two systems. Furthermore, better filling of the deep veins of the leg is obtained if an ankle tourniquet is employed which minimizes the preferential filling of the superficial system from the dorsal venous arch of the foot. Similarly, there is better demonstration of the veins in the venous phase of a leg arteriogram if an ankle tourniquet is employed. The tightness of the ankle tourniquet is adjusted during the injection of contrast medium, with television observation to ensure that deep venous filling occurs. Specific pressures for the tourniquets cannot be defined because their effect depends on the thickeness of the tissues and the width of the tourniquet. We use 2.5 cm wide self-fastening tourniquets which, being slightly radioopaque, can be identified on the radiographs. A narrow tourniquet, such as rubber tubing clamped with forceps, can be dangerous as it may occlude arterial flow if it is too tight. If, because of ankle ulceration or trauma, a tourniquet cannot be applied at the ankle it can be applied round the forefoot or higher up the leg, or deep venous filling can be encouraged by a steep foot-down table tilt alone. A tourniquet above the knee helps to delay emptying of the calf veins thus improving their filling. It also conserves contrast medium which is important if high cost, low osmolality medium is being used.

Technique When the tourniquets are in position the contrast medium is injected continuously by hand. Films are taken, under fluoroscopic control, from the foot to the lower inferior vena cava. Straight (postero-anterior with a fluoroscopy table) projections alone are sufficient to show the stem veins of the leg but lateral views, obtained by turning the patient's leg so that the side of the calf is flat on the table top, are desirable to display the foot veins and the muscle veins of the calf when looking for thrombus or minor post-thrombotic changes (Fig. 4.34). After films of the calf have been obtained, exposures are made of the femoral and iliac veins and lower inferior vena cava using hand compression of the calf muscles to improve filling.

The Valsalva manoeuvre The Valsalva manoeuvre can be very useful in ascending phlebography. If the manoeuvre is performed when the common femoral vein is filled with contrast medium, the deep femoral vein will be demonstrated as far as competent valves permit. Similarly, the internal iliac veins can be shown if a Valsalva manoeuvre is performed when the common iliac veins are filled (Fig. 4.35a and b). Venous valves are well shown during a Valsalva manoeuvre. Competent valves are seen as sharply defined bicuspid structures with hold up of contrast in each valve sinus (Fig. 4.35c. Also see Fig. 2.8b, page 30). This procedure may avoid

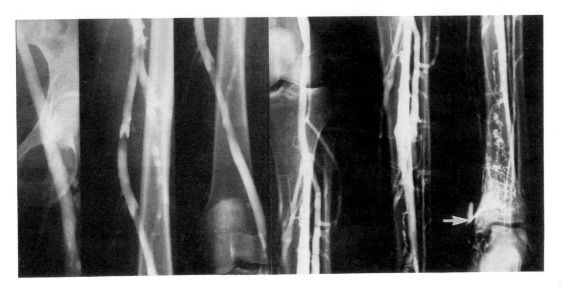

Fig. 4.33 An intraosseous phlebogram of the leg.
The intraosseous cannula has been introduced into the medial malleolus (arrow). The venous system in this example is normal. This technique is useful in an oedematous leg with no suitable vein for venepuncture. (See Fig. 18.7.)

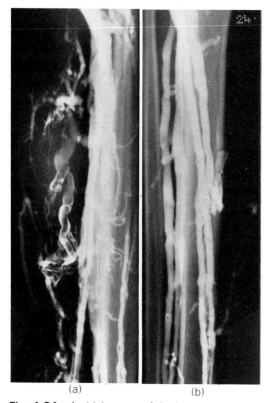

(a)   (b)

Fig. 4.34 A phlebogram of the lower leg. (a) In the lateral view there is a great deal of thrombus in the stem and muscle veins of the calf. (b) In the postero-anterior view only a little thrombus can be seen because of the overlying bone. This emphasizes the importance of taking a lateral view of the calf in all patients with suspected venous thrombosis.

the necessity for seperate descending phlebography. It is more effective to use a Valsalva manoeuvre in which the intrathoracic pressure is controlled and standardized. This is achieved by asking the patient to blow into the barrel of a 10 ml syringe connected to a mercury manometer to produce and maintain a pressure of 40 mmHg for 12 s.

Variations of ascending phlebography

The Bolus Technique Calf compression to produce a bolus of contrast medium improves the quality of ascending phlebograms. The technique is particularly useful when studying the iliac veins and inferior vena cava if access to the femoral veins is not possible because either they are occluded or the patient is obese.

A tourniquet is applied tightly above each knee and 50 ml of contrast medium are injected simultaneously into a vein in each foot. Calf compression is applied with the tourniquet still in place and, if necessary, repeated after they have been removed, and exposures are made of the proximal leg veins, the iliac veins and lower inferior vena cava. This simple method gives an adequate demonstration of the iliac veins and lower inferior vena cava in approximately 90 per cent of patients. In the remaining 10 per cent of patients separate femoral injections are required.[112]

Tilt phlebograhy This technique involves tilting the patient foot-down immediately after the injection of contrast in order to temporarily arrest its upward flow and reverse the hydrostatic gradient. This identifies the venous valves and gives an indication of their competence.[64,128] Similar information can be obtained by using a Valsalva manoeuvre during ascending phlebography as described above, or by descending phlebography.

Exercise phlebography This technique involves combining the foot-down posture with leg muscle exercise. The pumping action and the competence of communicating veins may be directly tested.[10,60]

Varicography

Varicography is the direct injection of varicose veins with contrast medium. It was first performed by McPheeters and Rice in 1929[135] using the oily medium lipiodol. Until the introduction of low osmolality contrast media, the technique was little used because early media almost invariably caused thrombophlebitis when injected into a varicose vein.[131]

With the patient standing, a varicose vein in the group of which the patient complains, is punctured with a 21 gauge 'butterfly' needle. The patient lies on a fluoroscopy table, prone or supine, depending on the position of the needle. Ideally, the table should be capable of being tilted 60° foot- or head-down. The examination is started with a steep (60°) foot-down table tilt. A hand injection of contrast is made under television control, and the passage of contrast is followed by fluoroscopy, cut films being taken at appropriate intervals. The examination is complete when the contrast medium reaches the region of the saphenous opening (or higher if tri-

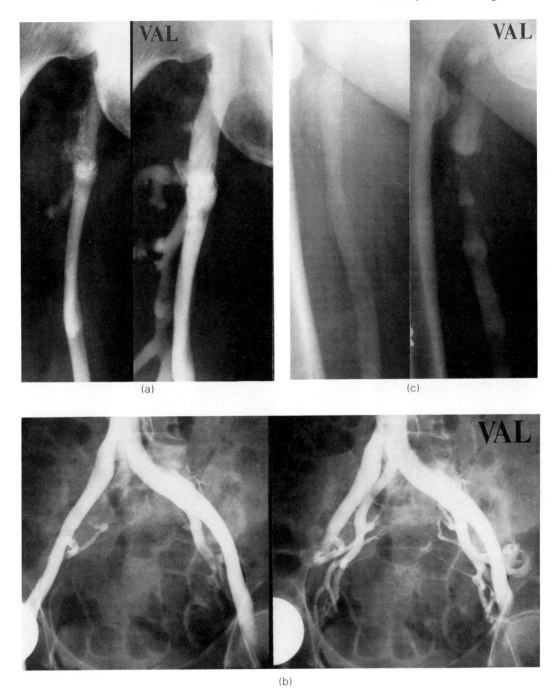

Fig. 4.35 Uses of the Valsalva manoeuvre in ascending phlebography.

(a) Much more of the deep femoral vein is shown during the Valsalva manoeuvre (right-hand panel).

(b) The right-hand panel shows how a Valsalva manoeuvre, performed when the common iliac veins are filled with contrast medium, causes contrast medium to reflux into the internal iliac veins.

(c) The left-hand panel shows an ascending femoral phlebogram without a Valsalva manoeuvre. The right-hand panel shows competent valves demonstrated by the Valsalva manoeuvre. In this situation a descending phlebogram to show competent valves is not necessary.

butaries pass towards the pelvis) or enters the deep veins of the leg through a thigh communicating vein. Films are taken to record the events observed by fluoroscopy. Several injections into different groups of varicose veins may be necessary to show all the connections. To show the short saphenous vein the patient is turned so that the knee is in a true lateral position and a further injection is made (Fig. 4.36a). Tourniquets are not normally applied for this technique because the aim is to watch the free flow of contrast medium from the varicose veins into connecting superficial and deep veins. If an incompetent communicating vein in Hunter's canal is suspected, it may be seen more clearly by applying a high thigh tourniquet above the suspected site.

A ruler with 1 cm metal markers placed beneath the leg helps to relate the site of any communicating veins to bony landmarks such as the knee (Fig. 4.36b). Varicography shows the extent of the varicosities and their superficial-to-deep connections (Fig. 4.36c and d).[52,109,117,122] The direction of blood flow during varicography cannot be used as a guide to valvular incompetence because the contrast medium follows the normal flow from the superficial to the deep systems. If, however, a communicating vein is dilated (more than 3 mm in diameter), it is likely to be incompetent. Incompetent communicating veins in the calf can

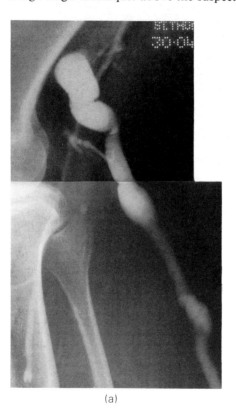

(a)

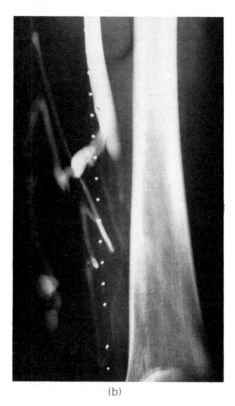

(b)

Fig. 4.36 Varicography. (a) Varicogram showing a varicose short saphenous vein. (b) This varicogram shows a dilated, almost certainly incompetent, communicating vein in the mid thigh (Hunter's canal). The ruler with metal markers allows the site of the communicating vein to be related to the knee joint.
(c) Recurrent varicose veins in region of the vulva. There are connections with the common femoral vein and with the internal pudendal vein (arrow). (d) Recurrent varicose veins in upper thigh and vulva. Varicose veins connect with the obturator vein and then into the internal iliac vein. (e) Medial lower leg (Cockett) communicating veins shown by varicography. Varicography is often a better way of showing the site of the incompetent communicating veins than ascending phlebography. The size and shape of these veins suggests that they are incompetent.

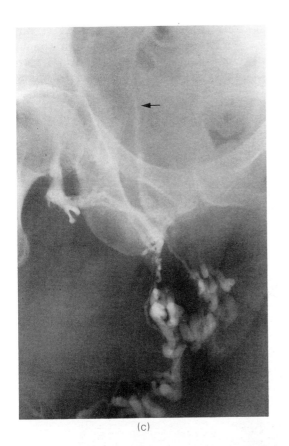

(c)

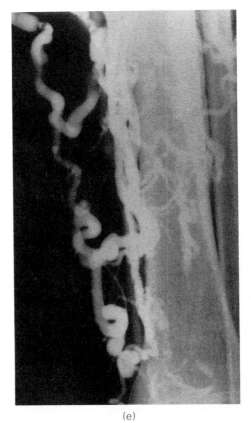

(e)

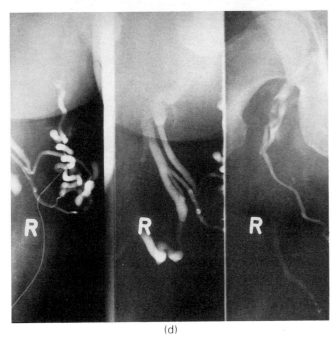

(d)

sometimes be more clearly shown by varicography than by ascending phlebography (Fig. 4.36e).[105]

Saphenography

The purpose of this investigation is to demonstrate the long saphenous vein, and occasionally the short saphenous vein, to assess their suitability for arterial bypass surgery. Until the advent of non-thrombogenic contrast media the examination could not be performed with safety because of the risk of thrombosis.

The patient lies supine on a tilting fluoroscopy table. Contrast medium is injected by hand through a 21 gauge 'butterfly' needle into the long saphenous vein at the ankle or, if this is not possible, into a superficial foot vein as close to the origin of the long saphenous vein as possible. Tourniquets are not used, except to distend the foot vein for the initial venepuncture, because they cause non-physiological distension of the vein and tend to divert the contrast medium into the deep veins. During the continuous injection of contrast medium the patient is tilted from the foot-down to the head-down position until the whole of the long saphenous vein has been visualized and spot films have been taken as a record (Fig. 4.37). Brief hand compression of the popliteal vein in the popliteal fossa, or of the common femoral vein at the groin, just before filming may help to show the complete long saphenous vein and any reduplications. This manoeuvre, by obstructing the deep veins, directs contrast into the long saphenous vein which may be bypassed if contrast medium passess preferentially through communicating veins into the deep system. To examine the short saphenous vein the patient is turned so that the calf and knee lie on the fluoroscopy table in the true lateral position.

A similar technique can be used to show the cephalic and basilic veins in the arm. To correct for magnification, ball-bearings of known diameter are placed on the anatomic course of the vein from which the true size of the veins can be calculated.[116]

Iliac phlebography and inferior vena cavography

Injection into femoral veins

The simultaneous injection of 50 ml of contrast

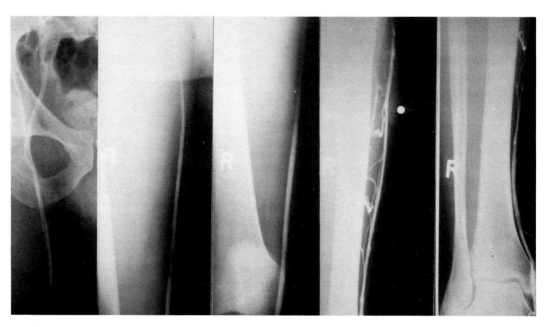

Fig. 4.37 Saphenography.
  Saphenogram performed before arterial bypass surgery. The vein has been demonstrated from the ankle to the groin and has a suitable diameter for bypass surgery. The ball-bearing (fourth panel) enables correction to be made for magnification.

medium by hand into both femoral veins when the patient is in the horizontal position produces excellent opacification of the femoral and iliac veins and inferior vena cava.

Each femoral vein is punctured with a 16 gauge Potts–Cournand needle medial to the maximum arterial pulsation at the groin. A Valsalva manoeuvre helps to distend the vein during puncture. Contrast medium is injected by hand and films are taken to show the iliac veins and inferior vena cava. The inferior vena cava is better shown by a 30° left anterior oblique projection so that its image is projected to the right of the vertebral column and is not obscured by bone. To show the internal iliac veins a Valsalva manoeuvre is carried out half-way through the injection of the contrast medium (see Fig. 4.35).

Vein walls are easily dissected and thrombus dislodged by the use of guide wires and catheters; we therefore prefer to avoid their use if possible.

The inferior vena cava can be demonstrated retrogradely from arm or neck veins with a guide wire–catheter system and television monitoring. Intrasosseous pertrochanteric injections are also useful to show the complete extent of an inferior vena caval occlusion.

Measurement of femoral vein pressures can be combined with femoral vein injections by connecting the intravenous cannula to a manometer.[147] Similarly, measurement of foot vein pressures can be combined with ascending phlebography of the legs.[40]

Intraosseous injections

Intraosseous injections are indicated when it is thought, or known, that the femoral veins are occluded. To facilitate bone puncture we use a cannula with a three-faceted drill tip which makes penetration of the cortex easier.[119] Bilateral simultaneous injections of 50 ml of contrast medium are made using pressure injectors set at a rate of 15 ml/s. A series of films are taken from the beginning of the injection for 30 s to allow sufficient time for the contrast medium to pass from the medullary cavity through any collateral veins.

It is better to use two pressure injectors rather than a 'Y' connection because there is a tendency for the contrast medium to pass into the bone with least resistance. Pertrochanteric intraosseous

phlebography has a particular advantage in inferior vena caval obstruction because the upper extent of the occlusion can be shown without resorting to retrograde phlebography (Fig. 4.38). A combination of a percutaneous femoral injection on the patent side and an intraosseous injection on the obstructed side can also be employed.

As contrast medium is hyperbaric, it fills the more dependent veins preferentially. This particularly applies to intraosseous phlebography

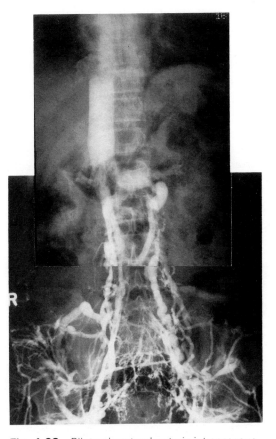

Fig. 4.38 Bilateral pertrochanteric intraosseous phlebography to show the iliac veins and inferior vena cava. The iliac veins are grossly narrowed by post-thrombotic changes. The inferior vena cava is totally occluded to just below the left renal vein. The collateral pathways are the ascending lumbar and azygos veins and the left gonadal vein. The advantage of intraosseous phlebography in this situation is that it often displays the vena cava above the obstruction so that separate retrograde phlebography is not required.

because of the slow passage of the contrast medium from the bone marrow into the veins. Better opacification of the external iliac veins is therefore obtained when the patient is in the prone position, whereas opacification of the internal iliac veins is better when the patient is in the supine position (Fig. 4.39).

Other sites of intraosseous phlebography to show the leg and pelvic veins include the malleoli or calcaneum (see Fig. 4.33), the tibial tubercle, the femoral condyles and the pubic rami.[122] The vertebral venous plexuses and the azygos veins can be visualized by injection of contrast into the spinous processes of a vertebra or into the posterior end of a rib. The veins of the arm can be demonstrated by injection into the lower end of the radius, the olecranon process or the acromion process.[176]

Indirect phlebography

The injection of contrast medium into an artery followed through into the venous phase is useful in certain situations where direct venous access is difficult. A notable example is the venous phase of a carotid arteriogram which displays the tributaries of the internal jugular vein. The overlap of superficial and deep veins in indirect phlebograms of the limbs makes interpretation difficult, and

direct phlebography is preferable. An example of the use of this technique in the demonstration of a vascular malformation is shown in Fig. 26.8, page 668.

Digital subtraction phlebography

Digital subtraction angiography enhances the opacification of vessels and so enables images to be obtained with much smaller volumes of dilute contrast medium. This advantage has to be balanced against the degradation of the image obtained compared with a screen – film phlebogram. The use of less contrast medium is safer and, if non-ionic contrast medium is used, much less expensive. The technique has, however, a limited place in phlebography because direct injections of veins are easy to perform, safe and produce far better phlebograms. Digital subtraction angiography can also be used to enhance the venous phase of an indirect phlebogram.

Descending phlebography

The usual method is to inject a bolus of contrast medium into the femoral vein when the patient is in an upright position with or without a Valsalva manoeuvre.[99,100] The amount of reflux towards

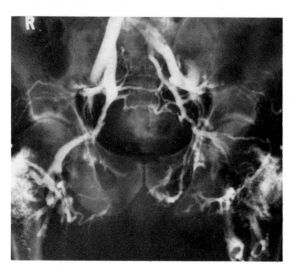 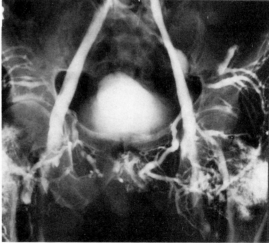

Fig. 4.39 Bilateral pertrochanteric intraosseous phlebograms of the pelvic veins. In the left-hand panel the patient is supine and, because contrast medium is hyperbaric, the more dependent internal iliac veins are well shown.

The right-hand panel shows the same patient examined in the prone position. In this position the external iliac veins are better demonstrated.

the periphery is graded from 0 to 4 (see Chapter 8).[3]

We prefer to examine the patient when he/she is in the supine position and to use a controlled, standardized Valsalva manoeuvre. The supine position is preferred by patients because vaso-vagal attacks do not occur, the needle or cannula in the groin is unlikely to be dislodged during the examination and a clearer cut off at normal valves is seen because a Valsalva manoeuvre closes the valves tightly. Furthermore, if the patient is in the upright position and a Valsalva manoeuvre is not used, the contrast medium tends to pass through normal valves exaggerating the degree of reflux.[110]

When the patient is supine on a fluoroscopy table the femoral vein is punctured in the groin with an 18 gauge Potts–Cournand needle which is threaded a short distance into the vein. The patient is then asked to perform a controlled Valsalva manoeuvre during which a bolus of 15 ml of contrast medium is injected. Films are taken of the upper thigh while the veins are observed on a television monitor. If reflux occurs below the thigh, the contrast medium is cleared from the veins with physiological saline and a further bolus is injected under similar conditions and films are taken at the knees and ankles (Fig. 4.40a–c).

Similarly, competence of popliteal valves can be shown by injecting a bolus of contrast directly into the popliteal vein (Fig. 4.40d).

Descending phlebography performed in this way is also useful when assessing long saphenous vein incompetence. Long saphenous vein reflux is not graded because any degree of reflux is abnormal (Fig. 4.40e). Descending phlebography is probably the most accurate method for assessing long saphenous vein incompetence.[104] Very occasionally, the needle puncture lies above a valve in the common femoral vein thus preventing reflux into the long saphenous vein but valves at this site are extremely rare and the valves can be seen on fluoroscopy and on the films.

Retrograde phlebography

This technique is a modification of descending phlebography and is often carried out after pulmonary angiography to detect thrombus in the large proximal veins or their tributaries.

A catheter is passed from the arm through the right atrium down the inferior vena cava and into the femoral vein. The catheter can also be positioned in the internal iliac vein. As the catheter is moved downwards under fluoroscopic control, small volumes of contrast medium are injected by hand at various levels and the state of the veins is recorded on spot films. In this way the whole of the inferior vena cava, the common iliac, external iliac and internal iliac veins can be demonstrated. There are no valves above the external iliac veins to impede the passage of the catheter.[65] An objection to the use of this method in venous thrombosis is that the guide wire and catheter may dislodge a thrombus thus causing pulmonary embolism. Retrograde phlebography has also been used to show the upper extent of an inferior vena caval obstruction (Fig. 4.41). In addition it has been employed to assess deep vein valve incompetence by injecting contrast medium at different sites in the femoral and popliteal veins.[187]

Artefacts in phlebograms

Artefacts are usually caused by underfilling of the veins, streaming of contrast medium along the vein walls, uneven mixing of the contrast medium with the blood, and entry of non-opacified blood from tributaries. They may also be produced by distortion of the veins by nearby normal or large anatomical structures, notably arteries (see Chapter 9), or by the position of the limb during examination (Fig 4.42a and b). Mixing artefacts may be mistaken for thrombus or post-thrombotic change (Fig. 4.42c–f). The incidence of artefacts can be minimized by using ample contrast medium, the bolus technique to improve filling and fluoroscopy to ensure that films are taken when the veins are fully opacified. Unlike thrombus, artefactual filling defects are inconstant in shape and position.[9,108]

Variations in technique according to clinical need

Deep vein thrombosis

A number of the non-invasive tests which have been developed to assist and improve the often clinically difficult diagnosis of lower limb thrombosis have been discussed earlier in this chapter. Contrast phlebography is, however, still the gold standard because of its ability to demonstrate

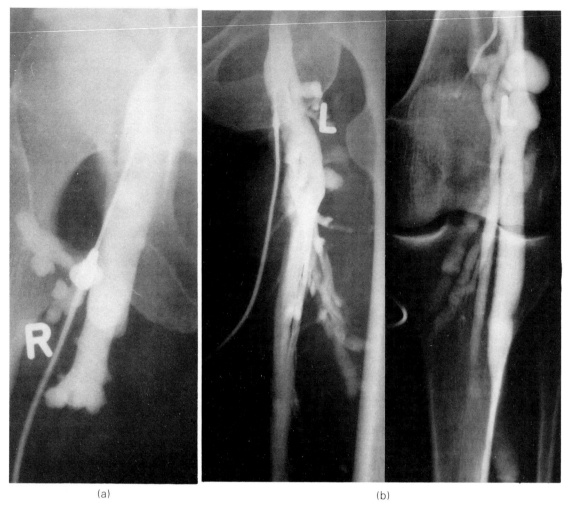

(a)   (b)

Fig. 4.40 (a) A normal descending phlebogram. There is Grade 1 deep vein reflux with a sharp cut-off at normal valves.

(b) In this descending phlebogram there is Grade 3 deep vein reflux; the contrast medium passes into the calf. The deep veins show post-thrombotic changes.

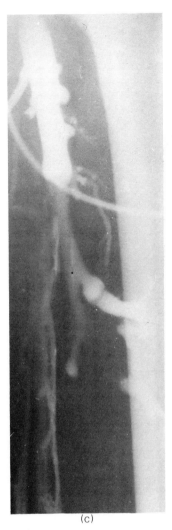

(c)

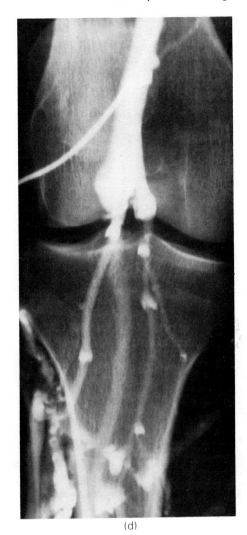

(d)

Fig. 4.40 (c) In this descending phlebogram there is a competent valve in the common femoral vein, though there are post-thrombotic changes in the superficial femoral vein below it. There are also competent valves in the deep femoral vein.

(d) A percutaneous popliteal vein descending phlebogram. The valves in the popliteal vein and the upper calf tributaries are normal.

This technique can be used if only the popliteal vein needs to be examined.

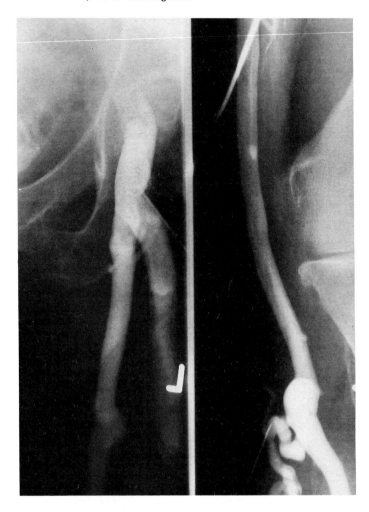

Fig. 4.40 (e) This descending phlebogram shows gross long saphenous vein reflux. This is probably the most reliable way of confirming long saphenous vein incompetence.

practically the entire deep venous system from the foot to the inferior vena cava. It yields immediate confirmation of the presence of a thrombosis and, at the same time, gives some indication of the nature of the thrombus and the likelihood of embolism. The accuracy of phlebography is approximately 95 per cent, approaching 100 per cent for large thrombi in the major veins.[168]

When ascending phlebography is undertaken to confirm the presence of deep vein thrombosis there should be special emphasis on the following.

- If the suspect limb contains thrombus, the other (clinically normal) limb should be examined as there is a 50 per cent chance that it will also contain thrombus. In practice both limbs should always be examined.

- The upper limit of any thrombus or occluded vein must be displayed, if necessary by per-femoral or intraosseous injections.
- More than one film must be taken of each part of the venous tree to confirm that any filling defects are persistent and of constant shape (i.e. not artefacts).
- As many calf and thigh veins as possible should be filled, especially any collateral veins which bypass occluded veins.
- The ankle tourniquet in ascending phlebography must not be so tight that the superficial veins are completely obstructed, otherwise superficial vein thrombosis can be missed.

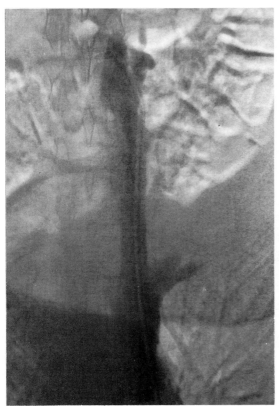

Fig. 4.41 A subtraction film of a retrograde phlebogram demonstrating occlusion of the inferior vena cava.

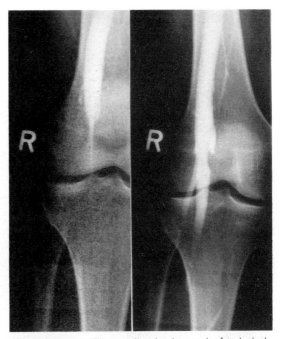

Fig. 4.42 (a) The popliteal vein can be occluded by hyperextension of the knee (left-hand panel).

With the knee slightly flexed the popliteal vein fills (right-hand panel). It is important that this appearance is not attributed to an organic obstruction.

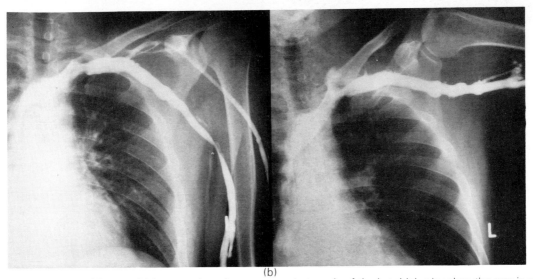

(b)

Fig. 4.42 (b) In this arm phlebogram there is an apparent stenosis of the brachial vein when the arm is at the side (left-hand panel). When the arm is abducted the narrowing is no longer present (right-hand panel). This abnormality, which is purely positional and caused by the axillary fold, should not be misinterpreted as a permanent stenosis. If the veins are examined in both positions, the nature of the artefact is obvious.

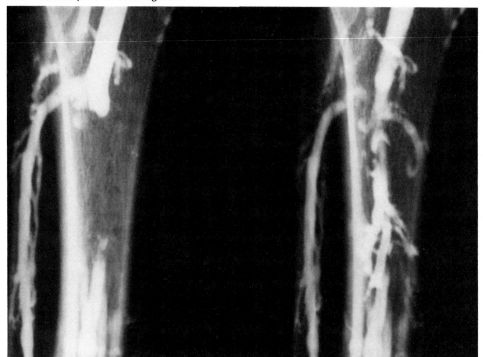

Fig. 4.42   (c) There is an unfilled segment of the peroneal vein (left-hand panel) which fills completely when more contrast medium is injected (right-hand panel). Underfilling should not be confused with obstruction by venous thrombosis. Often a little thrombus can be seen at either end of an unfilled segment if it is occluded by thrombus (see Fig. 4.43a).

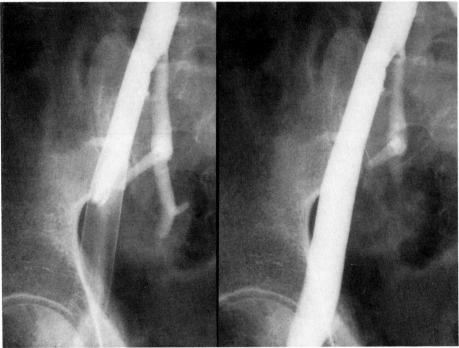

Fig. 4.42   (d) Streaming of contrast medium along the vein wall can closely mimic a recent thrombus (left-hand panel). The appearance is inconstant (right-hand panel).

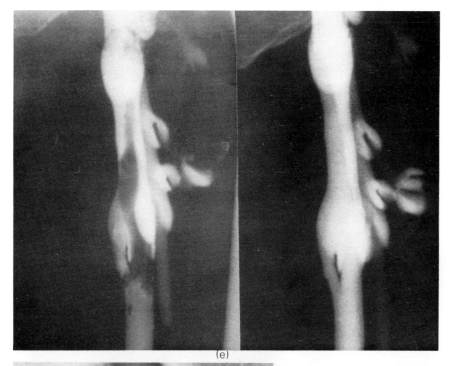

(e)

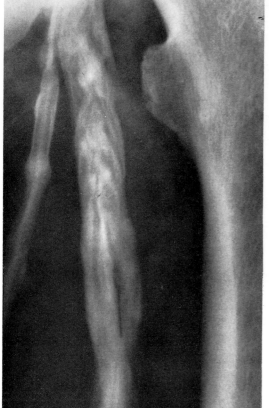

(f)

Fig. 4.42 (e) Streaming of non-opacified blood into a vein filled with contrast medium can closely resemble a thrombus (left-hand panel). It is inconstant in shape and position and disappears with better filling (right-hand panel).

(f) Incomplete mixing of hyperbaric contrast medium and blood produces mixing defects which may be confused with post-thrombotic changes. In this example the defects are present in the superficial femoral vein and also in the long saphenous vein. These changes are inconstant and, provided more than one film is taken of each segment of the venous system, should not cause confusion.

Phlebographic appearances of thrombus

Thrombus is seen as a constant filling defect in an opacified vein which is the same size and shape in at least two films taken with a brief time interval between them. For accurate diagnosis it is important to try to outline the thrombus itself and not rely solely on non-filling of veins. The ends of an unfilled vein should be carefully examined for a little thrombus projecting from one or other end (Fig. 4.43a). A constantly unfilled segment using a careful phlebographic technique is, however, suggestive of thrombus.

A fresh thrombus has a 'ground glass' appearance caused by a thin film of contrast medium surrounding it. If it is not adherent to the wall it appears as a translucent defect surrounded by contrast medium (Fig. 4.43b and c). Obliteration of this line indicates adherence of the thrombus to the wall (Fig. 4.43d). When thrombus completely occludes a vein there is no contrast around it but there is contrast medium above and below it and in the collaterals beside it (Fig. 4.43e). As thrombus ages it becomes smaller, a thicker layer of contrast medium surrounds it and its surface is more clearly defined (Fig 4.43f–h). The processes of adherence and retraction occur simultaneously.

An important feature of a thrombus is the nature of its proximal end. It may have a 'floating

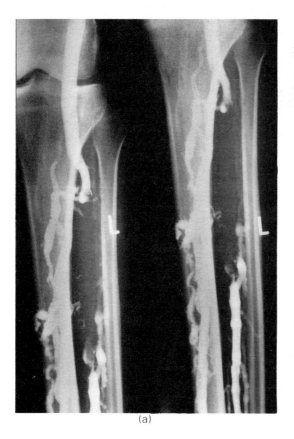
(a)

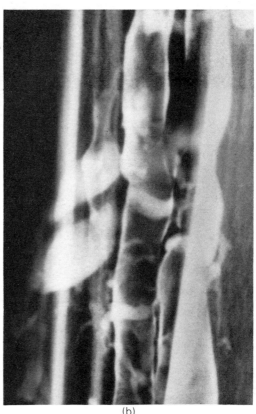
(b)

Fig. 4.43   (a) In this ascending phlebogram of the calf there is a segment of unfilled peroneal vein in both films taken at an interval. This is not caused by underfilling because close examination of each end of the unfilled segment shows a little recent thrombus. This phlebogram shows definite evidence of venous thrombosis.

(b) A close-up of recent thrombus in the muscle veins of the calf. The thrombus has a 'ground glass' appearance and is surrounded by a thin white line of contrast medium. This thrombus is loose and could become an embolus.

tail' which may become detached and embolize (Fig. 4.43i) or it may have a horizontal 'square cut' shape indicating that a portion has already broken off and embolized (Fig. 4.43j).

It is possible to estimate the age of a thrombus. In the first week the thrombus is smooth, almost filling the vein, with only a little contrast medium around it. Over the next 14 days the thrombus becomes adherent to the vein wall and retracts. Further retraction and organization over the next few weeks and months make the lumen of the vein irregular as the vein recanalizes.[114] An estimate of

the looseness or adherence of thrombus is important in the management of deep vein thrombosis because a loose thrombus is likely to embolize while an adherent thrombus is unlikely to do so. Non-adherent thrombus that is 'locked in' by adherent thrombus in veins proximal to it, cannot embolize. This feature is important when planning therapy (Fig. 4.43k).

A vein may remain totally occluded following thrombosis, return to normal, or recanalize with destruction of valves. It is not possible to predict the final outcome from the initial phlebogram.

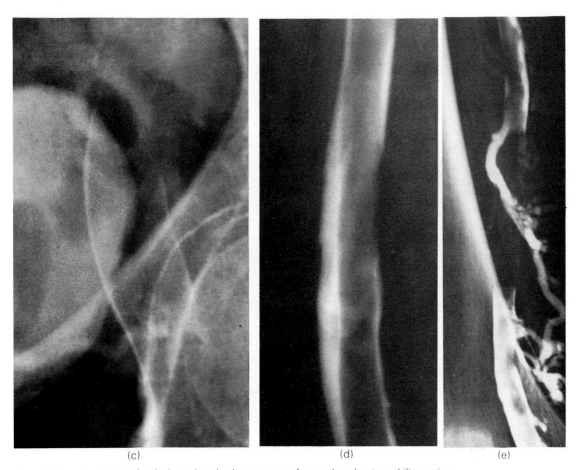

(c)　　　　　　(d)　　　　　　(e)

Fig. 4.43　(c) A loose fresh thrombus in the common femoral and external iliac veins.

(d) The thrombus in this femoral vein shows evidence of retraction and adherence. The contrast medium forms a thicker layer on the left-hand side of the vein and the surrounding layer of contrast medium is absent on the right side of the vein. This thrombus is about 10 days old and is becoming adherent to the vein wall.

(e) The thrombus in this example is occluding a long segment of the femoral vein in the adductor canal. The thrombus has been demonstrated above and below the occlusion, and the collaterals bridging the obstruction are filled with contrast medium. The thrombus above and below the occlusion shows evidence of some retraction.

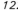

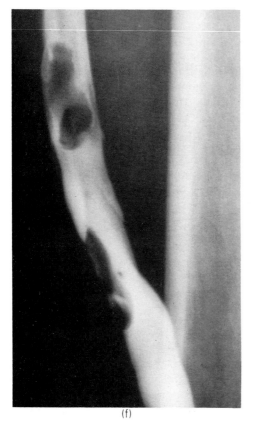

(f)

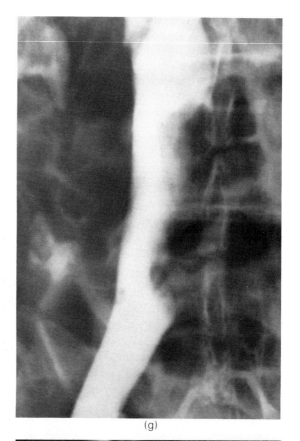

(g)

Fig. 4.43 (f and g) Examples of adherent thrombus. The thrombi are clearly defined with a sharp but irregular shape due to organization. They are unlikely to embolize.

(h) The left external and common iliac veins are shown to be totally occluded in this intraosseous pertrochanteric phlebogram. Thrombus is extending into the lower part of the inferior vena cava and narrowing its lumen. All this thrombus is adherent and is unlikely to embolize. The collateral pathways bypassing this major obstruction are the left internal iliac vein and the presacral plexus.

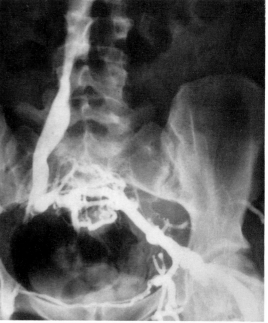

(h)

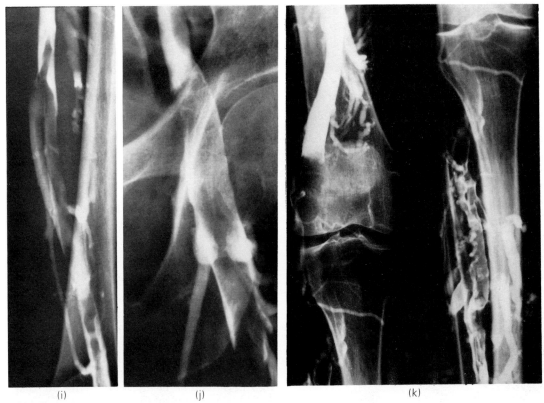

(i)   (j)   (k)

Fig. 4.43 (i) There is a 'loose tail' of thrombus extending above the major thrombus in the superficial femoral and popliteal veins. Such a 'loose tail' is likely to embolize but the embolus produced would probably be small and not clinically significant. It is important to consider the size and looseness of the entire thrombus when planning therapy.

(j) This shows a 'square cut' appearance of the upper end of a thrombus in the common femoral vein, indicating that a piece of the thrombus has already broken off and embolized.

(k) The loose thrombus in the calf veins of this patient (right-hand panel) cannot embolize because adherent thrombus is occluding the popliteal vein (left-hand panel). This patient has, in effect, an 'autoligation'.

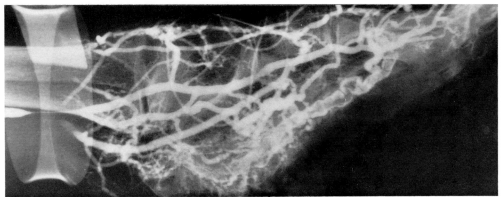

Fig. 4.44 There is a recent thrombus in the lateral plantar vein. The feet should always be examined in patients with suspected pulmonary embolism because though thrombi in the feet veins are small, they may cause repeated emboli. Venous thrombosis in the foot is also a cause of unexplained foot pain.

Recanalized or post-thrombotic veins are narrowed and irregular, with filling defects in the lumen representing organized thrombus. Valves are deformed or destroyed. Examples of phlebographic appearances seen in the post-thrombotic syndrome are shown in Chapters 11 and 12.

Pulmonary embolism

In the search for the source of pulmonary emboli, bilateral ascending phlebograms should always be performed. The bolus technique should be used to show the iliac veins and lower inferior vena cava and views of the feet should also be taken (Fig. 4.44).[115] If necessary, ascending phlebography should be supplemented by direct perfemoral phlebograms. If one femoral vein is occluded, the opposite vein should be injected to see if loose thrombus extends into the inferior vena cava from the occluded iliac vein. Occasionally, pertrochanteric intraosseous phlebography is necessary. Every attempt should be made to fill all the deep veins including the internal iliac veins.[107] Finally, right ventricular angiocardiography may rarely be required to exclude thrombus in the ventricle and pulmonary outflow tract.

Incompetent communicating veins

Ascending phlebography is modified by applying the ankle and the above-knee tourniquets tightly to completely occlude the superficial veins so that any reverse flow of contrast medium from the deep veins to the superficial veins through incompetent communicating veins can be seen on fluoroscopy.[113] If there is doubt as to which is a deep vein and which is a superficial vein, rotation of the leg will show that the deep veins remain close to the bones of the leg (Fig. 4.45a). A ruler with radio-opaque markers at 1 cm intervals placed beneath the leg is helpful in relating the position of incompetent communicating veins to bony landmarks such as the malleoli or knee joint. If ulceration is present, a tight tourniquet above and below the ulcer may help to demonstrate local incompetent communicating veins (Fig. 4.45b). Varicography can also be useful (see Fig. 4.36e).[105] A typical incompetent communicating vein is dilated (particularly at its outer end), valveless, and joins a varicose vein (Fig. 4.45c).

Congenital malformations

Direct injection of contrast medium through a fine 21 G needle into a suspected venous angioma confirms the diagnosis, shows the extent of the angioma, and shows its superficial and deep venous connections (see Fig. 4.47a). A tourniquet above the puncture site directs the contrast medium into the deep veins and their tributaries, thus helping to opacify the entire lesion. In the Klippel–Trenaunay syndrome the integrity or otherwise of the deep venous system must be shown by careful ascending phlebography or intraosseous phlebography. Varicography may be used to show the extent and termination of abnormal venous channels (see Chapters 23 and 26).

Operative and peri-operative phlebography

Simple television fluoroscopy and single film radiography are usually all that can be carried out in an operating theatre, timing of the film is therefore critical. A relatively large volume of contrast medium (50 ml) should be injected into the vein continuously and the film should be taken towards the end of the injection. In this way diagnostic results can be obtained with a minimum of delay by avoiding having to perform repeat injections because the critical phase has been missed. The value of on-table short saphenography before sapheno-popliteal ligation has been stressed by Hobbs.[81] Varicography can also be useful in recurrent varicose veins at unusual sites.

The aim of ilio-femoral thrombectomy is to prevent fatal pulmonary embolism and restore the patency of the ilio-femoral segment. The operation should always be controlled with peroperative phlebography. The contrast medium should be injected into the vein that has been cleared of thrombus and inspected with an image intensifier and recorded on a single cut film (see Fig. 18.9). Mavor and Galloway[129] recommend dividing the superficial circumflex iliac vein and preserving the portion leading to the long saphenous vein so that a catheter can be passed through it into the external iliac vein to facilitate post-operative phlebography.

Venous trauma

Trauma to the venous system is common but produces less dramatic effects than arterial trauma.

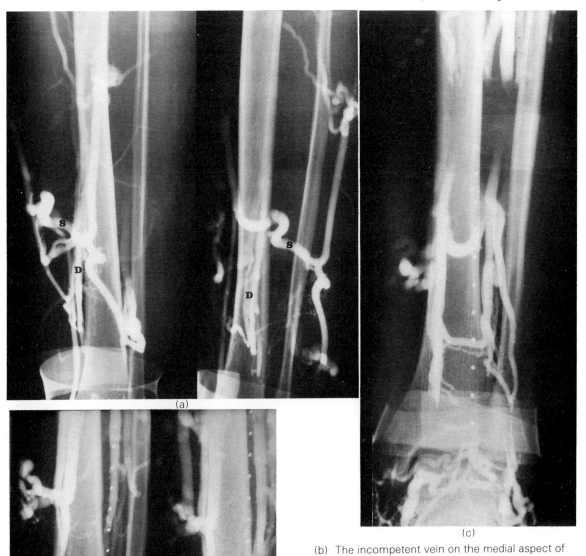

(a)

(b)

(c)

Fig. 4.45 The communicating veins.

(a) Sometimes the superficial and deep veins of the calf are difficult to distinguish on a phlebogram; rotation of the limb will make this clear. In the straight projection (left-hand panel) the superficial veins (S) and the deep veins (D) are superimposed. In the right-hand panel rotation of the limb separates the two sets of veins; the deep veins remain close to the bones.

(b) The incompetent vein on the medial aspect of the calf is beneath a venous ulcer. Tight tourniquets below and above the ulcer are helpful in demonstrating the causative incompetent communicating vein.

The ruler with metal markers enables the site of the communicating vein to be related to the medial malleolus.

(c) A medial incompetent communicating vein demonstrated by ascending phlebography. A tight ankle tourniquet occludes the superficial veins so that the contrast medium can be seen passing in the reverse direction from the deep veins to the superficial veins indicating incompetence. In addition to this abnormal flow an incompetent communicating vein is dilated, particularly at the outer end and connects with a varicose vein. The ruler with metal markers is used to relate the incompetent communicating vein to bony landmarks, in this case the medial malleolus.

For this reason, until recently, management was usually confined to tying off bleeding veins. Increased use of phlebography has drawn attention to the late sequelae of ligation of main veins, and interest has focused on immediate and late reconstitution procedures (see Chapter 25).

Phlebography may be used to assess the site and extent of acutely injured veins and, at a later stage, the results of the injury and emergency therapy.

The technique of phlebography must be tailored to individual circumstances. As injured patients are usually unable to stand or to be tilted on a fluoroscopy table, a tourniquet at the ankle or proximal to the site of injection must be used to direct contrast medium into the deep veins. If necessary, a single image (often in a single plane) of the injured region can usually be obtained with portable radiographic equipment in the Casualty Department or operating theatre (Fig 4.46a–d).[122]

Phlebography of the upper limbs

There is rarely any clinical indication for phlebographic demonstration of the veins of the hands and forearm except in the assessment of veins for bypass surgery or suspected or known venous malformations. A useful practical phlebographic method of demonstrating a venous malformation or tumour in the arm is by direct injection (Fig. 4.47a) or indirect phlebography by arterial injection with follow-through. The contrast image can

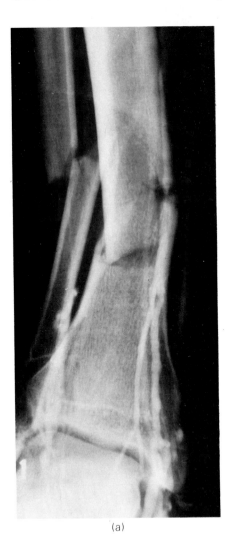

(a)

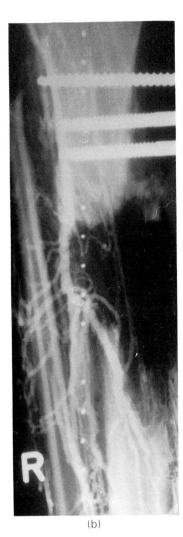

(b)

Fig. 4.46 (a) An ascending phlebogram in a patient with a fracture of the tibia and fibula. The posterior tibial vein is narrowed at the fracture site but there is no evidence of extravasation of the contrast medium. Single film phlebograms can be obtained with portable X-ray equipment in the casualty department.

(b) In this calf phlebogram there is a major bone defect in the tibia caused by a severe penetrating injury. The posterior tibial veins are totally disrupted but the venous return via the other stem veins is not affected.

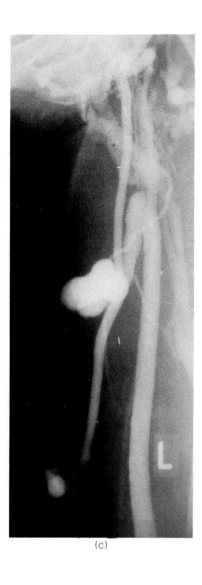

(c)

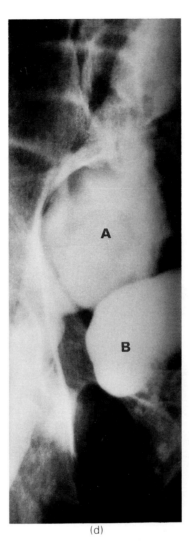

(d)

Fig. 4.46 (c) Following emergency treatment of trauma the late sequelae of both the trauma itself and the emergency therapy often need to be assessed phlebographically. In this example the common femoral vein has been ligated and a false aneurysm of the long saphenous vein has developed as a result of the initial injury, a penetrating wound of the left thigh.

(d) A right iliac phlebogram showing a large false aneurysm of the external iliac vein (A) following a fracture of the pelvis. The patient's bladder (B) is opacified below the aneurysm.

be enhanced by photographic or computerized digital subtraction (Fig. 4.47b).

Most venous abnormalities in the upper limb occur in the axillary, subclavian and innominate veins and the superior vena cava. The simplest way of demonstrating these large proximal veins is by injecting 50 ml of contrast medium through a large bore (16 FG) plastic cannula threaded into a vein in the anti-cubital fossa; injection by hand is usually sufficient. Tourniquets are not required; both the superficial and deep veins fill simultaneously (see Chapter 2, Fig. 2.32). Bilateral injections are required to show the superior vena cava (see Chapter 2, Fig. 2.33).

Ideally, the injections should be made into the basilic vein, as an injection into the cephalic vein bypasses the brachial vein, and an axillary vein lesion may be missed. If the basilic vein is not available, the cephalic vein may be injected provided a tourniquet is placed above the injection site to direct the contrast medium into the deep veins of the upper arm (Fig. 4.47c). The arm should be examined in the anatomical position (at the side) and in extreme abduction otherwise obstruction caused by position will be misinterpreted (Fig. 4.47d and e).

As with ilio-femoral phlebography, venous pressure can be measured by connecting a mano-

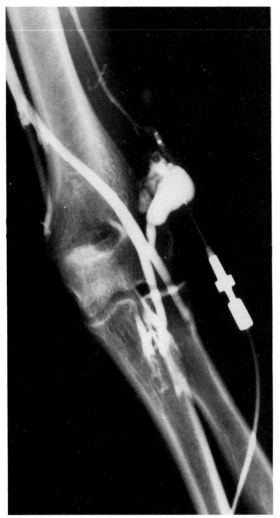

Fig. 4.47 (a) A phlebogram obtained by direct injection of contrast medium into a cavernous venous malformation which drains mainly into the median cubital vein.

meter to the intravenous cannula. After a baseline measurement the hand is exercised for 2 minutes. In a normal subject there is no rise in pressure; the pressure will increase, however, if there is significant outflow obstruction.[81]

When a suitable vein cannot be identified in the anti-cubital fossa, because of either oedema or obesity, 50 ml of contrast medium can be injected through a 21 G needle into a vein on the hand or wrist with a firm tourniquet applied above the elbow. When the tourniquet is released, the fore-

arm muscles compressed, and the arm elevated, a bolus of contrast medium opacifies the large central veins (Fig. 4.47d).

Alternatively, an intraosseous injection into the olecranon process or the greater tuberosity of the humerus can be used. Whatever method of phlebography of the upper limb is employed only a short rapid series of films and a few delayed films are necessary because, in the absence of obstruction, the venous flow is very rapid. Obtaining films with properly filled arm veins can be difficult and artefacts due to streaming are common. Catheterization techniques are advocated by some workers, both for proximal arm vein and superior vena cava visualization, but we feel that they should be avoided as far as possible because of the risk of damage to, or rupture of, the vein wall (see Chapter 25). If catheters are used, they should be introduced through the basilic vein, positioned with fluoroscopy, and tested with small injections of contrast medium before the main injection. If an obstruction is encountered, the catheter should be withdrawn for a few centimeters to minimize the risk of rupturing the vein. The cephalic vein joins the axillary vein almost at a right angle, and it is often impossible to negotiate this angle with a guide wire or catheter without damaging the vein; the cephalic vein is therefore less suitable for catheterization techniques.

Azygos, ascending lumbar and vertebral phlebography

Several techniques for opacifying these veins have been described. A needle or catheter may be introduced into either femoral vein, and contrast medium may be injected while the inferior vena cava is externally compressed. Other methods include direct catheterization of one or both ascending lumbar veins or retrograde catheterization of the azygos or hemi-azygos veins from the superior vena cava (see Chapter 2, Fig. 2.35).[2] Intraosseous phlebography by injecting a spinous process of a vertebral body in the lumbar region or the posterior end of a rib in the thoracic region will also demonstrate the azygos and vertebral venous systems (Fig. 4.48).[72]

There are very few indications for separate azygos, ascending lumbar or vertebral phlebography; most information is obtainable from inferior or superior vena cavography. The veins

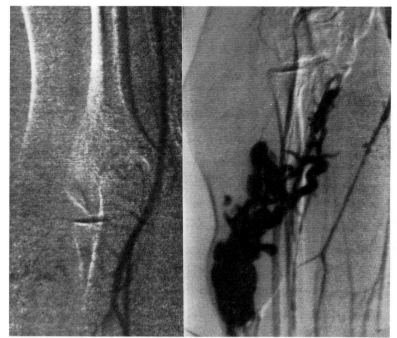

Fig. 4.47 (b) An intra-venous digital angiogram with follow through from the arterial phase (left-hand panel) to the venous phase (right-hand panel). The brachial artery is of normal size and the extensive venous malformation can be seen below the elbow in the left-hand panel. IV-DSA (intravenous digital subtraction angiography) is virtually non-invasive and can give useful information about the arterial supply and venous drainage of venous malformations. The image is degraded but is often sufficient for clinical management.

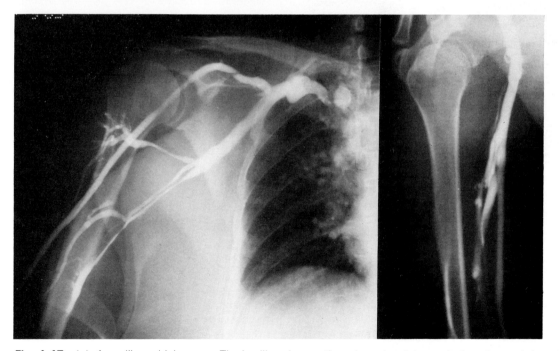

Fig. 4.47 (c) An axillary phlebogram. The basilic vein was thrombosed and the cephalic vein was injected with contrast medium. A tourniquet has been applied in the lower forearm above the injection site to direct the contrast medium into the deep veins; if this is not done, the cephalic vein bypasses the axillary vein and lesions may be missed. The apparent narrowing of the axillary vein in the region of the axillary fold is an artefact caused by the position of the arm.

The narrowing is not present when the arm is abducted (right-hand panel).

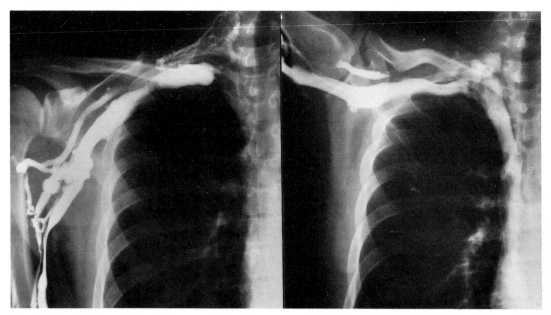

Fig. 4.47   (d) An axillary phlebogram. There is a very severe obstruction of the right innominate vein. When the arm is abducted (right-hand panel) the obstruction is shown to be less severe. It is important to carry out axillary phlebography in both adduction and abduction, otherwise a lesion may be missed.

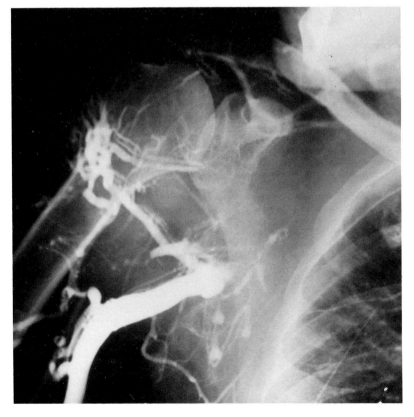

Fig. 4.47   (e) An axillary phlebogram showing total occlusion of the axillary vein, the so-called 'effort thrombosis'.

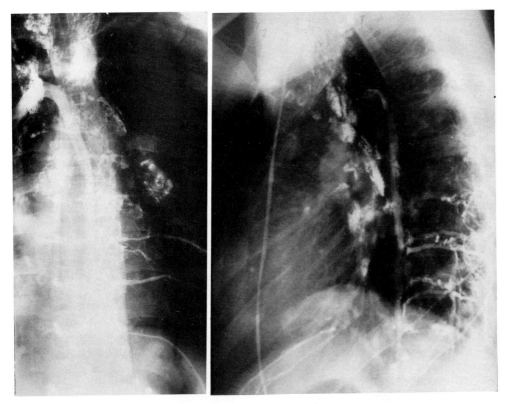

Fig. 4.48 A normal azygos vein shown by an intraosseous vertebral spinous process injection. This investigation is not often required. An alternative approach is selective catheterization of the azygos vein itself. In this example the patient has had a previous lymphangiogram.

may be displaced or invaded by mediastinal or thoracic masses, metastases, disc protrusions and para-spinal lymphadenopathy. In many of these situations computerized tomography, magnetic resonance imaging and myelography are easier to carry out and more useful in diagnosis and management. Unexplained cyanotic congenital heart disease can be caused by abnormalities of venous drainage which may be demonstrated by azygos phlebography.

Complications of phlebography

Systemic and idiosyncratic reactions

These reactions are not specific to phlebography but are caused by the contrast medium. Minor reactions such as nausea, vomiting, a feeling of heat and mild urticaria occur in 5 per cent of patients receiving conventional high osmolar contrast media. These reactions usually require no treatment and pass off rapidly. Severe reactions such as bronchospasm and glottic oedema may require treatment with oral antihistamines or intravenous hydrocortisone. Loss of consciousness, cardiac arrhythmias, cardiac arrest, pulmonary oedema, and myocardial infarction require immediate intensive therapy to prevent death. Severe reactions are unpredictable and inconstant. The response to a test injection is unreliable and such an injection is no longer used. Appropriate drugs and ventilators must be immediately available in a phlebography suite. There is evidence to suggest that idiosyncratic reactions are far less common with the low osmolar agents. The mortality of 1 in 40 000 injections[205] with conventional media is probably 1 in 250 000 or lower with low osmolality media. Patients with a history of severe allergy or with a history of a reaction to contrast medium should always receive non-ionic contrast media and, if there is no urgency, a course of hydrocortisone should be given 24–48 hours in advance.

Air embolism

This is a theoretical complication of phlebography but should not occur if all the connecting tubing and syringes are kept free of air and filled with either normal saline or contrast medium throughout the examination. If air embolus does occur, the injection should be immediately stopped and the patient turned onto the left side and tipped into a 20° head-down position so that air in the right ventricle floats away from the pulmonary outflow tract.

Pulmonary embolism

There have been very few reports of pulmonary embolism occurring before or during phlebography, even when recent thrombus has been demonstrated.[198] The use of calf compression to produce a bolus of contrast medium and the routine use of the Valsalva manoeuvre, both of which form part of our standard technique for ascending phlebography, can be criticized as being likely to dislodge thrombus; they should therefore probably not be employed if very loose thrombus is present. This theoretical risk should, however, be balanced against the advantage of showing all the deep veins of the leg, from the calf to the inferior vena cava, from foot injections alone. Manipulation of guide wires and catheters for selective phlebography of the branches of the superior and inferior vena cavae may dislodge an existing thrombus and new thrombus may form in and around catheters and then break free. Continuous flushing of the catheter with heparinized saline is advisable but emboli arising from catheter systems are likely to be small and not of clinical significance.

Cardiac arrhythmias

Manipulation of catheters in the right side of the heart is not part of phlebographic techniques but when catheterizing the superior vena cava or proximal end of the inferior vena cava, the catheter may inadvertently pass into the right ventricle and precipitate changes of cardiac rhythm. These

arrhythmias are short lived, provided the catheter is quickly withdrawn. Hyperosmolar contrast agents injected intravenously can cause arrhythmias but in the absence of pulmonary hypertension these are not usually significant.

Pulmonary hypertension

Phlebography is often requested for patients with pulmonary hypertension because the hypertension may be caused by massive or repeated pulmonary emboli. These patients are liable to develop cardiac arrhythmias and cardiac arrest which may be impossible to reverse. These complications are most likely to occur when the contrast medium is injected as a bolus but the risk is present which ever way it is injected. The pulmonary artery pressure should be monitored continuously throughout the examination, and appropriate drugs and support equipment must be available.

Rhythm disturbances following injections in the right side of the heart are caused by a sudden increase in pulmonary artery pressure – the patient dies of acute cor pulmonale. This is thought to be caused by hyperosmolar contrast agents producing red cell crenation which obstructs blood flow through the lungs and reduces systemic arterial pressure and coronary artery blood flow. This hypotensive complication is minimized by the intravenous administration of phenylephrine which constricts the arterioles and the infusion of plasma or plasma substitutes to help maintain the cardiac output. Even when these measures are used, phlebography in patients with pulmonary hypertension carries a significant morbidity. It has been demonstrated that low osmolality media cause a much less marked increase in pulmonary artery pressure,[8] and these media should therefore always be used for phlebography in patients with known or suspected pulmonary hypertension.

Local complications

Mild pain is the most common side-effect of phlebography of the leg or arm and is probably a direct effect of the contrast medium on the vein wall. It has been reported that mild pain occurs in 65 per cent of patients undergoing phlebography with conventional agents.[111] The pain appears to be related to the hyperosmolality of contrast media. Low osmolality media cause virtually no pain on injection.[106] Contrast agents cause an inflammatory reaction of the vein wall with venous thrombosis.[5] Post-phlebographic thrombophlebitis is said to occur in approximately one-third of all examinations carried out with hyperosmolar contrast media.[6] This incidence is, however, based on the ^{125}I fibrinogen uptake test which is very sensitive to endothelial damage and is non-specific; the clinical significance of these findings is therefore not clear. Nevertheless, it is certain that low osmolality contrast media are virtually non-thrombogenic[106,195] and are therefore the substances of choice for all phlebography. Whatever contrast medium is used every effort must be made to prevent thrombosis by clearing the contrast from the veins by injecting physiological saline and encouraging active movements at the end of the examination. Anticoagulation with heparin before, during and after

phlebography is not recommended routinely but should be used in patients with a high thrombotic tendency (e.g. patients with carcinomatosis and idiopathic recurrent thrombosis).

Extravasation of high osmolality media into the skin and soft tissues causes a chemical cellulitis which may progress to ulceration, soft tissue necrosis and even gangrene (Fig. 4.49).[120,178] Low osmolality contrast media do not cause pain when injected inadvertently into the soft tissues, and it is believed that they are much less likely to cause tissue necrosis because their osmolality is similar to that of tissue fluid. Nevertheless, great care should be taken with all contrast media to avoid extravasation. During the injection, the site of injection should be watched with the image intensifier. If extravasation occurs, the injection should be stopped and an attempt should be made to disperse the extravasated medium. This is best achieved by local massage, a wet warm towel, and

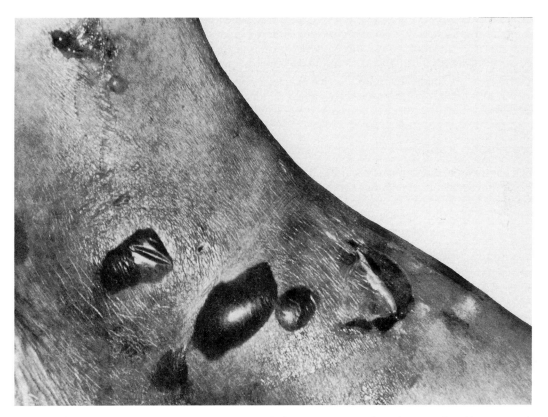

Fig. 4.49 Superficial skin necrosis and blistering following extravasation of conventional hyperosmolar contrast medium into the tissues. Although extravasation should be prevented, it seems likely that serious consequences such as this will not occur with low osmolality media because their osmolality approximates to that of tissue fluid.

perhaps dilution of the contrast medium in the tissues by injecting physiological saline. Hyaluronidase has been advocated, but the combination of this drug and contrast medium may increase the risk of tissue damage.[132]

Arteriovenous fistulae and *vein wall dissection* occur but are not common. Arteriovenous fistulae occur when a nearby artery is punctured as well as the vein, particularly at the groin or elbow. Vein wall dissection by guide wires and catheters is caused by faulty technique.

A number of complications are specific to intraosseous phlebography; they include accidental puncture of adjacent structures (e.g. aorta, spinal cord or pelvic viscera) and infection leading to osteomyelitis which is particularly likely to occur if the injection is made close to an ulcer. All intraosseous injections should be carried out under strict aseptic conditions. Fat embolism has been reported and should be suspected if the patient develops neurological symptoms a few hours after the procedure.[118]

It should be emphasized that the more serious complications of phlebography have been reported when using high osmolar conventional contrast media. Phlebography with low osmolar agents can be regarded as a very safe investigation.

Isotope phlebography

Although contrast phlebography is accurate, it is invasive, at times uncomfortable, has some complications (most of which can be avoided by using low osmolality contrast agents) and involves unavoidable radiation exposure; it is therefore not an ideal screening test.

Isotope phlebography outlines the pathways followed by technetium-99m (^{99m}Tc)-labelled microspheres which are injected into a peripheral foot vein or other vein.[62] This method detects abnormalities in venous flow in the major venous trunks but is much less reliable in the smaller veins (e.g. those in the calf). Furthermore, it is not specific for thrombosis, as similar changes in the venous blood flow may be caused by cardiac failure, extensive leg oedema, local soft tissue masses and reduced arterial inflow into the extremity. A negative test excludes deep vein thrombosis in the large proximal veins with an accuracy of approximately 90 per cent. False-negative results are explained by the occasional failure of even a large

thrombi to cause detectable obstruction.[168]

Technique A needle is inserted into a vein on the dorsum of each foot and tourniquets are applied above the ankles and knees to occlude the superficial veins. A bolus of 0.5 mCi ^{99m}Tc-labelled human albumin miscrospheres is injected simultaneously into each foot. The gamma scintillation camera image of both legs is recorded on polaroid photographs. The patient is positioned so that the veins from the abdomen to the foot are visualized. Adherent thrombus will cause segments of low radioactivity. The tourniquets are then released and the patient is asked to exercise by flexing the ankles. Further images are then photographed. Thrombus appears as a persistent area of radioactivity because by this time the isotope has diffused into and become trapped in the thrombus (Fig. 4.50a and b). The procedure is relatively safe but care should be taken when carrying out the technique in patients with reduced lung function in the same way that care is taken when perfusion lung scans are performed on these patients. The radiation of the examination is negligible. An advantage of using albumin macro-aggregates is that a lung scan can be obtained at the same time as the phlebogram. The ability to screen the limb for thrombus and obtain a lung scan from a single injection has obvious advantages.[62,121]

Computerized tomography

Computerized tomography (CT) has a limited role to play in the management of venous disease because transverse sections do not lend themselves to visualization of the largely longitudinal peripheral venous system. CT should not therefore be the primary investigation of a suspected abnormality of the venous system. In localized lesions such as venous tumours, tumours adjacent to veins, and venous malformations, enhanced computerized tomograms may help to show the extent of the lesion and indicate whether it is circumscribed, encapsulated or involves adjacent tissues (Fig. 4.51a and b) (see Chapters 23, 26). Primary vena caval thrombosis can also be shown (Fig. 4.51c) and can be confirmed by inferior vena cavography. To distinguish the vena cava from surrounding structures cuts should be taken before and after the injection of contrast medium to detect any enhancement. To show the superior vena cava, 100–150 ml contrast medium are infused through an arm vein; to show the inferior

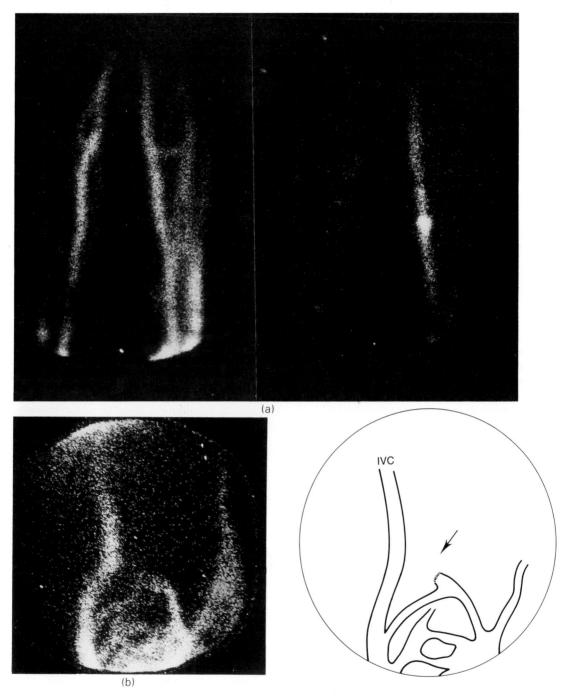

Fig. 4.50 (a) An isotope phlebogram. The left-hand panel shows the static phase and the right-hand panel shows the appearances after exercise. The accumulation of radioactivity in the calf in the right-hand panel remaining after exercise, indicates that this is likely to represent a thrombus rather than stasis below an obstruction.   (b) An isotope phlebogram of the pelvis and abdomen. The injection was made into the left foot only. There is an obstruction at the junction of the left common iliac vein with the inferior vena cava (arrowed). There are extensive pelvic collaterals filling the right iliac veins and inferior vena cava. This was an example of left common iliac vein obstruction caused by compression by the overlying artery (see Chapter 9).

vena cava a similar volume is infused through a foot vein. Additional bolus injections of 50–100 ml of contrast medium may be required in some examinations.

Anatomically the superior vena cava lies just to the right of the ascending aorta and just in front of the right main bronchus. It can thus be involved in diseases of the mediastinum, whether neoplastic or inflammatory, and particularly in carcinoma of the bronchus, with or without, enlarged lymph glands. The inferior vena cava is a long structure and has a variety of anatomical relations throughout its length. In its more proximal part it lies just behind the caudate lobe and the right lobe of the liver. Lower down it lies just antero-medial to the right kidney in front of its vascular pedicle. Identification of the inferior vena cava at these sites is important because lesions in the porta hepatis affect the former, and tumour thrombus extending from a renal carcinoma into a renal vein often grows along the wall of the inferior vena cava – this alters the surgical approach and prognosis.

Tumours arising from the kidney, or adjacent organs, will deform or invade the inferior vena cava (Fig. 4.51d). Collaterals around an iliac vein or inferior vena caval obstruction can also be seen on enhanced computerized tomography but are better demonstrated by angiographic techniques.

Magnetic resonance imaging

The role of magnetic resonance imaging in the diagnosis of venous diseases is uncertain. As it has highly sensitive densitometry characteristics, it will probably prove valuable in discriminating venous abnormalities from those in surrounding tissues. It may also enable measurement of venous blood flow, even in very small veins.

Lung scanning

Radioisotopic ventilation and perfusion lung imaging is a highly sensitive method of detecting pulmonary emboli and has become a routine procedure in the diagnosis of pulmonary embolism.[13,29,189,194]

Technique Usually, the ventilation study is followed immediately by a perfusion lung scan. Ventilation (V) studies are obtained in the posterior projection with the patient sitting up. An 'equilibrium' phase is obtained during the end of the wash-in phase while the patient re-breathes 10–20 mCi of xenon-133 (^{133}Xe). Sequential posterior washout images are obtained over 1 min intervals until the ^{133}Xe has cleared from the lungs or until 7–10 min have elapsed. More recently, labelled aerosols have been introduced in place of gases. For the perfusion scan (Q) approximately 2 mCi of technetium-99m (^{99m}Tc) labelled macro-aggregated albumin is injected intravenously. Images are obtained in anterior, posterior, both lateral and both posterior oblique positions.[155]

The V and Q images are reviewed together with a current chest radiograph. Images of ventilation are considered normal if the lungs exhibit uniform ^{133}Xe distribution and if all lung zones are cleared

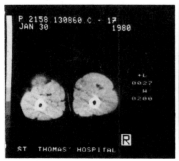 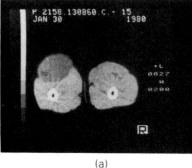 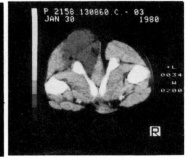

(a)

Fig. 4.51 Computerized tomography.
(a) A computerized tomogram of a mass in the anterior part of the left upper thigh extending into the pelvis. The mass is vascular because it uniformly enhances following injection of contrast media. It is circumscribed and not invading the tissues of the upper thigh.

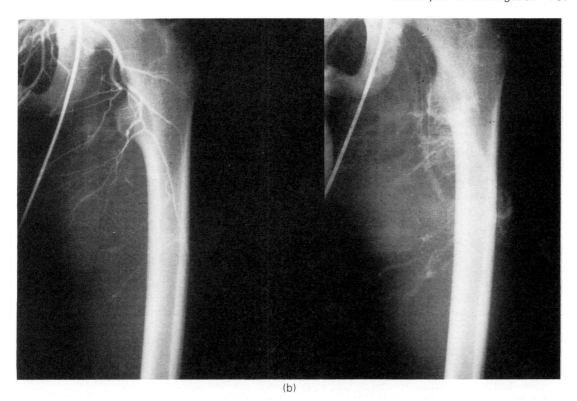

(b)

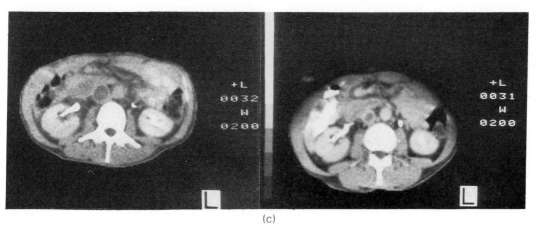

(c)

Fig. 4.51 (b) This indirect phlebogram, obtained by an injection of the femoral artery with follow-through, shows arteries of normal size and no evidence of early venous filling (left-hand panel) indicating that this abnormality is not an arteriovenous malformation. The late phase (right-hand panel) shows that it is a solely venous tumour.

(c) A computerized tomogram of the abdomen with contrast infusion. Films have been taken at 20 mm intervals and show extensive recent thrombosis obstructing the inferior vena cava (left-hand panel). A repeat examination 10 weeks later (right-hand panel) shows contraction of the thrombus. This is an example of idiopathic inferior vena cava thrombotic occlusion.

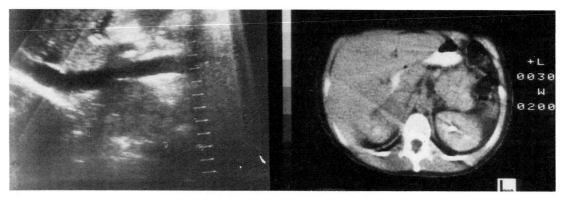

Fig. 4.51 (d) Ultrasound and tomography.
The left-hand panel is a sonogram of a longitudinal section through the inferior vena cava. It shows that the proximal end of the inferior vena cava is deformed by a mass which is posterior to it. A computerized tomogram (right-hand panel) confirms the presence of a mass in relation to the inferior vena cava which lies anterior to the upper pole of the right kidney. This was a phaeochromocytoma.

of the radionuclide in 3 minutes on washout images. Zones showing delayed washout indicate areas of obstructive pulmonary disease.

Perfusion scintigrams are evaluated for defects. When a perfusion defect is present, a comparison is made with the ventilation study to see if there is normal ventilation in the non-perfused region (V–Q mismatch) or abnormal ventilation in the same region (V–Q match) (Fig. 4.52a and b).[13] A perfusion defect is not specific for pulmonary embolus; other pulmonary diseases can cause perfusion abnormalities. The addition of ventilation images and the comparison between perfusion and ventilation abnormalities makes the diagnosis more specific.[7]

The probability of pulmonary embolism is high if there are multiple areas of mismatch.[13] A single large V–Q mismatch is suggestive of a pulmonary embolus but a direct pulmonary angiogram or digital subtraction pulmonary angiogram may be required to confirm the diagnosis. Small, matching ventilation perfusion defects are rarely due to pulmonary embolism and likely to be related to lung disease.

Pulmonary angiography

Pulmonary angiography is an invasive and potentially hazardous examination and should only be carried out by investigators who are familiar with cardio-pulmonary angiography and its potential complications. Equipment and drugs for cardio-

pulmonary resuscitation and an external cardiac defibrillator capable of synchronized cardioversion should be available. An intravenous line should be in place before the start of the procedure to facilitate blood sampling for blood gas analysis and for the intravenous administration of drugs.

Electrocardiographic and blood pressure monitoring is essential during pulmonary angiography. Patients with pulmonary hypertension are at greater risk during this procedure than during phlebography.

Two approaches to the pulmonary artery are used. A 'cut down' on to an arm vein and passage of a catheter, or a percutaneous entry into the femoral vein. The former is preferred because it eliminates the possibility of dislodgement of thrombus from the pelvic veins and inferior vena cava and can be used for retrograde phlebography. The non-selective techniques of pulmonary angiography have been superceded by digitial subtraction angiography.

Technique A 7 or 8 FG block-ended angiocatheter is passed from a cut down on the basilic vein, through the right atrium, right ventricle and across the pulmonary valve into the main pulmonary artery under television monitoring. The catheter is positioned with its tip in the main pulmonary artery, midway between the pulmonary valve and the bifurcation of the main pulmonary artery, and its position is checked by a test injection. A control film is taken for radiographic exposure, the film being slightly more penetrated than for a conventional chest radiograph. Fifty to sixty millilitres of Iohexol 350 are injected at 30 ml/s and serial films taken at 2–3/s for 4 s with a slower rate for a further 6 s. Antero-posterior radiographs alone are exposed, as in the lateral projections the two lungs are superimposed. During exposure of the films the patient holds his breath in deep inspiration because an inflated lung produces better detail of the pulmonary vasculature.[123] If a definite diagnosis is not made from a main pulmonary artery injection, selective right and left angiograms or selective injections of

doubtful areas are carried out with magnification radiography if available.

Interpretation of angiograms In a normal pulmonary arteriogram the arteries follow the distribution of the corresponding bronchi. The arteries are smooth and divide and taper as they approach the periphery of the lung fields. The veins follow the same anatomical pattern as the arteries (Fig. 4.53a). A definitive diagnosis of pulmonary embolism can be made if there are persistent intra-luminal filling defects in the arteries outlined by contrast medium (Fig. 4.53b–d). Contrast cut-off is also suggestive of pulmonary

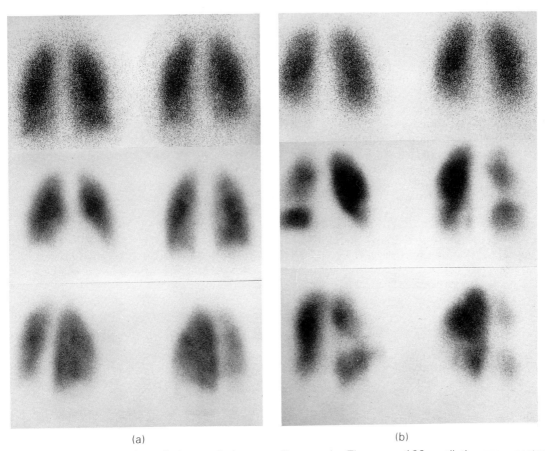

(a)   (b)

Fig. 4.52 (a) A normal ventilation–perfusion scan. Top panel – The xenon-133 ventilation scan, posterior view. Middle panel – The [99mTc] MAA perfusion scan, anterior and posterior views. Bottom panel – The [99mTc] MAA perfusion scan, right posterior and left anterior oblique views.

(b) Pulmonary embolism. There are segmental ventilation–perfusion mismatches in right upper and mid zones and in the left lower zone. Top panel – The xenon-133 ventilation scan, posterior view. Middle panel – The [99mTc] MAA perfusion scan, anterior and posterior views. Bottom panel – The [99mTc] MAA perfusion scan, right posterior and left posterior oblique views.

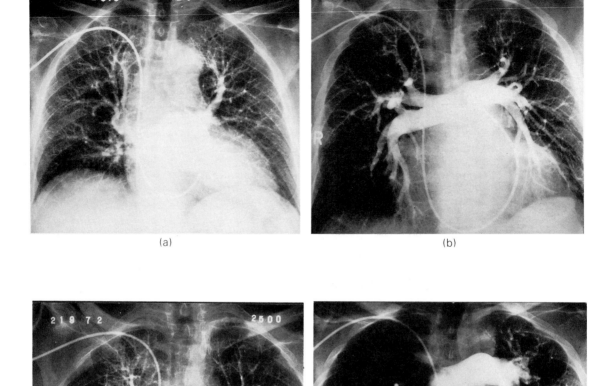

(a)   (b)

(c)   (d)

Fig. 4.53   (a) A normal pulmonary arteriogram. The branches of the main pulmonary arteries follow the distribution of the corresponding bronchi. The branches become narrower and divide as they approach the periphery.

(b) In this pulmonary angiogram there are undervascularized segments in the right upper zone and at the left base; attenuation and occlusion of the arteries are particularly noticeable at the right base. The left lung field appears normal.

(c) There are adherent emboli in both main pulmonary arteries and their proximal branches with marked oligaemia particularly in the right, mid, and lower zones with an occluded lower lobe artery. Similar, but less marked, changes are present on the left.

(d) There is a very large embolus almost completely occluding the right main pulmonary artery. There are less severe changes affecting the branches of the left pulmonary artery.

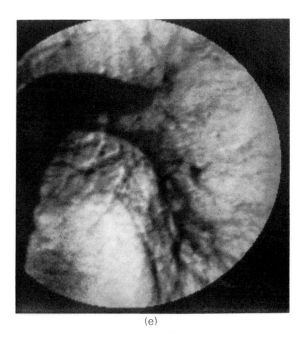

(e)

Fig. 4.53 (e) An intravenous digital subtraction pulmonary angiogram (IV-DSA). There is a large embolus in the left main pulmonary artery and smaller ones occluding the peripheral branches. IV-DSA is much less invasive than conventional pulmonary angiography. The image is degraded compared with screen film angiograms but is often sufficient for planning therapy. It carries the same risk as pulmonary angiography and phlebography in patients with severe pulmonary hypertension.

embolism but occlusion of small branches of the pulmonary artery is seen in other pulmonary diseases. Secondary features which are suggestive, but not diagnostic, of pulmonary embolism include: non-filling of the arteries, vascular pruning and tortuosity, decreased vascularity, asymetric and slow perfusion, and delayed venous return from affected segments. In these circumstances comparison with the chest radiograph and isotope lung scan may be required to reach a correct diagnosis (see Chapter 20).

Digital subtraction pulmonary angiography

Digital subtraction pulmonary angiography is increasingly used as a substitute for direct pulmonary angiography, though the poor images make it a less satisfactory diagnostic tool for pulmonary emboli. Its attraction is that less contrast medium is injected directly into the pulmonary vasculature and, if a bolus peripheral venous injection is used, it is less invasive and dangerous than cardiac catheterization angiography. Its major disadvantage is the loss of the measurement of pulmonary artery pressure before the contrast medium is injected, especially in patients with pulmonary hypertension.[136] The same precautions

should be taken as for conventional pulmonary angiography and phlebography. Low osmolality contrast media should always be used.

We use bolus injections of 50 ml of iopamidol 370 injected at 20 ml/s through a 16 FG catheter threaded into an anti-cubital vein. Both lungs can be included on a large field 14 inch intensifier, but with smaller intensifiers each lung is examined separately in anterior and oblique projections with separate injections for each view. Interpretation is the same as for pulmonary angiography but is more difficult because of overlap of the peripheral vessels. (Fig. 4.53e).

Comment

Although radionuclide lung scans have made a significant contribution to the understanding and treatment of pulmonary embolism, they frequently do not provide the diagnostic specificity which is necessary for therapeutic decisions. A normal V–Q scan is good, but not conclusive evidence, that the patient has not had a pulmonary embolus. An equivocal scan is often an indication for pulmonary angiography. Pulmonary angiography is indicated before using thrombolytic agents, interruption of the inferior vena cava, and before pulmonary embolectomy. In emergency situations, however, pulmonary embolectomy may have to be performed without confirmatory evidence.[138]

Although pulmonary angiography is the most definitive method of diagnosis, we find that ventilation perfusion scan plus lower limb phlebography is sufficient to establish a diagnosis of thromboembolism in 95 per cent of cases.

Commentary

The precise value of the tests described in this chapter are discussed in later chapters when distinct conditions are being described. In the following paragraphs we have drawn together our views of the value of these tests in the clinical context of venous thrombosis and chronic venous insufficiency.

Clinical application of the tests for deep vein thrombosis

The clinician needs answers to the following questions.

1. Does the patient have a venous thrombosis?
2. Where is the thrombus?
3. How big is it?
4. Is it fresh or old (i.e. is it likely to fragment or is it stable)?
5. Is it adherent to the vein wall or firmly fixed? (i.e. is it able to float away if it fragments?)

The majority of the tests described in this chapter answer the first and second questions, in part, but do not answer the other three.

Does the patient have a venous thrombosis?

Physical signs are notoriously unreliable – the absence of signs is more unreliable than the presence of positive signs. The clinician cannot, however, afford to ignore anything that suggests the possibility of a thrombus, and therefore even though it is known that 50 per cent of the patients with a tender calf do not have a thrombosis they must be investigated further.

Thermography, ultrasound flow detection, phleborheography, impedance plethysmography, phlebography and the fibrinogen uptake test can all be used.

The simple bed-side techniques of ultrasound flow detection, phleborheography and impedance plethysmography have serious limitations. Although they are good at detecting occlusive thrombi in major veins, they can miss non-occlusive thrombi in large veins and often miss small calf vein thrombi. It is not unreasonable to argue that it is the adherent thrombi in the large veins that cause serious debilitating post-thrombotic sequelae; it is, however, the non-adherent thrombi which are potentially lethal emboli, and even small calf vein thrombi can cause serious calf pump damage.

These techniques are therefore useful screening tests if the clinician performing them is aware of their deficiencies and provided they are repeated daily so that any missed calf vein thrombus that extends into the popliteal vein will be detected.

The clinician who wishes to detect thrombus in the calf veins must use the fibrinogen uptake test or phlebography. Those clinicians who wish to detect large vein non-adherent thrombi must use phlebography.

Where is the thrombus?

A test which does not provide an image cannot define the precise limits of a thrombus.

Most of the non-invasive methods can distinguish between popliteal vein and ilio-femoral vein occlusion but none reveals the exact anatomical position of the thrombus, or the presence of thrombus in other parallel veins.

Phlebography or venous imaging must be used to discover the exact site of the thrombus.

What is the nature of the thrombus?

The non-invasive methods do not reveal the size, nature, age or degree of adherence of a thrombus. Phlebography and ultrasound imaging will give some answers to these questions.

Comment

It is our considered view that the only method currently available in all hospitals that gives the maximum information about deep vein thrombosis is phlebography.

It would be impractical to X-ray every patient with minor leg or chest symptoms suggestive of thromboembolism. Screening methods must therefore be used. The simplest and most inexpensive method is the pocket Doppler flow detector but impedance plethysmography and phleborheography are more accurate. A patient who has only calf symptoms and a normal screening test can be monitored by repeated examinations. A positive test should be followed by a phlebogram.

If a patient has symptoms suggestive of pulmonary embolism, we believe phlebography is essential. No other investigation, except perhaps in the future ultrasound imaging, gives the information about the site and nature of a thrombus which is necessary to determine the appropriate treatment. Recurrent pulmonary embolism may be fatal. It must be treated urgently on the basis of the best information available – this means phlebography.

Clinical application of the tests of chronic venous insufficiency

The clinician needs the answers to the following questions about a patient's chronic venous insufficiency, a condition which he is usually able to suspect following clinical examination.

1. Is there chronic venous insufficiency?
2. Are the superficial veins incompetent?
3. Where are the incompetent superficial-to-deep vein connections?
4. Are the deep veins incompetent?
5. Are the deep veins occluded and obstructing blood flow?

Is there chronic venous insufficiency?

Any of the tests of overall calf pump function will answer this question – photoplethysmography, strain-gauge and isotope plethysmography, foot volumetry and foot vein pressures. In all patients with chronic venous insufficiency the fall of foot vein volume or pressure that should accompany exercise is reduced.

Although direct pressure measurement is the gold standard, photoplethysmography is the simplest qualitative method and foot volumetry is the simplest quantitative method.

Superficial veins

All the tests of leg vein blood volume or pressure can be used to test superficial vein valve incompetence by performing the test with and without superficial vein occluding tourniquets. The precise site of an incompetent communicating vein must be deduced by combining the information given by the non-invasive tests about the level of the abnormality and a knowledge of the known anatomical sites of communication.

Doppler flow detection may also be used to show incompetence of the superficial veins.

The anatomical display of superficial vein incompetence by seeing retrograde blood flow at phlebography is very accurate but not much better than the non-invasive technique. The visualization of retrograde blood flow in incompetent communicating veins at phlebography is a more accurate method of detection than the non-invasive techniques.

Isotope plethysmography can quantify this abnormality but this is rarely necessary in normal clinical practice.

Deep vein incompetence

All types of plethysmography can be used to detect deep vein incompetence from measurements of refilling times with and without superficial vein occlusion. Doppler flow studies of the femoral and popliteal veins are also helpful but the best demonstration of the full extent of deep vein reflux is obtained from a descending phlebogram.

Deep vein obstruction

This can only be shown by a physiological test. The presence of occluded veins on a phlebogram does not mean that the outflow from the leg is reduced; the collateral vessels may be more than adequate.

The physiological tests which reveal obstruction are the maximum venous outflow test (carried out by strain-gauge plethysmography), measurement of femoral vein pressures during exercise and foot volumetry during exercise. Femoral vein pressure studies give the best indication of iliac vein obstruction. Unfortunately, none of the other tests is able to detect mild or moderate degrees of obstruction below the groin.

In most patients the function of the calf veins can be assessed with one simple non-invasive test of calf pump function such as photoplethysmography or foot volumetry, backed up by careful clinical examination and, in selected patients, ascending and/or descending phlebography.

References

1. Abramowitz HB, Queral LA, Flinn WR, Nora PF, Peterson LK, Bergan JJ, Yao JST. The use of photoplethysmography in the assessment of venous insufficiency: A comparison to venous measurements. *Surgery* 1979; **86**: 434.

2. Abrams HL. The vertebral and azygos veins. In *Abrams' Angiography* 3rd edition. Boston. Little Brown. 1983.

3. Ackroyd JS, Lea Thomas M, Browse NL. Deep vein reflux: An assessment by descending phlebography. *Br J Surg* 1986; **73**: 31.

4. Adolfsson L, Nordenfelt I, Olsson H, Torstensson I. Diagnosis of deep vein thrombosis with ^{99m}Tc plasmin. *Acta Med Scand* 1982; **211**: 365.

5. Albrechtsson U, Olsson CG. Thrombosis after phlebography: A comparison of two contrast media. *Cardiovasc Radiol* 1979; **2**: 9.

6. Albrechtsson U, Olsson CG. Thrombotic side effects of lower limb phlebography. *Lancet* 1976; **1**: 723.

7. Alderson PO, Ruganavech N, Secker-Walker RH, McKnight RC. The role of ^{133}Xe ventilation studies in the scintigraphic detection of pulmonary embolism. *Radiology* 1976; **120**: 633.

8. Almen T, Aspelin P, Levin B. Effect of non-ionic contrast media on aortic and pulmonary arterial pressure. *Invest Radiol* 1975; **10**: 519.

9. Almen T, Nylander L. False signs of thrombosis in lower leg phlebography. *Acta Radiol* 1964; **2**: 345.

10. Almen, T, Nylander L. Serial phlebography of the normal lower limb during muscular contraction and relaxation. *Acta Radiol* 1962; **57**: 264.

11. Almen T. Contrast agent designs: Some aspects of the synthesis of water soluble contrast agents of low osmolality. *J Theor Biol* 1969; **24**: 216.

12. Anderson FA. Non-invasive quantification of the degree of venous outflow obstruction in the extremities by means of venous occlusion plethysmography. In Batel DL (Ed) *Advances in Bioengineering*. New York. American Society of Mechanical Engineers. 1983.

13. Anderson FA Jr, Li JM, Wheeler HB. Application of impedance plethysmography to the detection of venous insufficiency. *Bruit* 1983; **7**: 41.

14. Arnoldi CC. Venous pressure in patients with valvular incompetence of the veins of the lower limb. *Acta Chir Scand* 1966; **132**: 628.

15. Atkins P, Hawkins LA. Detection of venous thrombosis in the legs. *Lancet* 1965; **2**: 1217.

16. Barner HB, DeWeese JA. An evaluation of the sphygmomanometer cuff pain test in venous thrombosis. *Surgery* 1960; **48**: 915.

17. Barnes RW, Collicot RE, Hummell BA, Slaymaker EE, Maixner W, Reinertson JE. Photoplethysmographic assessment of altered cutaneous circulation in the post-phlebitic syndrome. *Proc Assoc Adv Med Instrum* 1978; **13**: 25.

18. Barnes RW, Collicott PE, Mozersky DJ, Sumner DS, Strandness DE Jr. Noninvasive quantitation of maximum venous outflow in acute thrombophlebitis. *Surgery* 1972; **72**: 971.

19. Barnes RW, Collicott PE, Mozersky DJ, Sumner DS, Strandness DE Jr. Noninvasive quantitation of venous reflux in the postphlebitic syndrome. *Surg Gynec Obstet* 1973; **136**: 769.

20. Barnes RW, Collicott PE, Sumner DS, Strandness DE Jr. Noninvasive quantitation of venous hemodynamics in the postphlebitic syndrome. *Arch Surg* 1973; **107**: 807.

21. Barnes RW, Hokanson DE, Wu KK, Hoak JC. Detection of deep vein thrombosis with an automatic electrically calibrated strain gauge plethysmograph. *Surgery* 1977; **82**: 219.

22. Barnes RW, Ross EA, Strandness DE Jr. Differentiation of primary from secondary varicose veins by Doppler ultrasound and strain gauge plethysmography. *Surg Gynec Obstet* 1975; **141**: 207.

23. Barnes RW. Doppler ultrasonic diagnosis of venous disease. In Bernstein EF (Ed) *Noninvasive Diagnostic Techniques in Vascular Disease*. St Louis. CV. Mosby. 1985.

24. Becker J. The diagnosis of venous thrombosis in the legs using I-labelled fibrinogen: An experimental and clinical study. *Acta Chir Scand* 1972; **138**: 667.

25. Beesley WH, Fegan WG. An investigation into the localization of incompetent perforating veins. *Br J Surg* 1970; **57**: 30.

26. Berberich J, Hirsch S. Die röntgenographische darstellung der Arterien und Venen ani lebeneden Menschen. *Klin Wochenschr* 1923; **2**: 2226.

27. Berge T, Berquist D, Efsing HO, Hallböök T. Local complications of ascending phlebography. *Clin Radiol* 1978; **29**: 691.

28. Bettman MA, Salzman EW, Rosenthal D, Clagett P, Davies G, Nebesar R, Rabinov K, Ploetz J, Skillman J. Reduction of venous thrombosis complicating phlebography. *AJR* 1980; **134**: 1169.

29. Biello DR, Mattar AG, McKnight RC, Siegel BA. Ventilation perfusion studies in suspected pulmonary embolism. *AJR* 1979; **133**: 1033.

30. Biland L, Hull R, Hirsh J, Milner M. The use of

electromyography to detect muscle contraction responsible for falsely positive impedance plethysmographic results. *Thromb Res* 1979; **14**: 811.

31. Bjordal RI. Pressure patterns in the saphenous system in patients with venous leg ulcers. *Acta Chir Scand* 1971; **137**: 495.
32. Bracey DW. Hazard of ultrasonic detection of deep vein thrombosis. *Br Med J* 1973; **1**: 420.
33. Bracey DW. Simple device for location of perforating veins. *Br Med J* 1958; **2**: 101.
34. Brodie BC. Lectures illustrative of various subjects in pathology and surgery. London. Longman. 1846.
35. Brodie TG, Russell AE. On the deterimination of the rate of blood flow through an organ. *J Physiol (Lond)* 1905; **32**: 47.
36. Brown JN, Polak A. Hazard of ultrasonic detection of deep vein thrombosis. *Br Med J* 1973; **1**: 108.
37. Browse NL, Clapham WF, Croft DN, Jones DJ, Lea Thomas M, Williams OJ. Diagnosis of established deep vein thrombosis with the ^{125}I-fibrinogen uptake test. *Br Med J* 1971; **4**: 325.
38. Browse NL. The ^{125}I-fibrinogen uptake test. *Arch Surg* 1972; **104**: 160.
39. Browse NL. Venous pressure measurements. In Bernstein EF (Ed) *Non-invasive Diagnostic Techniques in Vascular Disease*. St Louis. CV Mosby. 1985.
40. Burnand KG, O'Donnell TF, Lea Thomas M, Browse NL. The relative importance of incompetent communicating veins in the production of varicose veins and venous ulcers. *Surgery* 1977; **82**: 9.
41. Bygdeman S, Aschberg S, Hindmarsh T. Venous plethysmography in the diagnosis of chronic venous insufficiency. *Acta Chir Scand* 1971; **137**: 423.
42. Bynum LJ, Wilson JE, Crotty CM, Curry TS, Smitson HL, Non-invasive diagnosis of deep venous thrombosis by phleborheography. *Ann Intern Med* 1978; **89**: 162.
43. Challoner AVJ. Photoelectric plethysmography for estimating cutaneous blood flow. In Rolfe P (Ed) *Non-invasive Physiological Measurements* Volume 1. New York. Academic Press. 1979.
44. Chevrier L. De l'examin aux reflux veineux dans les varices superficielles. *Arch Gen Chir* 1908; **2**: 44.
45. Chilvers AS, Thomas MH. Method for the localization of incompetent ankle perforating veins. *Br Med J* 1970; **2**: 577.
46. Coelho JC, Sigel B, Ryva JC, Machi J, Rerigers SA. B Mode sonography of blood clots. *JCU* 1982; **10**: 323.

47. Comerota AJ, Cranley JJ, Cook SE, Sipple P. Phleborheography: results of a ten-year experience. *Surgery* 1982; **91**: 573.
48. Cooke ED, Bowcock SA. Investigation of chronic venous insufficiency by thermography. *Vasc Diag Ther* 1982; **3**: 25.
49. Cooke ED, Pilcher MF. Deep vein thrombosis. Preclinical diagnosis by thermography. *Br J Surg* 1974; **61**: 971.
50. Cooke ED. Thermography. In Nicolaides AN, Yao JST (Eds) *Investigation of Vascular Disorders*. New York. Churchill Livingstone. 1981; 416.
51. Cooperman M, Martin EW Jr, Satiani B, Clark M, Evans WE. Detection of deep venous thrombosis by impedance plethysmography. *Am J Surg* 1979; **137**: 252.
52. Corbett CR, McIrvine AJ, Aston NO, Jamieson CW, Lea Thomas M. The use of varicography to identify the sources of incompetence in recurrent varicose veins. *Ann R Coll Surg Engl* 1984; **66**: 412.
53. Cranley JJ, Flanagan LD, Sullivan ED. Diagnosis of deep vein thrombosis by phleborheography. In Bernstein EF (Ed) *Non-invasive Diagnostic Techniques in Vascular Disease*. St Louis. CV Mosby. 1985.
54. Cranley JJ, Gay AY, Grass AM, Simeone FA. A plethysmographic technique for the diagnosis of deep venous thrombosis of the lower extremities. *Surg Gynec Obstet* 1973; **136**: 385.
55. Cranley JJ. Air plethysmography in venous disease, the phleborheograph. In Bernstein EF (Ed) *Non-invasive Diagnostic Techniques in Vascular Disease*. St Louis. CV Mosby. 1985.
56. Cranley JJ. Phleborheography in the diagnosis of deep venous thrombosis. In Hershey FB, Barnes RW, Sumner DS (Eds) *Non-invasive Diagnosis of Vascular Disease*. Pasadena. Appleton Davies. 1984.
57. Cremer H. Über die registrierung mechnischer voranje auf electrischen veg.speziell mit hilfa des sait engalvonometers und saitendektromelers. *MMW* 1907; **54**: 1629.
58. Dahn I, Eiriksson E. Plethysmographic diagnosis of deep venous thrombosis of the leg. *Acta Chir Scand* (Suppl) 1968; **398**: 33.
59. Day TK, Fish PJ, Kakkar VV. Detection of deep vein thrombosis by Doppler angiography. *Br Med J* 1976; **1**: 618.
60. De Weese JA, Rogoff SM. Functional ascending phlebography of the lower extremity by serial long film technique. *AJR* 1959; **81**: 841.
61. Deacon JM, Ell PJ, Anderson P, Khan O. Technetium 99m plasmin: a new test for the detection of deep vein thrombosis. *Br J Radiol* 1980; **53**: 673.

62. Dean RH. Radionuclide venography and simultaneous lung scanning: Evaluation of clinical application. In Bernstein EF (Ed) *Noninvasive Diagnostic Techniques in Vascular Disease*. St Louis. CV Mosby. 1978.

63. Dodd H, Cockett FB. *The Pathology and Surgery of the Veins of the Lower Limb*. Edinburgh. Livingstone. 1965.

64. Dohn K. Tilt phlebography; retrograde phlebography by ascending injection. *Acta Radiol* 1958; **50**: 293.

65. Dow JD. Retrograde phlebography in major pulmonary embolism. *Lancet* 1973; **2**: 407.

66. Eiriksson E. Plethysmographic studies of venous diseases of the legs. *Acta Chir Scand* 1986; Suppl **398**.

67. Elem B, Shorey BA, Lloyd Williams K. Comparison between thermography and fluorescein test in the detection of incompetent perforating veins. *Br Med J* 1971; **4**: 651.

68. Evans DS. The early diagnosis of thromboembolism by ultrasound. *Ann R Coll Surg Engl* 1971; **49**: 225.

69. Fernandes FJ, Horner J, Needham T, Nicolaides A. Ambulatory calf volume plethysmography in the assessment of venous insufficiency. *Br J Surg* 1979; **66**: 327.

70. Fischer M, Wupperman Th. A new method of noninvasive estimation of ambulatory venous pressure. *Surgery* 1985; **97**: 247.

71. Fischer M, Wupperman Th. Vergleich der Wertigkeit der Phlebodynamometrie mittels unblutiger Infrarot-Photoplethysmographie und blutiger Druckmessung. *Phlebol Proktol* 1982; **11**: 259.

72. Fischgold H, Adam H, Ecoiffier J, Plquet J. Opacification of spinal plexuses and azygos veins by osseus route. *J Radiol Electrol Med Nucl* 1952; **33**: 37.

73. Flanagan LD, Sullivan ED, Cranley JJ. Venous imaging of the extremities using real-time B mode ultrasound. In Bergan JJ and Yao JST (Eds) *Surgery of the Veins*. Orlando. Grune & Stratton. 1985.

74. Flanc C, Kakkar VV, Clark MB. The detection of venous thrombosis of the legs using ^{125}I-labelled fibrinogen. *Br J Surg* 1968; **55**: 742.

75. Folse R, Alexander RH. Directional flow detection for localizing venous valvular incompetency. *Surgery* 1970; **67**: 114.

76. Froggatt DL, Tibbutt DA. Hazard of ultrasonic detection of deep vein thrombosis. *Br Med J* 1973; **1**: 614.

77. Gorney RL, Wheeler B, Belko JS, Warren R. Observations on the uptake of radioactive fibrinolytic enzyme by intravascular clots. *Ann Surg* 1963; **158**: 905.

78. Haeger K. Problems of acute deep venous thrombosis. 1. The interpretation of signs and symptoms. *Angiology* 1969; **20**: 219.

79. Hallböök T, Gothlin J. Strain gauge plethysmography and phlebography in the diagnosis of deep venous thrombosis. *Acta Chir Scand* 1971; **137**: 37.

80. Hallböök T, Ling L. Pitfalls in plethysmographic diagnosis of deep venous thrombosis. *J Cardiovasc Surg* 1973; **14**: 427.

81. Hemingway AF. Venography. In Grainger RG, Allison DJ (Eds) *Diagnostic Radiology*. Edinburgh. Churchill Livingstone. 1986.

82. Henderson HP, Cooke ED, Bowcock SA, Hackett ME. After-exercise thermography for predicting postoperative deep vein thrombosis. *Br Med J* 1978; **1**: 1020.

83. Hertzmann AB. The blood supply of various skin areas as estimated by the photo-electric plethysmograph. *Am J Physiol* 1938; **124**: 328.

84. Hobbs JT, Davies JWL. Detection of venous thrombosis with ^{131}I-labelled fibrinogen in the rabbit. *Lancet* 1960; **2**: 134.

85. Hobbs JT. Per-operative venography to ensure accurate sapheno-popliteal vein ligation. *Br Med J* 1980; **2**: 1578.

86. Hojensgard JC, Sturup H. Static and dynamic pressures in superficial and deep veins of the lower extremity in man. *Acta Physiol Scand* 1953; **27**: 49.

87. Holm JSE. A simple plethysmographic method for differentiating primary from secondary varicose veins. *Surg Gynec Obstet* 1976; **143**: 609.

88. Howe HR, Hansen KJ, Plonk GW. Expanded criteria for the diagnosis of deep vein thrombosis. Use of the pulse volume recorder and Doppler ultrasonography. *Arch Surg* 1984; **119**: 1167.

89. Huisman MV, Buller HR, Cate JW, Vrecken J. Serial impedance plethysmography for suspected deep venous thrombosis in out patients. *N Engl J Med* 1986; **314**: 823.

90. Hull R, Hirsh J, Sackett DL, Powers P, Turpie AG, Walker I. Combined use of leg scanning and impedance plethysmography in suspected venous thrombosis. An alternative to venography. *N Engl J Med* 1977; **296**: 1497.

91. Hull R, Hirsh J, Sackett DL, Taylor DW, Carter DW, Carter C, Turpie AG, Zielinsky A, Power SP. Gent M. Replacement of venography in suspected venous thrombosis by impedance plethysmography and ^{125}I-fibrinogen leg scanning: a less invasive approach. *Ann Intern Med* 1981; **94**: 12.

92. Hull R, Taylor DW, Hirsh J, Sackett DS, Powers P, Turpie AG, Walker I. Impedance plethys-

mography: The relationship between venous filling and sensitivity and specificity for proximal vein thrombosis. *Circulation* 1978; **58**: 898.

93. Hull R, van Aken WG, Hirsh J, Gallus AS, Hoicka G, Turpie AG, Walker I, Gent M. Impedance plethysmography using the occlusive cuff technique in the diagnosis of venous thrombosis. *Circulation* 1976; **53**: 696.

94. Hyman C, Winsor T. History of plethysmography. *J Cardiovasc Surg* 1961; **2**: 506.

95. Johnston KW, Kakkar VV. Plethysmographic diagnosis of deep vein thrombosis. *Surg Gynec Obstet* 1974; **138**: 41.

96. Kakkar VV, Nicolaides AN, Renney JT, Friend JR, Clarke MB. ^{125}I-labelled fibrinogen test adapted for routine screening for deep-vein thrombosis. *Lancet* 1970; **1**: 540.

97. Kakkar VV. The diagnosis of deep vein thrombosis using the ^{125}I-fibrinogen test. *Arch Surg* 1972; **104**: 152.

98. Kempczinski RF, Berlatzky Y, Pearce WH. Semiquantitative photoplethysmography in the diagnosis of lower extremity venous insufficiency. *J Cardiovasc Surg* 1986; **27**: 17.

99. Kistner RL. Surgical repair of the incompetent femoral vein valve. *Arch Surg* 1975; **110**: 1336.

100. Kistner RL. Transvenous repair of the incompetent femoral vein valve. In Bergan JJ, Yao JST (Eds) *Venous Problems*. Chicago. Year Book Medical Publishers Inc. 1978.

101. Kriessmann A. Ambulatory venous pressure measurements. In Nicolaides AN, Yao JST (Eds) *Investigation of Vascular Disorders*. New York. Churchill Livingstone. 1981.

102. Lambie JM, Mahaffy RG, Barber DC, Karmody AM, Scott MM, Matheson NA. Diagnostic accuracy in venous thrombosis. *Br Med J* 1970; **2**: 142.

103. Lawrence D, Kakkar VV. Venous pressure measurement and foot volumetry in venous disease. In Verstraete M. *Techniques in Angiology*. The Hague. Martinus Nijhoff. 1979.

104. Lea Thomas M, Bowles JN. Descending phlebography in the assessment of long saphenous vein incompetence. *Am J Roentgenol* 1985; **145**: 1255.

105. Lea Thomas M, Bowles JN. Incompetent perforating veins. Comparison of varicography and ascending phlebography. *Radiology* 1985; **154**: 619.

106. Lea Thomas M, Briggs GM. Low osmolality contrast media for phlebography. *Int Angiol* 1984; **3**: 73.

107. Lea Thomas M, Browse NL. Internal iliac vein thrombosis. *Acta Radiol* 1972; **12**: 660.

108. Lea Thomas M, Carty H. The appearances of artefacts on lower limb phlebograms. *Clin Radiol* 1975; **26**: 527.

109. Lea Thomas M, Keeling FP. Varicography in the management of recurrent varicose veins. *Angiology* 1986; **37**: 570.

110. Lea Thomas M, Keeling FP, Ackroyd JS. Descending phlebography: A comparison of three methods and an assessment of the normal range of deep vein reflux. *J Cardiovasc Surg* 1986; **22**: 27.

111. Lea Thomas M, MacDonald LM. Complications of ascending phlebography of the leg. *Br Med J* 1978; **2**: 317.

112. Lea Thomas M, MacDonald L. The accuracy of bolus ascending phlebography in demonstrating the ilio-femoral segment. *Clin Radiol* 1977; **28**: 165.

113. Lea Thomas M, McAllister V, Rose DH, Tonge K. A simplified technique for phlebography for the localization of incomplete perforating veins of the legs. *Clin Radiol* 1972; **23**: 486.

114. Lea Thomas M, McAllister V. The radiological progression of deep vein thrombosis. *Radiology* 1971; **99**: 37.

115. Lea Thomas M, O'Dwyer JA. A phlebographic study of the incidence and significance of venous thrombosis. *AJR* 1978; **130**: 751.

116. Lea Thomas M, Posniak HV. Saphenography. *AJR* 1983; **141**: 812.

117. Lea Thomas M, Posniak HV. Varicography. *Int Angiol* 1985; **4**: 475.

118. Lea Thomas M, Tighe JR. Death from fat embolism, a complication of intraosseous phlebography. *Lancet* 1973; **2**: 1415.

119. Lea Thomas M. An improved intraosseous phlebography cannula. *Br J Radiol* 1969; **42**: 395.

120. Lea Thomas M. Gangrene following peripheral phlebography of the legs. *Br J Radiol* 1970; **43**: 528.

121. Lea Thomas M. Phlebography of the limb veins. In Partridge JB (Ed) *A Textbook of Radiological Diagnosis*. Vol 2, 5th edition. London. HK Lewis. 1985.

122. Lea Thomas M. *Phlebography of the Lower Limb*. Edinburgh. Churchill Livingstone. 1982.

123. Lea Thomas M. Pulmonary angiography. In Dodd H, Cockett FB (Eds) *The Pathology and Surgery of the Veins of the Lower Limbs*. Edinburgh. Churchill Livingstone. 1976.

124. Lee BY, Kavner D, Thoden WR, Trainor FS, Lewis JM, Madden JL. Technique of venous impedance plethysmography for

quantitation of venous reflux. *Surg Gynec Obstet* 1982; **154**: 49.

125. Lowenberg RI. The sphygmomanometer cuff pain test. *Comm Med* 1958; **22**: 287.

126. Ludbrook J. *Aspects of Venous Function in the Lower Limbs*. Springfield. Charles C Thomas. 1966.

127. Lynn TN, Blakenship JB, Bottomley R. Semiquantified constriction of the leg; a test for deep venous thrombosis. *Geriatrics* 1963; **18**: 713.

128. Mathieson FR. Tilt phlebography of normal legs. *Acta Radiol* 1958; **50**: 493.

129. Mavor G, Galloway JMD. The ilio-femoral segment as a source of pulmonary emboli. *Lancet* 1967; **1**: 871.

130. May R, DeWeese JA. Surgery of the pelvic veins. In May R. *Surgery of the Veins of the Legs and Pelvic*. Stuttgart. Georg Thieme 1974.

131. May R. Thrombophlebitis nach Phlebographic. *Vasa* 1977; **6**: 169.

132. McAllister WH, Palmer K. The histological effects of four commonly used contrast media for excretory urography and an attempt to modify the response. *Radiology* 1971; **99**: 511.

133. McIrvine AJ, Corbett CCR, Aston NO, Sherriff EA, Wiseman PA, Jamieson CW. The demonstration of saphenofemoral incompetence. Doppler ultrasound compared with standard clinical tests. *Br J Surg* 1984; **71**: 509.

134. McLachlin J, Richards T, Paterson JC. An evaluation of clinical signs in the diagnosis of venous thrombosis. *Arch Surg* 1962; **85**: 738.

135. McPheeters HO, Rice CO. Varicose veins – the circulation and direction of the venous flow. *Surg Gynec Obstet* 1929; **49**: 29.

136. Meaney TF, Weinstein MA. Digital subtraction angiography. In Grainger RG, Allison DJ (Eds) *Diagnostic Radiology*. Edinburgh. Churchill Livingstone. 1986.

137. Mesereau WA, Robertson HR. Observations on venous endothelial injury following the injection of venous radiographic contrast media in the rat. *J Neurosurg* 1961; **18**: 289.

138. Meyers S, Neiman HL, Mintzer RA. Pulmonary angiography. In Neiman HL, Yao JST (Eds) *Angiography of Vascular Disease*. New York. Churchill Livingstone. 1985.

139. Miles C, Nicolaides AN. Photophlethysmography: principles and development. In Nicolaides AN, Yao JST (Eds) *Investigation of Vascular Disorders*. New York. Churchill Livingstone. 1981; 501.

140. Miles C, Nicolaides AN. Photoplethysmography: principles and development. In Nicolaides AN, Yao JST (Eds) *Investigation*

of Vascular Disorders*. New York. Churchill Livingstone. 1981; 516.

141. Miller SS, Foote AV. The ultrasonic detection of incompetent perforating veins. *Br J Surg* 1974; **61**: 653.

142. Milne RM, Gunn A, Griffiths JMT, Ruckley CV. Postoperative deep vein thrombosis, a comparison of diagnostic techniques. *Lancet* 1971; **2**: 445.

143. Molitor H, Kniajuk M. A new bloodless method for continuous recording of peripheral circulatory changes. *J Pharmacol Exp Ther* 1936; **57**: 6.

144. Mullick S, Wheeler H, Songster G. Diagnosis of deep venous thrombosis by measurement of electrical impedance. *Am J Surg* 1970; **119**: 417.

145. Nachbur B. Die periphere Venendruckmessung: Eine Methode zur Bestimmung der venösen Leistungsreserve der unteren Extremitäten. *Zentralbl Phlebol* 1971; **10**: 224.

146. Nanson EM, Palko PD, Dick AA, Fedoruk SO. Early detection of deep venous thrombosis of the legs using human fibrinogen. A clinical study. *Ann Surg* 1965; **162**: 438.

147. Negus D, Cockett FB. Femoral vein pressures in post-phlebitic vein obstruction. *Br J Surg* 1967; **54**: 522.

148. Negus D, Pinto DJ, Le Quesne LP, Brown N, Chapman H. ^{125}I-labelled fibrinogen in the diagnosis of deep vein thrombosis and its correlation with phlebography. *Br J Surg* 1968; **55**: 835.

149. Negus D, Edwards JM, Kinmonth JB. The iliac veins in relation to lymphoedema. *Br J Surg* 1969; **56**: 481.

150. Nicholas GG, Loreny RP, Botti JJ, Chez RA. The frequent occurrences of false positive results in phleboreography during pregnancy. *Surg Gynec Obstet* 1985; **161**: 133.

151. Nicolaides AN, Fernandes JF, Schull K, Miles C. Calf volume plethysmography. In Nicolaides AN, Yao JST (Eds) *Investigation of Vascular Disorders*. New York. Churchill Livingstone. 1981.

152. Nicolaides AN, Fernandes JF, Zimmerman H. Doppler ultrasound in the investigation of venous insufficiency. In Nicolaides AN, Yao JST (Eds) *Investigation of Vascular Disorders*. New York. Churchill Livingstone. 1981.

153. Nicolaides AN, Olsson CG. The [99mTc] plasmin test. In Bernstein EF (Ed) *Non-invasive Diagnostic Techniques in Vascular Disease*. St Louis. CV Mosby. 1985.

154. Nicolaides A, Hoare M, Miles C. The value of ambulatory venous pressure in the assessment

of venous insufficiency. *Vasc Diag Ther* 1982; **3**: 41.

155. Nielson PE, Kirchner PT, Gerber GH. Oblique views in lung perfusion scanning; Clinical utility and limitations. *J Nucl Med* 1977; **18**: 967.

156. Noble J, Gunn AA. Varicose veins. Comparative study of methods for detecting incompetent perforators. *Lancet* 1972; **1**: 1253.

157. Norgren L. Functional evaluation of chronic venous insufficiency by foot volumetry. *Acta Chir Scand* 1973; Suppl **444**.

158. Norris CS, Beyrau A, Barnes RW. Quantitative photoplethysmography in chronic venous insufficiency: A new method of noninvasive estimation of ambulatory venous pressure. *Surgery* 1983; **94**: 758.

159. Palko PD, Nauson EM, Fedornk SO. The early detection of deep venous thrombosis using ^{131}I tagged human fibrinogen. *Can J Surg* 1964; **7**: 215.

160. Partsch H. Simultane venendruckmessung und plethysmographie. am Fuss. In May R, Kriessmann A (Eds) *Periphere Venendruck-messung*. Stuttgart. Georg Thieme 1978.

161. Patil KD, Williams JR, Lloyd Williams K. Thermographic localization of incompetent perforating veins in the leg. *Br Med J* 1970; **1**: 195.

162. Pearce WH, Ricco J-B, Queral LA, Flinn WR, Yao JST. Haemodynamic assessment of venous problems. *Surgery* 1983; **93**: 715.

163. Perthes G. Über die Operation der Unterschenkelvaricen nach Trendelenburg. *Dtsch Med Wochenschr* 1895; **21**: 253.

164. Pilcher R. Postoperative thrombosis and embolism. *Lancet* 1939; **2**: 629.

165. Pochaczevsky R, Pillari G, Feldman F. Liquid crystal contact thermography of deep venous thrombosis. *AJR* 1982; **138**: 717.

166. Pollack AA, Taylor BE, Myers TT, Wood EH. The effect of exercise and body position on the venous pressure at the ankle in patients having venous valvular defects. *J Clin Invest* 1949; **28**: 559.

167. Pollack AA, Wood EH. Venous pressure in the saphenous vein at the ankle in man during exercise and changes in posture. *J Appl Physiol* 1949; **1**: 649.

168. Rabinov K, Paulin S. Venography of the lower extremities. In Abrams HL (Ed) *Abrams' Angiography* 3rd edition Boston. Little Brown. 1983.

169. Ritchie WGM, Lynch RR, Stewart GJ. The effect of contrast media on normal and inflamed canine veins. *Invest Radiol* 1974; **9**: 444.

170. Ritchie W, Lapayowker MS, Soulen RL. Thermographic diagnosis of deep venous thrombosis. Anatomically based diagnostic criteria. *Radiology* 1979; **132**: 321.

171. Rosenberg ER, Trought WS, Kirks DR, Sumner TE, Grossman H. Ultrasonic diagnosis of renal vein thrombosis in neonates. *AJR* 1980; **134**: 35.

172. Rosenberg N, Marchese FP. Perforator vein localization by heat emission detection. *Surgery* 1963; **53**: 575.

173. Sandler DA, Martin JF. Liquid crystal thermography as a screening test for deep vein thrombosis. *Lancet* 1985; **2**: 665.

174. Satiani B, Paoletti D, Henry M, Burns R, Smith D. A critical appraisal of impedance plethysmography in the diagnosis of acute deep venous thrombosis. *Surg Gynec Obstet* 1985; **161**: 25.

175. Schanzer H, Lande L, Premus G, Pierce EC III. Non-invasive evaluation of chronic venous insufficiency. Use of foot mercury strain-gauge plethysmography. *Arch Surg* 1984; **119**: 1013.

176. Schobinger RA. *Intraosseous Phlebography*. New York. Grune & Stratton. 1960.

177. Sigel B, Felix WR, Popky GL, Ipsen J. Diagnosis of lower limb venous thrombosis by Doppler ultrasound technique. *Arch Surg* 1972; **104**: 174.

178. Spigos DG, Thane TT, Capek V. Skin necrosis following extravasation during peripheral phlebography. *Radiology* 1977; **123**: 605.

179. Strandness DE, Sumner DS. Ultrasonic velocity detector in the diagnosis of thrombophlebitis. *Arch Surg* 1972; **104**: 180.

180. Strandness DE. Doppler ultrasonic techniques in vascular disease. In Bernstein EF (Ed) *Non-invasive Diagnostic Techniques in Vascular Disease*. St Louis. CV Mosby 1985.

181. Sturup H, Hojensgard IC. Venous pressure in varicose veins in patients with incompetent communicating veins. *Acta Chir Scand* 1950; **99**: 518.

182. Sullivan ED, Peter DJ, Cranley JJ. Real-time B-mode venous ultrasound. *J Vasc Surg* 1984; **1**: 465.

183. Sullivan ED, Reece CI, Cranley JJ. Phleborheography of the upper extremity. *Arch Surg* 1983; **118**: 1134.

184. Sumner DS, Baker DW, Strandness DF. The ultrasonic velocity detector in a clinic study of venous disease. *Arch Surg* 1968; **97**: 75.

185. Sumner DS. Diagnosis of deep venous thrombosis by Doppler ultrasound. In Nicolaides AN, Yao JST (Eds) *Investigation of Vascular Disorders*. New York. Churchill Livingstone. 1981.

186. Sumner DS. Strain gauge plethysmography. In Bernstein EF (Ed) *Non-Invasive Diagnostic Techniques in Vascular Disease*. St Louis. CV Mosby. 1985.

187. Taheri SA, Lazar L, Elias S, Marchand P, Heffner R. Surgical treatment of postphlebitic syndrome with vein valve transplant. *Am J Surg* 1982; **144**: 221.

188. Talbot SR. Use of real-time imaging in identifying deep venous obstruction: A preliminary report. *Bruit* 1982; **6**: 41.

189. Taplin GV, Johnson DE, Dore EK. Suspensions of radioalbumin aggregates for photoscanning of the liver, spleen, lung and other organs. *J Nucl Med* 1964; **5**: 259.

190. Taylor DW, Hull R, Sackett DL, Hirsch J. Simplification of the sequential impedance plethysmograph technique without loss of accuracy. *Thromb Res* 1980; **17**: 561.

191. Thulesius O, Norgren L, Gjores JE. Foot volumetry, a new method for objective assessment of oedema and venous function. *Vasa* 1973; **2**: 325.

192. Trendelenburg F. Über die Unterbindung der Vena saphena magna bei Unterschenkelvaricen. *Beitr Z Klin Chir* 1891; **7**: 195.

193. Tyson MD, Goodlett WC. Venous pressures in disorders of the venous system of the lower extremities. *Surgery* 1945; **18**: 669.

194. Wagner HN, Sabiston DC, McAfee JG. Diagnosis of massive pulmonary embolism in man by radioisotope scanning. *N Engl J Med* 1964; **271**: 377.

195. Walters HL, Clemenson J, Browse NL, Lea Thomas M. [125]I fibrinogen uptake following phlebography of the leg. *Radiology* 1980; **135**: 619.

196. Warren R, White EA, Beicher CD. Venous pressures in the saphenous system in normal, varicose and post phlebitic extremities. Alterations following femoral vein ligation. *Surgery* 1949; **26**: 435.

197. Webb IJ, Berger LA, Sherlock S. Greyscale ultrasonography of portal vein. *Lancet* 1977; **2**: 675.

198. Werner H, Otto K. Hazards and complications in roentgenological venous diagnosis. *Fortschr Roentgenstr* 1962; **96**: 655.

199. Wheeler HB, Anderson FA. The diagnosis of venous thrombosis by impedance plethysmography. In Bernstein EF (Ed) *Non-invasive Diagnostic Techniques in Vascular Disease*. St Louis. CV Mosby. 1985.

200. Wheeler HB, Mullick SC, Anderson JN, Pearson D. Diagnosis of occult deep vein thrombosis by a non-invasive bedside technique. *Surgery* 1971; **70**: 20.

201. Wheeler HB, O'Donnell JA, Anderson FA, Penney BC, Penra RA, Benedict CJP. Bedside screening for venous thrombosis using occlusive impedance phlebography. *Angiology* 1975; **26**: 199.

202. Whitehead SM. Quantitative assessment of calf pump function using [99m]Technetium labelled red blood cells. *Br J Surg* 1981; **68**: 366.

203. Whitehead S, Clemenson G, Browse NL. The assessment of calf pump function by isotope plethysmography. *Br J Surg* 1983; **70**: 675.

204. Widmer LK. *Peripheral Venous Disorders. Basle Study III*. Berns. Hans Huber. 1978.

205. Witten DM, Hirsch FD, Harman GW. Acute reactions to urographic contrast medium. *AJR* 1973; **119**: 823.

206. Wojciechowski J, Holm J, Zachrisson BT. Thermography and phlebography in the detection of incompetent perforating veins. *Acta Radiol (Diag) (Stockh)* 1982; **23**: 199.

207. Wupperman T, Exler U, Mellman J, Kestila M. Noninvasive quantitative measurement of regurgitation in insufficiency of the greater saphenous vein by Doppler ultrasound. A comparison with clinical examination and phlebography. *Vasa* **10**: 24.

5

Varicose veins: pathology

Definitions

The World Health Organisation[82] defines varicose veins as:

'Saccular dilatation of the veins which are often tortuous.'

This definition specifically excludes:

- dilatation of small intradermal subcutaneous veins called 'venectasis'
- any tortuous dilated veins that are secondary to previous thrombophlebitis or an arteriovenous fistula.

The Basle study[22,26,106] separated varicose veins into:

1. dilated saphenous veins (stem veins)
2. dilated superficial branches (reticular veins)
3. dilated venules (hyphenwebs)

We would agree that groups 1, and 2, of the Basle definition are varicose veins but, like the WHO, would exclude group 3, though it is difficult to define when a small vessel is a venule rather than a vein.

It has been suggested[39] that a varicose vein is defined as a subcutaneous surface vein in which the valves have become incompetent. While this definition may be etymologically satisfactory, valvular incompetence of a superficial vein is difficult to detect on clinical examination, and in this book the descriptive definition of varicose veins will be used (i.e. veins which have become excessively tortuous and dilated) because, though this definition is imprecise and open to consider-

able observer variation, it has the major advantage of simplicity (Figs. 5.1a and b).

Epidemiology

The incidence of a condition is the estimated number of patients in whom the condition has developed in a specified time period.

The prevalence of a condition is the estimated

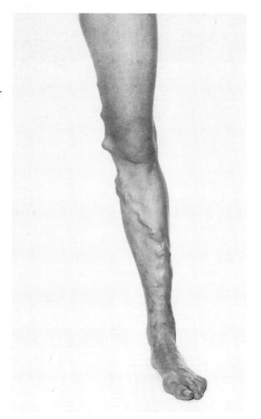

Fig. 5.1 (a) A number of tortuous dilated 'varicose' veins, all tributaries of the long saphenous vein.

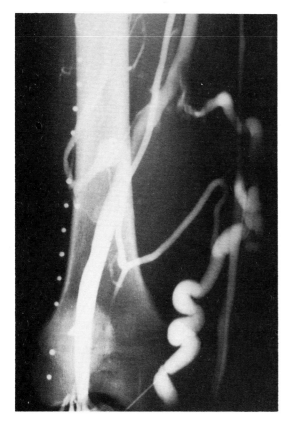

Fig. 5.1 (b) A varicogram showing tortuous dilated tributary veins draining into a long saphenous vein of normal size.

number of patients in whom the condition exists at a specified time or within a specified interval of time.

The prevalence of varicose veins (the incidence in the whole population) has been studied in a number of national surveys and by three local population surveys.[12]

The US National Survey of 1961–1963[103] This was based on interviews conducted by non-medical personnel. It produced an estimated rate (prevalence) of 2.25 patients with varicose veins per 100 of the population per year, comprised of 0.8 per cent in men and 3.5 per in women.

The UK Survey of Sickness (England and Wales 1950)[33] This was also based on interviews conducted by non-medical personnel, and showed that 1.41 per cent of men and 3.74 per cent of women had varicose veins. It was estimated that 2.25 per cent of the population had varicose veins.

The Sickness Survey of Denmark 1952–

1953[92] This survey of patients attending hospital with varicose veins found an incidence of 1.7 per cent of males and 2.0 per cent females attending in 1 year.

The Canadian Sickness Survey 1950–1951[41] This survey showed a lower incidence of varicose veins than the others (0.53 per cent overall), but was poorly organized and is of doubtful value.

Summary All these surveys were conducted by questionnaire, administered by untrained non-medical personnel, and therefore probably underestimate the prevalence of varicose veins.

Regional surveys

There have been five major regional surveys.

The first by Gjöres[34] in Sweden, using a questionnaire administered to the population of a town in Sweden, revealed that 2.21 per cent had a clinical history of deep vein thrombosis and that 70 per cent of these patients had developed varicose veins within 5 years and 85 per cent within 10 years of the thrombosis.

Arnoldi[5] carried out a survey, in Denmark, on the families of patients over 25 years of age with varicose veins. He found that 38 per cent of the female relatives and 18.4 per cent of the male relatives had varicose veins.

Bobeck et al.,[11] surveyed a defined population over the age of 15 years in Czechoslovakia using a questionnaire and a medical examination. He found an incidence of varicose veins of 14 per cent in women and 6.6 per cent in men.

Widmer et al.,[106] in a survey carried out in 1974 in Basle, Switzerland, showed that 4.2 per cent of 4376 chemical workers had evidence of severe varicose veins. They found that 5.2 per cent of the men and 3.2 per cent of the women were affected. Widmer's team took photographs of all the subjects in the survey which was carried out entirely by medical personnel. The Basle study showed that 10 per cent of the population between the ages of 25 and 34 years had varicose veins, while 50 per cent of those between the ages of 64 and 75 years were affected.

Beaglehole et al.,[8] looked at the prevalence of varicose veins in New Zealand in 1976. They showed that 36.3 per cent of Maori men and

47.4 per cent of Maori women had varicose veins. In the white population the incidence was 21.5 per cent in men and 40.4 per cent in women, after standardizing the prevalence for the ages of the two races.

Comment In both Europe and North America the national surveys have shown a remarkably consistent prevalence of varicose veins of approximately 2 per cent. Local surveys have showed a greater prevalence with levels varying between 4 and 15 per cent. The problem with all these surveys is the varying diagnostic criteria and knowledge of the observers. The Basle study is the only survey in which the prevalence of severe varicose veins was found to be higher in males than in females; though females had a minimally greater incidence of all types of veins, however small, were included.

If it is accepted that 2 per cent of the population has varicose veins and that a proportion of these subjects will develop problems that need treatment, the size of the problem on an international or even a national basis is enormous.

Aetiology of varicose veins (Table 5.1)

Valvular deficiency

The concept that varicose veins are caused by descending valvular incompetence was the rationale for performing a high saphenous vein ligation for long saphenous vein incompetence. Trendelenburg[101] suggested that the venous valves normally protect the wall of the vein below each valve from the pressure in the vein above it. He believed that varicose veins began when the highest valve in the long saphenous vein gave way and that if the vein was ligated and divided, preventing reflux of blood downwards, the saphenous vein would regain its former dimensions

and the varicosities in the tributaries would regress.

Anatomical studies[7,28,79] on the distribution of venous valves in cadavers have shown that between 20 and 40 per cent of apparently 'normal' individuals have an absent valve in and above the common femoral vein on one or both sides (Fig. 5.2). These studies suggested that an absence of the ilio-femoral valves exposes the highest valve in the long saphenous vein to thoraco-abdominal pressures and that on standing upright the hydrostatic pressure produced by the vertical column of venous blood between the groin and the heart would be resisted only by this single important upper valve. Basmajian[7] however, failed to show a convincing association between the absence of ilio-femoral valves and the presence of long saphenous incompetence.

The greater incidence of left-sided varicose veins that has been reported by some workers[62] may be related to left common iliac vein compression because the venous return from the leg is always partially impeded where the right common iliac artery compresses the left common iliac vein in front of the sacral promontary.[19,62]

One study in the 1950s suggested that almost

Table 5.1 Aetiology of varicose veins

Valvular deficiency
Vein wall weakness
Incompetent communicating veins
Arteriovenous fistulae
Increased venous pressure (erect stance or tight clothing)

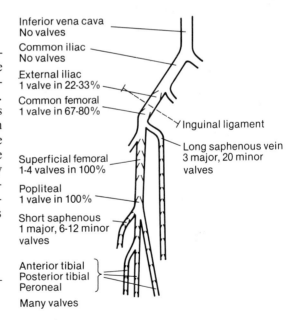

Fig. 5.2 Diagram of the distribution of the valves in the veins of the lower limb and pelvis collated from the cadaver dissection studies of Eger and Casper,[28] Powell and Lynn,[79] and Basmajian.[7]

half the patients with varicose veins had defective valves in the deep veins.[67] The technique by which the absence of the deep venous valves was judged was, however, disputed,[70] and our own recent studies of descending phlebography in patients with varicose veins contradict these earlier findings.[1]

In 1963 Ludbrook[58] re-examined the validity of the theory of descending incompetence by trying to discover if valvular incompetence in the long saphenous vein preceded the development of its varicose tributaries. He investigated the fall of foot vein pressure during exercise with and without thigh tourniquets in eight normal subjects, five subjects with gross saphenous varicosities, and eight subjects with very mild varicosities of the lower leg. He found the pressure falls on exercise were equally poor in patients with both severe and mild varicose veins. He interpreted these findings as evidence that incompetence of the long saphenous valve preceded the development of severe distal varicosis.

There are a number of flaws in this argument. The pressure falls found in the patients with long saphenous incompetence were in fact significantly worse than those found in the patients with mild disease, in whom no attempt was made to exclude the presence of long saphenous incompetence. Incompetence of the long saphenous valve could just as well be the result as the cause of venous dilation – a fact that the author did not address. It is difficult to quantify the degree of varicosity in the main vein and its tributaries, as the method used is open to observer error and bias. There was no evidence that the patients with the 'minor varicosities' and pressure abnormalities ever went on to develop 'full blown' saphenous vein incompetence. It is possible that an abnormal venous pressure profile in the presence of minor varicosities could be the result of abnormalities in the deep veins, which were not investigated in this study.

In order to prove that the descending valvular incompetence theory is correct, an attempt must be made to show that ligating the long saphenous vein reverses the changes in existing varicose veins and prevents the development of new varicose veins. Our clinical experience indicates that neither of these events occurs. Varicograms, descending phlebography and Doppler examinations show that tributary veins can become vari-

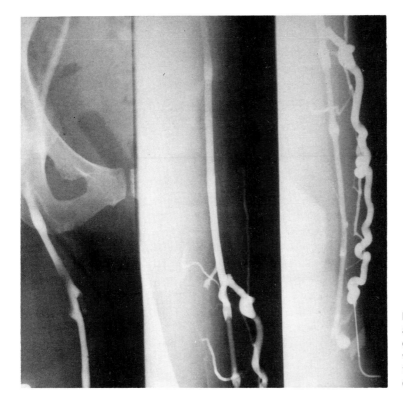

Fig. 5.3 A varicogram showing a long saphenous vein of normal calibre containing normal valves, with an obviously varicose tributary that is tortuous and dilated.

cose and incompetent before there is any evidence of long saphenous incompetence. (Fig. 5.3).

Ludbrook's paper is the last study to be published that has seriously attempted to support the descending theory of valvular incompetence which is thought to result from congenital valvular absence or an acquired valvular defect.[47,109]

There are a few patients who have a congenital absence of all venous valves[54,55] who often do develop severe secondary varicose veins. These patients may also have an absence of valves in their arm and other veins (see Chapter 23, Fig. 23.7).

It is interesting to note that Williams' dissections of the forelimbs and hind limbs of cats, dogs and monkeys,[107] showed that while the valves are equally distributed in the fore- and hind limbs of the cat and the dog, the hind limbs of the monkey contain distinctly fewer valves. As the monkey (*Rhesus macaca*) is often known to adopt the semi-upright position, while the other animals do not, the role of the valves as an anti-gravity mechanism is open to doubt. Williams' conclusions were similar to Jager's,[42] namely that 'the function of venous valves is to protect the capillaries and venules from sudden excessive rises in pressure during muscular exercise'. As Foote,[31] in his monograph on varicose veins, comments that he was unable to find any evidence of the existence of varicose veins in any members of the animal kingdom, except possibly in one donkey, it appears that varicose veins are a human condition unrelated directly to the presence or absence of venous valves.

Defective structure of the vein wall

It is difficult to know who first suggested that a defect in the tissues of the wall of the vein was responsible for the development of varicosity. In an influential article written in 1950 King[46] made the following points.

- Varicose veins usually make their first appearance as a sharply circumscribed group of veins which communicate with other veins of normal calibre. These varices often communicate with a saphenous vein of normal calibre in which there is no evidence of valvular incompetence (Fig. 5.3).

  (This is our own experience and makes Ludbrook's observations of doubtful validity).

- The early 'swelling' of the vein is distal not proximal to the valve, making the position of the dilation difficult to explain by the theory of 'back-pressure'.
- The extent of the varicosities may vary from time to time without any obvious mechanical alteration. The veins may be larger on some occasions and smaller on others.
- Histological examination of the vein wall in the early stages of varicosis shows it to be thickened with hypertrophy of the muscle coat and increased vascularity of the adventitia.

Having made these observations, King did not suggest a local abnormality of the vein wall but instead proposed that the venous dilatation was caused by a haemodynamic alteration in blood flow brought about by a chemical stimulus. All his observations could, however, be explained on the basis of an abnormality of the vessel wall.

The position of the dilatation in relation to the valve is of critical importance in refuting the theory of descending valvular incompetence. The site of dilatation has been addressed by several investigators (Table 5.2).

In 1961 Cotton[20] published a detailed study of the relationship between the venous dilation and the valves. He examined saphenous veins which had been removed by stripping at operation, veins removed from cadavers and the whole venous system in amputated limbs. The veins were either opened to inspect the valve distribution or resin casts were made of the whole system.

Table 5.2 Site of dilatation in varicose veins[20]

Dilatation proximal to the valve
    Callender 1862[17]
    Rindfleisch 1867[85]
    Bennett 1890[9]

Proximal and distal to the valve
    Löwenstein 1908[56]

No relation to the valve
    Schwartz 1934[90]

Below the valve
    Trendelenburg 1891[100]
    Slavinski 1899[94]
    Ledderhose 1906[53]
    Hasebroek 1916a and b[36, 37]

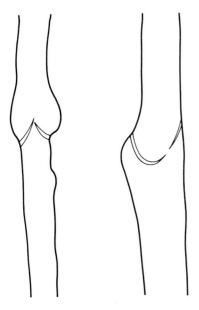

Fig. 5.4 Diagram of the eccentric dilatation found by Cotton[20] beneath the valve in casts taken of varicose veins. A normal valve is shown for comparison.

Inspection of the veins was carried out at operation and venograms were also obtained. From these studies Cotton drew the following conclusions.

1. The number of valves in varicose long saphenous veins was significantly less than the number found in normal long saphenous veins.

2. There was no evidence of primary valvular disease to be found on naked eye inspection.

3. The number of valves did not diminish with age.

4. Prominent dilations occurred below the cornua of the valve cusps (Fig. 5.4).

5. The long saphenous vein showed little evidence of lengthening while the varicose tributaries were greatly elongated and tortuous.

6. The varicose tributaries showed saccula-

tions projecting from alternate sides of the vein (Fig. 5.5).

7. Tributaries joining communicating veins were also very tortuous (Fig. 5.6).

8. There were no varicosities in the deep veins of the leg.

Points 1 and 2 of Cotton's conclusions appear to be contradictory, though the quantity and quality of the valves may be independent features. He did, however, definitely show that the site of dilatation was below rather than above the valves, though this had previously been disputed by others (see Table 5.2), but he also pointed out that this cannot be taken as unequivocal evidence of a wall abnormality as opposed to a valvular defect, because valvular incompetence might allow regurgitant blood to impinge on the wall of the vein below the valve and so weaken it and cause it to dilate. This would be akin to the post-stenotic dilation seen beyond a narrowed artery. Arguing against this hypothesis, Cotton indicated that the dilatation of varicose veins is always eccentric (see Figs. 5.4 and 5.5) whereas the cusps are always concentric making the possibility of dilatation from valvular reflux less likely.

Rokitansky[86] suggested that venous valves 'increase to a certain degree with dilatation of the vein but, after a time, cease to increase and are no longer capable of closing the enlarged vessel'. Edwards and Edwards[27] also described separation and shortening of the valves cusps as a result of venous dilatation. Cotton proposed that the venous dilatation so increased the tension in the valves that it led to sclerosis and contraction of the valve cusps with the eventual disappearance of the whole valve. All these studies supported the hypothesis that the valvular incompetence followed rather than preceded a change in the vein wall.

Collagen, elastin and hexosamine content In 1963 Svejcar *et al.*,[96,97] analysed the content of the vein wall in terms of collagen, elastin, muscle, and hexosamine. They assumed that because of the association between varicose veins and flat fleet, hernias and haemorrhoids, there was likely to be a connective tissue abnormality. They took veins

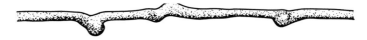

Fig. 5.5 Diagram of the spiral arrangement of the dilatations found along the course of a varicose long saphenous vein. (After Cotton.)[20]

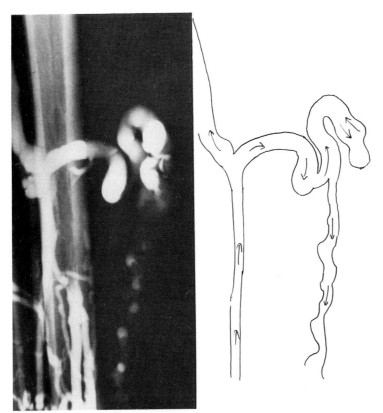

Fig. 5.6 A dilated surface varicosity lying directly over and connected to an incompetent communicating vein. The diagram shows the direction of blood flow.

from normal subjects and compared them with varicose veins and 'normal' veins from a group of patients with varicose veins at other sites. This last group they called 'potential varicose veins'.

They found the following.

- The collagen content was significantly lower in the varicose veins and 'potential varicose veins' than in normal veins.
- Varicose veins contained relatively more muscle than normal veins.
- The hexosamine content was significantly higher in actual and potential varicose veins than in normal veins.
- There was a much greater variation of water and hexosamine content in different segments of varicose veins when compared with different segments of normal veins which showed relatively little variation.

From these results Svejcar *et al.*, proposed the hypothesis that the similarity between varicose veins and potential varicose veins might be the result of an inherited abnormality of collagen metabolism.

This is a very important study but is heavily dependent upon the methods used to assess the constituents of the vein wall. Barbaro *et al.*,[6] repeated this work and reported completely different results, but Andreotti *et al.*,[4] in a later study confirmed a significantly lower content of collagen and elastin in varicose veins compared with controls.

The presence of a localized dilatation at one area of the vein wall has suggested to Rose[87] that a local fault must be present because back pressure would be likely to produce uniform dilatation.

Rose has made certain clinical observations which support the concept of a defect in the vein wall.[87]

- Sixty per cent of varicose veins occur below a competent saphenous valve (not all investigators would agree with this observation).
- A normal saphenous vein inserted as an

arterial substitute has no difficulty in withstanding arterial pressure without becoming varicose.

- When varicose veins are used as a conduit or patch they invariably dilate or develop localized aneurysms.
- *In situ* saphenous vein bypass grafts in which all the valves have been deliberately destroyed before they are attached to the arterial system do not show any increased evidence of aneurysmal dilation.

All these clinical 'experiments' make the theory of descending valvular incompetence as a cause of varicose veins untenable.

A recent study in our department on the mechanical properties of vein wall and valves[2] showed that the valve cusps have twice the strength of the vein wall, again indicating that the venous valve is less likely to give way under pressure than the venous wall.

Haemodynamic effects

Varicose veins definitely develop upstream of an arteriovenous fistula.[40] We regularly observed this response after deliberately forming arteriovenous fistulae in the hind-limb of a dog to produce venous hypertension.[15]

In 1916 Hasebroek[36,37] made a vein model using a thin-walled latex tube containing three single flap non-return valves. He then attached this model to a pulsatile fluid pump at pressures which were comparable to those within the venous system. He showed that 'blow outs' occurred in the side of the latex tubing at certain critical frequencies of pulsation. He asserted that arterial pulsation transmitted through the venae comitantes of the legs might induce varicosities in the surface veins. Cotton[20] attempted to repeat these experiments but failed unless the tubing was deliberately narrowed at the 'valve sites'. He concluded that reflection of the pulse waves at the sites of valvular narrowing might be responsible for the development of dilatation. Nylander[74] has shown that varicosities assume the shape of a sine wave which is the wave form that results from an increase in blood flow.

Pigeaux[77] was the first person to observe that blood in varicose veins may be as red as that found in arteries, and he noted that an arterial pulsation could occasionally be felt over the veins. Pratt[80] also suggested that some primary varicose veins could be felt to pulsate, and he called these 'arterial varices'; it is possible, however, that Pratt was looking at limbs with the Parkes–Weber syndrome.

Raised oxygen tensions have been found in blood taken from varicose veins as compared with blood taken from normal veins;[13,83] this suggested that arteriovenous shunts might be responsible for the development of varicose veins. There is, however, little evidence for the existence of functioning pathological arteriovenous shunts in every patient with varicose veins. Recent work has shown a lower oxygen content of blood samples from saphenous varicosities when compared with popliteal blood from the same level.[84] The only conceivable possibility is that the arteriovenous shunts which are normally present in the skin to allow temperature regulation open intermittently in response to changes in temperature or venous pressure.[49,88]

It has been suggested that venous reflux through incompetent valves in the ankle communicating veins causes turbulent flow in the superficial system,[29,30] an asymmetrical fine jet of high velocity retrograde flow affecting the overlying vein wall. There is no experimental or clinical evidence to support this hypothesis.[38] Although the concept of an increased blood flow giving rise to turbulence which in turn causes venodilatation is an attractive hypothesis, more studies are required.

Secondary aetiological factors (Predisposing factors) (Table 5.3)

Age   The surveys which have been described in the section on epidemiology have all shown that the prevalence of varicose veins increases with age. There appears to be a peak frequency between 50 and 60 years of age[22] with a declining frequency in old age. This latter observation may, however, be incorrect because elderly patients

Table 5.3   Predisposing factors

Age	Bowel habit
Sex	Occupation
Race	Heredity
Weight	Alcohol
Height	Clothes
Pregnancy	Erect stance
Diet	

with varicose veins are rarely referred for surgery. Varicose veins are unusual in subjects less than 20 years of age and are most common in people between 45 and 65 years of age.

Sex The Basle Survey[106] is the only study that shows a male to female preponderance. Studies on patients presenting to doctors for treatment are biased because women are more likely to complain of 'unsightly veins' (especially in those parts of the world where they expose their legs by wearing dresses) than men.[31] All the other large surveys show a female to male excess of between 2:1 and 4:1 (Fig. 5.7).

Pregnancy This factor is obviously closely associated with the difference in sex incidence of varicose veins. Lake *et al.*,[50] examined the preva-

lence of varicose veins in a group of 536 employees, all over 40 years of age, in a New York department store. They found an increased incidence in women who had been pregnant compared to the nulliparous group (Table 5.4).

When they compared the male and female employees they found a greater prevalence of varicose veins in the women but even when a correction was made for sex, the effect of pregnancy persisted. This suggests that pregnancy and gender influence the development of varicose vein independently.

The incidence of varicose veins developing during pregnancy varies between 8 and 20 per cent.[24,45,72] In a group of 405 women with varicose veins Mullane[68] found that 13 per cent were primaparous, 30 per cent were secundiparous, 57 per cent were multiparous; Donato and Nejamkin[25] found similar rates, and Berge and Feldthusen[10], who reviewed 908 pregnancies, found that the risk of developing varicose veins after two or more pregnancies was significantly greater than the risk after the first pregnancy.

It is possible that the development of varicose veins during pregnancy is related to the changing hormone levels particularly oestrogens which encourage venous distension by causing smooth muscle relaxation.[63] Compression of the iliac veins by the enlarging uterus may also contribute to their development.

This review of the published work makes the Basle survey[106] which failed to confirm any relationship between childbirth and the prevalence of varicose veins both interesting and inexplicable.

Race, diet and bowel habit It is easier to consider these factors together. The figure for the overall prevalence of varicose veins of 2 per cent is based on the European and American surveys. A comparison between German and Japanese soldiers, however, showed a sixfold increase in varicose veins in the Germans.[66] It was suggested

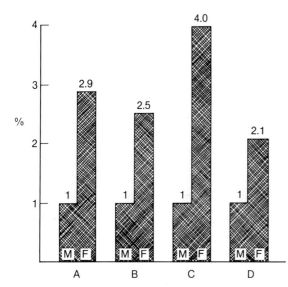

Fig. 5.7 Prevalence rates for varicose veins in both sexes found in four surveys with the prevalence in males standardized to 1 per cent.

	Actual rates (%)	
	M	F
(a) The Sickness Survey of Denmark 1951–1954	8.7	25.3
(b) England and Wales: Morbidity statistics for General Practice 1955–1956	6.5	16.4
(c) US National Health Survey 1961–1963	8.8	35.3
(d) Bobeck *et al.* Klator District of Czechoslovakia 1961–1962	6.6	14.1

(Redrawn from Borschberg.)[12]

Table 5.4 Prevalence of varicose veins related to parity

	Total	With varicose veins	%
Nulliparous	133	89	66.9
Multiparous	98	78	79.5

Adapted from Lake *et al.*, 1942.[50]

that this difference in prevalence was caused by a difference in height.

Both Pirner[78] and Foote[31] stated that varicose veins are uncommon in Africans, and Dodd[23] found only three cases of varicose veins in 11 000 inpatient admissions in a tribal reserve in Zululand. Dodd also reported that black people living in Eastern Africa in Western conditions developed varicosities as often as their white counterparts.

Cleave[18] suggested that a lack of fibre in the Western diet causes faecal arrest which results in compression of the iliac veins by the distended sigmoid colon and caecum, but Burkitt[14] claimed that the lack of fibre combined with straining at defaecation on Western style lavatory seats raises the venous pressure. He suggested that the squatting position and the relative ease of defaecation achieved by the African on a high fibre diet protected him from the ill effects of a raised abdominal venous pressure. As it now seems likely that descending valvular incompetence is not the cause of varicosities, this hypothesis is probably incorrect.

Two investigators actually measured venous pressures in the sitting and squatting position during straining[61] and showed that the squatting position was no more effective than the sitting position in preventing the transmission of intra-abdominal pressure to the veins of the lower leg.

Alexander[3] has re-examined the published work concerning the influence of race on varicose veins. He felt that there was good evidence that the prevalence is greater in Western than in Eastern communities, and is very low in both Africa and India.

The influence of race is probably multi-factorial and cannot easily be separated from genetic factors, dietary factors, body build and other extraneous factors such as clothing and occupation. We do not subscribe to Cleave and Burkitt's hypothesis that dietary fibre is a major aetiological factor.

Height and weight Both excessive height and increased weight have been thought to be associated with a greater risk of developing varicose veins. In 1913 Miyauchi[66] originally suggested that the high prevalence of varicose veins in German soldiers compared with their Japanese counterparts was a result of their greater height. Dodd, however, noted a very low incidence in the Zulus who are an excessively tall race.[23] There is a

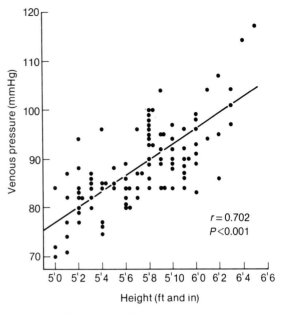

Fig. 5.8 The relationship between height (feet and inches) and the resting venous pressure measured in the foot (mmHg) of 100 subjects. There is a highly significant correlation between height and foot vein pressure.[16]

significant correlation between the height of the individual and the resting venous pressure[16] (Fig. 5.8) but it is doubtful if this correlation is of any clinical importance. Widmer[106] found that 4.5 per cent of the very tall people in his survey developed varicose veins compared with 5 per cent of the very short people, indicating little effect of height.

Both Myers[71] and Ludbrook[57] found that patients with varicose veins were heavier than age and sex matched controls without varicose veins, but the Basle study[106] again failed to reveal any significant differences in the mean weight of patients with or without evidence of varicose veins. Widmer did find evidence of an increased prevalence of dilated intradermal venules in obese women but no association with subcutaneous vein varicosities. It has been recently claimed[91] that there is an inverse relationship between the waist/hips and waist/thigh fat ratios and the incidence of varicose veins, suggesting that fat storage in the hips and thighs might increase the risk of varicose veins.

Occupation, posture and clothing In the same way that the height of the patient was thought to influence the development of varicose veins so occupations which involve prolonged periods of standing were also considered to increase the risk of varicose veins. Policemen and shop assistants, in addition to surgeons, were regarded as high risk occupations. Santler *et al.*,[89] reviewed 2854 patients with varicose disease and found 6.3 per cent were required to walk in their occupation, 29.2 per cent spent their time sitting, and 64.5 per cent stood still at work. Lake *et al.*,[50] in their New York department store survey, found that 74 per cent of the employees who stood had varicose veins compared with 57 per cent who sat. In one of the analyses of the Basle study[106] a weak correlation was found between the type of occupation, standing or sitting, and the risk of varicose veins.

Mekky *et al.*,[65] reported a different incidence of varicose veins in two matched populations of cotton workers in Egypt and England. The prevalence of the condition was much higher in the English workers than in the Egyptians, and this was significantly related to age, parity, bodyweight, type of corsetry, and occupation (namely standing at work).

Taken together, these studies suggest that occupations which involve prolonged standing may carry an increased risk of varicose veins. The case against tight corsetry requires further support!

Heredity Foote[31] reported that the majority of patients who sought medical attention for their varicose veins proffer information that 'one or other of their parents was a sufferer'. Virchow[104] recognized the influence of heredity in the development of varicose veins, and Gay[32] reported two affected families in some detail. Ottley[75] examined 50 families with varicose veins and claimed that inheritance was of a simple dominant type. The prevalence of relatives affected in eight studies up to 1950 is given in Table 5.5.

Table 5.5 Incidence of a positive family history in patients with varicose veins

1921, Magnus[59]	50–75%
1927, Nicholson[73]	55%
1930, de Takat's and Quint[21]	65%
1932, Jensen[43]	50%
1936, Payne[76]	50%
1943, Larsen and Smith[51]	43%
1946, McPheeters and Anderson[64]	6–10%
1950, Pratt[81]	80%

A more recent review by Gundersen and Hauge in 1963[35] found that 43 per cent of the relatives of women and 19 per cent of the relatives of men had varicose veins. Although this prevalence is higher than that expected in the general population, it is far less than that expected from a true dominant inheritance. These authors conclude that the inheritance of varicose veins is polygeneric. Recently, Munn *et al.*,[69] have reported a family history of varicose veins of almost 80 per cent in their patients admitted for surgery for long saphenous vein incompetence. Surprisingly, we have been unable to find any evidence in the medical literature of the incidence of varicose veins in twins, where detailed studies might help to elucidate the mechanism of inheritance.

Summary of factors responsible for primary varicose veins

Inherited structural weakness with a possible but as yet unidentified haemodynamic factor appears to be the main cause of primary varicose veins. Age, female sex, parity, race and occupation may all contribute to the development of varicose veins. A much weaker case exists for the role of height, weight, alcohol, and tight underclothes.

Secondary varicose veins are caused by post-thrombotic damage, pelvic tumours, especially pregnancy, congenital abnormalities (Klippel-Trenaunay syndrome, and congenital valvular agenesis) and acquired (Fig. 5.9) or congenital arteriovenous fistulae (Fig. 5.10).

The pathology of varicose veins

Histological studies on varicose veins[87,109] have shown that the most striking change is an increase in fibrous tissue which invades the media, breaking up the smooth muscle layers into a number of separate bundles. Collagen and fibrous tissue also accumulate in the subintima, and the elastic fibres tend to be spread throughout the layers of the vein wall instead of being restricted to the internal and external elastic laminae (Fig. 5.11). All these changes have a patchy distribution.

On electron microscopy the smooth muscle cells are seen to contain excessive numbers of granules but the significance of these granules is not known. It has been suggested[87] that the granules contain collagenase and elastase which, when secreted by the smooth muscle cells, may

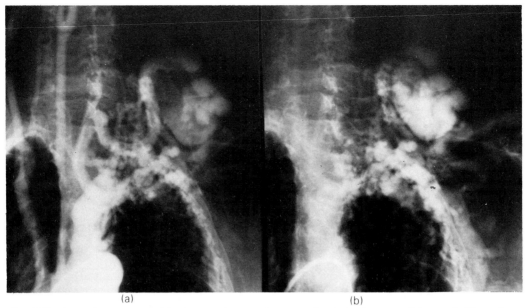

(a)   (b)

Fig. 5.9   An arch aortogram (a) of a massive arteriovenous fistula in the root of the neck. The venous phase (b) shows a large mass of secondary varicose veins.

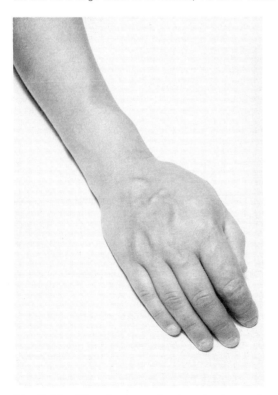

Fig. 5.10   Dilated tortuous 'varicose' veins on the back of the hand secondary to a congenital arteriovenous fistula.

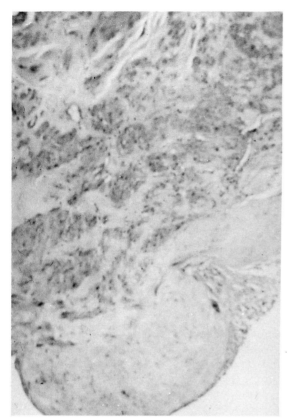

Fig. 5.11 A photomicrograph of the wall of a varicose vein showing collagen fibres extending throughout all layers of the wall breaking up the muscle of the media.

(We are indebted to Mr S Rose for this illustration.)

cause weakening of the wall which in turn leads to dilatation. The loss of muscle cells and their replacement by connective tissue appears to be the main pathological process associated with varicosity.

Smooth muscle hypertrophy has also been found in the wall of varicose veins. Histochemical studies performed on varicose veins with smooth muscle hypertrophy suggest that the hypertrophic muscle depends on anaerobic glycolysis for its metabolic requirements.[105] When, however, the reaction of venous smooth muscle to distension was studied in the walls of normal and varicose veins no significant differences could be found.[99] This appears to exclude a primary abnormality of the smooth muscle as a cause of varicosity.

Valves

The valves of varicose veins become stretched and, in the later stages of vein distention, atrophic.[20] In grossly dilated varices there is often evidence of thrombosis on the valve cusps which may become calcified.

The anatomical distribution of the varices

Although the long saphenous system of veins is most frequently affected, the main trunk (stem) vein only rarely becomes varicose, and it is the tributaries of the long saphenous vein that dilate (Fig. 5.12). The long saphenous vein itself may be protected by its well-developed muscular media and a layer of fibrous tissue which binds it to the deep fascia.[99]

The tributaries of the long saphenous vein contain relatively less muscle in their walls and lie unsupported in the subcutaneous fat close to the skin. This combination of a lack of support with relative weakness of the muscle wall probably explains the frequency with which the tributaries dilate.

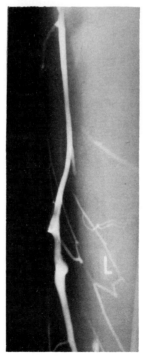

Fig. 5.12 A varicogram showing dilatation and tortuosity of the long saphenous vein itself, a relatively unusual finding.

The cause of tortuosity

The explanation for the development of tortuosity as opposed to dilatation is obscure. Many rivers follow a course that is remarkably similar to a tortuous varicose vein, and it has been argued that the changes in flow that are responsible for the meanders and curves of a river also cause tortuosity in veins. Nylander[74] has argued that venous dilatation and tortuosity are caused by an increased blood flow but the transmural pressure may also be relevant. Turbulent flow has also been incriminated,[29] and it is possible that localized dilatation produces turbulent flow which in turn is responsible for the development of tortuosity.[95] Haemodynamic influences may not be involved at all. If the vein wall is weak enough to allow dilatation, it will also allow elongation. The tortuosity may just be further evidence of wall weakness allowing stretching to occur both in a circumferential and longitudinal direction.

Changes in the muscle layers

Venous muscle is arranged as a thin outer circular layer which surrounds a thicker longitudinal muscle layer whose fibres turn outward to interdigitate with the inner layers of the circular muscle.[87] The circular muscle consists of cells arranged in regular whorls between a fine connective tissue matrix. There is also a poorly developed outer longitudinal muscle layer whose fibres extend out into the adventitia. All these layers are spirally arranged, so it is possible that as the vein wall stretches it may take on a serpiginous appearance. Cotton,[20] in his casts of long saphenous veins, found that many of the varices were distributed along the length of the vein in a spiral configuration often with the varices projecting from alternate sides of the vein. He suggested that when a vein becomes varicose, it twists, rotating the valves and that this is responsible for the spiral appearances of the varices. These observations bring to mind Hasebroek's experiments[36,37] on the ability of pulsatile flow to induce varicosities in a latex tube which Cotton was able to reproduce when he inserted a stenosis into the tube.

The intima and adventitia

Deposition of collagen has been observed[87] in the deeper layers of the intima and media, and collagen fibrils have been seen within intimal smooth muscle cells which is indicative of collagen phagocytosis. This may be a possible mechanism for collagen breakdown and remodelling of the vein wall.[44]

Enzymatic changes in the wall   The alteration of hexosamine production by the vein wall has already been discussed (see p. 156). Collagenase, elastase, maleate dehydrogenase, non specific esterases, adenosine triphosphate and 5-nucleotidases[96,97] are all said to be reduced in varicose veins when compared with normal veins, while acid phosphatase and lactic dehydrogenase have been found to be elevated.[102]

Plasminogen activator   The level of tissue plasminogen activator is reduced in varicose veins compared with normal controls (Fig. 5.13),[52,108] and recently it has been shown that monoclonal and polyclonal plasminogen activator antibodies localize to the smooth muscle of vein wall in addition to the endothelial cells.[52] The reduction in plasminogen activator levels found in varicose veins may therefore be the result of poor activator production by defective or damaged smooth muscle cells. It is unlikely that low levels of activator are the cause of varicosities.

Prostacyclin   Prostacyclin causes contraction

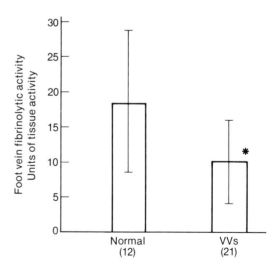

*Significantly different from normal ($P = 0.006$)

Fig. 5.13   The fibrinolytic activity of the foot veins of 21 patients with varicose veins (VVs) compared with 12 control normal subjects. Varicose veins are shown to contain significantly less plasminogen activator in the vein wall than normal veins.

of the smooth muscle of both normal and varicose veins.[93] It is conceivable that a deficiency in prostacylin production might be involved in the development of varicose veins.

Lysozymes It has been suggested that an increase in lysosomal enzymes[48] may dissolve ground substance and so cause varicosity. Blood levels of proteoglycans have been found to be raised in the serum of patients with varicose veins compared with the levels in normal controls.

Changes in the calf muscle Makitie[60] has found changes in the striated muscle of the calf pump in patients with varicose veins. He has not shown whether these changes are primary or secondary to the varicose veins.

The complications of varicose veins

The pathology of the complications such as superficial thrombophlebitis, eczema, pigmentation, lipodermatosclerosis, haemorrhage, ulceration and an increased risk of deep vein thrombosis are discussed in detail in Chapters 12, 16, and 22.

References

1. Ackroyd JS, Lea Thomas M, Browse NL. Deep vein reflux: an assessment by descending phlebography. *Br J Surg* 1986; **73**: 31.
2. Ackroyd JS, Pattison M, Browse NL. A study of the mechanical properties of fresh and preserved human femoral vein wall and valve cusps. *Br J Surg* 1985; **72**: 117.
3. Alexander CJ. The epidemiology of varicose veins. *Med J Aust* 1972; **1**: 215.
4. Andreotti L, Cammelli D, Banchi G, Guarnieri M, Serantoni C. Collagen, elastin and sugar content in primary varicose veins. *Ric Clin Lab* 1978; **8**: 273.
5. Arnoldi CC. The heredity of venous insufficiency. *Dan Med Bull* 1958; **5**: 169.
6. Barbaro G, Guerrina G, Traverso G, Vota L. Determinazione quantitativa del collagene e delle frazioni del connettivo nella varice idiopatica. *Pathologica* 1967; **59**: 871.
7. Basmajian JV. The distribution of valves in the femoral, external iliac and common iliac veins and their relationship to varicose veins. *Surg Gynec Obstet* 1952; **95**: 537.
8. Beaglehole R, Salmond Clare E, Prior IAM. Varicose veins in New Zealand. Prevalence and severity. *NZ Med J* 1976; **84**: 396.
9. Bennett WH. Congenital sacculations and cystic dilations of veins. *Lancet* 1890; **1**: 788.
10. Berge TH, Feldthusen U. Varicer hos kvinner. Faktorer av betydelse för deras uppkomst. *Nord Med* 1963; **69**: 744.
11. Bobek K, Cajzl L, Cepelak V, Slaisova V, Opatrny K, Barcal R. Etude de la fréquence des maladies phlébologiques et de l'influence de quelques facteurs étiologiques. *Phlébologie* 1966; **19**: 217.
12. Borschberg E. *The Prevalence of Varicose Veins of the Lower Extremity.* Basle. S Karger 1967.
13. Brewer AC. Arteriovenous shunts. *Br Med J* 1950; **2**: 270.
14. Burkitt DP. Varicose veins, deep vein thrombosis, and haemorrhoids: epidemiology and suggested aetiology. *Br Med J* 1972; **2**: 556.
15. Burnand KG, Clemenson G, Whimpster I, Gaunt J, Browse NL. The effect of sustained venous hypertension on the skin capillaries of the canine hind limb. *Br J Surg* 1982; **69**: 41.
16. Burnand KG. *Studies on the Cause of Venous Ulceration.* London University MS Thesis. 1981.
17. Callender GW. Diseases of the veins. In: Holmes T (Ed). *System of Surgery.* London. Parker and Bourn 1862.
18. Cleave TL. *On the Causation of Varicose Veins and their Prevention and Arrest by Natural Means.* Bristol. Wright 1960.
19. Cockett FB, Lea Thomas M, Negus D. Iliac vein compression: its relation to ilio-femoral thrombosis and the post thrombotic syndrome. *Br Med J* 1967; **2**: 14.
20. Cotton L. Varicose veins: gross anatomy and development. *Br J Surg* 1961; **48**: 589.
21. de Takats G, Quint H. The injection treatment of varicose veins. *Surg Gynec Obstet* 1930; **50**: 545.
22. DeSilva A, Widmer LK, Martin H, Mall TH, Glaus L, Schneider M. Varicose veins and chronic venous insufficiency. *Vasa* 1974; **3**: 118.
23. Dodd HJ. The cause, prevention and arrest of varicose veins. *Lancet* 1964; **2**: 809.
24. Dodd H, Wright HP. Vulval varicose veins in pregnancy. *Br Med J* 1959; **1**: 831.
25. Donato VM, Nejamkim J. Varices y embarazo. Su tratamiento. *Prensa Med Argent* 1952; **43**: 551.
26. Duchosal F, Allemann H, Widmer LK, Breil H, Leu HJ. Varikosis – Alter – Körpergewicht. *Z Kreislaufforsch* 1968; **57**: 380.
27. Edwards JE, Edwards EA. The saphenous valves in varicose veins. *Am Heart J* 1940; **19**: 338.
28. Eger SA, Casper SL. Etiology of varicose veins from an anatomic aspect based on dissections of 38 adult cadavers. *JAMA* 1943; **123**: 148.
29. Fegan WG, Kline AL. The cause of varicosity in

superficial veins of the lower limb. *Br J Surg* 1972; **59**: 798.

30. Fegan WG. Anatomy and pathophysiology of varicose veins. In: *Venous Diseases Medical and Surgical Management*. Montreux. Foundation International Corporation, Medical Sciences 1974.

31. Foote RR. *Varicose Veins*. London. Butterworths 1954.

32. Gay J. *On Varicose Diseases of the Lower Extremities. The Lettsomian lectures of 1867*. London. Churchill 1868.

33. General Register Office: *Studies on medical and population subjects. Number 12. The survey of sickness 1943–52*. Logan WPD, Brooke EM. London 1957.

34. Gjöres JE. The incidence of venous thrombosis and its sequelae in certain districts of Sweden. *Acta Chir Scand* (Suppl) 1956; **206**.

35. Gundersen J, Hauge M. Hereditary factors in venous insufficiency. *Angiology* 1969; **20**: 346.

36. Hasebroek K. Über die Bedeutung der Arterienpulsationen für die Strömung in den Venen und die Pathogenese der Varicen. *Pflügers Arch Ges Physiol* 1916; **163**: 191.

37. Hasebroek K. Eine physikalisch-experimentell begründete neue Auffassung der Pathogenese der Varicen. *Deutsche Ztschr Chir* 1916; **136**: 381.

38. Hobbs J. Surgery and sclerotherapy in the treatment of varicose veins. A random trial. *Arch Surg* 1974; **109**: 793.

39. Hobsley M. *Pathways in Surgical Management*. 2nd edition London. Edward Arnold. 1986; 196.

40. Holman EF. Development of arterial aneurysms. *Surg Gynec Obstet* 1955; **100**: 599.

41. *Illness and Health Care in Canada. Canadian Sickness Survey 1950–1951*. The Department of National Health and Welfare and the Dominion Bureau of Statistics. Ottawa 1960.

42. Jager A. Venenklappen und muskelkontraktion. *Pflügers Arch Ges Physiol* 1936; **238**: 508.

43. Jensen DR. Varicose veins and their treatment. *Ann Surg* 1932; **95**: 738.

44. Jurukova Z, Milenkov C. Ultrastructural evidence for collagen degradation in the walls of varicose veins. *Exp Mol Pathol* 1982; **37**: 37.

45. Kilbourne NJ. Varicose veins in pregnancy. *Am J Obstet Gynecol* 1933; **25**: 104.

46. King ESJ. The genesis of varicose veins. *Aust NZ J Surg* 1950; **20**: 126.

47. Klotz K. Untersuchungern, über die Saphena Magna beim Menschen besonders zücksichtlich ihrer Klappenverhältnisse. *Arch Anat Physiol (Lpz)* 1887; **3**: 159.

48. Kreysel HW, Nissen HP, Enghofer E. A possible role of lysosomal enzymes in the pathogenesis of varicosis and the reduction in their serum activity by Venostasin. *Vasa* 1983; **12**: 377.

49. Kulka JP. In: Hill AGA (Ed) *Modern Trends in Rheumatology*. Vol 1. London. Butterworths 1966.

50. Lake M, Pratt GH, Wright IS. Arteriosclerosis and varicose veins: Occupational activities and other factors. *JAMA* 1942; **119**: 696.

51. Larsen RA, Smith FL. Varicose veins: evaluation of observations in 491 cases. *Proc Mayo Clin* 1943; **18**: 400.

52. Layer GT, Pattison M, Evans B, Davies DR, Burnand KG. Tissue fibrinolytic activity is reduced in varicose veins. In Negus D, Jantet G (Eds) *Phlebology '85*. London. John Libbey 1986.

53. Ledderhose G. Studien über den Blutlauf in der Hautvenen unter physiologischen und Pathologischen Bedingungen. *Mitt Grenzgeb Med Chir* 1906; **15**: 355.

54. Lindvall N, Lodin A. Congenital absence of venous valves. *Acta Chir Scand* 1962; **124**: 310.

55. Lodin A, Lindvall N, Gentele H. Congenital absence of venous valves as a cause of leg ulcers. *Acta Chir Scand* 1959; **116**: 256.

56. Löwenstein A. Über die Venenklappen und Varicenbildung. *Mitt Grenzgeb Med Chir* 1907; **18**: 161.

57. Ludbrook J. Obesity and varicose veins. *Surg Gynec Obstet* 1964; **118**: 843.

58. Ludbrook J. Valvular defect in primary varicose veins. Cause or effect? *Lancet* 1963; **2**: 1289.

59. Magnus G. Zirkulationsverhältnisse in varicen. *Dtsch Z Chir* 1921; **162**: 71.

60. Makitie J. Muscle changes in patients with varicose veins. *Acta Pathol Microbiol Scand* (A) 1977; **85**: 864.

61. Martin A, Odling-Smee W. Pressure changes in varicose veins. *Lancet* 1976; **1**: 768.

62. May R, Thurner J. The cause of the predominately sinistral occurence of thrombosis of the pelvic veins. *Angiology* 1957; **8**: 419.

63. McCausland AM. Influence of hormones upon varicose veins. *West J Surg* 1943; **51**: 199.

64. McPhetters HO, Anderson JK. *Injection Treatment of Varicose Veins and Haemorrhoids* Philadelphia. Davis 1946.

65. Mekky S, Schilling RSF, Walford J. Varicose veins in women cotton workers. An epidemiological study in England and Egypt. *Br Med J* 1969; **2**: 591.

66. Miyauchi K. Die Häufigkeit der varizen am unterschenkel bei Japanem und der Erfolg einiger operativ beihandelter Fälle. *Arch Klin Chir* 1913; **100**: 1079.

67. Moore HD. Deep venous valves in the aetiology of varicose veins. *Lancet* 1951; **2**: 7.

68. Mullane DJ. Varicose veins of pregnancy. *Am J Obstet Gynecol* 1952; **63**: 620.

69. Munn SR, Morton JB, Macbeth WAAG, McLeish AR. To strip or not strip the long saphenous vein? A varicose vein trial. *Br J Surg* 1981; **68**: 426.

70. Murley RS. Deep venous valves in the aetiology of varicose veins. *Lancet* 1951; **1**: 176.

71. Myers TT. Varicose veins. In: Barker, Hines (Eds) *Barker and Hines's Peripheral Vascular Diseases* 3rd edition. Philadelphia, Saunders 1962.

72. Nabatoff RA. Varicose veins of pregnancy. *JAMA* 1960; **174**: 1712.

73. Nicholson BB. Varicose veins etiology and treatment. *Arch Surg* 1927; **15**: 351.

74. Nylander G. Meanders of the great saphenous vein. *Angiology* 1969; **20**: 587.

75. Ottley C. Heredity and varicose veins. *Br Med J* 1934; **1**: 528.

76. Payne RT. The treatment of varicose diseases of the lower limbs. *Br Med J* 1936; **1**: 877.

77. Pigeaux ALJ. *Traite Practique des Maladies des Vaisseaux Contenant des Recherches Historiques Speciales*. Paris. Labe et Rouvier 1843.

78. Pirner F. *Der variköse Symptomen-komplex*. Stuttgart 1957.

79. Powell T, Lynn RB. The valves of the external iliac, femoral and upper third of the popliteal veins. *Surg Gynec Obstet* 1951; **92**: 453.

80. Pratt GH. Arterial varices: a syndrome. *Am J Surg* 1949; **77**: 456.

81. Pratt GH. Differential diagnosis and treatment of pathologically enlarged veins. *Med Clin N Amer* 1950; **34**: 897.

82. Prerovskly I. *Diseases of the Veins*. World Health Organization, internal communication. MHO-PA 10964.

83. Puilacks P, Vidal Barraquer F. Pathogenic study of varicose veins. *Angiology* 1953; **4**: 59.

84. Reikeras O, Sorlie D. The significance of arteriovenous shunting for the development of varicose veins. *Acta Chir Scand* 1983; **149**: 479.

85. Rindfleisch E. *Lehrbuch der Pathologischen Gewebelehre* 6th edition. Leipzig. Engelmann 1867.

86. Rokitansky C. *A Manual of Pathological Anatomy*. Vol 4. London, Sydenham Society 1852.

87. Rose SS, Ahmed A. Some thoughts on the aetiology of varicose veins. *J Cardiovasc Surg* 1986; **27**: 534.

88. Ryan TJ, Copeman PWM. The microvascular system. *Br J Dermatol* 1969; **81**: 563.

89. Santler R, Ernst G, Weiel B. Statistisches über der varikösen symptomenkomplex. *Hautarzt* 1956; **10**: 460.

90. Schwarz E. Die Krampfadern der unteren Extremität mit besonderer Berücksichtigung ihrer Entstehung und Behandlung. *Ergebn Chir Orthop* 1934; **27**: 256.

91. Seidell JC, Oosterlee A, Deurenberg P, Hautvast JGAJ. What causes varicose veins? *Lancet* 1986; **1**: 321.

92. *The Sickness Survey of Denmark*. The committee on the Danish national morbidity survey. Copenhagen. 1960.

93. Sinzinger H, Fitscha P. Prostacyclin (PGI$_2$) contracts normal and varicose human saphenous veins. *Vasa* 1984; **13**: 228.

94. Slawinski Z. Przyczynek do anatomii zylaków konczyny dolnej; o umiejscowieniu rozszerzen woreczkowatych zyly podskornej uda wielkiej. *Gaz Lek Warsz* 1899; **19**: 1355.

95. Somerville J, Byrne P, King D. Turbulence in the causation of varicose veins. *Br J Surg* 1973; **60**: 311.

96. Svejcar J, Prerovsky I, Linhart J, Kruml J. Content of collagen, elastin, and water in walls of the internal saphenous vein in man. *Circ Res* 1962; **11**: 296.

97. Svejcar J, Prerovsky I, Linhart J, Kruml J. Content of collagen, elastin and hexosamine in primary varicose veins. *Clin Sci* 1963; **24**: 325.

98. Tannyol A, Menduke H. Alcohol as a possible etiological agent in varicose veins. *Angiology* 1961; **12**: 382.

99. Thompson H. The surgical anatomy of the superficial and perforating veins of the lower limb. *Ann R Coll Surg Engl* 1979; **61**: 198.

100. Thulesius O, Gjöres JE. Reactions of venous smooth muscle in normal men and patients with varicose veins. *Angiology* 1974; **25**: 145.

101. Trendelenburg F. Über die unterbindung der vena saphena magna bie unterschenkel varicen. *Beitr Klin Chir* 1891; **7**: 195.

102. Urbanova D, Prerovsky I. Enzymes in the wall of normal and varicose veins. Histochemical study. *Angiologica* 1972; **9**: 53.

103. US Department of Health, *Education and Welfare: National Health Survey 1935–1936*. Washington DC. 1938.

104. Virchow R. *Cellular Pathology*. London. Churchill 1860.

105. Wegmann R, El Samannoudy FA, Olivier C, Rettori R. Histochemical studies on the wall of human varicose veins: the saphenous varicose vein. *Ann Histochim* 1974; **19**: 285.

106. Widmer LK. *Peripheral Venous Disorders. Prevalence and Socio-medical Importance. Observations in 4529 apparently Healthy Persons. Basle III Study*. Bern. Hans Huber 1978.

107. Williams AF. A comparative study of venous valves in the limbs. *Surg Gynec Obstet* 1954; **99**: 676.

108. Wolfe JHN, Morland M, Browse NL. The fibri-

nolytic activity of varicose veins. *Br J Surg* 1979; **66**: 185.

109. Zancani A. Über die Varicen der unteren Extremitäten; experimentelle und klinische Untersuchungen. *Arch Klin Chir* 1911; **96**: 91.

110. Zwillenberg LO, Laszt L, Zwillenberg H. Die Fienstruktur der Venenwand bei Varikose. *Angiologica* 1971; **8**: 318.

6

Varicose veins: diagnosis

The symptoms caused by varicose veins

The major symptoms caused by varicose veins are summarized in Table 6.1; other conditions which may give similar appearances are listed in Table 6.2.

Unsightliness

Many patients with varicose veins complain of the unsightliness produced by tortuous dilated veins

Table 6.1 Symptoms caused by varicose veins

Unsightliness
Aches and pains
Mild ankle oedema
Superficial thrombophlebitis
Haemorrhage
Eczema
Pigmentation
Lipodermatosclerosis
Ulceration

Table 6.2 Differential diagnosis of varicose veins

Visible veins
Post-thrombotic collateral veins
Klippel–Trenaunay syndrome
Parkes–Weber syndrome
Arteriovenous fistula or fistulae (congenital or acquired)
Avalvular disease of the deep veins (congenital absence)
Dilated cutaneous venules
Pelvic tumours causing venous obstruction
Venous angiomata
Herniation of the anterior tibial muscle through the fascia
Dilated veins of pregnancy

in their lower limbs. Women are more aware of varicose veins than men, because even today, with the exception of a few countries, men tend to cover their legs with long trousers while women expose their legs by wearing skirts. The desire to have legs without blemish, whether for personal 'body-image' or sexual motives, is the main cause of the increasing demand for the treatment of varicose veins.

Patients concerned with the unsightly appearance of their varicose veins often complain of discomfort but the severity of this discomfort is difficult to assess and does not seem to be related to the size of the varices.[7] Massive varicosities in men often cause few symptoms while minor varicosities in women may be the source of intractable pain. Perhaps patients wishing treatment for cosmetic reasons assuage their conscience by convincing themselves that they are suffering pain, or perhaps pain is unrelated to the size of the varicosities.

Some patients without any obvious tortuosity or elevation of their subcutaneous veins ask for treatment, and it is sometimes difficult to decide when a 'visible vein' becomes a 'varicose vein' (Fig. 6.1). These patients often state on the day when they attend the clinic that the veins have 'gone down' and do not represent their true appearance. In women the size of the varices may alter with the menstrual cycle and varices may also increase in size in very warm weather. It is best to ask such patients to return for review in 3–6 months when the veins may have become more obvious.

The other group of patients who complain of severe disfigurement are those with dilated intradermal venules ('spider veins', 'venous stars', 'sunburst veins', or 'cutaneous arborizing telangiectases') (Fig. 6.2, Colour plate 1). These are

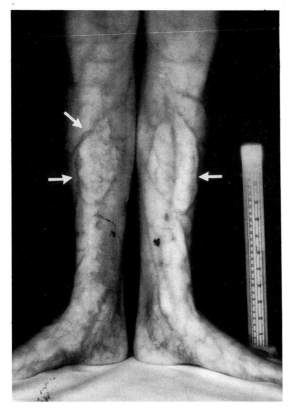

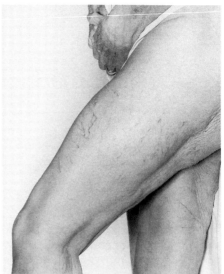

Fig. 6.2 Cutaneous telangiectases in the skin of the thigh. These dilated skin venules are more common in women than in men and may develop during pregnancy. They have been called 'spider veins', 'venous stars' and 'sunburst veins' and a number of other descriptive terms including 'birch-twigs'.

Fig. 6.1 An infrared photograph which shows many visible but straight subcutaneous veins. One vein on the front of the left shin is dilated but straight (arrowed) whereas another on the right shin (arrowed) is tortuous but not dilated. Varicose veins are both tortuous and dilated.

not true varicose veins. They are frequently associated with varicose veins but are a separate, distinct, independent entity. They often develop during pregnancy or at the menopause which suggests that they may be caused by a change in hormone levels. They are far more common in women and may extend to cover the whole leg, turning the skin a deep blue–purple colour. Their exact cause remains obscure.

Aches and pains

This is the most common symptom to accompany the complaint of unsightliness and has already been discussed. Many patients will admit, on close questioning, that their pain is minor and infrequent and that the real reason for consultation is because they dislike the appearance of their legs.

Many patients do, however, experience considerable discomfort which is sometimes localized to the main varices, but is often a diffuse dull ache felt throughout the leg which gets worse as the day passes and is exacerbated by prolonged standing.

Pain that is present at rest or in bed is unlikely to be caused by varicose veins, and another source must be sought. The typical description of 'venous' pain is an 'ache' or 'discomfort'. The presence of a sharp or acute pain should suggest an alternative diagnosis.

Relief of the discomfort by wearing an elastic stocking provides good circumstantial evidence that the pain is of venous origin. We sometimes use this as a diagnostic test when uncertain if varicose veins are the cause of leg pain. Elevation of the legs, bedrest and walking all relieve venous pain, while standing still for prolonged periods invariably makes it worse.

A history of a bursting pain during exercise (venous claudication) may indicate venous outflow obstruction but is a rare symptom in patients with uncomplicated varicose veins.

Night cramps are a common complaint but appear to be particularly frequent in patients with

Table 6.3 Some of the causes of discomfort in the leg which must be differentiated from varicose vein pain

Osteoarthritis of the hip
Osteoarthritis of the knee
Sciatica and spinal claudication
Sarcomata of soft tissue or bone
Osteomyelitis
Osteoid osteoma
Tears of the menisci of the knee joint
Achilles tendonitis
Torn Achilles tendon
Rheumatoid arthritis
Intermittent claudication (arterial)
Venous claudication
Cramp
Myalgia
Peripheral neuropathy
Meralgia paraesthetica
Neuromas
Lymphoedema

varicose veins, especially after a long day of standing without exercise.

Table 6.3 lists the other causes of leg pain that may be incorrectly ascribed to varicose veins. A careful history of the nature of the leg pain, followed by a meticulous clinical examination will often help to indicate its cause. Some leg pains, however, defy all attempts at diagnosis in spite of phlebography, arteriography, radiculography, electromyography and computerized tomography.

Ankle oedema

Oedema is not a common or prominent feature of varicose veins. It is usually mild and only becomes noticeable at the end of the day. If there is marked oedema and the patient complains of swelling of the lower leg as well as the ankle, other causes of oedema such as deep vein obstruction or lymphatic obstruction must be excluded.

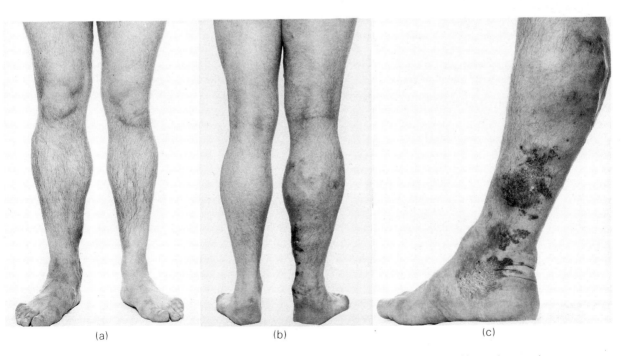

(a)   (b)   (c)

Fig. 6.3 (a–c) These photographs show swelling of the right calf and ankle caused by varicose veins. Swelling is not a common symptom of uncomplicated varicose veins. (a) A few dilated veins can just be seen on the anterior view of the swollen right leg. (b) The posterior view shows lipodermatosclerosis and the swelling. (c) The medial view shows skin pigmentation and dilated calf varicosities caused by incompetent communicating veins in the medial calf.

Table 6.4   Causes of ankle oedema

Local
Acute deep vein thrombosis
Post-thrombotic deep vein damage
Venous obstruction
Venous valvular agenesis
Lymphoedema
Lipodystrophy
Hemihypertrophy

General
Cardiac failure
Nephrotic syndrome
Hypoalbuminaemia
Fluid overload
Fluid retention syndromes

Incompetence of the lower leg communicating veins in isolation or in association with post-thrombotic damage of the deep veins can cause moderate oedema of the ankle and lower leg (Fig. 6.3), especially in elderly obese patients who take little exercise.

Table 6.4 lists the causes of ankle swelling. Lymphoedema is the condition most commonly misdiagnosed as venous oedema (Fig. 6.4). Isotope or radiographic contrast lymphangiography is often needed to confirm a diagnosis of lymphoedema, and the general causes of oedema must not be forgotten. Fat does not pit with digital pressure (Fig. 6.5). Hemihypertrophy, which may be suspected when the limb and foot are enlarged, can be confirmed by computerized tomography.

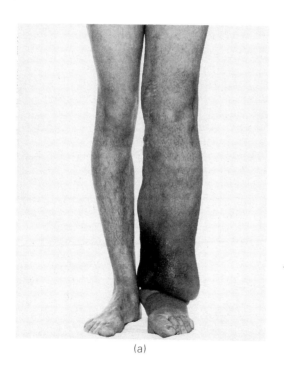

(a)

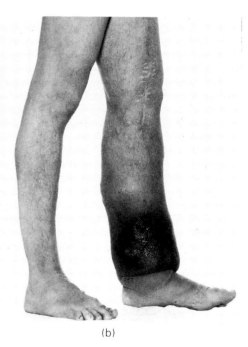

(b)

Fig. 6.4 (a and b)   This swollen limb shows evidence of lipodermatosclerosis (pigmentation, induration and inflammation).
   A few varicose veins are visible, but phlebography was essentially normal. Radiographic lymphography showed peripheral lymphatic obliteration. All the visible changes were caused by the lymphoedema.

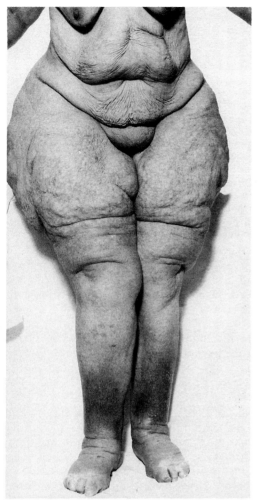

Fig. 6.5 A lady with marked lipodystrophy. This is an abnormal and excessive deposition of fat in the lower half of the body causing apparent swelling, in this patient mainly of the thighs and buttocks. There is mild secondary lymphoedema and lipodermatosclerosis. Fat does not pit on pressure.

Superficial thrombophlebitis

This is a common complication of varicose veins but must be differentiated from superficial thrombophlebitis caused by other conditions (see Chapter 22). Thrombophlebitis usually presents as a tender hot red thickening on the course of a varicose vein. Patients usually know that they have varicose veins, and they may have had previous episodes of thrombophlebitis. The attack may be initiated by an episode of minor trauma or a period of bedrest but in many instances no predisposing cause is found, other than the presence of a varicose vein. The inflamed vein is usually extremely painful and tender, and the patient may be pyrexial and feel unwell.

Haemorrhage

A varicose vein may bleed after injury and can occasionally bleed spontaneously. Large veins are easily knocked or cut and, if this occurs, they can bleed profusely for a short time. Despite their apparent vulnerability, it is surprising how well the overlying skin protects most varicose veins from injury.

'Spontaneous' rupture of a varix may cause bleeding from the skin surface or into the subcutaneous tissues. Elderly patients with thin-walled veins are particularly at risk. The bleeding usually comes from one of the small intradermal veins near the ankle and may be profuse and even life-threatening. The high venous pressure at the ankle during standing is presumably responsible for a 'true' spontaneous rupture of a surface varix but minor trauma is invariably involved. The patient may be unaware of the rupture until they feel a sensation of 'wetness' as blood runs down the leg or they begin to feel faint.

Subcutaneous bleeding in elderly people with weak veins, causing bruises and petechiae, is common but rarely of clinical importance, though it may frighten and distress the patient.

Ulcers overlying subcutaneous varicosities near the ankle can bleed in a similar manner to the spontaneous variceal rupture already described,[23] and it has been suggested that local steroidal medications applied to the ulcer may increase the risk of bleeding.[18] It is important to ensure that another lesion on the leg is not responsible for the bleeding and to exclude any haematological abnormality which could be responsible for a bleeding tendency. These patients are usually old and, if they are unfortunate enough to faint in a sitting position, the bleeding continues, whereas if they fall to the ground, so lowering the venous pressure, the bleeding usually stops spontaneously. The mistaken application to the leg of a tourniquet which is not tight enough to occlude the arteries but which is sufficient to cause venous congestion may enhance rather than reduce the rate of bleeding.

In a survey published in 1971,[23] 23 deaths were

reported as the result of haemorrhage from varicose veins.

Eczema, pigmentation, lipodermatosclerosis and ulceration

These complications of varicose veins are discussed in detail in Chapters 12 and 14 on the post-thrombotic syndrome and venous ulceration.

It is important to ask patients if they have ever had a deep vein thrombosis or leg ulcer and to also question them about the duration of skin discoloration or induration around the ankle. Many patients who complain of varicose veins may fail to notice minor skin changes in the lower leg which should be detected on physical examination.

Family history

The age of onset of the varicosities should be recorded and any family history of varicose veins noted. Varicose veins occurring in a patient under 20 years of age suggests the possibility of a congenital abnormality such as the Klippel–Trenaunay syndrome, valvular agenesis, or a congenital arteriovenous fistula (see Chapter 23). More than a third of the patients presenting with varicose veins have relatives who are also affected (see Chapter 5).

Past history

All patients presenting with varicose veins must be closely questioned about the possibility of a previous *deep vein thrombosis*. It is often necessary to ask additional direct questions about leg swelling after childbirth, previous operations, injuries (including fractures), or prolonged periods of bedrest. A history of chest pain, haemoptysis, or anticoagulant therapy provides good circumstantial evidence of a previous thrombosis but confirmation by phlebogram or lung scan obtained at the time of the event is even better.

Previous episodes of haemorrhage, superficial thrombophlebitis, acute lipodermatosclerosis, skin irritation and ulceration must also be recorded.

All past treatments for varicose veins and their complications must be documented with the dates and places where the treatment was given.

All past operations, serious injuries and ill-nesses must be noted together with a history of previous medication and known allergies.

General health

It is essential to enquire about the patient's general health and fitness as this will be important if surgical treatment of the varicose veins is contemplated, and it may also influence the method of treatment that is selected.

Comment

The history is of critical importance both in detecting conditions masquerading as varicose veins and in drawing attention to other systems that deserve examination. The overall picture of the patient's present and past health may have considerable bearing on the method of treatment that is selected. If the history suggests previous thromboembolism, particular care must be taken to record this in a prominent place so that the need for antithrombosis prophylaxis will not be forgotten if the patient is admitted to hospital.

Physical signs of varicose veins

A general examination of the patient, paying special attention to any system which the history indicates might be abnormal, is followed by a detailed examination of the lower limbs. This examination is best described in the traditional manner of 'inspection', 'palpation', 'percussion' and 'auscultation', but most clinicians quickly develop their own technique for examining varicose veins which does not necessarily follow this rigid pattern.

The examination should take place in a warm and well lit room which should preserve the privacy and respect the modesty of the patient.

A vaginal or rectal examination must always be performed, especially if there is ankle oedema or any suspicion of a pelvic tumour.

Inspection

The legs should be examined with the patient standing on a low stool or platform, suitably undressed to expose the whole of both lower limbs from the groins to the toes. Shoes, socks, stockings, trousers, dresses, skirts, shirts or

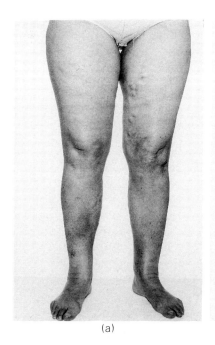

(a)

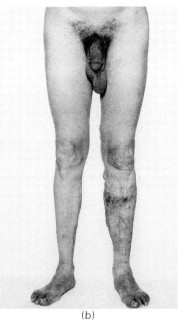

(b)

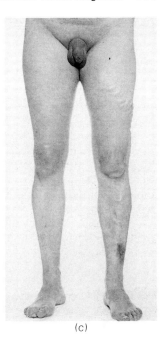

(c)

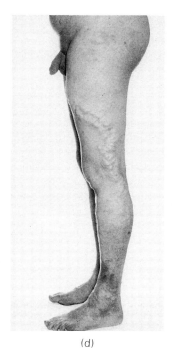

(d)

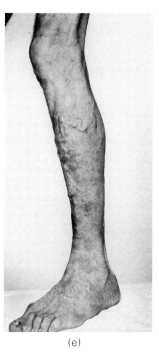

(e)

Fig. 6.6 (a–e) The common distribution of varicose veins.

(a) A varicose tributary lying over the course of the long saphenous vein on the medial side of the thigh. Varicosities in this position suggest long saphenous incompetence.

(b) This photograph also shows varicosities over the course of the long saphenous vein, mainly visible above and below the knee but not in the upper thigh.

Varicosities are also present over the front of the calf. The pigmentation and slight swelling suggests there may also be some incompetent medial calf communicating veins.

(c and d) A varicose antero-lateral thigh vein which is one of the two major tributaries of the long saphenous vein that join it near its termination. This tributary may become varicose without any evidence of long saphenous incompetence.

(e) Simple tributary varicosities on the front of the lower leg in a limb *without* evidence of incompetence of the long or short saphenous veins.

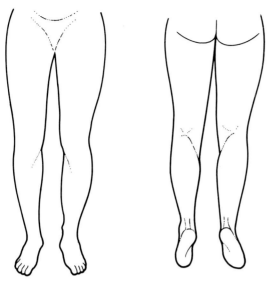

Fig. 6.7 Outline 'stamps' of the legs used in our clinic to record the distribution of the varicosities.

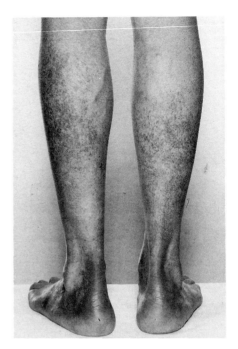

Fig. 6.9 Diffuse telangiectases over the back of both calves. Varicose veins are not present in either limb.

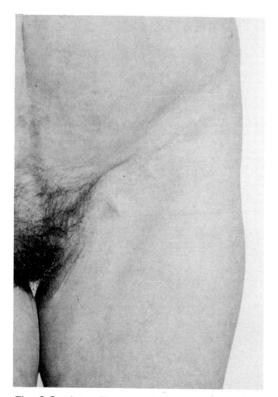

Fig. 6.8 A swelling over the termination of the long saphenous vein. The swelling disappeared on lying down and had a marked 'cough impulse'. A saphena varix.

blouses must be removed to ensure adequate exposure of the lower limbs.

The presence or absence of the following abnormalities should be recorded.

1. The distribution of all major subcutaneous varicosities (Fig. 6.6a–e).

Both limbs must be inspected from all aspects to ensure varicosities in the short saphenous territory are not missed. The distribution of the varicosities should be recorded on stamps or outline drawings of the leg, showing both the anterior and the posterior surfaces (Fig. 6.7). Particular note should be made of varicose veins in unusual positions (e.g. a large vein on the lateral side of the limb is often present in the Klippel–Trenaunay syndrome [Chapter 23, Fig. 23.12]).

2. The presence of a saphena varix (Fig. 6.8).
3. The presence of a capillary naevus (Chapter 23, Fig. 23.11).
4. The presence of dilated intradermal venules ('spider veins', or 'venous stars') (Figs. 6.2 and 6.9).

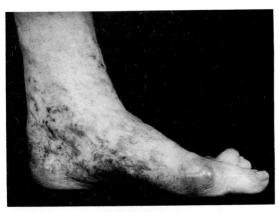

Fig. 6.10 An 'ankle flare' of dilated small venules in the skin beneath the malleolus. There are large varicose veins in the calf and there is early lipodermatosclerosis. This suggests persistant venous hypertension probably associated with incompetent calf communicating veins which are often the result of post-thrombotic damage. The ankle flare of dilated capillaries is also called the 'corona phlebectatica'.

5. The presence of any angiomatous malformations (Chapter 26, Fig. 26.2).
6. The presence of ankle oedema or limb swelling (Figs. 6.3 and 6.4).
7. The presence of an 'ankle flare' (corona phlebectatica) (Fig. 6.10, Colour plate 4).
8. The presence of large varicosities, 'blowouts', over known sites of communicating veins (Fig. 6.11).
9. The presence of acute and chronic lipodermatosclerosis (Colour plates 7 and 8).
10. The presence of eczema (Fig. 6.12, Colour plate 5).
11. The presence of ulceration (Fig. 6.13, Colour plates 10 to 13).
12. The presence of atrophie blanche or livedo reticularis (Fig. 6.14, Colour plate 9).
13. An increase in the length or circumference of the limb (Chapter 23, Figs. 23.13, 23.16 and 23.17).
14. Shortening of the limb or muscle wasting (Chapter 23, Fig. 23.25).
15. Evidence of swollen or deformed knee or hip joints (Chapter 23, Fig. 23.13).

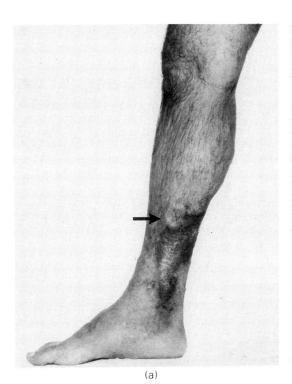

(a)

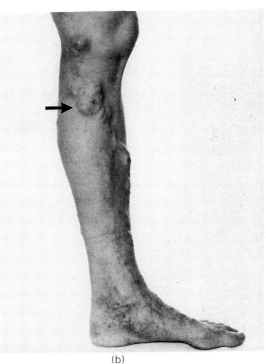

(b)

Fig. 6.11 (a) A limb with lipodermatosclerosis; a large 'blow-out' is situated just above the abnormal skin. This is over Cockett's 'middle calf' communicating vein.
(b) A limb with dilated varicosities overlying Boyd's communicating vein.

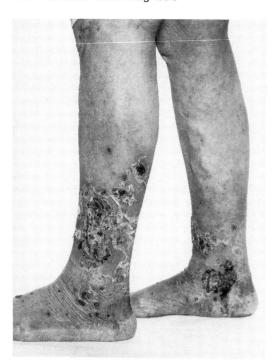

Fig. 6.12 Marked venous eczema over both gaiter regions. Varicosities can be seen on the medial surface of the right leg.

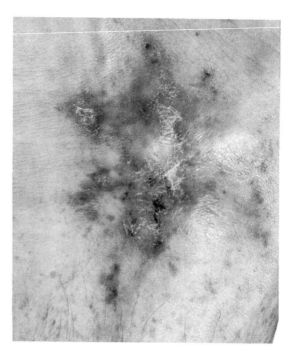

Fig. 6.14 An area of 'atrophie blanche' which appears as a 'white scar' often in an area of chronic lipodermatosclerosis and pigmentation.

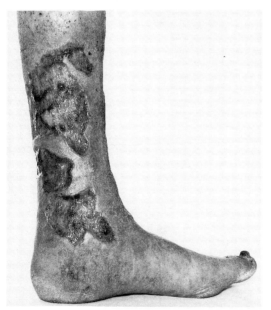

Fig. 6.13 A large irregularly shaped venous ulcer situated over the gaiter region of the leg.
There is marked lipodermatosclerosis in the skin around the ulcer; an 'ankle flare' is just visible beneath it.

16. Evidence of distended veins in the groin, pubic region or abdominal wall (Fig. 6.15).

It is helpful to have either a specially designed record card with a printed outline of the front and back of a pair of lower limbs, or re-usable ink stamps, of the same design, that can be stamped on the records and on which the distribution of the abnormalities found by inspection can be noted (Fig. 6.7). Individual varicosities and their connections (see Fig. 6.6a–f) should be accurately recorded on these charts.

Palpation and percussion

Some varicose veins are more easily felt than seen. For example, the upper end of a dilated long saphenous vein can often be felt along its course in the thigh between the groin and a lower dilated visible varicose tributary, even when it cannot be seen. A dilated short saphenous vein is invariably easier to feel than to see because it lies beneath the layer of fascia covering the popliteal fossa. The short saphenous vein is easier to palpate if the knee is slightly flexed to relax the deep fascia.

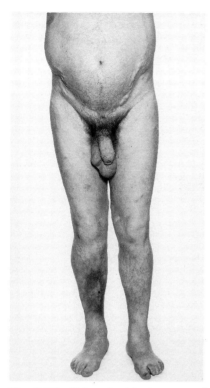

Fig. 6.15 This patient had an area of lipodermatosclerosis in the right calf but dilated superficial inferior epigastric veins suggested a diagnosis of ilio-caval obstruction, which was confirmed on phlebography.

After palpating the terminal segments of the long and short saphenous veins, the hand should be gently passed over the inner side of the thigh and leg and up the posterior surface of the calf to detect other sites of venous dilatation that might not have been detected on inspection.

Any difference in the temperature of the two limbs should also be recorded, and any firm subcutaneous cords, which are usually felt if there have been past episodes of superficial thrombophlebitis, should be noted.

Palpation of the 'gaiter' region may confirm the edge of plaque of indurated subcutaneous fat in an area of lipodermatosclerosis. This is not always obvious on inspection and may only be found by careful palpation. The degree of tenderness should also be recorded.

The cough impulse test[16] A visible or palpable venous expansion that occurs on coughing indicates the absence of competent valves between the right atrium and the vein under examination.

When this sign is detected in the groin over a large saphena varix (Fig. 6.8) it indicates long saphenous incompetence and may be accompanied by a palpable 'thrill' indicating turbulent retrograde flow. The presence of a 'thrill' is clear evidence of reflux, but patients who jerk or cough overvigorously can make the detection of an expansile venous cough impulse extremely difficult. A cough impulse is very difficult to detect in the very obese.

The percussion test (Schwartz test)[12,16,22] This consists of 'tapping' a varix with the finger-tip of one hand while the other hand palpates the termination of the long or short saphenous veins. The vein must be distended with blood for the impulse (or shock wave) to travel up the vein. The test should then be repeated in the opposite direction with the tap applied to the main vein and the examining hand placed over the varices. The vein must be incompetent for the impulse to be conducted down through the valves.

Palpation of fascial defects Cockett[14] originally suggested that large 'blow-out' veins in the calf indicated underlying incompetent communicating veins. The site at which a dilated communicating vein pierces the deep fascia can sometimes be felt as a 'gap' or 'defect' in the deep fascia.[31] This is an inaccurate method of locating incompetent communicating veins (see Tables 6.5, 6.6, 7, 6.8, 6.9, 6.10). Many of the palpable 'defects' are simply depressions or spaces in thickened subcutaneous fat occupied by a varix.

Sliding finger control Both Hobbs and Fegan[4,19,26] have suggested that incompetent communicating veins should be suspected if the veins, which have been emptied by leg elevation, can be prevented from refilling by one or more fingers placed over the suspected sites of communicating vein incompetence. The sites of incompetence can be confirmed by showing rapid venous refilling when the fingers are slid away from the 'points of control'; control should be regained when the fingers are slid back to their original positions.

This test is difficult to perform and interpret, and it only achieves acceptable accuracy when complete control is achieved by pressure at one site, indicating a single incompetent communicating vein.

Table 6.5   A comparison of the methods used to detect incompetent ankle communicating veins

	Method	Limbs	Suspected	Found	Mean no ICV*/limb
Miller & Foote[35]	Doppler	69	165	135	2.11
Foote et al.[21]	Doppler	30	106	94	3.13
Beesley & Fegan[4]	Clinical	32	90	46	1.44
Beesley & Fegan[4]	Thermography	32	102	40	1.25
Beesley & Fegan[4]	Phlebography	32	67	34	1.06
Patil et al.[43]	Clinical	66	83	50	0.78
Patil et al.[43]	Thermography	66	91	79	1.23
Chilvers & Thomas[13]	Fluorescein	27	54	50	1.40
Townsend et al.[51]	Clinical	46	112	72	1.50
Townsend et al.[51]	Phlebography	46	109	96	2.08
Nobel & Gunn[40]	Clinical	44	73	135	3.10
Nobel & Gunn[40]	Thermography	44	86	135	3.10
Nobel & Gunn[40]	Fluorescein	44	63	135	3.10
Callum et al.[9]	Clinical	45	78	51	2.40
Callum et al.[9]	Fluorescein	45	79	41	2.40
Callum et al.[9]	Phlebography	45	83	73	2.40
O'Donnell et al.[41]	Clinical	39	64	33	1.40
O'Donnell et al.[41]	Phlebography	39	40	33	1.40
O'Donnell et al.[41]	Doppler	39	83	39	1.40
Lamont et al.[27]	Clinical	47	45	123	2.50
Lamont et al.[27]	Doppler	47	48	123	2.50
Lamont et al.[27]	Combination	47	58	123	2.50
Massell & Ettinger[33]	Clinical	40	39	133	3.30
Massell & Ettinger[33]	Phlebography	40	92	133	3.30

*ICV = Incompetent communicating vein

Table 6.6   Compilation of 11 studies on locating incompetent calf communicating veins

Method	Number of studies	Number of studies with false-positive results	% of false-positive results* (range)	Number of studies with false-negative results	% of false-negative results† (range)
Clinical	8	5	16–95%	3	46–70%
Doppler	3	3	12–50%	1	52%
Fluorescein	3	2	8–92%	1	53%
Thermography	3	2	15–150%	1	36%
Phlebography	5	3	13–97%	2	27–30%

* $\dfrac{\text{Number of positive tests} - \text{Number of true positives}}{\text{Number of true positives}} \times 100$

† $\dfrac{\text{Number of true positives} - \text{Number of test positives}}{\text{Number of true positives}} \times 100$

Table 6.7   Accuracy of tests in predicting the presence or absence of incompetent communicating veins in 39 limbs[41]

	Present	Absent	False-positive	False-negative
Operation	31	8	0	0
Clinical examination	31	0	8	0
Phlebography	25	7	1	6
Ultrasound	31	2	6	0

Table 6.8 Accuracy of tests in predicting the site of incompetent calf communicating veins in 39 limbs[41]

Test	Total number predicted	Number correctly predicted	False-negatives	False-positives
Operation	55	55 (100%)	0	0
Clinical examination	64	33 (60%)	22 (40%)	31
Phlebography	40	33 (60%)	22 (40%)	7*
Ultrasound	83	34 (62%)	21 (38%)	49*

*The difference between these two figures is significant ($\chi^2 = 18.8$, $P = 0.00025$).

Table 6.9 Accuracy of a combination of tests in predicting the site of incompetent communicating veins in 39 limbs[41]

Test	Total number predicted	Number correctly predicted	False-negatives	False-positives
Operation	55	55 (100%)	0	0
Clinical examination and phlebography	83	48 (58%)	7 (8%)	35
Clinical examination and ultrasound	108	48 (45%)	6 (6%)	59
Ultrasound and phlebography	98	48 (49%)	7 (9%)	50
All three tests combined	115	53 (22%)	2 (2%)	62

Table 6.10 Methods used for investigating varicose veins

1. Ultrasound
   (a) Direction of flow
      • Superficial vein reflux*
      • Communicating vein reflux
      • Deep vein reflux*
   (b) Duplex imaging – the direction of flow in the deep, superficial and communicating veins

2. Contrast phlebography
   (a) Varicography – site, extent and connections of varices*
   (b) Ascending phlebography – state of deep veins and detection of incompetent communicating veins*
   (c) Descending phlebography – function of deep vein valves and long saphenous incompetence
   (d) Dynamic cine phlebography – direction of blood flow during exercise
   (e) Percutaneous femoral phlebography – anatomy of iliac veins and vena cava
   (f) Intraosseous phlebography – anatomy of iliac veins and vena cava
   (g) Retrograde caval phlebography – anatomy of the inferior vena cava above an iliac or caval occlusion and the function of femoral vein valves

   (h) Intra-operative venography – sites of superficial to deep communication

3. Foot volumetry – calf pump function*
4. Foot vein pressure measurements – calf pump function
5. Strain gauge, impedance, isotope or photoplethysmography – calf pump function
6. Thermography – sites of incompetent communicating veins
7. Fluorescein angiography – site of incompetent communicating veins

*Tests commonly used to assess varicose veins by the authors.

Auscultation

A bruit coming from a superficial vein usually indicates the presence of an arteriovenous fistula in the limb. When either a single fistula or multiple fistulae are present the veins can often be seen to pulsate if they are carefully observed.

The Tourniquet test (The Brodie–Trendelenburg test)[5,52] (Chapter 4, page 74)

This simple bed-side test was designed to assess

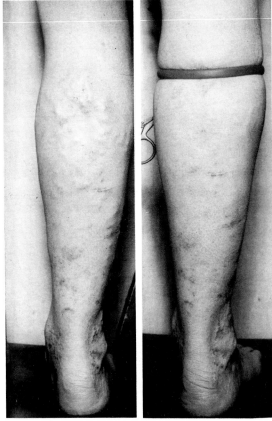

Fig. 6.16 (a and b)   The tourniquet test.
    Large calf varicosities (a), which were not
controlled by a thigh tourniquet, are controlled by a
below knee tourniquet (b).

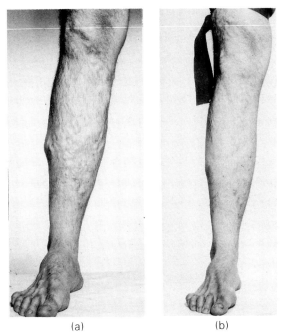

(a)   (b)

Fig. 6.17 (a and b)   The tourniquet test.
    Large varicosities in the lower leg (a) which have
been controlled by a thigh tourniquet (b).

the direction of blood flow and the source of refilling of the superficial veins. Its accuracy depends upon the skill of the investigator who performs the test, and the results improve with experience.

The patient must be laid flat on the couch or bed and the limb elevated to at least 45° to empty all the subcutaneous veins. This may be helped by stroking the limb with the hand from the foot upwards along the course of the major veins. When the veins have been emptied a narrow rubber tourniquet is applied around the thigh as close to the groin as possible.

We use a simple piece of 1 cm diameter red rubber tubing or a short length of rubber bandage and a strong pair of artery forceps or fingers to hold it in place (Fig. 6.16). Sapheno-femoral

incompetence is indicated if the varices remain collapsed for between 15 and 30 seconds after the patient stands up and rapidly refill when the tourniquet is removed (Fig. 6.17). The test should be repeated if the results are equivocal.

Errors result from inadequate venous emptying, releasing the tourniquet too soon, and failure to appreciate that natural venous refilling always occurs; natural venous refilling is more obvious after periods of exercise or in hot weather. If the tourniquet is applied too tightly, it can cause pain, but if it is not applied tightly enough, saphenous reflux will not be controlled and the test will give incorrect results. Venous reflux may be particularly difficult to control in fat limbs.

When sapheno-femoral incompetence is associated with other sites of superficial incompetence, the varices quickly refill on standing but the venous distension may still increase when the tourniquet is released. This additional refilling can best be detected by palpating the increased tension in the varices on release of the tourniquet.

If the high thigh tourniquet fails to control venous refilling, the tourniquet should be placed just above the patella, to exclude an incompetent mid-thigh communicating vein, and then below the knee to detect sapheno-popliteal incompetence. Incompetence of individual lower leg communicating veins may be detected by applying the tourniquet around the lower leg, but the lower the level, the fewer the varices that are controlled and the more difficult it is to interpret the results. The presence of incompetent communicating veins in the lower leg should be suspected if a below-knee tourniquet fails to control the varices. Tourniquet testing is a poor way of discovering the precise sites at which incompetent lower leg communicating veins pierce the deep fascia.[33]

Ochsner and Mahorner[42] advocated a triple tourniquet test, with tourniquets placed around the upper thigh, the lower thigh and below the knee. This test sometimes helps to distinguish between sapheno-femoral and sapheno-popliteal incompetence when both are present, but usually gives no more information than repeated single tourniquet tests at different levels.

Foote described a modification (a double tourniquet test) in which the tourniquets are placed above and below a collection of prominent varices while they are full of blood.[22] Emptying of the varicosities when the leg is elevated implies that there is a superficial to deep communication between the two tourniquets. If the leg is lowered and the veins between the tourniquets refill, this communicating vein must be incompetent. This test is often difficult to interpret and is rarely used because there are more accurate methods of identifying the site of incompetent communicating veins.

Perthes suggested that, if a tourniquet was placed below the knee and the patient either walked or heel-raised on the spot, the veins would collapse if the communicating veins and the deep veins were competent and unobstructed.[44] Failure of the superficial veins to empty may be caused by incompetence of valves in the communicating or deep veins or by deep venous obstruction. This test is an inaccurate but simple way of detecting a deep vein abnormality, and it may be used as a screening test to reveal a severe deep venous abnormality.

Summary

After taking the history and completing the physical examination (including the tourniquet tests) the clinician should know the answers to the following questions, and this will dictate the patients' further management.

1. Are the varicose veins the cause of the patient's symptoms?

If the history or the physical signs fail to convince the examiner that the varicose veins are the cause of the patients symptoms, additional examination and tests of the spine, abdomen, hip and knee joints, peripheral arteries and nervous system may be indicated.

2. If the varicose veins are the cause of the symptoms, are they primary varicose veins or secondary to another condition?

The history and examination may reveal the possibility of a post-thrombotic syndrome, a congenital venous abnormality or a pelvic tumour, when further investigations are required.

3. If the patient has primary varicose veins which are responsible for the symptoms, which veins are dilated and incompetent?
The possibilities are:

- sapheno-femoral incompetence
- sapheno-popliteal incompetence
- incompetence of lower leg communicating veins
- mid-thigh communicating vein incompetence
- gastrocnemius communicating vein incompetence
- tributary varicosity without major superficial vein incompetence

An attempt should be made to categorize the cause of the varicose veins under one or more of these headings. Sapheno-femoral incompetence is by far the most common abnormality. Sapheno-popliteal incompetence is said to be responsible for only 6–14 per cent of all varicosities,[24,38] but it has been suggested that these figures are underestimations.[25,47] If categorization is difficult or impossible on the basis of clinical evaluation, additional tests are required.

4. Has the patient any associated diseases that will prejudice or influence treatment?

The patient's general health may preclude active treatment. Unsightly varicose veins in a 90-year-old with heart failure, are best left untreated! Varicose veins in a leg which is ischaemic should not be treated, and the long saphenous vein should not be stripped out of a lymphoedematous limb.

5. Has the patient developed any complications as a result of the varicose veins that make treatment imperative?

Lipodermatosclerosis, incipent or past ulceration, haemorrhage or recurrent attacks of superficial thrombophlebitis are all indications for active treatment.

6. Does the patient need any treatment at all?

Intradermal spider veins or very small visible veins in women are often best treated by reassurance.

7. Is the available information sufficient to plan treatment?

If not, further investigations are necessary.

Special investigations

The techniques that are available for investigating varicose veins have been described in Chapter 4. The indications and accuracy of the special investigations which are of value in the further management of varicose veins are discussed below and listed in Table 6.10.
NB The majority of patients with straightforward varicose veins require nothing more than a full history and the careful examination described above.

Tests for saphenous reflux

Directional Doppler ultrasound (Chapter 4, page 80)

Confirmation of sapheno-femoral or sapheno-popliteal reflux using a simple handheld 8-mHz directional Doppler ultrasound probe in the clinic is a valuable adjunct to clinical examination.[10,21,25,28,34,35,36,37,45,55]

Comparisons have been made between the clinical tests of reflux during a Valsalva manoeuvre and after tourniquet release and the same tests with the Doppler flow detector. The results have been compared with reflux provoked by positive pressure ventilation before and after operative division of the long saphenous vein.[10,25,34] These studies have shown a better correlation between operative valvular incompetence and the Doppler tests of reflux than any of the clinical tests of sapheno-femoral incompetence. Reflux at open operation is, however, a poor 'gold standard' for assessing sapheno-femoral incompetence, and in a recent study in which the Doppler test was compared with clinical examination, descending phlebography, varicography, and intra-operative testing, we found the Doppler ultrasound test gave a number of false-positive and false-negative results (Fig. 6.18).[8]

The Doppler ultrasound test of long saphenous incompetence is, however, quick and easy to perform and helpful when clinical tests are equivocal. If this test is to be considered a valuable guide to management, it must be shown to help avoid operations that would have been performed had it not been used, and to detect valvular incompetence that would have been missed by simple clinical examination. Finally, the 'expected' improvement in patient management should result in a lower rate of recurrent varicose veins after treatment. A massive prospective study would be needed to assess this improvement because the end point is so diffuse. Clinicians must therefore act on their clinical impression that Doppler testing of superficial vein reflux is of value, particularly in fat legs.

The directional Doppler ultrasound flow detector may also be used to detect sapheno-popliteal reflux down the short saphenous vein,[25,45,47] and it has been used to determine the exact site of the sapheno-popliteal junction[45] which may vary considerably in position (see Chapter 2). Short saphenous incompetence is confirmed if retrograde flow after calf squeezing is abolished by digital or tourniquet compression which occludes the short saphenous vein.

Additional tests of saphenous reflux

When in doubt about sapheno-femoral reflux we perform foot volumetry and measure refilling times ($t_{1/2}$) with and without a high thigh tourniquet to occlude the long saphenous vein (Chapter 4, page 97). A marked increase in the half refilling time ($t_{1/2}$) produced by the tourniquet is indicative

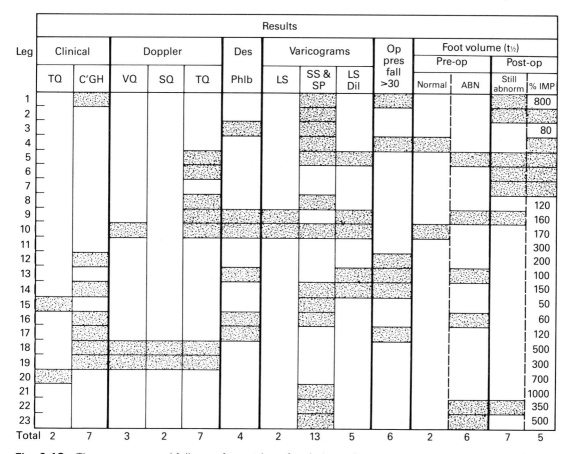

Fig. 6.18 The successes and failures of a number of techniques for diagnosing long saphenous vein incompetence in 23 patients thought to have long saphenous incompetence on clinical examination.

Clinical tests
TQ = tourniquet control of all varicosities
C'GH = a positive cough impulse in the groin

Doppler ultrasound tests
VQ = reflux heard over the long saphenous vein during a Valsalva manouevre
SQ = a 'biphasic' signal on calf squeezing over the long saphenous vein
TQ = reflux heard over the long saphenous vein on tourniquet release

Descending phlebography (Des Phlb) Reflux of contrast down the long saphenous vein seen on descending phlebography.

Varicograms
LS = long saphenous communications alone seen
SS and SP = additional communications to the short saphenous and calf communicating veins seen
LSDil = varices connected to an obviously dilated long saphenous vein

Operative pressure fall (Op pres fall > 30)
When the long saphenous vein was connected to a pressure monitor at operation a rapid fall from 100 mmHg to 0 mmHg was seen if the valves were incompetent. It was considered that the vein must contain some functioning valves if it took longer than 30 s for the pressure to fall.

Foot volumes taken pre-operatively and postoperatively showed that some limbs had a normal $t_{1/2}$ (half return time) before operation, and in some limbs a high thigh tourniquet failed to correct an abnormal $t_{1/2}$.

Postoperative foot volumes still remained abnormal in a number of patients after sapheno-femoral ligation which failed to improve the $t_{1/2}$ in five limbs.

The stippled areas represent individual tests that did not 'fit' clinical long saphenous vein incompetence. It can be seen that tourniquet and ultrasound Doppler tests did not always correlate. Descending phlebography is not a gold standard, and varicograms often showed unexpected communications. There is no perfect test at present for long saphenous vein incompetence.

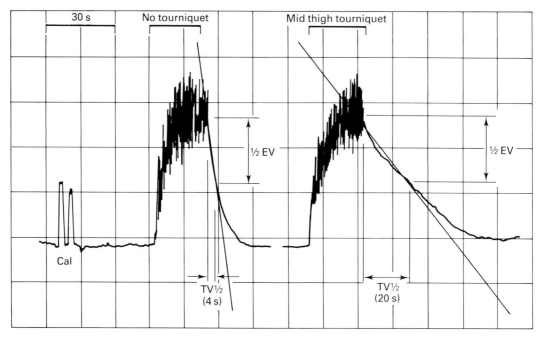

Fig. 6.19   This shows a foot volume tracing of a patient with long saphenous incompetence. The time taken for 1/2 the foot volume to be regained on completion of exercise is rapid at first but returns to normal when a tourniquet is placed around the thigh to stop blood refluxing down the long saphenous vein.

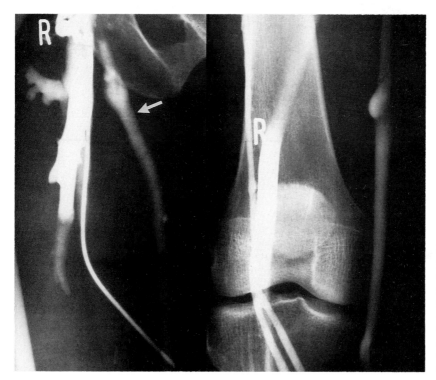

Fig. 6.20   A descending phlebogram showing contrast rapidly refluxing down a dilated long saphenous vein (arrowed) to the knee where it re-enters the deep veins through a gastrocnemius communicating vein.

of sapheno-femoral incompetence (Fig. 6.19).

If this test is equivocal we perform descending phlebograms ensuring that the needle is in the upper common femoral vein well above the termination of the long saphenous vein (Fig. 6.20). Many clinicians would regard this investigation as unnecessary and would work on the policy that it is better to ligate a few normal sapheno-femoral junctions than to leave sapheno-femoral incompetence untreated.

Tests to detect incompetent lower leg communicating veins

Although some investigators have claimed an 80 per cent accuracy[21,35] for simple directional Doppler detection of incompetent communicating veins, other workers have not been able to achieve this high level of accuracy,[27,41] probably because blood refluxing through incompetent communicating veins then passes some distance

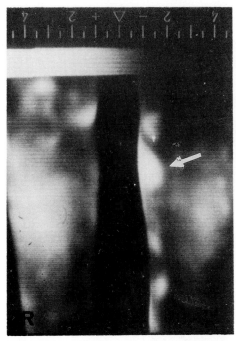

Fig. 6.21 A thermogram taken with the superficial veins of the left leg occluded by a tourniquet above the knee. The veins below the knee are refilling through an incompetent communicating vein just below the right knee (Boyd's communicating vein)—arrowed.

(We are indebted to Dr E Cooke for providing this illustration.)

along incompetent superficial veins making it difficult to define the exact site at which that the communicating vein pierces the deep fascia (see Chapter 4).

None of the other techniques which include thermography[40,43,53] (Fig. 6.21), fluorescein dye injection[9,13,32,40] and isotope plethysmography[54] (see Chapter 4) is any better at determining the exact sites of incompetent calf communicating veins; calf pump function tests simply indicate their likely presence (see Tables 6.5, 6.6, 6.7, 6.8, 6.9).[2]

Consequently, we rely heavily on phlebography to diagnose both the presence and position of incompetent calf communicating veins, knowing that its specificity is good, though its sensitivity is poor. It is unusual for phlebography to fail to detect any incompetent communicating veins when more than one is present (Fig. 6.22).

The detection of one incompetent communicating vein in a patient with lipodermatosclerosis or ulceration is an indication to explore all the known sites of incompetent calf communicating veins through a long incision. The importance of this approach can be seen from a study in which we compared the accuracy of clinical, ultrasound and ascending phlebography,[41] in 39 patients who were thought to have incompetent calf communicating veins on clinical testing, against operative exploration and intra-operative testing of incompetence (Fig. 6.23). Phlebography proved to be the most accurate test but failed to detect a number of communicating veins that would also have been missed by a selective surgical approach.

In limbs without skin changes or ulceration accurate pre-operative localization of incompetent calf communicating veins may allow a selective exploration of suspected sites to be made. If a selective approach is followed, it must be recognized that in more than one-third of the limbs managed in this way, communicating veins will pass undetected and will therefore be untreated.

Duplex ultrasound (Doppler and Grey Scale ultrasound) assessment

Duplex ultrasound scanners are capable of imaging the superficial and deep veins of the leg and the communications between these two systems.[46,49,50] Directional Doppler signals can then be obtained from specific anatomical locations, during Valsalva manoeuvres and calf squeezing,

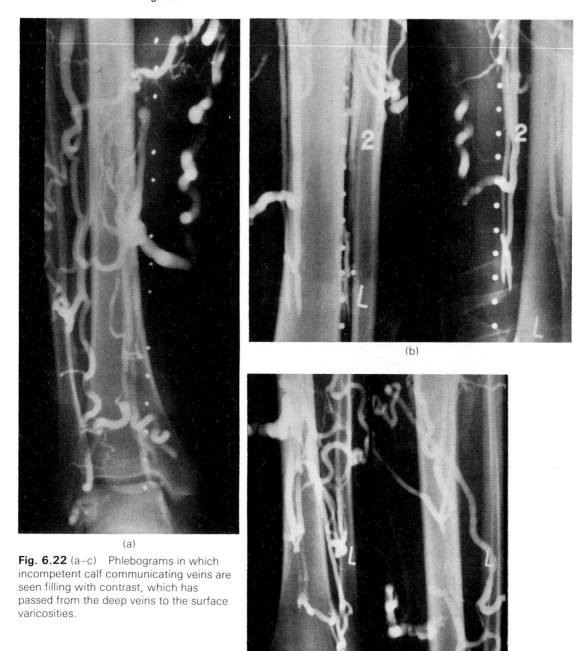

(a)

(b)

(c)

Fig. 6.22 (a–c)   Phlebograms in which incompetent calf communicating veins are seen filling with contrast, which has passed from the deep veins to the surface varicosities.

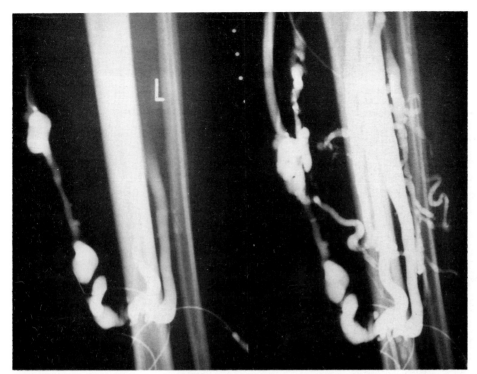

Fig. 6.22 (d) This varicogram shows a large calf communicating vein. It is not possible to know if this vein is incompetent as the contrast medium in a varicogram passes from the superficial to the deep veins.

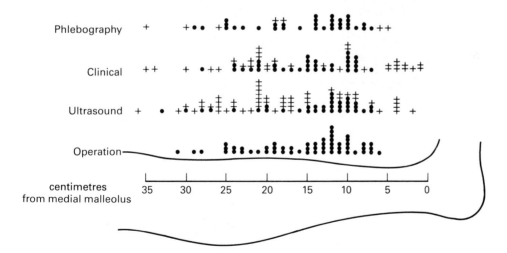

Fig. 6.23 The results of a study we performed in 1977, which compared the accuracy of clinical examination, phlebography and directional Doppler ultrasound testing to localize incompetent calf communicating veins (ICVs) in 39 legs.

Each symbol corresponds to a positive test results. ● = incompetent communicating vein found at operation; + = no communicating vein found. It can be seen that phlebography was the most accurate test but even this test failed to detect some ICVs which were found and confirmed to be incompetent at operation. Doppler testing had poor sensitivity.

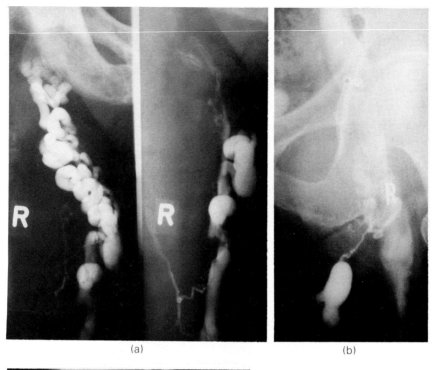

(a)   (b)

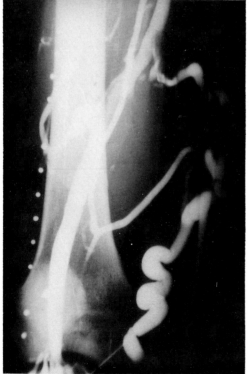

(c)

Fig. 6.24   (a) A varicogram showing a large mass of veins reconnecting a previously divided long saphenous vein to the femoral vein.

(b) A varicogram showing a minute vein reconnecting a previously divided long saphenous vein to the femoral vein.

(c) A varicogram showing a residual long saphenous vein, which has been divided at the groin, draining into the superficial femoral vein through a dilated incompetent Hunterian communicating vein.

and the presence of venous reflux in different veins can be determined (see Chapter 4). This represents a considerable advance over the simple handheld Doppler flow detector because it is often very difficult to know exactly from which vessel the reflected ultrasound is coming. This is very important in the groin and popliteal fossa, where the deep and superficial systems meet, and also in the calf if ultrasound is used to assess incompetence of the communicating veins and to localize their position. The value of duplex scanning in localizing communicating veins and confirming valvular incompetence awaits further assessment (see Chapter 4, Fig. 4.12).

Definition of the extent and connections of varicosities

Varicography is the direct injection of contrast medium into surface varicosities followed by screening and radiographs to determine their connections (see Chapter 4). This investigation is particularly useful in assessing recurrent varicose veins (Fig. 6.24).[3,6,11,15,17,29,48] We have also found it to be of value in examining veins which cannot be classified by clinical examination and the tourniquet tests (Fig. 6.25).[6] It can also be used to determine the exact position of the termination of the short saphenous vein (Fig. 6.26).

The information obtained from a varicogram does, however, depend upon the site chosen for the injection. One injection will not reveal all the sites of the superficial to deep venous connections, and we sometimes perform three or four injections in one study.

Varicograms show the superficial connections, the communicating veins,[30] the tortuosity, the dilatation and the extent of the varicose veins (Fig. 6.27) but they do not give any information about valve function or venous reflux which must

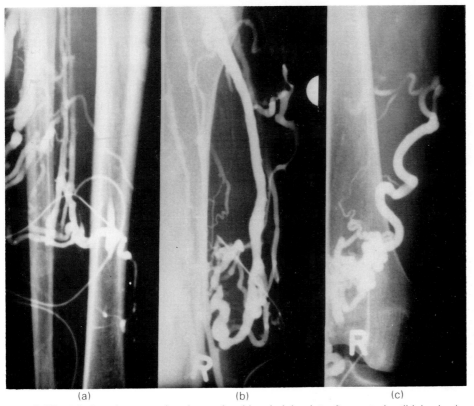

(a)   (b)   (c)

Fig. 6.25 (a) A varicogram showing varicosities draining into the posterior tibial veins by a large (and probably incompetent) communicating vein.

(b) The same varicosities also connect to a large gastrocnemius communicating vein and (c) to a communicating vein in Hunter's canal. All these sites must be ligated or sclerosed if the veins are to be prevented from recurring.

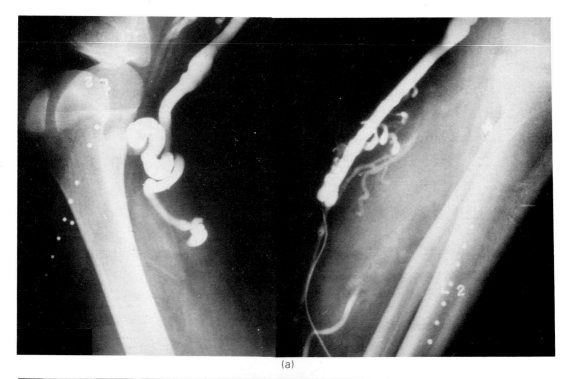

(a)

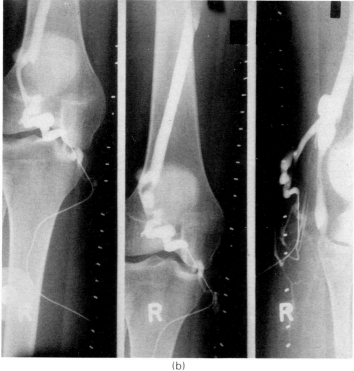

(b)

Fig. 6.26   (a) A varicogram
showing a dilated tortuous
termination of the short saphenous
vein.
 (b) A varicogram showing dilated
varicosities connected to the short
saphenous vein near its termination,
which is situated high in the
popliteal fossa.

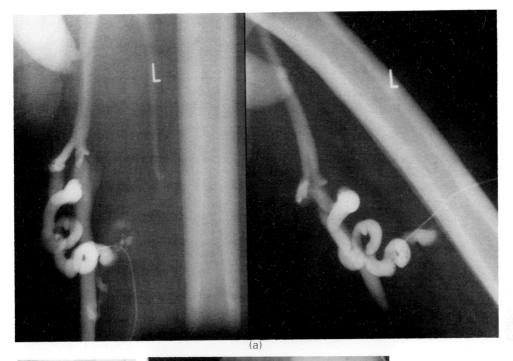

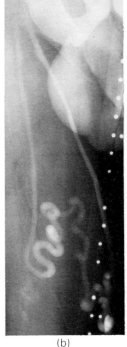

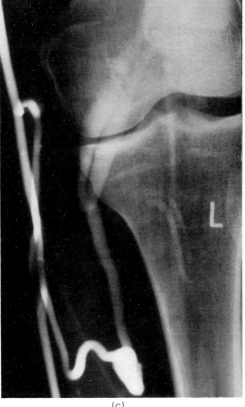

(a)

(b)

(c)

Fig. 6.27 (a–f)   A selection of varicograms showing different connections.

(a) Varicosities connecting with a 'normal' long saphenous vein in the thigh which contains valves of normal appearance.

(b) Varicosities connecting an 'undilated' long saphenous vein to an antero-lateral thigh vein, which is dilated.

(c) Varicosities connecting the long saphenous vein to a paired gastrocnemius communicating vein. An undilated short saphenous vein can be seen passing up behind the tibia.

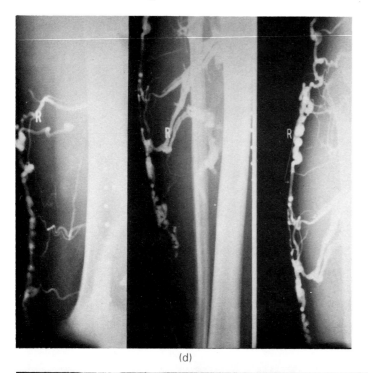

(d)

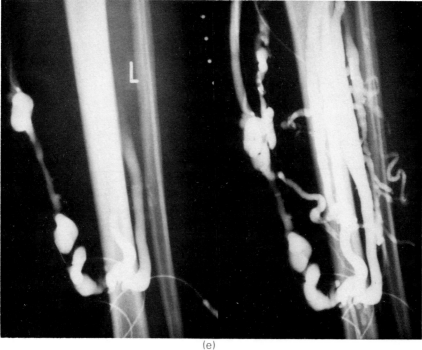

(e)

Fig. 6.27 (d) A varicose vein passing up on the lateral side of the calf and thigh which is connected by a series of paired communicating veins to the peroneal veins, the superficial femoral vein and the deep femoral vein. (e) A large, and probably incompetent, communicating vein on the medial side of the calf connecting subcutaneous varicosities to the posterior tibial veins.

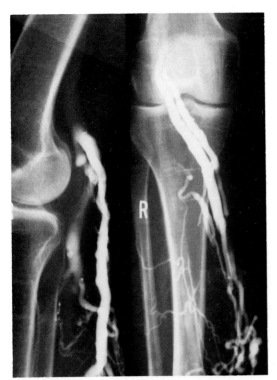

Fig. 6.27 (f) Varicosities connected to a pair of medial gastrocnemius veins.

Descending phlebography

This is the best method of demonstrating venous reflux if 'Duplex' ultrasound imaging is not available (see Chapter 4 and Chapter 8).[1]

Venous obstruction

This can only be demonstrated by a test of venous function. The presence of a venous occlusion on a phlebogram should not be equated with functional obstruction. Obstruction must be confirmed by detecting an increase in distal venous pressure or venous volume during exercise or reactive hyperaemia, by measuring the venous pressure directly or with some form of plethysmography.

Detection of post-thrombotic deep vein damage

If we suspect that a patient's varicose veins are secondary to deep vein damage, we routinely

be assessed by ascending and descending phlebography or directional Doppler ultrasound testing.

Deep vein obstruction and incompetence

Directional Doppler ultrasound

Some investigators have found that this test of deep vein reflux is accurate[20,39] but we have found that it does not correlate well with reflux demonstrated by descending venography.[1]

The combination of venous ultrasound imaging with Doppler flow detection

This allows the operator to identify the source of the flow signal. Individual valves may be visualized and the direction of venous flow observed; this should greatly improve the detection and measurement of venous reflux (see Chapter 4).[46,49,50]

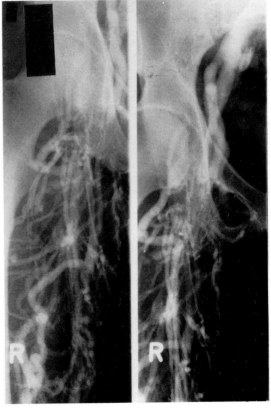

Fig. 6.28 The ascending phlebogram of a young male who was stabbed in the groin and sustained a total femoral vein occlusion during the surgery which was required to stop the haemorrhage.

obtain ascending phlebograms (Fig. 6.28) and perform foot volumetry to establish the anatomy and functional severity of the damage. Foot vein pressure measurements and the other forms of plethysmography are alternative and equally efficacious tests. We find foot volumetry the most simple and reliable quantitative method; photoplethysmography is just as simple but is only qualitative.

Suggested diagnostic pathways

After a thorough clinical examination, including the tourniquet tests, it is usually possible to place the patient into one of several categories. The diagnostic pathway is then complete and treatment can begin. The following section summarizes our use of the special investigations in patients who have been placed in one of these clinical categories, when the information available from clinical examination is not sufficient to proceed with treatment.

1. Sapheno-femoral incompetence with long saphenous vein tributary dilatation

No lipodermatosclerosis, ulceration, or ankle flare. All the veins controlled by a high thigh tourniquet. Perthes' test shows superficial veins empty with exercise.
Action
   (a) Confirmation of sapheno-femoral reflux with the Doppler test is *optional*.
   (b) No further tests are required – proceed to treat.

(NB This is the most common situation seen in a vein clinic)

2. Sapheno-popliteal incompetence with short saphenous vein tributary dilatation

No clinical evidence of sapheno-femoral incompetence. No lipodermatosclerosis, ulceration or ankle flare. All varicosities controlled by a below-knee tourniquet. Perthes' test shows superficial veins empty with exercise.
Action
   (a) Confirm sapheno-femoral competence with Doppler test.
   (b) Confirm sapheno-popliteal incompetence with Doppler test.
   (c) Varicogram to define the anatomy of sapheno-popliteal junction (optional but valuable

if the termination of the short saphenous cannot be easily felt).
   (d) Ultrasound imaging may be used as an alternative method of detecting the site of the sapheno-popliteal junction.
   (e) Proceed to treat.

3. Sapheno-femoral and sapheno-popliteal incompetence with tributary dilatation of both saphenous veins

No lipodermatosclerosis, ulceration or ankle flare. All varicosities controlled by a below-knee tourniquet. Perthes' test shows superficial veins empty with exercise.
Action
   (a) Confirm sapheno-femoral and sapheno-popliteal incompetence with Doppler test.
   (b) Varicogram to confirm that varices connect to both saphenous systems and to define the anatomy of the sapheno-popliteal junction (optional).
   (c) Proceed to treat.

4. Sapheno-femoral or sapheno-popliteal incompetence or both but varices below the knee not controlled by a below-knee tourniquet

No lipodermatosclerosis or ulceration. An ankle flare may be present. No past history of deep vein thrombosis. Perthes' test shows veins remain distended during exercise.
Action
   (a) Clinical examination of the sites of possible incompetent communicating veins in the lower leg.
   (b) Confirm presence of sapheno-femoral and sapheno-popliteal incompetence with Doppler flow detector.
   (c) Test for popliteal reflux with directional Doppler flow detector.
   (d) Varicography of superficial veins to examine the communications of the superficial veins (optional).
   (e) Assess function of deep veins and define site of incompetent communicating veins with foot volumetry (or photophlethysmography) and ascending phlebography.
   (f) Proceed to treat.

5. Sapheno-femoral or sapheno-popliteal incompetence or both, but varices below the knee not controlled by a below-knee tourniquet

with skin changes, ankle flare,
lipodermatosclerosis, past or present ulceration

History of deep vein thrombosis unreliable. Perthes' test shows superficial veins remain distended during exercise.
Action – as above.

6. Skin changes and calf varices with no clinical evidence of long or short saphenous incompetence

No history of deep vein thrombosis.
Action
    (a) Test the competence of sapheno-popliteal and sapheno-femoral junctions with the directional Doppler flow detector.
    (b) Varicography of the superficial veins (optional).
    (c) Ascending phlebography.
    (d) Foot volumetry.

7. Varicosities of tributary veins but no evidence of sapheno-femoral or sapheno-popliteal incompetence

No lipodermatosclerosis, ankle flare or ulceration.
Action
    (a) Confirm competence of sapheno-femoral and sapheno-popliteal junction with directional Doppler flow detector.
    (b) Varicograms if mid-thigh communicating vein or gastrocnemius communicating vein is suspected (optional).
    (c) Proceed to treat.

8. Recurrent varicose veins after previous surgery

If clinical examination does not clearly indicate the cause of the recurrence (e.g. the site of the superficial to deep vein incompetence), both ascending phlebography and varicography are very helpful investigations followed by calf pump function studies (foot volumetry) if the ascending phlebogram shows any deep vein damage.

References

1. Ackroyd JS, Lea Thomas M, Browse NL. Deep vein reflux: An assessment by descending phlebography. *Br J Surg* 1986; **73**: 31.
2. Anon. The hidden perforating veins. *Br Med J* 1970; **1**: 186.
3. Barabas AP, MacFarlane R. The use of varicography to identify the sources of incompetence in recurrent varicose veins. *Ann R Coll Surg Engl* 1985; **67**: 208.
4. Beesley WH, Fegan WG. An investigation into the localization of incompetent perforating veins. *Br J Surg* 1970; **157**: 30.
5. Brodie B. *Lectures Illustrative of Various Subjects in Pathology and Surgery*. London. Longmans 1846.
6. Burnand KG. Intérêt de la varicographie dans l' appréciation des varices essentielles des membres inférieurs. In: *Phlebologie '83*. Brussels. Medical Media International 1984; 269.
7. Burnand KG. Management of varicose veins of the legs. *Nursing Mirror* 1977; **144(11)**: 45.
8. Burnand KG, Pattison M, Powell S, Lea Thomas M, Browse NL. Can we diagnose long saphenous incompetence correctly? In Negus D, Jantet G (Eds) *Phlebology '85*. London. John Libbey 1986.
9. Callum KG, Gray LJ, Lea Thomas M. An evaluation of the flourescein test and phlebography in the detection of incompetent perforating veins. *Br J Surg* 1973; **60**: 699.
10. Chan A, Chisholm I, Royle JP. The use of directional Doppler ultrasound in the assessment of saphenofemoral incompetence. *Aust NZ J Surg* 1983; **53**: 399.
11. Chant ADB, Jones HO, Townsend JCF, Williams JE. Radiological demonstration of the relationship between calf varices and sapheno-femoral incompetence. *Clin Radiol* 1972; **23**: 519.
12. Chevrier L. De l'examin aux reflux veinaux dans les varices superficielles. *Arch Gen Chir* 1908; **2**: 44.
13. Chilvers AS, Thomas MH. Methods for the localization of incompetent ankle perforating veins. *Br Med J* 1970; **2**: 577.
14. Cockett FB. Diagnosis and surgery of high pressure venous leaks in the leg. A new overall concept in the surgery of varicose veins and venous ulcer. *Br Med J* 1953; **2**: 1399.
15. Corbett CR, McIrvine AJ, Aston NO, Jamieson CW, Lea Thomas M. The use of varicography to identify the sources of incompetence in recurrent varicose veins. *Ann R Coll Surg Engl* 1984; **66**: 412.
16. Dodd H, Cockett FB. *The Pathology and Surgery of the Veins of the Lower Limb*. London. Churchill Livingstone 1976.
17. Doran FS, Barkat S. The management of recurrent varicose veins. *Ann R Coll Surg Engl* 1981; **63**: 432.

18. Evans GA, Evans DMD, Seal RME, Craven JL. Haemorrhage from varicose veins. *Lancet* 1973; **2**: 1359.

19. Fegan WG. *Varicose Veins: Compression Sclerotherapy*. London. Heinemann 1967.

20. Folse R, Alexander RH. Directional flow detection for localizing venous valvular incompetency. *Surgery* 1970; **67**: 114.

21. Foote AV, Miller SS, Grossman JA. The ultrasonic detection of incompetent perforating veins. *Br J Surg* 1971; **58**: 872.

22. Foote RR. *Varicose Veins*. London. Butterworths 1954.

23. Harman RRM. Haemorrhage from varicose veins. *Lancet* 1974; **1**: 363.

24. Helmig L, Stelzer G. Haufigkeit der operativen Behandlung der insuffizienten Vena saphena parva. *Vasa* 1983; **12**: 159.

25. Hoare MC, Royle JP. Doppler ultrasound detection of saphenofemoral and saphenopopliteal incompetence and operative venography to ensure precise saphenopopliteal ligation. *Aust NZ J Surg* 1984; **54**: 49.

26. Hobbs J. Surgery and sclerotherapy in the treatment of varicose veins. A random trial. *Arch Surg* 1974; **109**: 793.

27. Lamont P, Bavin D, Woodyer A, Ruston N, Butler J, Terry T, Dundas D, Dormandy J. Accuracy of clinical versus Doppler examination for detecting incompetent perforating veins. *Br J Surg* 1986; **73**: 493.

28. Large J. Doppler testing as an important conservation measure in the treatment of varicose veins. *Aust NZ J Surg* 1984; **54**: 357.

29. Lea Thomas M, Keeling FP. Varicography in the management of recurrent varicose veins. *Angiology* 1986; **37**: 570.

30. Lea Thomas M, Bowles JN. Incompetent perforating veins: Comparison of varicography and ascending phlebography. *Radiology* 1985; **154**: 619.

31. Lofgren KA. Management of varicose veins: Mayo Clinic Experience. In: Bergan JJ, Yao JST (Eds) *Venous Problems*. Chicago. Year Book Medical Publishers 1971.

32. Lofqvist J, Jansson I, Thomsen M, Elfstrom J. Evaluation of the fluorescein test in the diagnosis of incompetent perforating veins. *Vasa* 1983; **12**: 46.

33. Massell TB, Ettinger J. Phlebography in the localization of incompetent communicating veins in patients with varicose veins. *Ann Surg* 1948; **127**: 1217.

34. McIrvine AJ, Corbett CRR, Aston NO, Sherriff EA, Wiseman PA, Jamieson CW. The demonstration of saphenofemoral incompetence; Doppler ultrasound compared with standard clinical tests. *Br J Surg* 1984; **71**: 509.

35. Miller SS, Foote AV. The ultrasonic detection of incompetent perforating veins. *Br J Surg* 1974; **61**: 653.

36. Miller SS. Investigation and management of varicose veins. *Ann R Coll Surg Engl* 1974; **55**: 245.

37. Myers KA. Special investigations prior to surgery for varicose veins. *Aust NZ J Surg* 1983; **53**: 394.

38. Nabatoff RA. 3000 stripping operations for varicose veins on a semi-ambulatory basis. *Surg Gynec Obstet* 1970; **130**: 497.

39. Nicolaides AN, Fernandes JF, Zimmerman H. Doppler ultrasound in the investigation of venous insufficiency. In: Nicolaides AN, Yao JST (Eds) *Investigations of Vascular Disorders*. Edinburgh. Churchill Livingstone 1981.

40. Noble J, Gunn AA. Varicose veins: Comparative study of methods for detecting incompetent perforators. *Lancet* 1972; **1**: 1253.

41. O'Donnell TF, Burnand KG, Clemenson G, Lea Thomas M, Browse NL. Doppler examination vs clinical and phlebographic detection of the location of incompetent perforating veins: a prospective study. *Arch Surg* 1977; **112**: 31.

42. Ochsner A, Mahorner HR. The modern treatment of varicose veins. *Surgery* 1937; **2**: 889.

43. Patil KD, Williams JR, Lloyd-Williams K. Thermographic localization of incompetent perforating veins in the leg. *Br Med J* 1970; **1**: 195.

44. Perthes G. Über die Operation der Unterschenkel varicen nach Trendelenberg. *Deutsch Med Wochenschr* 1895; : 253.

45. Roberts AK, Hoare MC, Royle JP. The detection of sapheno-popliteal incompetence using Doppler ultrasound and operative venography. *J Cardiovasc Surg* 1985; **26**: 400.

46. Semrow C, Ryan TJ, Buchbinder D, Rollins DL. Assessment of valve function using real-time B-mode ultrasound. In: Negus D, Jantet G (Eds) *Phlebology '85*. London. John Libbey 1986.

47. Sheppard M. Sapheno-popliteal incompetence. *Phlebology* 1986; **1**: 23.

48. Starnes HF, Vallance R, Hamilton DNH. Recurrent varicose veins: a radiological approach to investigation. *Clin Radiol* 1984; **35**: 95.

49. Sullivan ED, David JP, Cranley JJ. Real-time B-mode venous ultrasound. *J Vasc Surg* 1984; **1**: 465.

50. Szendro G, Nicolaides AN, Zukowski AJ, Christopoulos D, Malouf GM, Christodoulou C, Myers K. Duplex scanning in the assessment of deep venous incompetence. *J Vasc Surg* 1986; **4**: 237.

51. Townsend J, Jones H, Williams JE. Detection of incompetent perforating veins by venography at operation. *Br Med J* 1967; **3**: 583.

52. Trendelenberg F. Über die Unterbildung der Vena saphena magna bei unterschenkel Varicen. *Beitr Klin Chir* 1891; **7**: 195.

53. Vuori J, Inberg MV, Koskinen R, Rasanen O, Vanttinen E. Pre-operative localization of incompetent perforating veins. *Ann Chir Gynaecol* 1972; **61**: 22.

54. Whitehead SM, Clemenson G, Browse NL. The assessment of calf pump function by isotope plethysmography. *Br J Surg* 1983; **70**: 675.

55. Zelikovski A, Zamir B, Hadar H, Urea I. Saphenofemoral valve insufficiency in varicose veins of the lower limb. *Angiology* 1981; **32**: 807.

7

Varicose veins: natural history and treatment

The natural history and treatment of varicose veins

The natural history of untreated and uncomplicated varicose veins

It is tacitly assumed that if varicose veins are left untreated they will continue to enlarge and the 'varicose process' will spread to involve other previously 'normal' veins. It is reasonable to make these assumptions if the pathological abnormality is an inherited structural defect of the vein wall (see Chapter 5), but without knowing more about this abnormality it is not possible to estimate the rate of progression.

There is some anecdotal evidence that long saphenous vein incompetence can regress. This certainly seems to occur after pregnancy,[50,75,124] and regression of thigh vein varices may follow the injection of incompetent lower leg communicating veins,[46] though this latter claim has been disputed.[65,66] Other investigators have observed that simple ligation and division of the sapheno-femoral junction causes regression of distal varices.[91]

The influence of prolonged external elastic compression on the natural history of varicosities has not, to our knowledge, been specifically examined, but it is interesting to note that many patients with primary varicose veins who have been given elastic stockings to wear while they await operation, subsequently decline hospital admission for surgery on the grounds that they are so much better that they no longer require treatment.[23]

It is obvious that we know little about the rate of progression of varicose veins or about the factors which modify this, but we agree with Watts[145] that the propensity to develop varicose veins is a progressive incurable disease that can be satisfactorily palliated, *but not cured*, by a number of different techniques.

The skin complications of primary varicose veins

It is frequently argued that varicose veins must be treated to prevent the development of skin changes but little is known about the magnitude of the risk that patients with uncomplicated varicose veins have of developing the skin changes that lead to ulceration.

Some authors[47,56,109,110] have suggested that all patients with skin changes or venous ulceration in the 'gaiter' area of the leg have incompetent lower leg communicating veins, and Haegar[56] has stated that 'No venous ulcer can exist without perforator incompetence'; this is unlikely to be true. Hoare detected evidence of incompetent communicating veins with Doppler ultrasound in only a small proportion of a large series of patients with venous ulceration,[60] and Bjordal[12,13,14,15,16] has shown that incompetence of the calf communicating veins has a smaller effect on calf pump function than incompetence of the saphenous vein; we have confirmed his findings.[20] Cockett found no evidence of incompetent calf communicating veins at operation in only 18 out of 54 limbs with skin changes and long saphenous incompetence,[39] and we too have explored legs looking for incompetent communicating veins and found no major veins crossing the deep fascia in some patients with grossly abnormal venous pressures and healed venous ulcers.

The problem with all these studies and observations is the definition of communicating vein incompetence. The accepted gold standard for proof of communicating vein incompetence is significant back bleeding on transection of the suspect vein during forcible foot dorsiflexion at the time of operative exploration. This is called the Turner–Warwick bleed back test.[25,86,143] This test does not take account of the diameter of the communicating vein. Although a large vein of 4–5 mm diameter, which bleeds profusely when divided, is obviously significant, a small vein which only just bleeds on forcible dorsiflexion is of doubtful clinical importance. Nevertheless, a small vessel that is shown to reflux is considered to be significant, even though the vein is so small that the quantity of blood that is capable of refluxing through it is of no haemodynamic significance (though of course it may be of hydrostatic significance). The method of division of the vessel and forcible dorsiflexion of the foot varies from surgeon to surgeon, and reflux may be abolished if there is traumatic venospasm caused by clumsy dissection and division of the vein. The very act of opening the deep fascia and dissecting the vein away from the surrounding tissues that may normally hold it open, may render an incompetent vein competent or vice versa. Finally, a surgeon who has made an extensive incision in the leg has a bias in favour of finding incompetent communicating veins, as have junior surgeons instructed by their consultants to "ligate this patient's incompetent communicating veins".

A satisfactory method for diagnosing incompetent communicating veins and measuring their effect on calf pump haemodynamics is needed urgently. Until we can do this satisfactorily, we cannot investigate the precise role of superficial and communicating vein incompetence in the genesis of skin changes and venous ulceration. We have to rely on our clinical experience which suggests that a small number of patients with simple long saphenous incompetence will develop skin changes and ulceration.

We must therefore either advise all patients with varicose veins to have treatment in the hope of avoiding this risk or watch these patients carefully and treat them if, or when, early skin changes appear. Large prospective studies of the natural history of varicose veins, documented with anatomical and physiological, as well as clinical, measures are required so that the true relationship between the presence of varicose veins, their progression and the development of skin changes can be elucidated.

Fletcher and Tibbs,[49] using dynamic phlebo-graphy, have been able to distinguish between two groups of incompetent communicating veins. One group allows re-entry of blood refluxing down the saphenous vein; in the other group the direction of blood flow is chiefly outward. The first group of veins does not appear to be related to skin changes; the second group of veins does seem to be related to skin changes.

Not every incompetent communicating vein is associated with proof of post-thrombotic damage in deep veins,[19] and we find it difficult to accept that a localized thrombosis can occur on so many occasions solely within a communicating vein, to account for all the patients whose communicating veins have become incompetent. It is conceivable that communicating vein incompetence is part of the involvement of these veins in the generalized inherited varicose process.[39,49,69] Confirmation of this hypothesis awaits the development of better tests for assessing incompetence of the calf communicating veins. The magnitude of the risk of developing skin changes and ulceration from primary varicose veins can only be assessed by well organized prospective long-term studies.

Should varicose veins be treated?

Yes – if the patient wishes to be treated for symptomatic or cosmetic reasons
No – if the patient does not wish to be treated and has perfectly normal skin
Yes – when changes appear in the skin of the lower leg however minor
No – if the object of treatment is solely to stop progression of varicosis and to avoid treatment later

Can we cure varicose veins?

No – every patient should be told that all treatment is palliative not curative

Treatment

Clinical objectives of treatment

The treatment of varicose veins has five main objectives.

1. Satisfactory cosmesis
2. Relief of symptoms
3. Relief of complications

4. Prevention of complications
5. Prevention of recurrence

1. Satisfactory cosmesis

If all varices were removed without leaving visible evidence of this removal and at the same time any future recurrences were prevented, a perfect cosmetic result would have been achieved. Neither of these aims has, however, been realized though some remarkably low 5-year and 10-year recurrence rates have been claimed for surgical treatment.[78,122]

2. Relief of symptoms

All forms of treatment that successfully eradicate or compress varicose veins have been claimed to relieve pain and discomfort.[23,39,46,119] but it has been pointed out, in a report of a comparative trial of sclerotherapy and surgical treatment,[22] that the level of agreement on the severity of symptoms within a group of observers varied between 50 per cent and 70 per cent. This lack of correlation has been confirmed by other investigators.[119] A score based on the number of symptoms and signs may give no indication of the severity of the discomfort or disability experienced by the patient. Symptom relief is almost impossible to quantify, requests for additional treatment may be a better indication of a patient's dissatisfaction. The results of clinical trials based on symptomatology must be viewed with considerable scepticism.

3. Relief and prevention of complications

The major complications of varicose veins are skin changes, ulceration, haemorrhage and superficial thrombophlebitis. When there is definite evidence of communicating vein incompetence, treatment should relieve symptoms and reverse some of the skin changes (see Chapter 15). We do not know whether the treatment of saphenous vein incompetence prevents the development of skin changes, though eradication of surface varices does prevent haemorrhage and superficial thrombophlebitis (see below).

4. Prevention of complications

Skin changes and ulceration The role of varicose vein surgery in preventing and alleviating skin changes and ulceration is discussed in detail in Chapter 15.

Superficial thrombophlebitis This is common in patients with varicose veins (see Chapter 22), and removal of varicose subcutaneous veins prevents its development. Once thrombophlebitis has occurred it can usually be treated conservatively by support and analgesia, followed later, if the veins remain visible, by elective surgery to prevent further attacks. Surgical ligation of the long saphenous vein or short saphenous vein is indicated to prevent the development of deep vein thrombosis if the superficial thrombophlebitis is extending upwards towards the femoral or popliteal veins. If an acute attack of superficial thrombophlebitis fails to resolve, symptomatic relief may be provided by expelling the intravascular thrombus through a small incision or needle puncture into the vein.

5. Prevention of recurrence

This is the second main aim of treatment. Reports of success following sclerotherapy vary from approximately 80 per cent at 2–3 years[23,42] to 50 per cent at 3 years[105] and to as little as 8 per cent at 5 years.[66] Eighty-five per cent success at 10 years and 93 per cent success at 6–10 years postoperatively have been claimed by Larsson *et al.*[78] and Rivlin[122] respectively. In these studies the assessment was through the subjective and unacceptable method of 'surgeons' appraisal', which was not submitted to any form of external audit.

Physiological methods of relieving symptoms

1. Eradication of all visible varices by excision or obliteration
2. Disconnection of the connections between the superficial veins and the deep veins
3. Reduction of transmural pressure by external elastic compression

1. Eradication of all visible varices by excision or obliteration

Chapter 2 which discusses the anatomy of the venous system shows that the superficial drainage of the lower leg is extensive and cannot be

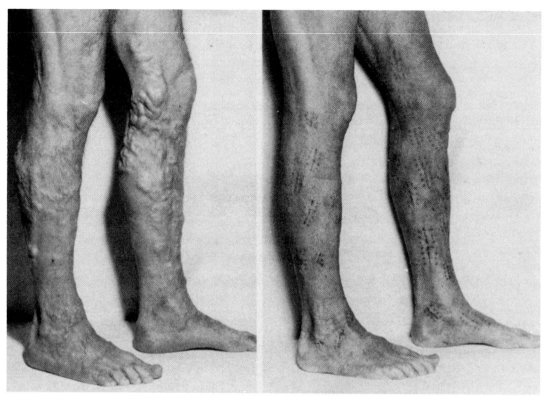

Fig. 7.1 Lofgren's method[90] of radical excision of superficial varicosities. It can be seen that this method, though very effective at eradicating the varicose veins, leaves many large scars, some of which are unsightly. We therefore prefer to remove surface varicosities through multiple minute stab incisions. (Reproduced from Lofgren KA with kind permission.)[90]

completely removed, though Lofgren's[90] post-operative pictures show that this can almost be achieved at the cost of multiple extensive incisions (Fig. 7.1).

Stripping, direct excision, avulsion, sclerotherapy, diathermy coagulation and infra-red coagulation are methods which have been used to eradicate or obliterate surface varices. These techniques will be discussed in detail in the subsequent sections.

2. Eradication of the connections between the superficial and deep veins

This forms the basis of surgical treatment and sclerotherapy which are both designed to occlude the connections between the superficial and deep veins. Some investigators believe that this eradication prevents descending valvular incompetence,[91] and other workers think that it prevents

transmission of high pressure in the deep veins to the superficial veins.[25,46,86] Although primary valvular incompetence may not be the cause of varicose veins (see Chapter 5), once it has developed it must be stopped to prevent recurrence of varicose veins.

3. Reduction of the transmural pressure with external elastic compression

The role of elastic compression is discussed in detail in chapters 12 and 15. Support stockings have been recognized for many years as an alternative method of relieving symptoms in patients with varicose veins;[39,50] it has also been suggested that elastic support may produce a prolonged reduction in ambulatory venous pressure.[136] This study needs further confirmation before it can be accepted as only 12 patients were evaluated. Elastic stockings are so effective that some patients will voluntarily withdraw themselves from surgical waiting lists for varicose vein surgery, preferring to continue with external support.[23]

No treatment

One-third of all patients attending a varicose vein clinic are said to require no treatment,[98] and certainly there is a group of patients who have visible veins, spider veins or varicose veins of such small proportions that active treatment would be inappropriate. Some patients may be considered too old or unfit to be treated by any method other than elastic support and in other patients the symptoms may be the result of another abnormality.

Surgical treatment of varicose veins

Most varicose vein operations are performed under general anaesthesia. These operations have a low mortality and morbidity but there are some contraindications and these are listed in Table 7.1. The different types of operation are given below and are discussed in this chapter.

1. Flush ligation of the sapheno-femoral junction, also called high saphenous ligation
2. Stripping of the long saphenous vein
3. Sapheno-popliteal junction ligation, also called short saphenous ligation
4. Stripping of the short saphenous vein
5. Ligation of the medial lower leg communicating veins
6. Ligation of other communicating veins (i.e. gastrocnemius, lateral calf, Hunterian and miscellaneous veins)
7. Avulsion of varicosities, ligation of tributaries and local excision of tributaries
8. Operations on recurrent varicose veins

Table 7.1 Contraindications to varicose vein surgery

General ill health affecting fitness for anaesthesia
Arterial ischaemia of the lower limb
Pregnancy
Contraceptive pill ingestion
Severe co-existent skin infection
Lymphoedema
Bleeding diatheses

Ligation and division of the long saphenous vein and its tributaries at the sapheno-femoral junction

Although a number of surgeons suggested ligation of the long saphenous vein near its termination, it was Homans[68] not Trendelenburg[142] who first suggested that this vein and its tributaries should be ligated *flush* with the femoral vein in the groin. This prevents the reflux of blood into the origin of the long saphenous vein and any of the four or five tributaries that join it near its termination. Recurrent varicose veins are common if the saphenous vein is ligated below these tributaries or if they are left untied. The additional procedure of stripping the long saphenous vein was introduced by Mayo,[102] and refined by Babcock[6] and Myers,[106] with the introduction of better intraluminal and flexible strippers.

Pre-operative preparation If the operation is being performed under general anaesthesia, the patient's general fitness must be confirmed by a full history and clinical examination. The skin of the groin and leg must be shaved before the operation, and the sites of all the prominent varicosities must be carefully marked on the skin with an indelible pen (Fig. 7.2).

The sites of incompetent superficial-to-deep connections are also carefully located and marked. Care must be taken to ensure that these marks are not removed or obliterated before the patient reaches the operating theatre. Some surgeons seal the marks with a plastic wound dressing to prevent their removal, but this is not necessary if a pen with waterproof ink is used.

Anaesthesia We prefer to use general anaesthesia because we invariably combine sapheno-femoral ligation with long saphenous vein stripping and multiple avulsions, but local anaesthesia[107] and regional anaesthesia[11] are preferred by others. If the sapheno-femoral ligation is the sole procedure, local anaesthesia is more than adequate.

Position The patient lies supine with each leg abducted by 20–30°, and with the heels supported on a padded vein board (Fig. 7.3). The leg veins are emptied by 15–30° of head down-foot up tilt which reduces intra-operative haemorrhage. Dale[31] recommends additional elevation of the legs on a slotted rack attached to the end of the operating table, but we have not used this tech-

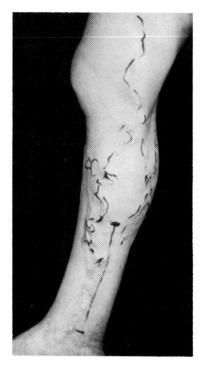

Fig. 7.2 A leg that has been 'marked-out' before varicose vein surgery. An indelible, black felt-tip pen is used to mark the course of the subcutaneous varicose veins on the overlying skin. Separate marks (crosses inside circles) maybe used to indicate specific sites for exploration for incompetent communicating veins. This patient had a full-length Linton exploration.

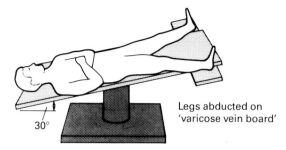

Legs abducted on 'varicose vein board'

Fig. 7.3 Diagram to show the position of the patient on the operating table for long saphenous vein surgery. Note the 'foot-up' tilt of the operating table and the use of a padded board to allow abduction of both lower limbs. The 'foot-up' tilt reduces venous engorgement and therefore haemorrhage. The abduction of both limbs allows easier access to the medial side of the leg for long saphenous vein stripping, multiple avulsions and exposure of the medial calf communicating veins.

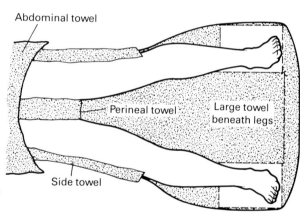

Fig. 7.4 The positions of the sterile towels used to cover all the nonsterile skin and still provide a sufficiently wide sterile field for access to the whole limb.

nique. A diathermy electrode is placed under the patient's buttocks.

Skin preparation and drapes All surfaces of the limb from the heel to the groin, including the anterior surface of the abdomen and pubis to the level of the umbilicus, are prepared with chlorhexidene in spirit. Two per cent iodine may be used as an alternative but this occasionally produces skin reactions and the colour tends to obscure the pre-operative markings. When the limb has been fully painted, with the exception of the foot which is being held by an unsterile assistant, large sterile towels are placed beneath one or both legs on the surface of the operating table (Fig. 7.4). The surgeon or the assistant then holds each limb in turn, supporting it with a sterile swab or towel placed beneath the prepared skin of the calf. The skin of the foot and heel is then prepared, taking care to 'paint up' all parts of the

foot and toes and especially between the toes. Alternatively, the foot can be wrapped in a towel or covered with a sterile surgical glove, taking care not to contaminate the outer surfaces of the glove when it is applied. It is important to remove the glove after the operation, as if the wrist ring is accidentally left around the foot it can cause ischaemia of the toes. Sterile towels are then laid over the abdomen and chest and on either side of the patient to screen off the abdomen and buttocks (Fig. 7.4). A narrow towel is placed

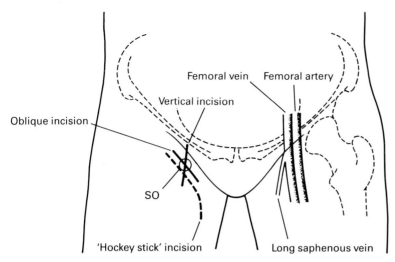

Fig. 7.5 The incisions that can be used to approach the sapheno-femoral junction which lies approximately 2 cm below and lateral to the pubic tubercle. The relationship of the sapheno-femoral junction to the other anatomical structures is also shown. We favour the oblique incision placed just below the groin crease centred over the sapheno-femoral junction.
FA = femoral artery. FV = femoral vein.
LSV = long saphenous vein. SO = saphenous opening.

between the legs to cover the unsterile skin of the genitalia and perineum (Fig. 7.4).

Incision An oblique incision is made just below the crease of the groin, centered over the sapheno-femoral junction which is 2.5 cm lateral to and below the pubic tubercle. The incision should be straight or curved slightly downwards at its medial end to improve the exposure of the upper end of the long saphenous vein. We have not found vertical incisions, or the long 'hockey stick' incision[38] suggested by Dodd helpful (Fig. 7.5). These incisions do not follow Langer's lines (Fig. 7.37) and do not give as good a scar as an incision which is placed parallel to but just below the groin crease. The edges of an incision placed exactly in the groin crease tend to 'invert' easily and are more susceptible to superficial infection.

The length of this incision has been the subject of much debate.[31,39,94,101,107] Although it is desirable for cosmetic reasons that the length of the incision should be kept to a minimum, adequate exposure is essential and must not be compromised. It is important to be able to see the anatomy of the subcutaneous veins so that a satisfactory operation can be performed. The size of the leg and the thickness of the subcutaneous fat are factors that must be considered when deciding on the length of the incision. We usually make a

4–6 cm incision but reduce this length in a thin, young subject, or increase it to as much as 10 cm in a very obese patient. Incisions are rarely placed too high, and the majority of errors occur when the incision is placed too low or is made too short.

Procedure The subcutaneous tissues are divided with a scapel through both the fatty and fibrous layers until the first large vein is seen; this is often the long saphenous vein itself. The skin and subcutaneous tissues are then swept upwards and downwards with a swab to improve the exposure (Fig. 7.6a). This dissection is extended by inserting a self-retaining retractor (Cockett's, Traver's, or West's retractors are ideal) into the subcutaneous fat and opening its blades as far as the skin will allow. It is then left in place, retracting the edges of the wound.

Any remaining subcutaneous tissue covering the veins is then divided until the trunk of the long saphenous vein is found running in a vertical direction towards the sapheno-femoral junction. The trunk of the vein is traced upwards using both sharp and blunt dissection until its junction with the femoral vein is found (Fig. 7.6b). This dissection is simple and bloodless if the correct plane of cleavage is found between the subcutaneous fat and the adventitia of the vein. This plane is easy to recognize because until it is opened the veins are held down flat and compressed by the subcutaneous tissue. Once this fascia has been divided the veins bulge out and are easy to dissect. If the incision has been placed too low, or if the patient is very fat, the upper edge of the incision may need to be retracted by an assistant using an additional right-angle retractor as the vein is traced upwards.

The main trunk of the vein should *never* be divided until the sapheno-femoral junction has been clearly seen (Fig. 7.6b). It is possible to mistake the femoral vein or artery for the long saphenous vein[44,92] with disasterous consequences if either of these vessels is divided. The only foolproof method of avoiding such complications is

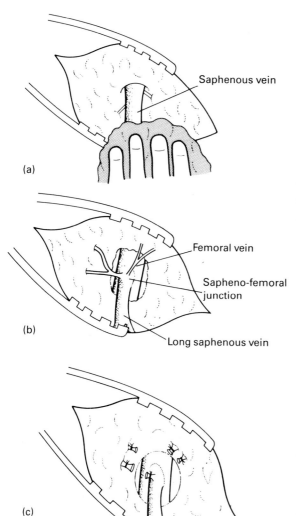

(a)

(b)

Saphenous vein

Femoral vein

Sapheno-femoral junction

Long saphenous vein

(c)

to display the whole anatomy of the long saphenous vein, its tributaries and its junction with the femoral vein, before any large vessels are divided or ligated.

The surgical anatomy of the sapheno-femoral junction A variable number of tributaries join the long saphenous vein as it approaches the femoral vein. The normal anatomy, the anomalies, and their approximate incidences are shown in Figs. 7.7–7.11. These diagrams are derived from two studies of the normal anatomy found in a series of cadaver dissections and a comparable number of operations.[33,59] It can be seen that the 'normal' anatomy described in the 'student textbook' is found in less than one-third of the dissections. Few sapheno-femoral junctions are similar, and this makes knowledge of the possible variations very important before undertaking operations in this area. Tortuosity and sacular dilatation of the termination of the tributaries sometimes makes them appear more prominent than the long saphenous vein itself, for which they may be mistaken, thus making the dissection even more difficult.

There are six named veins that join the long saphenous vein, near its termination (Fig. 7.7), but they are variable in both number and position. The postero-medial and antero-lateral veins of the thigh enter the long saphenous vein on its medial and lateral side respectively at various points

Fig. 7.6 (a) After the skin and subcutaneous tissues have been incised the subcutaneous fat is separated by blunt dissection or is pushed gently apart by two gauze swabs to reveal the long saphenous vein passing up towards the sapheno-femoral junction.

Tributaries can be seen entering the vein from either side. A self-retaining retractor is inserted into the wound and is opened widely to provide a better view of the vein.

(b) The long saphenous vein is traced upwards until the sapheno-femoral junction is clearly identified. Neither the main trunk of the vein nor any of its major tributaries should be divided until this junction has been clearly identified. Small tributaries can be ligated and divided if they interfere with the dissection.

(c) Once the sapheno-femoral junction has been identified, all the tributaries of the long saphenous vein are ligated and divided. Small veins joining the femoral vein near the sapheno-femoral junction are also ligated and divided.

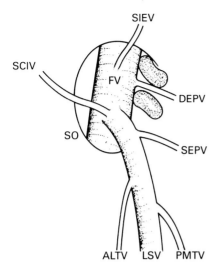

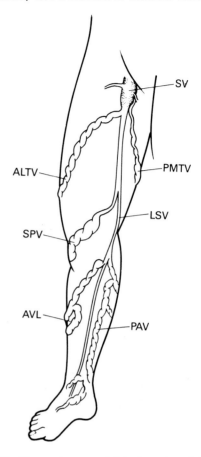

Fig. 7.7 The 'normal' anatomical arrangement of tributaries that are found near the sapheno-femoral junction. *All* these vessels must be defined, ligated and divided at the time of a saphenous vein ligation. SIEV = superficial inferior epigastric vein. SEPV = superficial external pudendal vein. SCIV = superficial circumflex iliac vein. ALTV = antero-lateral thigh vein (lateral accessory saphenous vein). PMTV = postero-medial thigh vein, (Medial accessory saphenous vein). LSV = long saphenous vein. FV = femoral vein. SO = saphenous opening.

Fig. 7.8 The major superficial tributaries of the long saphenous vein which become varicose. Note that the long saphenous vein itself rarely becomes varicose.

SV = saphena varix. ALTV = anterolateral thigh vein. PMTV = postero-medial thigh vein. SPV = suprapatellar vein. PAV = posterior arch vein. AVL = anterior vein of leg (accessory saphenous vein). LSV = long saphenous vein.

between 0 and 20 cm below its termination (Figs 7.7 and 7.8). The superficial inferior epigastric, the superficial circumflex iliac and the superficial external pudendal veins usually join the long saphenous vein just before its termination, but all the variations shown in Fig. 7.9 are frequently encountered. The deep external pudendal vein usually joins the medial side of the femoral vein near the sapheno-femoral junction, but this vein quite often joins the saphenous vein at its termination.

Independent terminations of the antero-lateral and postero-medial thigh veins into the femoral vein may give the appearance of a double saphenous vein (Fig. 7.10), or the long saphenous vein may be truly double with one channel joining the femoral vein lower down the leg, below the level of the real saphenous opening (Fig. 7.11). This is the variation that even an experienced surgeon is likely to miss. It is an important cause of excessive bleeding during vein stripping and

may be responsible for the early recurrence of varicose veins.

The other structure that is encountered during the dissection of the sapheno-femoral junction is the external pudendal artery which may pass either in front or behind the saphenous vein (Fig. 7.12). Care should be taken to avoid damaging this vessel, as the resulting haemorrhage can be annoying. If this vessel is inadvertently damaged, it can be ligated and divided with impunity.

Once all the tributaries of the saphenous vein have been clearly displayed they can be doubly

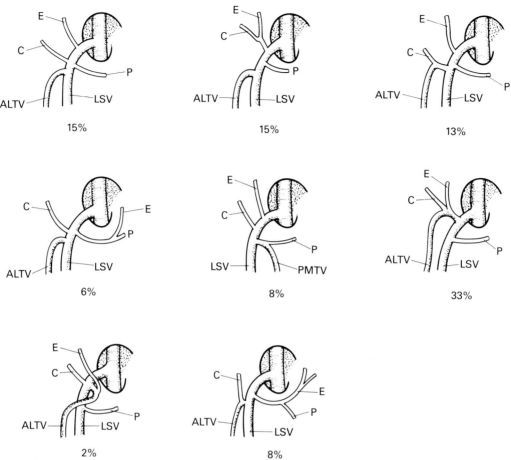

Fig. 7.9   The different appearances and terminations (and their incidences) of the long saphenous vein and its main tributaries that were found by Daseler *et al.*[33] and Hilty[59] at operation and at autopsy dissections. (Modified from Foote).[50]

E = epigastric. C = circumflex iliac.
P = pudendal. LSV = long saphenous vein.
ALTV = antero-lateral thigh vein. PMTV = postero-medial thigh vein.

ligated in continuity with fine chromic catgut (or polyglycolic acid absorbable sutures) and divided. Division of each tributary between artery forceps is an alternative method but is more likely to cause damage and lead to haemorrhage. It is important to re-emphasize that *no major branches should be divided before the site of the sapheno-femoral junction has been clearly identified.*

Both sides of the femoral vein should then be dissected free for 2 cm above and below the sapheno-femoral junction. The deep external pudendal vein and any other tributaries joining the femoral vein must be ligated and divided. The long saphenous vein itself can then be ligated, in continuity, with absorbable or non-absorbable

ligatures, and divided. If the vein is particularly large, we doubly ligate the proximal stump and use a transfixion stitch for the second ligature (Fig. 7.13). If these ligatures are placed between the sapheno-femoral junction and some of the divided tributaries, there is less chance of them slipping off (Fig. 7.13). Care should be taken to ensure that all the tributaries are ligated and divided between the long saphenous stump and its ligature, as any tributaries that are left intact may be responsible for recurrence (Fig. 7.14).

The distal segment of the long saphenous vein is dissected downwards for 5–10 cm. A right-angled retractor is inserted under the lower skin flap to expose the saphenous vein more clearly. If the

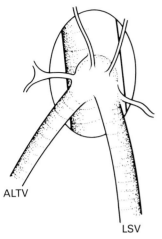

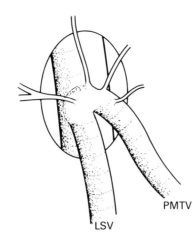

ALTV

LSV

PMTV

LSV

Fig. 7.10   Dilatation and a high termination of either of the two main thigh tributaries, the antero-lateral (ALTV) or the postero-medial (PMTV) thigh veins, may be mistaken for the long saphenous vein, or raise the suspicion that there is a bifid or double long saphenous vein (LSV).

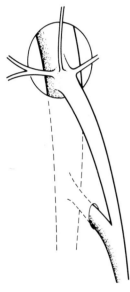

Fig. 7.11   A bifid termination of the long saphenous vein. One division joins the femoral vein in the normal position, the other division joins the femoral vein lower down the thigh. If this anomaly is not detected, considerable haemorrhage may follow stripping, or, if only the upper vein is ligated, varicosities may rapidly recur because of the missed lower branch.

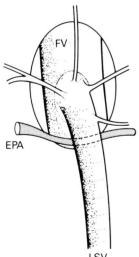

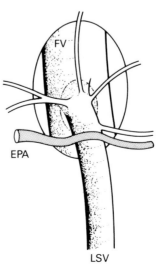

FV

EPA

LSV

FV

EPA

LSV

Fig. 7.12   The relation of the external pudendal artery (EPA) to the sapheno-femoral junction. This vessel normally passes between the termination of the long saphenous vein (LSV) and the femoral vein (FV), but it sometimes passes in front of the long saphenous vein, making it more susceptible to damage during the dissection.

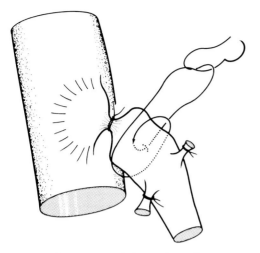

Fig. 7.13 Ligation of the sapheno-femoral junction. After all the branches of the long saphenous vein have been ligated and divided, the long saphenous vein is itself ligated in continuity, and is divided. Two ligatures are usually placed on the proximal end as a precautionary measure. If the vein is exceptionally large a transfixion suture may be used for the second ligature. It is important to place these ligatures between the junction and all the major tributaries of the saphenous vein. The stumps of the tributaries then prevent the ligature from 'rolling off'.

antero-lateral and postero-medial thigh veins can be seen, they should be freed, doubly ligated and divided, even if the saphenous vein is not going to be stripped out. At least 5–10 cm of the long saphenous vein should be resected if a sapheno-femoral ligation is the only operation to be performed.

Care must be taken to:

1. avoid damaging the femoral vein or tearing off small tributaries that enter this vein;
2. ligate all small tributaries entering the femoral vein directly (particularly the deep external pudendal vein);
3. make sure that all sutures are properly tied and do not come undone or slip off the long saphenous vein or its tributaries;
4. ensure that the long saphenous vein is tied flush with the femoral vein without narrowing the femoral vein;
5. avoid dividing any vein assumed to be the long saphenous vein until its junction with a normal femoral vein has been confirmed.

Closure The incision should be closed using

catgut sutures to approximate the fatty layers and fine nylon or an intradermal absorbable suture to close the skin. The latter sutures may be used in conjunction with adhesive tapes.

Technical problems

Bleeding Sudden massive bleeding from a slipped ligature or direct damage to a major vein should be controlled by applying direct pressure to the bleeding point with a finger or swab. If a junior surgeon is doing the operation, he should obtain help from an experienced senior colleague (preferably one who has had vascular training). After applying pressure for several minutes (a minimum of 2 min) the swabs or finger may be gently removed. The bleeding is usually much reduced, and the damaged vein can be closed with a direct vascular suture aided by wound suction to remove the blood and provide a clear view of the bleeding point.

If the bleeding cannot be controlled in this way, pressure should be reapplied and the wound should be enlarged to allow the femoral vein to be exposed some distance above and below the saphenous opening. Direct digital compression of the femoral vein above and below the saphenous junction will always control the bleeding, allowing further dissection of the damaged vein and the placement of sutures to close the defect. It is only necessary to apply clamps to the femoral vein when it has been severely damaged and requires some form of reconstruction. In these circumstances the anticoagulant heparin should be given to the patient before the vein is clamped. A vein patch may be used to repair the femoral vein if necessary (see Chapter 25).

Artery forceps must never be applied to a bleeding point without a good view of the damaged vessel and should never be applied to a side hole in a large vein – such unthinking precipitous action will often make the venous injury worse.

Damage to the femoral artery The femoral artery should not be injured during straightforward varicose vein surgery; if, however, it is damaged, and the damage is recognized, it should be repaired by direct suture, a vein patch or a vein graft. The three common ways of injuring the femoral artery are: tearing off a small side branch, inadvertent ligation and inadvertent stripping.

Damage to the femoral vein Damage to the

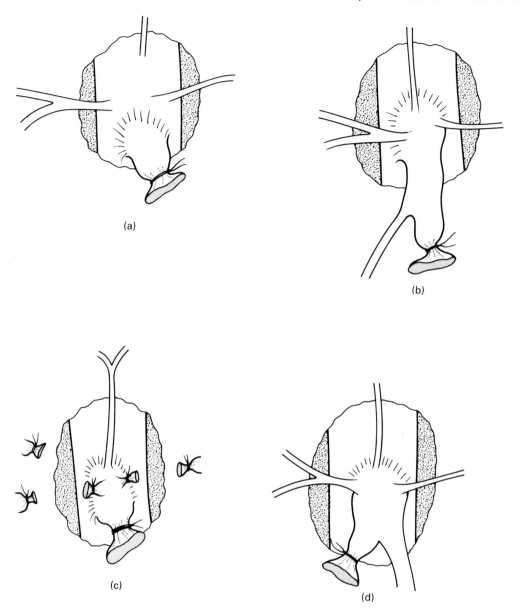

Fig. 7.14   Reasons for the development of recurrent connections between the deep and superficial veins at the saphenous opening.

(a) Failure to ligate 'normal' tributaries of the long saphenous vein which join the common femoral vein directly.

(b) A low ligation of the long saphenous vein, which produces the same circumstances as (a).

(c) Failure to ligate all the tributaries. Usually, either the superficial inferior epigastric or the superficial external pudendal veins are not ligated.

(d) Ligation of the antero-lateral or postero-medial thigh vein in the mistaken belief that it is the long saphenous vein, thus leaving the long saphenous vein intact.

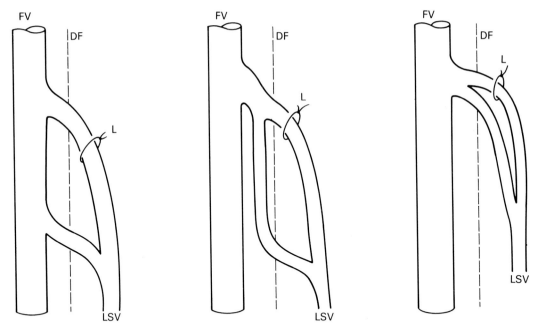

Fig. 7.14   (e) Placement of the ligature below one limb of a bifid termination of the long saphenous vein.
FV = femoral vein. LSV = long saphenous vein. DF = deep fascia. L = site of ligature.

femoral vein which causes bleeding is discussed above. The femoral vein may also be inadvertantly ligated, and if this is recognized, the ligature should be carefully removed and the vein wall should be inspected (see Fig. 25.5, page 647). If there is a circumferential disruption of the intima, the vein may have to be resected and repaired with an end-to-end anastomosis or an interposition vein graft (see Chapter 25).

Stripping the long saphenous vein

We routinely strip the long saphenous vein to a point just below the knee to prevent recurrence developing through the Hunterian communicating veins[28] and to remove a vein in the thigh which is difficult to treat later by sclerotherapy. Vascular surgeons have recently complained that unnecessary stripping of the long saphenous vein removes a potential vascular conduit[27,67] but other surgeons have pointed out that a grossly distended incompetent long saphenous is probably of little use in bypass surgery.[89] Both arguments are probably valid but most authorities agree that a combination of a high saphenous ligation with long saphenous stripping reduces the incidence of upper thigh recurrences.[31,39,78,90,106,107,122] We only

strip the long saphenous vein to just below the knee to avoid damaging the saphenous nerve whose branches are close to the vein in the lower leg. This leaves a reasonable length of vein below the knee for use by the cardiac surgeons at a later date.[7]

Technique   After ligating and dividing the long saphenous vein (as described above), a long silk ligature is passed around the lower part of the vein and a transverse venotomy is made in the vein above the ligature (Fig. 7.15). The ligature is 'held up' to occlude the vein and prevent haemorrhage from the venotomy, but it is not tied down until the stripper has been inserted.

A flexible intraluminal stripper is chosen, preferably from a selection with 'olives' of differing sizes. We prefer a flexible wire stripper (Fig. 7.16) because we find that it is easier to direct through the kinks and lateral sacculations of a varicose vein; other workers, however, prefer the modern stiff plastic disposable strippers with reversible heads (Fig. 7.17).

The blunt pointed tip of the stripper (Fig. 7.16) is inserted into the venotomy and pushed downwards. The ligature is then tied down to prevent bleeding from around the stripper, and an artery forceps is placed on the proximal end of the

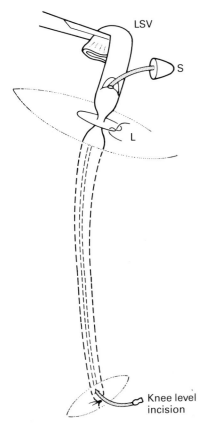

Fig. 7.15 The insertion of the stripper. After the long saphenous vein (LSV) has been ligated and divided, the distal end of the vein is freed from the surrounding subcutaneous tissues for several centimetres and the termination of both the antero-lateral and postero-medial thigh veins are ligated and divided. An artery forceps is placed on the end of the vein for counter-traction, and a ligature (L) is passed around the vein and pulled taut to prevent bleeding when the venotomy is made. The stripper (S) is then inserted and manipulated down to the knee. The stripper is retrieved from the vein at the knee level, through a small incision, to allow the vein to be avulsed from above downwards.

tion on the divided vein, while the surgeon uses his free hand to feel and direct the stripper head down the main vein and, by applying gentle external pressure over its tip; prevent it passing into varicose tributaries. The passage of the stripper may be facilitated at knee level by flexing and extending the knee joint with external pressure applied over the tip of the stripper, accompanied by further rotation of the stripper wire and intermittent insertion and withdrawal. As the surgeon's experience of the use of the stripper increases, more successful passages of the stripper to the knee will be achieved.

When the stripper has successfully negotiated the vein beyond the level of the knee joint a short oblique incision is made in the direction of Langer's lines, (Fig. 7.37) over the palpable tip. The vein containing the stripper (it may be the long saphenous, the anterior leg vein, or the posterior arch vein) is isolated by blunt dissection, and the distal end of the vein is ligated with catgut. A venotomy is then made and the stripper is extracted from the lumen of the vessel. A further ligature is passed around the proximal part of the vein containing the stripper wire and the vein is divided.

A handle is attached to the stripper and the vein is removed by steady firm traction applied in the long axis of the vein. The vein and its tributaries are avulsed as it concertinas up against the under-surface of the mushroom-shaped olive on the end of the stripper (Fig. 7.18). The incision at the knee must be long enough to allow the mass of vein on the stripper to pass through it, but if a small incision is required at knee level, the stripper head can be pulled back up its track by attaching a silk ligature to the head[73,125] and removed, with the vein, through the groin incision. The plastic disposable strippers have removable heads, which can be attached at either end, thus the direction of stripping is optional.

If the stripper will not pass down the vein, an incision must be made just below the medial condyle of the tibia to expose the long saphenous vein, which is always quite deep at this point, lying on the deep fascia. A segment of vein is dissected out and suitably ligated and the stripper is passed up to the groin (Fig. 7.19). Upward passage of the stripper is unavoidable in some operations. We prefer to strip the vein downwards, not simply because it allows a smaller incision below the knee, but also because greater lengths of tributary

divided vein to allow counter traction to be exerted on the vein as the stripper is advanced down the limb. On many occasions the stripper will pass without difficulty to below the knee but if resistance is met during insertion, the stripper should be withdrawn a few centimetres and then reinserted while a rotatory movement is applied to the free portion which is still protruding outside the vein. The passage of the stripper may be made easier if an assistant takes over the counter trac-

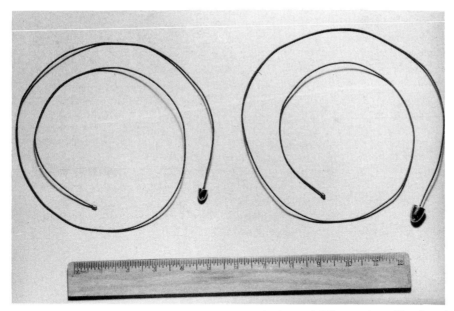

Fig. 7.16 Two flexible Myers' wire strippers with olives of different sizes. The tips also come in different shapes and sizes. These strippers must be carefully handled and stored to avoid kinking the wire.

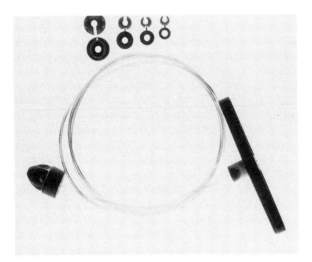

Fig. 7.17 A disposable, flexible, intraluminal, plastic stripper with removable heads of different sizes (shown above) and handle.

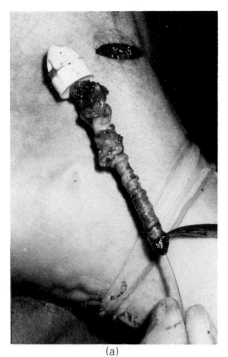

(a)

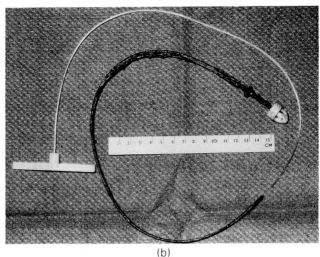

(b)

Fig. 7.18 Stripping the long saphenous vein.

(a) As the stripper head is pulled through the leg the vein 'concertinas up' on the wire below the olive so that when the stripper is removed from the lower incision, the concertina'd vein appears to be quite short.

(b) The vein should be pulled out, to check that the full length of the long saphenous vein and short lengths of its tributaries have been removed.

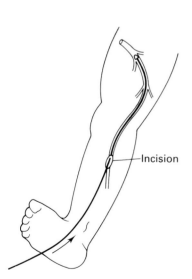

Fig. 7.19 Passage of the stripper through the long saphenous vein from the knee upwards. The long saphenous vein is isolated near the knee and, after it has been ligated distally, the stripper is inserted and passed up to the groin.

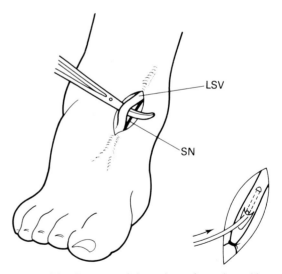

Fig. 7.20 Passage of the stripper from the ankle. The vein is isolated where it crosses the anterior aspect of the medial malleolus, taking care to separate it from the saphenous nerve. The stripper is inserted into the vein and then passed up to the groin. (insert).

(LSV = long saphenous vein. SN = saphenous nerve.)

veins are usually avulsed when the stripper is pulled downwards rather than upwards, and there is a lower incidence of saphenous nerve damage when the stripper is pulled downwards.[29]

May[101] has emphasized the dangers of passing a stripper from the ankle to the groin to help to locate the sapheno-femoral junction; he pointed out that the stripper may enter the deep veins through a communicating vein in the thigh or an accessory low sapheno-femoral junction (Fig. 7.11), thus making inadvertent ligation or stripping of the femoral vein more likely. He has also suggested that thrombus can form on a stripper which is left in place for a long time during the groin dissection. Small pulmonary emboli may then occur, if the long saphenous vein is not ligated early in the dissection. The only advantage of passing a stripper from the ankle is the ease with which the vein can be found as it crosses the subcutaneous surface of the medial malleolus and the fact that it will pass up to the groin unimpeded in 90–95 per cent of cases (Fig. 7.20). The disadvantages, which have already been mentioned, are the loss of a potentially useful normal vein below the knee which might be used as an arterial graft at a later date[27,67] and an increased risk of skin anaesthesia secondary to saphenous nerve damage.[29]

Stripping the long saphenous vein below the knee does *not* correct any lower leg communicating vein incompetence as most of these veins do not drain directly into the long saphenous vein (see Chapter 2), whereas the Hunter Canal communicating vein in the thigh does drain directly into the saphenous vein. Furthermore, the long saphenous vein below the knee is often normal in size with competent valves, even when the upper thigh segment is dilated and incompetent. For these reasons (lack of abnormality and no worthwhile physiological effect) we do not normally strip the long saphenous vein below the knee. We have not found problems with retrograde passage of the stripper to the knee, because if the operation is being done for the correct indications there should be few if any competent valves to obstruct its passage. Nevertheless, we do not persist for a prolonged time with our attempts at retrograde passage; if any difficulty is experienced, we cut down, find the vein below the knee and pass the stripper upwards.

Technical problems

Failure to pass the stripper Occasionally, varicosities of the long saphenous vein itself (Fig. 7.21) prevent the passage of a stripper in both directions. If this happens two strippers are passed, one from above and one from below, to the point of obstruction (Fig. 7.22). An incision is made at this point and the tips of both strippers are extracted before both segments of the vein are avulsed. Alternatively, the heads of the strippers can be tied together so that either one can be used to guide the other stripper through its segment of vein. Occasionally, all these manoeuvres fail and the vein has to be stripped 'piecemeal' through a number of separate incisions. These incisions should be as small as possible, and they should be placed in the direction of Langer's lines (Fig. 7.37).

Haemorrhage from the track Stripping of the vein can be left to the end of the operation. The limb may be then bandaged as the stripper is removed in an attempt to minimize haematoma formation in the track. Alternatively, stripping can be performed at an early stage so that any collections of blood can be expelled by gentle compression produced by rolling a gauze swab, made into a ball, up and down the leg along the course of the vein. If the leg is elevated, the

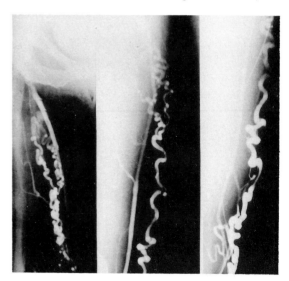

Fig. 7.21 This varicogram shows a double long saphenous vein. One vein is straight and the stripper would pass along it easily (this is the normal finding). The other vein is so tortuous that the stripper would not pass through it.

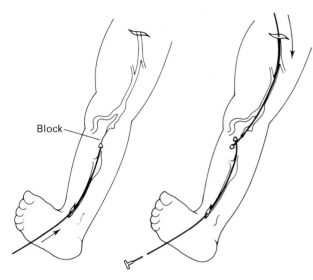

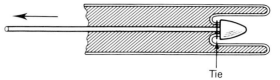

Fig. 7.23 Inversion of the vein by the stripper. This happens when the olive that has been selected is too small for the diameter of the vein being stripped. The vein often breaks when this happens.

Fig. 7.22 A narrow portion or a varicosity on the long saphenous vein may prevent the passage of the stripper. In these circumstances it may be helpful to pass the stripper from the opposite direction to the level of the block. The second stripper may occasionally pass through the block and down the full length of the vein but if this does not happen, a cut-down should be made over the obstruction to allow the strippers to be tied together and pulled through the full length of the vein or the vein should be stripped out in two halves.

haemorrhage soon stops, providing the uppermost major branches (the antero-lateral and postero-medial thigh veins) have been ligated before the vein was stripped. Severe bleeding can invariably be controlled by external pressure and increased elevation of the leg. It is very seldom necessary to explore the track of a stripped vein to arrest bleeding; if it is necessary, an arterial injury or a co-incidental bleeding diathesis must be suspected.

Inversion of the vein If the olive of the stripper that is selected is too small, it may pass into the lumen of the vein which is then invaginated as the vein is stripped (Fig. 7.23). Usually, the vein can still be delivered satisfactorily from below by gentle traction, but if this fails, the silk ligature threaded through the olive may be used to pull the stripper back so that a stripper with a larger olive may be substituted.

Perforation of the vein If the stripper cannot be passed (despite the techniques described above) and excessive force is used during its insertion, the tip may pierce the vein wall before passing down the leg in a false passage alongside rather than inside the vein. This is recognized when the cut-down over the tip finds the stripper lying outside the lumen of the vein. If an attempt is made to strip the vein, the whole of the vein may be satisfactorily avulsed but often only part of the vein is stripped out. It is wiser to pass a second stripper from below, by the method described above, and to strip the vein upwards or use the lower stripper to guide the upper stripper down the correct path (Fig. 7.22).

Damage to the saphenous nerve This is a well-recognized complication when the long saphenous vein is stripped to the ankle,[29] but it seldom occurs if the vein is only stripped to just below the knee. Care must be taken to avoid damaging the saphenous nerve below the knee, where it can easily be caught in the ligature placed around the vein to fix it to the stripper. The nerve must be carefully dissected off the vein before the ligature is passed, particulary if the stripper is inserted at the ankle. Stripping below the knee should always be carried out in a downward direction; stripping at this level serves little purpose and should be avoided.

Skin closure Small incisions on the leg, whether for stripping or for avulsion, can be closed with fine nylon sutures or adhesive skin tapes. Adhesive skin tapes give the best cosmetic results. The legs should be bandaged firmly from toe to groin.

Contra-indications to stripping

Patients with *bleeding problems* are best treated by high saphenous ligation without stripping the long saphenous vein, unless the bleeding problem can be overcome before operation.

In patients with *lymphoedema* ankle swelling can be exacerbated by stripping, perhaps as a result of damage to the lymphatics which lie around the vein. If lymphoedema and bleeding problems coexist, the veins should be treated by ligation without stripping.

In patients with varicose veins and *arterial insufficiency* a sapheno-femoral ligation alone should be carried out, if the veins really need to be treated, leaving the vein for possible future use as an arterial conduit. The surgeon should avoid making incisions in the lower leg which may not heal satisfactorily.

Postoperative management

Patients should be encouraged to get up and walk as soon as possible (e.g. the same evening or the following morning) and they can be discharged from hospital the following day, unless there are social contraindications to discharge or they develop complications. Mild oral analgesic drugs are provided for the first few days. Sutures are removed 5–7 days after the operation, but firm compression bandages should be worn at all times during the first week, and for the next 3 weeks they should only be removed at night. These bandages reduce postoperative bruising and oedema, and may also reduce the risk of deep vein thrombosis.[146,147] We use a combination of Elastocrepe bandages covered with Tubigrip stockinette because the heavier Blue or Red Line[10] bandages tends to slip down after a few hours of activity. Alternatively, all patients could be provided with elastic stockings but these stockings are expensive and patients find them painful to put on and difficult to wear when they have tender incisions on the legs. The newer elastic bandages which have recently come on the market may be better but they require further evaluation.

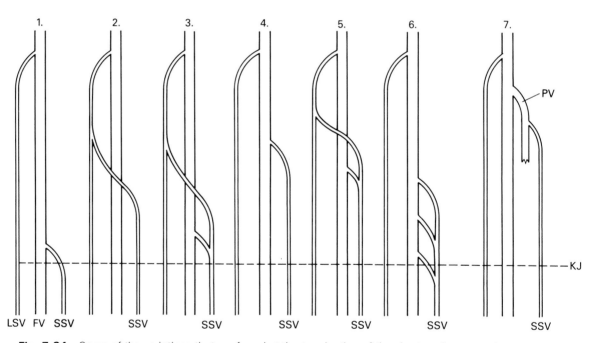

Fig. 7.24   Some of the variations that are found at the termination of the short saphenous vein.
   1. The 'normal' (only found in 60 per cent of all short saphenous terminations) termination
   2. The short saphenous vein drains into the long saphenous vein rather than into the popliteal vein
   3. A connection between the short saphenous vein and long saphenous vein
   4. A high termination
   5. A high termination and a connection with the long saphenous vein
   6. Multiple terminations and connections, at different levels, with the femoro-popliteal vein
   7. The short saphenous vein may be connected to a tributary of the deep femoral vein or may terminate in the deep femoral vein[103]

KJ = level of knee joint. LSV = long saphenous vein. SSV = short saphenous vein. FV = femoral vein. PV = deep femoral vein.

Ligation and division of the sapheno-popliteal junction and stripping of the short saphenous vein

The position of the sapheno-popliteal junction is extremely variable (see Chapter 2); a summary of the anatomical variations is shown in Fig. 7.24. Haeger[57] and Kosinski[77] have shown that the short saphenous vein joins the popliteal vein a few centimetres above the level of the knee joint in 57 per cent of all limbs. In approximately one-third (33 per cent) of limbs, the short saphenous vein has a high termination joining either the long saphenous vein or connecting with one of the inter-muscular communicating veins to empty into the deep femoral vein.[103] In 10 per cent of limbs the short saphenous vein has a low termination joining either the long saphenous vein in the calf or one of the deep veins in the centre of the calf.[100,104] Some surgeons advocate routine stripping of the short saphenous vein; other surgeons think the short saphenous vein should be disconnected and never stripped. If a long saphenous vein operation is to be performed under the same anaesthetic, the short saphenous vein operation should be carried out first.

Pre-operative preparation Particular care must be taken to identify the termination of the short saphenous vein. Clinical examination is notoriously inaccurate; better information can be provided by the Doppler flow detector,[61] varicography,[21,79] or intra-operative phlebography.[62]

Position If the operation is to be performed under a general anaesthetic the patient must be intubated, before being placed in a prone position on the operating table. Two pillows are placed under the patient's hips and chest to prevent abdominal compression and to allow free movement of the diaphragm. Abduction of the limbs is not essential but is often quite helpful.

Skin preparation and towelling When the patient has been placed in a prone position on the operating table an assistant grasps the foot and bends the knee to 90°, to allow the lower part of the leg (with the exception of the foot) to be painted with Hibitane in spirit (1 in 10,000) or iodine (2 %). The assistant then lifts the whole leg off the table so that the knee and anterior surface of the thigh can be painted. A large towel is slipped beneath the knee to cover the upper surface of the operating table. The surgeon grasps the painted area of the calf in a swab before painting the foot with antiseptic or enclosing it in a towel or glove. The upper part of the limb is covered by another large sterile towel. The operating table is placed with a 15–30° head-down tilt to reduce venous congestion and lessen bleeding.

Short saphenous vein stripping We routinely strip the short saphenous vein because there are communicating veins which drain directly into it, and the presence of the stripper within the vein helps us to indentify the vein in the popliteal fossa. We begin by making a short vertical incision midway between the Achilles tendon and the lower part of the fibula over the lower end of the short saphenous vein (Fig. 7.25). The vein is found in the subcutaneous tissue deep to this incision. Care must be taken to define the sural nerve which is occasionally mistaken for the vein and is always closely applied to it. Careful inspection will reveal that the nerve is composed of a number of nerve bundles without branches, whereas the vein usually receives one or two tributaries at this level.

When the vein has been separated from the nerve, a catgut ligature is tied around the distal end of the vein. Another ligature is passed around the vein, proximally, but is not tied. A transverse venotomy is then made in the vein between the two ligatures; the upper ligature is held taut to prevent back-bleeding, and a flexible wire stripper

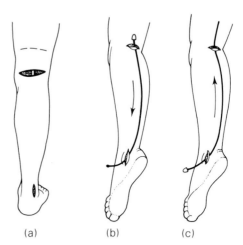

(a) (b) (c)

Fig. 7.25 Short saphenous vein stripping.
(a) The incisions used for stripping the short saphenous vein. A second incision, higher in the popliteal fossa, may be required if there is a high termination of the vein.
(b and c) The vein may be stripped upwards or downwards.
Modified from May.[101]

is inserted into the vein, as for long saphenous vein stripping. After the stripper has been passed a short distance the upper ligature is tied to prevent back-bleeding. The stripper is then gently passed up the vein from below in a manner similar to that already described in long saphenous vein stripping (see page 214).

If the sapheno-popliteal junction has been defined by one of the methods already described and if the stripper passes easily up to the expected level, the popliteal incision can be made directly over the sapheno-popliteal junction but if pre-operative localization of the junction has not been attempted, careful palpation of the stripper tip as it enters the popliteal fossa may help to define the level of the junction. The short saphenous vein can pass beneath the deep fascia at any point as it ascends the leg (Fig. 7.26)[104] but it bends sharply (90 °) inwards where it turns to join the popliteal vein. The stripper tip can often be felt to disappear at this point and it may give a little kick or jump as it enters the popliteal vein. This is a useful indication (but no more than an indication) of the site of the termination of the short saphenous vein, and it can be used if other methods of sapheno-popliteal localization are not available.

As short saphenous incompetence is relatively rare[107] (see Chapter 6), we prefer to perform pre-operative varicograms on all patients with short saphenous incompetence to confirm the diagnosis and ascertain the exact anatomy (Fig. 7.27). Intra-operative venography, as suggested by Hobbs,[62]

provides a satisfactory alternative but does add time to the operation. The vein is stripped after the sapheno-popliteal junction has been dissected and divided.

Exploration of the popliteal fossa

A transverse incision is made over the termination of the short saphenous vein. This incision will vary in length according to the size of the patient and the amount of subcutaneous fat surrounding the limb, but it should always err on the generous side and should be at least 5–8 cm long.

The subcutaneous fat is split beneath the line of the incision down to the deep fascia which is also opened in a similar direction; care must be taken because the vein and the sural nerve may occasionally lie within the layers of fascia rather than deep to it. A self-retaining retractor is inserted to open the skin, fat and the deep fascia (Fig. 7.28). The short saphenous vein should be found passing vertically upwards. It can easily be felt if it contains the stripper, but *great care must be taken to ensure that the stripper is not in the popliteal vein having entered it through a connecting vein in the lower calf.*

The stripper is withdrawn to allow dissection of the short saphenous vein which should be traced to its junction with the popliteal vein. The short saphenous vein should never be ligated until the surgeon has clearly seen its junction with the popliteal vein (Fig. 7.28). Sometimes this dissection is difficult, especially when the short saphenous vein dips down into a deep and fatty popliteal fossa. Visability can sometimes be improved by inserting two Langenbeck retractors to pull the fat and the heads of the gastrocnemius muscle apart.

A large tributary commonly joins the short saphenous vein from above, before it turns deeply to join the popliteal vein or one of the paired venae comitantes that pass up on either side of the popliteal artery. This tributary must be carefully divided between ligatures before the short saphenous vein is ligated flush with the popliteal vein. Dodd and Cockett[39] recommend flexion of the knee during dissection of the popliteal fossa to relax the popliteal fascia, but we have not found this to be of any particular benefit. The popliteal dissection is, however, difficult, and it is essential that the popliteal vein is not damaged because this can have disasterous consequences.

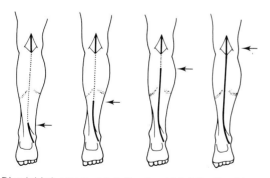

Distal third   Middle third   Proximal third   Popliteal fossa
    7%   51.5%   32.5%   9%

Fig. 7.26 The positions where the short saphenous vein may pierce the deep fascia at it ascends the leg. The relative incidences are based on Moosman *et al.*[104]

Modified from May.[101]

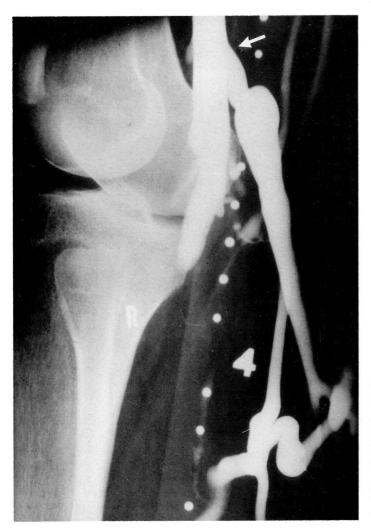

Fig. 7.27 A varicogram showing a dilated short saphenous vein with a termination (arrowed) 4 cm above the knee joint. The metal ball-bearings (1 cm apart) are incorporated in a plastic ruler which is placed on the surface of the leg. There are varicose veins connecting the long and short saphenous veins. The caliber of the long saphenous vein is normal.

Large veins from the gastrocnemius muscle and other large tributaries may also join the undersurface of the short saphenous vein near its termination making the anatomy difficult to define. All the tributaries of the short saphenous vein must be carefully ligated. A young surgeon in training is advised to look at an anatomical dissection of the popliteal fossa before undertaking this operation, as this provides a salutary reminder of the important structures within the popliteal fossa that can be damaged by inexpert dissection (Fig. 7.29). It is better to leave a stump of short saphenous vein, rather than damage the popliteal vein while attempting to perform a perfect flush ligation, but if a small stump of vein is left, it may

allow recurrent incompetent veins to develop which can be extremely difficult to manage.

If the popliteal incision is too low a second incision may be required at a higher level, which may be gauged by pulling down on the vein and seeing where this produces a dimple in the skin. After ligating and dividing the short saphenous vein in the popliteal fossa, it is also divided at the ankle and stripped out.

The fascia of the popliteal fossa is closed with 2/0 chromic catgut and the skin is closed with interrupted 4/0 nylon stitches or a subcuticular suture with adhesive skin strips.

If no other procedure is to be performed, the foot and lower leg are firmly bandaged. Alterna-

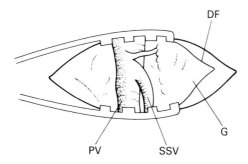

tively, after the short saphenous incisions have been covered by sterile gauze and the leg has been wrapped in a sterile towel to prevent contamination, the patient can be turned onto their back for long saphenous vein ligation and stripping.

Postoperative care This is identical to that following the long saphenous operation.

Fig. 7.28 The dissection of the termination of the short saphenous vein in the popliteal fossa.

(a) The short saphenous vein is usually found lying beneath the deep fascia (see Fig. 7.26) and can be traced to its termination in the popliteal vein.

All the tributaries joining the short saphenous vein should be ligated and divided once the site of the sapheno-popliteal junction has been confirmed. The vein may then be stripped out, if stripping is indicated.

PV = popliteal vein. SSV = short saphenous vein. DF = deep fascia. G = gastrocnemius muscle.

Technical problems

The problems associated with this operation are similar to those already described for the long saphenous vein operation, except that the popliteal artery, vein and nerve are all at risk during the popliteal fossa dissection. The sural nerve is easily damaged if it is not dissected free from the vein at the ankle and if it is not found and preserved in the popliteal fossa.

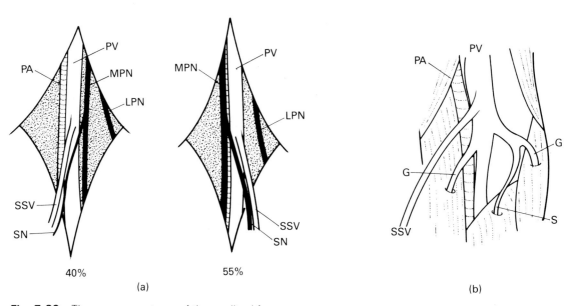

Fig. 7.29 The venous anatomy of the popliteal fossa.

(a) There is a close relationship between the short saphenous vein and the medial popliteal nerve in the popliteal fossa. The vein can lie either medial or lateral to the nerve.

PV = popliteal vein. SSV = short saphenous vein. LPN = lateral popliteal nerve. MPN = medial popliteal nerve. SN = sural nerve. PA = popliteal artery.

(b) The 'normal' venous anatomy. The gastrocnemius veins may join the short saphenous vein before it joins the popliteal vein.[101]

PV = popliteal vein. PA = popliteal artery.
SSV = short saphenous vein. G = medial and lateral tributaries from gastrocnemius muscle.
S = tributaries from the soleus muscle.

Ligation of the medial lower leg communicating veins

Surgery for these veins is usually required in patients with lipodermatosclerosis or ulceration, but as Fletcher and Tibbs have shown[49] (see Chapter 6) some 're-entry' communicating veins may exist with superficial venous incompetence. Failure to ligate these veins may account for recurrence despite satisfactory saphenous surgery, and Sherman,[133] Massel,[99] and May[101] have all emphasized the value of accurate 'perforator' surgery in preventing recurrent varicosities. In order to prevent the unsightly scar of a full ankle communicating operation (see below), 'on-table'[99,101] or pre-operative varicography[21,80] may allow local ligations to be carried out.

A full exploration should be carried out in patients with venous skin complications; this is described below.

Subfascial ligation of the medial communicating veins (Linton's operation)[86]

The patient is prepared and positioned as if for long saphenous vein surgery which has been described above. The suspected sites of 'communicating vein incompetence' are carefully marked on the skin with an indelible pen in a manner which distinguishes them from the other marks placed over the superficial varices that are to be avulsed.

A vertical incision is made 2 cm (1 inch) behind the posterior border of the subcutaneous surface of the tibia from the tip of medial malleolus to a point at least three hand's breadths above the malleolus which is usually just above the mid-point of the leg (Fig. 7.30).

Some surgeons perform this operation in a bloodless field (having expelled the blood with an Esmarch bandage and inflated an arterial occlusion tourniquet above the knee),[126,127] but we have not found it necessary to adopt this technique.

The incision should pass straight down through the subcutaneous tissues to the deep fascia which is vertically incised in line with the skin incision. The subcutaneous fat is often sclerotic and contains many large veins, which may bleed copiously when they are divided; this bleeding can, however, be controlled by digital pressure on either side of the incision or by applying an artery forceps to the deep fascia and everting it over the

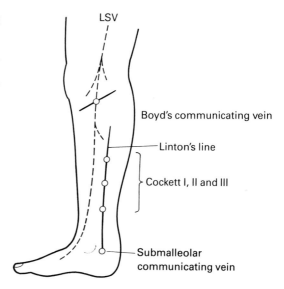

Fig. 7.30 The common sites of the medial calf communicating veins and the incision used to explore them (Linton's line) LSV = long saphenous vein.

edge of the wound. Small curved artery forceps can then be directly applied to the cut ends of the divided subcutaneous veins which are then carefully ligated with 2/0 or 3/0 chromic catgut.

Alternatively, the veins in the subcutaneous fat can be dissected and clamped before they are divided. This is possible if the fat is relatively soft and pliable but can be very difficult if it is fibrotic. The veins can be under-run with fine catgut sutures if the surrounding tissues are too firm to allow the veins to be picked up with artery forceps. It is important not to undercut or dissect beneath the skin but to make a vertical incision down to the deep fascia to avoid damaging the blood supply of the skin.

After the deep fascia has been incised and the bleeding has been controlled, artery forceps are placed on the cut edges of the fascia to help elevate it from the underlying muscles which are gently dissected free with a gauze swab or by a gentle sweep of an index finger. As the muscles are separated from the deep surface of the fascia, the communicating veins will be seen crossing the subfascial plane, between the flexor digitorum longus and the free border of the soleus muscle, to enter the under surface of the deep fascia (Fig. 7.31). These veins should be isolated, doubly ligated and divided. If the Turner–Warwick test[143] is to be performed, the

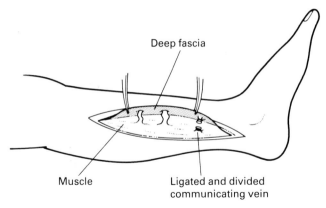

Deep fascia

Muscle

Ligated and divided
communicating vein

Fig. 7.31 Subfascial ligation of incompetent medial calf communicating veins.[20] A long vertical incision is made through the skin and subcutaneous fat down to the deep fascia, approximately 1 cm behind the subcutaneous posterior border of the tibia. Any subcutaneous veins that are divided are ligated. The deep fascia is incised in the same line as the skin incision and is held open gently with a self-retaining retractor. As the subfascial space is opened, leashes of communicating vessels (usually two veins and one artery) can be see passing from the posterior tibial vessels between the muscles to the under-surface of the deep fascia. These vessels are isolated, divided and ligated. If necessary, their incompetence can be tested by a Turner–Warwick test.[43] When all the communicating veins have been ligated, the deep fascia and skin are carefully approximated.

deep end of the vein should be clamped and divided leaving a good stump of vein protruding from the muscle. The deep stump will bleed if the valve of the communicating vein is incompetent. This may be made more obvious if the ankle is forcibly dorsiflexed. The distance of the communicating vein above the tip of medial malleolus and the presence or absence of venous reflux should be recorded.

The subfascial dissection should continue until all the subfascial space has been explored and all the vessels which cross it, between the subcutaneous border of the tibia and the mid-line posteriorly, have been ligated and divided. The communicating veins most likely to be missed are those which come out in front of flexor digitorum longus, close to the posterior border of the tibia and any vein which comes out below the level of the medial malleolus.

When the dissection is complete, a finger must be pushed up beneath the deep fascia under the upper end of the incision to explore the subfascial space to the level of the medial condyle of the tibia. Sometimes other large communicating veins may be found in this area and these must be ligated and divided. The positions of the main calf communicating veins are shown in Fig. 2.31 (page 46). Further small communicating vessels may be found in other positions[118,144] but these are almost

all indirect communicating veins which are of doubtful clinical significance.

When the whole of the subfascial space on the medial side of the leg has been separated from the muscles and cleared of communicating veins, haemostasis is achieved and the deep fascia is closed with an interrupted or continuous 2/0 chromic catgut suture. The skin is closed with a minimum of carefully placed nylon mattress stitches or simple sutures, between adhesive skin tapes or with adhesive tape alone. Although closure with a subcuticular suture may produce a more satisfactory result cosmetically; it should be resisted because it increases the chances of skin necrosis.

Postoperative care After subfascial communicating vein ligation, the patient should be kept in bed with the leg bandaged and elevated to 30° for 24 hours. The patient may be mobilized but this must be done gradually as the leg is painful and skin healing is slow. Patients may be discharged after 4 or 5 days if the wound is healing satisfactorily but the sutures are left in place for 10 days. If the wound becomes infected or the skin edges look unhealthy, the patient should be kept in hospital until the infection is under control and the incision is showing signs of healing. The scar of the incision will eventually become almost invisible (Fig. 7.32).

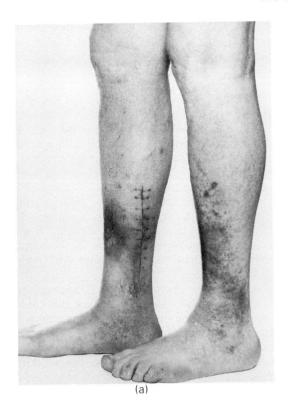

(a)

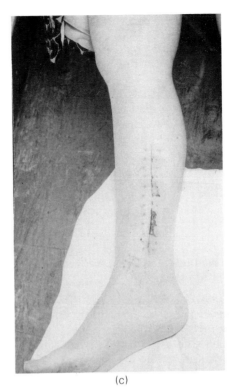

(c)

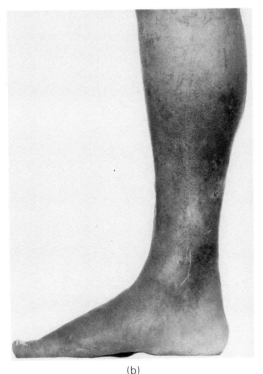

(b)

Fig. 7.32 The scars of communicating vein exploration.

　(a) A young (1 month) wound that is healing well.

　(b) An old (5 years) wound that is just visible as a thin white line in the pigmentation.

　(c) A recent (3 weeks) wound, the edges of which have become necrotic. The necrosis is usually the result of undercutting the skin edges or pulling the skin sutures too tight. Sometimes the skin is so unhealthy that any wound made within it will heal badly.

Extra-fascial ligation of the medial communicating veins (Cockett's operation)[136]

In patients who have had venous ulceration or in those that have severe lipodermatosclerosis this operation is more difficult to perform than the subfascial operation because the sclerosis of the subcutaneous fat makes dissection of the subcutaneous layer extremely difficult.

　The initial preparation and incision are the same as for the subfascial procedure, but when the deep fascia is reached the skin and subcutaneous tissues are stripped from it by blunt dissection. The communicating veins are found as they appear through defects in the fascia and can be tested for incompetence by the bleed-back test (see above). Care must be taken to prevent the deep end of the vein retracting beneath the fascia when it is tested for incompetence. An area of deep fascia should be exposed which is of similar size to that undermined in the subfascial procedure. Skin closure and postoperative care is identical to that for the subfascial ligation operation.

As this operation is more difficult to carry out than the subfascial procedure and is, in our experience, associated with a higher incidence of skin necrosis, we advise against its use and hardly ever use it ourselves.

Alternative methods of ablating the medial lower leg communicating veins

The stocking-seam incision Dodd[37,38,40] recommends that a vertical incision should be made down the back of the calf – the 'stocking-seam' incision. Subfascial flaps are then elevated on both sides of the calf to expose the medial and lateral communicating veins.

This incision has two possible advantages. Both sides of the lower leg can be explored through a single incision and, because the tissues on the back of the leg are often healthier, there may be a lower incidence of wound edge necrosis.[39,109,110] In our experience, however, the incidence of wound edge necrosis is not decreased, and the scar of the procedure is often more obvious and unsightly than a medial incision. In addition, the operation has to be carried out with the patient in the prone position, making it less convenient to combine it with the long saphenous vein operation and, in our experience, incompetence of the lateral communicating veins is uncommon and seldom of clinical importance. We therefore do not use this approach.

Multiple transverse incisions De Palma[34] recommends an extra fascial exploration through three or four oblique incisions placed in the direction of Langer's lines (Fig. 7.33) to reduce the incidence of wound edge necrosis. We have not found that the appearance of the resulting scars is any better than that following a vertical incision, and we commonly find that the communicating veins lie between rather than under each incision. This method has not received widespread support but may be selected for a limited exploration of

the medial side of the lower leg in patients without skin changes or ulceration. This type of selective approach, after localization of the incompetent medial calf communicating veins by one of the techniques described in Chapter 6, will probably fail to ligate up to one-third of all the communicating veins that are present.

Subfascial shearing Albanese,[1,2] Edwards,[43] and Petrov and Pennin[115] have all invented blunt instruments to cut through or 'shear off' the communicating veins. Albanese[1,2] uses a series of chisels, Petrov and Pennin[115] use a 'communicatome' and Edwards[43] uses a 'phlebotome' (Fig. 7.34). The advantage of this approach is that the skin can be incised some distance from the area of lipodermatosclerosis or previous ulceration, which reduces chance of poor healing.

A transverse or oblique incision is made on the medial side of the upper calf, below the knee, often at the site of the lower incision used for stripping the long saphenous vein. The deep fascia is incised and the subfascial space is opened by gentle finger dissection. The 'chisel' or 'shearer' can then be inserted and pushed down beneath the deep fascia to the level of the malleolus to separate the fascia from the muscle; this should open up the same area of subfascial space as that explored

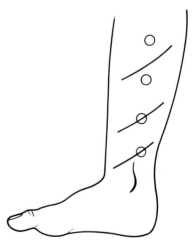

Fig. 7.33 An alternative approach to the medial calf communicating veins. De Palma[34] has suggested using multiple oblique incisions as an alternative to the long vertical incision. If ulcers are present, skin grafts can be applied to them simultaneously.

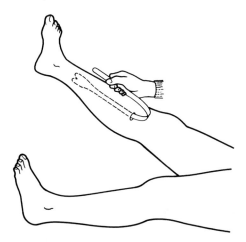

Fig. 7.34 Technique for avulsing calf communicating veins.

The Edwards' phlebotome (this is similar to the phlebotome of Petrov and Pennin.)[115] The instrument is inserted beneath the deep fascia[43] and is then pushed down to the ankle in the subfascial space to divide any veins that are crossing this space. The blade must be held up against the deep fascia to avoid damaging the muscles and the posterior tibial vessels.

(Modified from Edwards).[43]

in the standard open operation. Several thrusts must be made with the shearer to ensure that all the communicating veins are divided. Considerable bleeding usually appears from the track of the shearer when large incompetent perforating veins are divided. Care must be taken to keep the instrument close against the deep fascia to avoid damaging the posterial tibial vessels which lie near to the surface at the ankle.

There is no objective evidence that these methods do divide all the communicating veins, and no long-term results of their efficacy have been published. We have seen shearing cause extensive bruising of the lower leg and skin necrosis and therefore doubt the claims that these devices abolish the incidence of 'wound' complications. As these techniques are imprecise and must often 'miss' dividing veins that are close to the tibia or fascial septae, we do not use them in patients who have a history of ulceration, but they can be used as an alternative method for dividing the communicating veins in limbs with healthy skin.

Complications of communicating vein ligation

Necrosis of the wound edges This is the most common and troublesome complication of both the subfascial and extrafascial operations. We believe that it occurs more frequently after the extrafascial operation but we have no hard evidence to support this impression. If the skin edges are not undercut and if trauma to the skin edges is kept to a minimum, the incidence of this complication is reduced; a suturing technique in which care is taken not to overtighten the skin sutures also helps. More than 50 per cent of the wounds following the Linton operation heal within 14 days of surgery, but some wounds take more than 6 weeks to heal.[48] Prolonged healing of this degree usually occurs where there has been ulceration and extensive fibrosis. Haeger[56] quotes a wound infection and skin necrosis rate of 15 per cent but in our opinion, if careful attention is paid to the details discussed above, this should be less than 5 per cent.

Haemorrhage This may occur if the posterior tibial vessels are damaged during the dissection of the lowermost communicating veins. The foot may become ischaemic if the posterior tibial artery is inadvertently tied; this is extremely rare, unless there is pre-existing arterial insufficiency. A large subfascial haematoma may cause considerable pain and make walking difficult. If the haematoma is not evacuated, the skin becomes stretched, oedematous and more ischaemic. If the tension is not relieved, the risk that the wound will break down is increased.

Operations to ligate other communicating veins

Raivió[118] and Van Limborgh[144] have shown that more than 150 veins cross the deep fascia in every lower limb. Most of these veins are, however, considered unimportant. Some authors make a distinction between direct and indirect communication.[26,81] Direct communicating veins pass directly from the superficial veins to the main trunks. Indirect communicating veins pass from a superficial vein to a vein within a muscle before draining to a deep vein.

The sites of the direct communicating veins on the medial side of the leg are shown in Fig. 2.31 (page 46). The communicating veins discussed below are of clinical significance and must be ligated if they become incompetent.

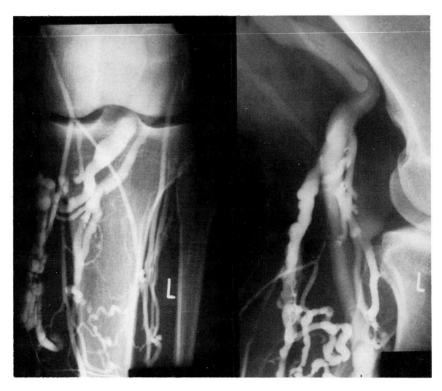

Fig. 7.35 A varicogram showing superficial varicosities connecting to a medial gastrocnemius communicating vein.

Boyd's vein The vein known as Boyd's communicating vein[18] joins the termination of the posterior arch vein or the long saphenous vein just below the knee (Fig. 6.11b). It is relatively constant and connects the superficial veins with the posterior tibial vein.

Lateral communicating vein There is a single constant large lateral[26] communicating vein which joins the short saphenous vein to the peroneal vein. Occasionally, there is a second smaller communicating vein which joins the same veins a little lower down the calf.

Mid-calf communicating vein This is an inconstant vein which joins the tributaries of the short saphenous vein to the soleal muscle sinusoids.

Gastrocnemius communicating veins Varicosities close to the popliteal fossa may drain into the veins in the bellies of the gastrocnemius muscle and then into the popliteal vein, often via the termination of the short saphenous vein (Fig. 7.35). These veins have been underestimated and are an important cause of recurrent varicosities. They are, strictly speaking, indirect communicating veins but their course and length

within the muscle is so straight and short that they are, in effect, direct communications.

Hunterian communicating veins (Dodd's communicating veins)[37,38] These veins connect the long saphenous vein with the femoral vein as it lies in the lower part of Hunter's subsartorial canal. These veins are often multiple (Fig. 7.36), but occasionally a single vein or a pair of vessels is found on varicography (Fig. 2.30c, page 45).

Operations

Each of the veins described above can be ligated and divided through an incision placed directly over the point where the vein traverses the deep fascia. The vein should subsequently be traced to its deep connection and ligated.

The Boyd and the Hunterian communicating veins are usually avulsed during long saphenous vein stripping. The lateral communicating vein is avulsed when the short saphenous vein is stripped, and the mid-calf communicating vein is rarely important.

The gastrocnemius communicating veins should be ligated on the superficial surface of the gastrocnemius and again where they appear from the deep surface of the gastrocnemius muscle to join the short saphenous vein, before it enters the popliteal vein. A full popliteal exploration for recurrent varices caused by an incompetent gastrocnemius communicating vein may require a vertical incision in the popliteal fossa to allow the anatomy to be properly displayed. The site of these unusual communicating veins must be precisely defined by phlebography or varicography before an operation is undertaken.

Avulsion, ligation or excision of varicose veins

Lofgren[90] makes a vast number of large incisions to excise superficial varicosities (see Fig. 7.1). This is a very effective method of extirpating all the varicose veins and preventing recurrence but it invariably leaves some unsightly scars. Many surgeons have independently developed a technique whereby the tributaries are exposed and then avulsed or ligated through multiple minute (2–3 mm long) incisions. With meticulous marking, careful planning and great perseverance, it is possible to remove virtually all the subcutaneous varicosities of a leg through these tiny incisions. The incisions should be made carefully in the direction of Langer's lines to ensure good healing (Fig. 7.37). The incisions are made with a fine blade or narrow scalpel, the vein is then gently freed by lifting it through the wound with very fine pointed artery forceps and clearing the surrounding fat with a second pair of forceps (Fig. 7.38). The loop of vein which appears through the wound is then doubly clamped and divided (Fig. 7.38). Each end of the vein is gently teased out through the incision as the areolar tissue on its surface is dissected off using another pair of forceps (Fig. 7.38). As the vein is

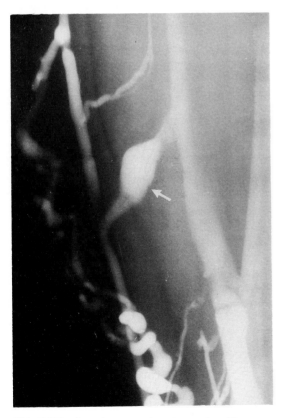

Fig. 7.36 A varicogram showing varicosities connecting to a normal size long saphenous vein which is connected to the femoral vein by three Hunterian communicating veins. One of these communicating veins (arrowed) is large and obviously abnormal.

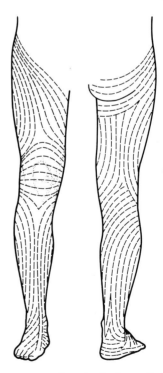

Fig. 7.37 Langer's lines in the lower limb. Whenever possible, skin incisions should be placed parallel to these lines to achieve the best cosmetic result. This is particularly important when multiple incisions are being made for local avulsions.

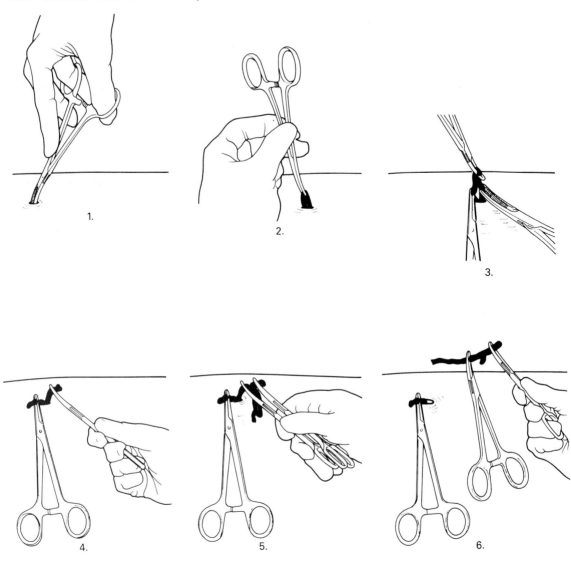

Fig. 7.38   The technique of varicose vein avulsion.

1. A small incision (2–3 mm) is placed in Langer's lines over a varicosity and is gently enlarged by inserting fine artery forceps and opening the blades to expose the varix lying in the subcutaneous fat. Careful pre-operative marking is important if the vein is to be easily found.

2. A loop of the vein is pulled out of the wound.

3. Once a sufficient length of vein has been delivered, the vein is divided between forceps.

4. Both ends of the divided vein are gradually pulled out of the wound by gentle traction and rotation of the forceps.

5. As the vein appears, the forceps are reapplied close to the wound to allow traction to be applied on the stronger piece of vein close to the incision.

6. The vein eventually tears off. The spasm caused by stretching and tearing the vein reduces the haemorrhage. Alternatively, the vein can be ligated with very fine catgut before it tears.

The other end of the vein is then avulsed towards the next cut-down incision.

delivered, new forceps are placed upon it, near the wound, to prevent it breaking (Fig. 7.38). A gentle circular motion on the forceps sometimes helps to free the vein from the tethering areolar tissue and delivers a longer length of vein.

If the veins are thick-walled and appear 'white' they avulse well, but if they are thin-walled and 'blue' they often tear easily and the operation is frustrating and often quite bloody. When the vein is strong it can be rolled around the jaws of the forceps by twisting the handles. The forceps are then pulled down onto the wound and a longer length of vein is obtained without stretching the skin incision.

When a suitable length of vein has been freed, another incision may be placed 5–10 cm further along its course through which the intervening length of vein may be successfully teased out. The distance between incisions should be reduced if the veins are thin-walled and tear easily. This technique can be used to remove a long unsightly vein through three or four small incisions; this gives satisfaction to the surgeon and provides a very acceptable cosmetic result for the patient.

The varicosities avulsed by this technique are usually major tributaries of one of the saphenous veins, which will require stripping at the same operation. The lower end of the vein can be ligated with fine catgut to prevent excessive bleeding. Some surgeons prefer to ligate each segment of vein, other surgeons reduce bleeding by performing the avulsions after the limb has been exsanguinated by using a tourniquet.[126,127] In most patients the bleeding that occurs after avulsion can be controlled by firm external pressure applied by an assistant.

The tiny stab incisions can be left unsutured or may be closed with a subcuticular stitch, adhesive skin strips, or a single 4/0 nylon suture.

The cosmetic results of this method of removing varices are very good, providing it is accompanied by appropriate surgery to the saphenous veins if these are incompetent. It can be used as an alternative to injections for varicosis of a single tributary.

Comment Many limbs in which there are varicose veins have a combination of long saphenous, short saphenous and calf communicating vein incompetence with multiple varicosities all over the leg. Often both lower limbs are affected. Careful pre-operative evaluation of the physiological abnormalities followed by careful marking of all the major sites of superficial-to-deep incompetence and of all surface varicosities is essential. Varicosities cannot be seen when the patient is anaesthetized and the leg veins are collapsed. We always try to treat all the veins in both limbs at one operation, though this is sometimes extremely time consuming. Occasionally, it is advisable to treat legs with large numbers of varicose veins at separate operations.

It is easiest to start with the patient in the prone position and to treat short saphenous incompetence or varicosities on the posterior surface of the limb first. When the surgery on these veins has been completed, the patient is turned over so that the long saphenous vein, the calf communicating veins and the varicosities in the anterior aspect of the leg can be excised.

Very occasionally, it is necessary to replace the blood loss from bilateral, multiple, combined operations. A blood sample should be taken pre-operatively for blood grouping and the serum should be saved for cross matching. During the last 30 years we have not had to give a blood transfusion during a varicose vein operation, except to two patients who were anaemic before surgery.

Recurrent varicose veins

It is important to distinguish between residual veins and recurrent veins.

Residual veins These are veins that were not treated at the original operation, because they were not detected pre-operatively, not found during the operation or were deliberately left untreated. Residual veins can be treated by further surgery or sclerotherapy. Surgery is relatively straightforward because it is unhampered by the scar tissue that complicates the surgery of recurrent veins. A failure to remove the full length of a tortuous tributary is the most common cause of residual varicosities, but short saphenous vein incompetence may only become obvious when long saphenous vein incompetence has been treated, especially if it has not been carefully excluded before the first operation.

Recurrent varicose veins

Recurrent varicose veins are veins which have become varicose after the original treatment, having been 'normal' at the time of that treatment. This occurs when all the visible varicosities were treated but the underlying physiological abnormality was not corrected; the remaining 'normal' veins therefore continue to be subjected to abnormal pressures and subsequently dilate. Failure to correct the physiological abnormality is caused by:

- an inadequate or incorrect original operation;
- failure to occlude an 'incompetent' superficial-to-deep communication;
- the development of new sites of superficial-to-deep incompetence – often as a result of a deep vein abnormality.

It is easy to treat an incompetent superficial-to-deep communication once the site of the communication has been diagnosed. Similarly, new sites of superficial-to-deep incompetence can be easily corrected if the new abnormality is in a site previously untouched by surgery. Surgical problems arise from the first category, and sometimes from the third category, when the recurrence is at the site of a previous operation.

Sapheno-femoral recurrence

Incompetent communications between the femoral vein and the superficial veins in the upper thigh may cause recurrent varicose veins under the following conditions.

- The original long saphenous ligation was not made 'flush' with the femoral vein.
- Terminal tributaries of the saphenous vein were left intact (Fig. 7.11).
- There were two terminations of the long saphenous and only one was ligated (Fig. 7.14).
- There were two separate long saphenous veins and only one was ligated.
- The long saphenous vein was tied but not stripped so that recurrence develops from dilatation of the Hunterian communicating veins (Fig. 7.36).
- After simple ligation of the long saphenous vein, collaterals may develop to reconnect the common femoral vein with the long saphenous veins (Fig. 6.24).

It is not clear which of these causes of recurrence is the most common. Sheppard[132] reported that 90 per cent of 204 legs that developed recurrent varicose veins had recurrent

sapheno-femoral incompetence as a result of new collateral veins. He suggested that neovascularization of granulation tissue around the sapheno-femoral junction leads to the formation of new channels between the saphenous stump on the femoral vein and the residual saphenous vein or its tributaries, even when the original surgery has been correctly performed. Sheppard proposed that to prevent this happening a flap of pectineus fascia should be sutured over the stump of the long saphenous vein to separate the femoral vein from the superficial veins after sapheno-femoral ligation (Fig. 7.39). Unfortunately, there is no prospective data to show whether this modification is worthwhile, but there is some support for Sheppard's theory in a report by Glass[53] who found that recurrent varicose veins that developed after a sapheno-femoral ligation connected with the femoral vein through vessels with a 'primitive' structure. Similar primitive vessels were found bridging sections of locally excised saphenous

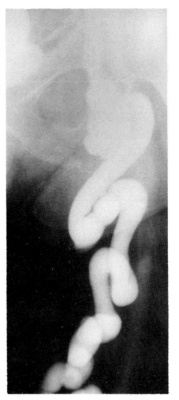

Fig. 7.39 A varicogram showing a large groin recurrence reconnecting the superficial veins to the site of a previously ligated sapheno-femoral junction.

vein at the knee level. Glass concluded that recurrences would be less frequent if the ligated sapheno-femoral junction was covered by fascia or a synthetic mesh.

Lofgren and Lofgren,[88] however, have suggested, on the basis of their clinical experience, that the main cause of recurrence in the groin is improperly performed initial surgery.

A trial in which the incidence of recurrent varicosities was compared in patients who had been randomly treated either by sapheno-femoral ligation alone or by ligation combined with long saphenous vein stripping[105] showed that recurrences were reduced by the addition of the vein stripping. This suggests that the development of incompetence in the Hunterian communicating vein may be an important cause of recurrent varicosities after sapheno-femoral ligation without stripping.

Diagnosis If the old scar is found to be some distance from the groin crease, a proper flush ligation of the long saphenous vein was probably not performed at the first operation, and a groin recurrence is therefore a strong possibility.

The likelihood of sapheno-popliteal incompetence must also be considered in any patient with new varices after a sapheno-femoral ligation.

A cough impulse or thrill can rarely be felt in the groin when it is scarred but the varicosities are often seen extending up towards the groin. If a high thigh tourniquet controls all the varicosities in the limb, clinical suspicions are confirmed.

We always attempt to confirm the diagnosis by obtaining varicograms (Fig. 6.24); these demonstrate single or multiple connections between a residual segment of long saphenous vein or one of its major tributaries and the femoral vein, and thus help to clarify the abnormal anatomy before the subsequent dissection.

Re-exploration of the groin We favour the direct approach in which the old scar is excised and usually extended both medially and laterally. The femoral vein can then be approached from either the medial[82] or the lateral side (Fig. 7.40).[58] If the incision is deepened laterally through relatively normal tissues, the femoral artery can be found first and the scar tissue can be dissected from its anterior surface before the femoral vein is found lying on the medial side of artery. The dissection can then continue over the front of the vein to expose the sapheno-femoral junction. The stump of the long saphenous vein is usually

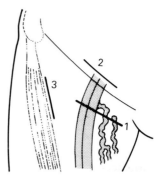

Fig. 7.40 The three approaches that can be used to explore recurrent sapheno-femoral varicosities.
1. The approach of Li.[82]
2. The approach of Luke.[93]
3. The lateral approach, now rarely used.
(Modified from May.[101]

found entering the anterior surface of the femoral vein. This stump is freed on all surfaces until a Lahey forceps can be passed around it, followed by a strong ligature (Fig. 7.41). Once the sapheno-femoral junction has been tied off, the main tributary veins are dissected and individually ligated and divided. If the incision is deepened medially down to the fascia covering the pectineus muscle, the medial aspect of the femoral vein can be identified just before its anterior aspect is cleaned to expose the sapheno-femoral junction.

An alternative approach (Fig. 7.40) is to make an incision above the previous groin incision down to the lower edge of the external oblique aponeurosis before dissecting downwards to find the anterior surface of the femoral vein immediately below the inguinal ligament.[39,93] This approach may be awkward if the original scar is high, but it does allow the femoral vein and artery to be found and protected before the difficult dissection of the small recurrent branches attached to the sapheno-femoral junction is undertaken and it avoids dividing any lymphatics.

Second operations are always more difficult, and if the anatomy is not displayed first, it is easy to damage the major vessels. Care must be taken not to damage the femoral nerve during the lateral approach.

Two particular problems may follow a second extensive dissection. A lymphocele or lymph fistula may appear in the early postoperative period and lymphoedema of the leg may, very occasionally, appear months later.

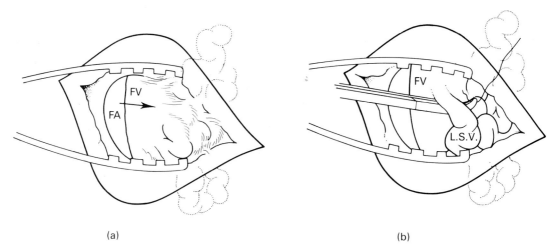

(a)   (b)

Fig. 7.41   The ligation of groin recurrences using the approach of Li.[82]
  (a) The lateral end of the incision is deepened to find the femoral artery (FA). The dissection then continues in the direction of the arrow over the front of the femoral vein.
  (b) When the stump of the long saphenous vein is found on the front of the femoral vein, a ligature is passed around the stump and tied. This can be carried out using an aneurysm needle or by passing a Lahey forceps behind the stump as shown.
  When the upper ligature has been tied the mass of small varices draining into the stump can be ligated. (Modified from Li.)[82]

It is important not to disturb the lymphatic channels during the dissection. May[101] has recommended that patent blue–violet dye should be injected subcutaneously in the thigh to reveal the lymphatics before beginning the dissection. The lateral approach is more likely to damge lymphatics than the medial approach.

Lymphocele (Fig. 7.42) and lymph fistulae usually resolve spontaneously but occasionally they have to be aspirated or excised.

Lymphoedema probably only occurs if there is a pre-existing congenital or acquired lymphatic deficiency. Acquired lymphatic deficiency is common in geographical areas where the people do not wear shoes and get repeated subclinical episodes of cellulitis and lymphadenitis. It may be

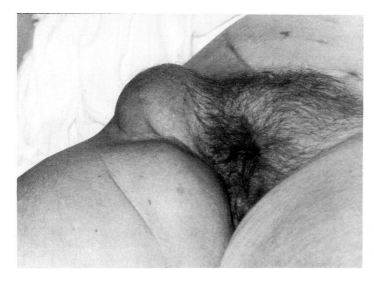

Fig. 7.42. A lymphocele in the groin which developed after the re-exploration of the groin for a recurrent hernia.

possible to treat severe lymphoedema caused by a localized lymphatic obstruction by an entero-mesenteric bridge operation.[71,76]

Sapheno-popliteal recurrence

Although recurrent short saphenous vein incompetence in the popliteal fossa is less common than groin recurrence (because of the lower frequency of primary sapheno-popliteal incompetence), when it does occur it is as difficult, if not more difficult, to correct than sapheno-femoral recurrence. The same factors that cause recurrences in the groin cause recurrences in the popliteal fossa, but because of the variable entry of the short saphenous termination, technical errors are much more common. Recurrences develop from collaterals in the scar tissue, trans-gastrocnemius communicating veins which were not ligated at the initial operation, and muscle communications that connect short saphenous tributaries with an incompetent long saphenous vein system.

The diagnosis is usually suspected on clinical grounds, confirmed by tourniquet testing and defined by varicography.

Re-exploration of the popliteal fossa is best carried out through a vertical or S-shaped incision. The popliteal vein and artery are found well above the previous scarring and are traced down until the stump of the short saphenous vein and any other vessels connecting to the superficial veins are found and ligated. All the tributaries of the short saphenous vein in the popliteal fossa are then dissected, ligated and divided.

Communicating vein recurrence

This is discussed in detail in Chapter 15. Some patients definitely develop recurrent varicose veins from incompetent communicating veins that were missed at the initial operation. Also, some previously competent communicating veins may later become incompetent. The clinical diagnosis should always be confirmed by varicography and ascending phlebography. A second subfascial exploration with ligation of the incompetent vein or veins is then performed through the original incision.

Isolated recurrent superficial varicosities

Most recurrent varicosities are the result of missed or new superficial-to-deep communicating vein

incompetence, but they can also develop as a result of localized venous dilatation in a previously normal subcutaneous vein. If there is no evidence of new superficial-to-deep incompetent connections, recurrent varicosities can either be avulsed through multiple small incisions under local or general anaesthesia or be treated by injection sclerotherapy. Recurrences in the lower part of the leg are best treated by injection compression; recurrences within the thigh are best avulsed.[50,101,107]

Comment Not all recurrences are caused by inadequate operations. Perhaps one in every two recurrences is the result of poor technique (the surgeon sometimes fails to ligate the saphenous vein itself) but in nearly half the cases the second exploration of the groin or popliteal fossa reveals abnormal veins that have clearly developed since the first operation. An accurate knowledge of the anatomical variations that can exist, combined with a careful exploration of the common sites of superficial-to-deep connections, will undoubtedly reduce the incidence of recurrent varicosities. The role of the separation of the deep veins from the subcutaneous tissues with a layer of fascia, which is aimed at reducing the incidence of recurrence, has yet to be established.

Short saphenous vein incompetence is often overshadowed by a more obvious long saphenous vein incompetence and will only be found if the surgeon searches diligently for it; the same is true for communicating vein incompetence.

All the possible sites of superficial-to-deep communication must be carefully re-examined in patients with recurrent varicosities. Phlebography and varicography are extremely helpful investigations for the assessment of these patients.

A deep vein abnormality must be considered a possibilty in all patients who have recurrent varicose veins after apparently satisfactory primary surgery. Clinical suspicion may be confirmed by physiological tests of calf pump function, or by bipedal ascending phlebography (see Chapter 4).

Recurrent varicose veins in the presence of a deep vein abnormality are best treated by elastic compression. Further surgery may be beneficial but should not be expected to be curative and must always be followed by life-long elastic compression.

General complications of varicose vein surgery

The complications which are specific to each operation have been discussed under the headings of individual operations. They include:

Recurrence (page 233), haemorrhage (page 212), damage to the deep veins – femoral, popliteal, crural (page 212), damage to the arteries – femoral, popliteal and posterior tibial (page 212), damage to the superficial nerves – saphenous or sural (page 219), wound necrosis (page 229), haematoma formation (page 229), lymphoedema and lymphocele (page 236), unsightly or keloid scars and recurrent ulceration (Chapter 15).

Chest infection   Chest infection rarely occurs after varicose vein surgery, even though some operations are lengthy, because most patients are fit, many are young, the level of anaesthesia is light and there are no wounds which restrict chest movement.

Wound infection   Infection of the groin wound is uncommon. Some obese patients have intertrigo, and in these patients it is worthwhile treating the skin pre-operatively to reduce the risk of sepsis. Lower leg wounds may become infected if they are in the vicinity of an open ulcer. In general, infection is more often a sequel of haematoma formation than an event in its own right.

Deep vein thrombosis and pulmonary embolism   Deep vein thrombosis seldom occurs after varicose vein surgery. Cockett and Dodd[39] observed one case of pulmonary embolism in 204 varicose vein operations at St Thomas's Hospital performed between 1949 and 1954, and Keith[74] reported that three deep vein thromboses occurred in 544 operations, an incidence of 0.6 per cent. Lofgren *et al.*[87] reported 16 patients out of 4000 who were suspected on clinical grounds, to have had a pulmonary embolism, a risk of 0.39 per cent. Some deep vein thromboses undoubtedly pass undetected but the incidence of pulmonary embolism does appear to be very low. The bandages that are used to reduce haematoma and swelling and the early mobilization of patients that is encouraged after operation may be important prophylactic factors.

Our own practice includes many patients who have varicose veins which complicate the post-thrombotic syndrome. We give these patients 5000 units of heparin subcutaneously, twice daily, starting on the day of their admission. Before beginning this routine, we saw a number of these patients develop deep vein thrombosis, not only postoperatively but even during the pre-operative period.

General postoperative care

The special aspects of aftercare have been discussed with the individual operations. The general aspects of postoperative care are summarized here.

Compression bandages   The legs are elevated to 20° or 30° and compression is maintained by elastocrepe bandages. This reduces the incidence of haematoma formation and may reduce the incidence of deep vein thrombosis.

Analgesia   Opiates may be needed during the first 24 hours after surgery but milder oral analgesics (e.g. soluble aspirin, Panadol, DF118, Co-Proxamole or codeine) will usually suffice thereafter.

Mobilization   Patients should be encouraged to get up and walk[108] as soon as they are wide awake, which is usually within 4–6 hours of surgery unless they have had a full exploration of the medial leg communicating veins, when they should rest in bed for at least 24 hours. When the patient gets up an additional supporting bandage (Blue line, Bisgaard, Elastocrepe, Tensopress or Thusane) must be worn over the bandages which were put on in the operating theatre. The patient must either walk or sit with the legs elevated when not in bed. Standing still or sitting with dependent legs is discouraged.

Duration of admission   Most patients can be discharged the day after the operation, though if surgery is performed under local anaesthesia, they may go home on the day of the operation.

Patients who have had an exploration of the medial calf communicating veins must stay in hospital longer. They can usually be discharged after 5–7 days but if the skin is red and tender or if the wound shows any signs of slow healing (e.g. a serous discharge) the patient should be treated as if he/she had a venous ulcer and should be confined to bed until the wound is dry and the inflammatory response has subsided. Strong supporting bandages should be applied, sometimes Calaband or Viscopaste, and the patient should be told to rest as much as possible and only increase daily exercise when the leg feels comfortable.

After discharge from hospital The sutures should be removed from the multiple tiny avulsion incisions, and from the groin and popliteal incisions 5–7 days after the operation, unless absorbable subcutaneous sutures or adhesive skin strips have been used. At least 10 days should elapse from the time of operation before the sutures are removed from the vertical incisions used to ligate the medial leg communicating veins. If the healing of these wounds is slow, they may be wrapped in an impregnated bandage and covered by an elastic compression bandage for 2 weeks.

Elastic bandages or stockings should be worn for at least 1 month after surgery. If ankle oedema develops when the bandages are discarded, they should be reapplied.

Review Patients should be seen 1 month after the operation to review the state of the wounds, to look for oedema and to record the presence of any residual varices. A second review at 3 months allows a more complete examination when the wounds have fully healed and the bruising has disappeared; residual varices are easily detected at this review. Recurrent varices may be obliterated by injection sclerotherapy or by local excisions. If the results satisfy both the surgeon and the patient, we discharge the patient back to his family doctor with the advice that the patient should return if new varicosities develop. Patients are not encouraged to return with minor varicosities, and we do not recommend long-term elastic compression stockings to patients with normal skin, as the purpose of the surgery is to eradicate the veins and to obviate the necessity for wearing stockings permanently.

Injection sclerotherapy

The invention of the hypodermic syringe[70] in the 1840s allowed Chassaignac[24] in 1855 to try to obliterate varicose veins by injecting a solution of ferric chloride. Foote[50] lists a series of clinicians who attempted to sclerose veins with ferric chloride, iodotannin, phenol, mercury bichloride, alcohol and Lugol's iodine.

Surgical ligation was, at one stage, combined with a distal injection of sclerosant to obliterate varices,[128,139] and in 1916 Linser[83,84,85] described the use of compression bandages after the injection of hypertonic saline; this probably makes Linser the father of modern compression sclerotherapy. Unfortunately, his choice of sclerosant did not prove ideal, as it caused considerable pain and, if injected outside the vein, gave rise to a severe inflammatory reaction which often resulted in skin necrosis.

A number of safer sclerosants were developed after the First World War. A mixture of quinine and urothane was introduced by Génévrier,[52] sodium salicylate was first used by Sicard,[134] and Maingot[97] injected both these substances using a twin injection technique. Sodium morrhuate[123] and monoethanolamime oleate[9] were introduced in the 1930s, and at the same time, Tournay[140,141] in Paris began to use sodium tetradecyl sulphate (STD). STD is still the most popular sclerosant in use; it is essentially a detergent which produces a local chemical phlebitis with minimal systemic complications.[121] All sclerosants are, however, toxic if given in large quantities; they cause haemolysis and renal damage. Sclerosants also cause catastrophic thrombosis if they are injected by mistake into an artery, and they all cause local skin necrosis if a sufficiently large quantity is injected between a vein and the overlying skin.

Some newer sclerosant solutions have recently been introduced, for example Aethoxysclerol 1%, Variglobin 0.5% (a sodium iodide solution) and Sclerovein 1–2%. The exact concentration at which each sclerosant is used varies between 0.5% and 5% depending upon the size and type of vein that is being sclerosed.

Aim of treatment

The aim of compression sclerotherapy is to produce a sterile inflammation on the inner surface of the vein wall. Clinicians who believe that compression is an essential part of the treatment[45,46,64,65,114,125] think that it occludes the lumen by making opposing surfaces stick together without any intervening thrombus. The vein is theoretically converted into a thin fibrosed cord (the sclerosis), not a vein full of red thrombus which can recanalize. The evidence that this always occurs is poor. Many veins do recanalize, and some clinicians consider that prolonged compression is unnecessary and have abandoned it altogether. In our opinion the effectiveness of sclerotherapy depends upon the intensity of the inflammatory response. A severe response causes venospasm and vein wall swelling; both these effects reduce the size of the lumen thus reducing the quantity of intraluminal thrombus. We have considerable doubts that external compression always achieves this, though fully agree that a superficial vein which becomes full of red thrombus will almost certainly recanalize.

Some radiographic investigations[17] have suggested that sclerosants which are injected into the superficial veins quickly disperse into the deep veins; this casts doubt on the effectiveness of sclerotherapy and implies that injections increase the risk of deep vein thrombosis. Other studies[72] have shown that sclerosants can remain in the superficial veins for a considerable time. These variations make the results of injection sclerotherapy less reliable than the results of surgery.

Indications

Many advocates of injection sclerotherapy use it to treat all types of varicose veins. The French school[32,114] even inject sclerosant directly into the uppermost portion of the long saphenous vein to obliterate its termination. The British school[22,46,64,65] concentrate on the distal veins of the limb and treat sapheno-femoral and sapheno-popliteal incompetence by surgical ligation. We support the later approach, as we are very concerned that deep vein thrombosis may be initiated if sclerosant is injected into the upper part of the long saphenous vein. Compression sclerotherapy is ideal for solitary varicose tributaries in the absence of main saphenous vein incompetence. It is also ideal for obliterating small varicose veins that were not avulsed at the time of saphenous surgery. We do not consider compression sclerotherapy to be suitable or effective for the treatment of incompetent lower leg communicating veins. It is the treatment of choice for patients who are very old or unfit, or for those who refuse operation. Intradermal spider veins can also be treated by injection sclerotherapy.

Contra-indications to sclerotherapy

Sclerotherapy is contra-indicated under the following circumstances.

- Women on the contraceptive pill
- Pregnancy
- Patients with a strong history of allergy, especially if this has been to previous sclerosant injection
- Foot veins should not be injected because of the risk of intra-arterial injections
- Patients with very fat legs, because compression is very difficult

Technique

We use a modification of the technique described by Hobbs,[65] rather than that of Fegan.[45,46]

After a decision has been taken to treat the varicose veins by compression sclerotherapy, the patient is re-examined standing on a stool in a good light. The surface varices are carefully marked with an indelible pen. The patient then lies down horizontally on a couch. A sufficient number of 2 ml syringes fitted with 25 gauge (16 mm) needles are filled with 0.5 ml of STD to cater for the number of injections that are planned (Fig. 7.43). The maximum volume of STD that can be given during one treatment is 20 ml but many clinicians would regard this as excessive.[95] The skin is cleaned with chlorhexidene and venepunctures are made at approximately 5 cm intervals along the course of each vein, beginning at either end. A total of 10–15 injections can be given into one, or both limbs, at one time. If many more injections are required, it is best to treat one leg at a time.

When the patient is lying on the couch the veins are partially collapsed but are not completely empty. This allows the surgeon to confirm the position of the needle by withdrawing blood into the syringe. The simplest technique is to transfix the vein with the needle and then gradually pull it back through the vein whilst simultaneously withdrawing the plunger of the syringe (Fig. 7.44a and b). When the tip of the needle is located in the lumen of the vein, blood will appear in the barrel of the syringe. At this moment the fingers of the injector's free hand empty the vein by gentle simultaneous movement, on either side of the needle away from the needle, combined with downward pressure so that the sclerosant is injected into an 'empty' vein. When the injection has been completed, an assistant presses the compression dressing on to the injection site as the needle is withdrawn. We use dental rolls held on with Micropore tape for compression, and we have not encountered any problems with blistering. Cotton wool balls, which are recommended by Hobbs,[65] are a satisfactory alternative. We do not use the foam rubber pads advocated by Fegan, except occasionally over the course of the long saphenous vein if the injections are put close to, or into this vein at knee level or in the lower thigh.

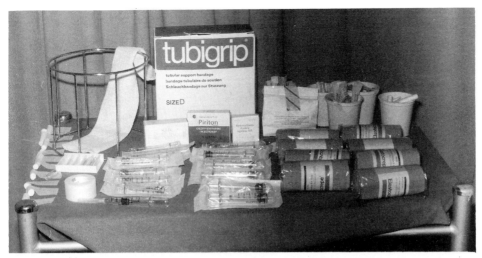

Fig. 7.43 The trolley we use for sclerotherapy. The syringes, needles, dental rolls, and sclerosant (STD) are shown. Hydrocortisone, adrenaline and Piriton are kept on the trolley to treat anaphylactic shock.

When all the injections have been completed, the leg is bandaged with Elastocrepe and covered with Tubigrip. Many other bandaging methods and elastic stockings are equally effective.[130] The patient is encouraged to walk immediately afterwards to clear any sclerosant from the deep veins and thus reduce the risk of thrombosis.

Fegan originally recommended[45,46] that the bandages should be worn for 6 weeks but two recent studies[8,51] have suggested that shorter periods of compression give identical results. Hobbs has argued that the compression time should vary with the size of the legs and veins injected (e.g. longer periods of compression for large varices in fat legs than for those in thin legs).[63]

In the absence of any firm evidence to guide us, we ask our patients to wear their bandages for 3 weeks. Patients are instructed not to remove or loosen their bandages and to keep the legs dry when bathing by putting them on the rim of the bath or covering them with a plastic bag. On the weekend before they return to the clinic they are asked to remove the bandages and dental rolls and have a full normal bath; this allows the legs to be examined without bandage marks or compression dents. The legs are carefully inspected and palpated and untreated varices or failed injection sites are re-injected.

Extra-vascular haematoma and veins full of red thrombus are evacuated by making a minute puncture into the vein with a pointed scalpel blade or a large needle and expelling the thrombus by gentle finger pressure.[65,135] It is important to do this to avoid skin discoloration and to prevent the thrombus persisting as a tender palpable or sometimes visible thickened cord. The veins of the opposite leg may be injected at this time, if this was the original intention. Throughout the whole period of treatment the patient is encouraged to work and walk normally.

Alternative techniques of injection sclerotherapy

Sigg[135] inserts a number of needles into the veins that are going to be injected with the patient standing. The positions of the needles are confirmed by allowing blood to drain from them. The patient then lies down and the leg is elevated before syringes are attached to the needles and the injections are made. Sigg uses up to 15 injections of 0.5 ml of Variglobin (4%) in one session.

Fegan[45,46] inserts needles which are already attached to syringes with the patient sitting on a couch. When blood can be sucked back into the syringe, the syringe is taped to the leg. The leg is then elevated, the vein is occluded above and below the site of injection with the ring and index fingers, and the sclerosant is injected. The syringe is then withdrawn but the fingers are kept in place to hold the sclerosant in the isolated segment of vein. The free hand immediately applies a bandage over a sorbo-rubber pad which is placed over the course of the injected vein; further turns of the bandage are applied over the pad and along the leg until the next site of injection is reached. Fegan recommends that injections should be

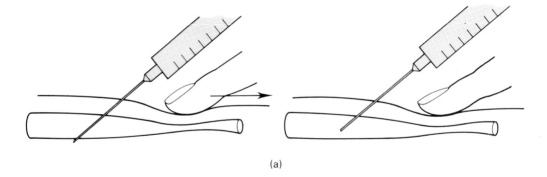

(a)

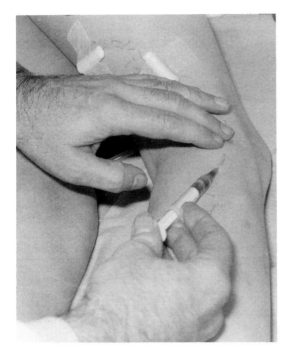

Fig. 7.44 (a and b) The technique of injecting a varicose vein. The varicosity is transfixed. The needle is then slowly withdrawn while exerting suction through the needle by pulling on the plunger of the syringe. When blood appears in the syringe, the sclerosant is injected. The vein is kept as empty as possible by the fingers of the free hand, which also stretches the vein to prevent it from kinking. The vein is compressed as the needle is withdrawn. Dental rolls are used to keep the vein compressed beneath the bandage.

started distally to avoid the development of venous congestion as a result of the bandaging. Each injection site is bandaged in an identical manner until all the veins which have been injected have been compressed. Fegan inspects the leg after 3 weeks, and gives further injections if required. He uses multiple injections and gives up to 1 ml of sodium tetradecyl sulphate in each injection.

Davy and Ouvry[32,114] give only one or two injections at each session and spend many weeks treating a single limb. They inject the long saphenous vein right up to its termination, and they have reported few problems (e.g. venous thrombosis) from their high thigh vein injection technique.

Comment Sigg's technique is time consuming and upsetting to the patient, and carries a high risk of vaso-vagal attacks. Fegan's technique is more difficult to use than Hobbs' method, because the needles often slip out of the vein as the patient changes position. Although Fegan's method keeps the veins empty at the time of injection, the number of injections is limited by the instant application of the bandage. We have not yet been bold (or foolish) enough to try injecting the upper end of the long saphenous vein.

Complications of sclerotherapy[96]

Vaso-vagal attacks Fainting during the venepuncture is reported to occur in 1 in every 100 patients.[150] It is much more frequent when using the technique of Fegan or Sigg[45,46,135] in which the needles are inserted while the patient is sitting or standing.

Allergic or anaphylactic reactions These reactions are reported to occur in 2 of every 1000 patients treated[150] but only one fatality has been recorded in a series of over one million patients injected with sodium tetradecyl sulphate.[96] MacGowan attributes allergic reactions to over-dosage (more than 5 ml per sitting) but also recommends care in patients with a long history of allergy.[96] Piriton (chlorpheniramine maleate), adrenaline, hydrocortisone and salbutamol should be kept on the injection trolley to treat these reactions instantly if they occur.

Toxic reactions These reactions consist of shivering, loin pain and haematuria; they are usually caused by the haemolysis of red cells. Such reactions rarely occur if less than 5 ml of sclerosant is used[95] but they are occasionally seen with smaller doses.

Skin necrosis and ulceration There are no published statistics that indicate how often this complication occurs. Skin necrosis and ulceration should be suspected when the patient complains of severe pain after a course of injections. When the bandages are removed there is usually an inflammatory reaction and signs of skin necrosis. Large ulcers may follow a misplaced injection and are difficult to treat and slow to heal; they are the main source of the medico-legal problems asso-ciated with injection sclerotherapy.[96]

Venous thrombosis Although Winstone[150] claimed that the incidence of this complication is low (1 in 1000 treatments), other investigators[148] found evidence of thrombosis in 9 out of 67 extremities treated by sclerotherapy. The former estimate, based on clinical evidence, is definitely too low, the latter estimate, based on impedence phlethysmography which is not a very sensitive method of detecting calf vein thrombosis, may be more accurate. A definitive study is required to ascertain the true incidence of thrombosis after sclerotherapy.

Pulmonary embolism This complication is reported to occur in 8 out of every 10,000 patients (0.1 per cent);[55] this is a lower incidence than that reported after operations on varicose veins.

Intra-arterial injection Five examples of this complication had been reported to the Medical Defence Union in Great Britain by 1985.[95] At least two of these patients had to have part of the leg amputated. MacGowan reported that injections around the posterior part of the ankle were parti-cularly dangerous, with the posterior tibial artery being especially at risk.[95] The anterior tibial artery may also be inadvertently punctured when injec-tions are made on the front of the lower leg and ankle. If the upper end of the long saphenous is injected, the femoral artery may be at risk.

An accidental intra-arterial injection causes severe burning pain, often with tingling sensa-tions in the foot.[96] Patients should always be asked if the injection is causing pain as the injec-tion is being given and, if it is, the injection should be stopped immediately, *but the needle should not be withdrawn*. Blood should be drawn back into the syringe to empty the needle of sclerosant, then the syringe should be removed and replaced with a syringe containing 10,000 units of heparin which should be injected slowly into the artery. The needle should then be removed and the leg watched carefully for 2 or 3 hours. If the pulses remain palpable and the skin of the leg remains warm, the patient can be allowed to go home, but if there is any suggestion of arterial thrombosis or distal ischaemia, the patient must be admitted to hospital for full anticoagulation and observation.

Injection of a nerve The saphenous and sural nerves may be injected with sclerosant. This is very painful, and if continued may cause anaesthesia and sometimes a permanent interrup-tion of nerve function.

Skin discoloration This is a common side-effect of injection sclerotherapy. Every patient should be warned that they may develop some brown pigmentation over a thrombosed vein. The pigment is haemosiderin and is caused by the peri-venous inflammatory response. Hobbs[65] con-siders that discoloration is caused by the injection of too much sclerosant at a single site but it can occur after a perfect injection of a small amount of sclerosant. It usually fades after 1–2 years.

Alternative treatments of varicose veins

Out-patient percutaneous ligation[129,149]

This is an alternative to sclerotherapy or excision of local varices under local anaesthesia. There is no evidence to suggest that it is any better than other established techniques.

Diathermy sclerosis[111,112]

This is another way of producing a vigorous thrombophlebitis. A fine electrode is threaded down the vein to allow endovenous percutaneous diathermy destruction of the intima. It can be used as an alternative to sclerotherapy. O'Reilly has reported diathermy skin burns after this form of treatment, and it has not been widely adopted.

Light coagulation[113]

The equipment for light coagulation is expensive, and the technique has only been used in a few patients.

Pharmacological palliation

A number of studies have investigated the benefit of rùtosides on the symptoms of varìcose veins. These drugs do not reduce the size of the varicosities but, by altering capillary permeability, they are said to relieve the aching, swelling and nocturnal cramps that are commonly experienced by patients with varicose veins. The scientific evidence supporting these claims is slender, principally because symptoms such as aching are impossible to measure accurately. Some controlled trials have shown a significant improvement in symptoms in patients taking the active drug compared with patients taking a placebo,[117] but this form of treatment can only be regarded as palliation because there is no effect on the veins themselves. Rutosides may be of value in patients who decline other methods of treatment or who continue to complain of symptoms after other treatments have eradicated the veins. There are no controlled trials which compare the effect of elastic compression with the effect of rutosides on symptom relief.

Results of treatment

Measurement of recurrence

The measurement and classification of recurrence is extremely difficult because there is always a considerable difference of opinion between observers on what constitutes a recurrence.[22,119] Very few patients, if any, have a totally perfect, 'normal' leg 1 year after treatment, let alone after 20 years. Some new varicose veins invariably develop but these may not require further treatment. Probably the best way of determining the success of treatment is to count the number of patients who have further treatment,[32] but it is difficult to follow patients for 10 or 20 years, because many move house and have second and

third courses of treatment elsewhere. Almost every published long-term study lacks credibility because of the large proportion of patients who cannot be followed up and the absence of a clearly defined anatomical or physiological assessment by an *independent* observer.

The first aim of treatment must be the eradication of the veins that exist when the patient presents. The second aim is to prevent recurrence. Proof that the first aim has been achieved needs a careful extensive documentation of the site and size of the original varices – this is rarely done. Proof that the second objective has been achieved needs a 100 per cent independant follow up and even then it will depend upon the length of the follow up. It might be better to express recurrence as a yearly rate rather than as an absolute number.[32,108]

Surgery

Lofgren's 10-year review[90] of radical surgical obliteration of the veins (the ligation of sites of superficial-to-deep incompetence and the removal of subcutaneous varicosities) showed that 44 per cent had excellent results, 41 per cent had good results and 15 per cent had a fair result. No patients reported poor results. These results were obviously open to considerable observer bias, as 15 per cent had definite recurrences requiring further treatment which most clinicians would classify as poor results.

Rivlin[122] claimed that only 7 per cent of patients developed residual or recurrent varicosities between 6 years and 10 years after operation, but these results have not been confirmed by any form of external audit, and they may also be affected by observer bias.

Sclerotherapy

Fegan[45,46] claimed that 82 per cent of his patients were satisfied with the result of sclerotherapy. Similar results have been published by Strother *et al.*[138] in a study of 348 legs. Strother claimed 89 per cent success between 1 year and 4 years and 68 per cent success at 3–4 years.

Reid and Rothnie[120] treated 1080 legs with primary varicose veins and claimed that 90 per cent had good results at 1 year.

Dejode[35] treated 146 patients and followed them for between 1 year and 5 years. The results were very good in 83 per cent but in 3 per cent the veins were not improved.

Raj and Makin[119] found that 80 per cent of patients had good results at 6 weeks, as assessed by the surgeon, but there was only a 40 per cent agreement between the surgeon and the patient as to what constituted a good result!

Sigg,[135] Davy,[32], Ouvry,[114], Nabatoff[108] and Dale[31] all recognized that a significant number of recurrences occur after sclerotherapy and they recommend regular follow-up examinations with further courses of injections whenever these are indicated.

Comparisons between sclerotherapy and surgery

In 1968 Hobbs[64] reported the 2-year results of a controlled trial comparing compression sclerotherapy against surgery. This showed that all the veins in the legs could be treated by injection sclerotherapy but Hobbs felt that patients with sapheno-femoral incompetence were best treated by surgery because the recurrence rate after sclerotherapy was greater. Injections below the knee cured 60 per cent and improved 40 per cent

of patients and were more effective than surgery. By 1974, however, the 5-year results[66] showed that the sclerotherapy 1-year 'cure' rate of 82 per cent had fallen to only 7 per cent and only 30 per cent were still improved (Fig. 7.45). In contrast 20 per cent of the surgical group remained 'cured' and 80 per cent were still improved at 5 years.

In a randomized study of 155 patients treated by injection compression sclerotherapy compared with 100 patients treated surgically (Fig. 7.46) Chant *et al.* found that 14 per cent of the surgical group and 22 per cent of the injection group required further treatment by 3 years.[22] This difference was not found to be statistically different, and patients were said to express a preference for injection compression therapy.

In 1973 Seddon[131] also showed no statistically significant differences between the results of surgery and sclerotherapy, 12–18 months after treatment.

In 1975 Doran and White[42] concluded that the long-term results of Fegan's method were uncertain but suggested that the cost saving was so great that it should always be used as a first procedure. Piachaud and Weddell[116] had already commented

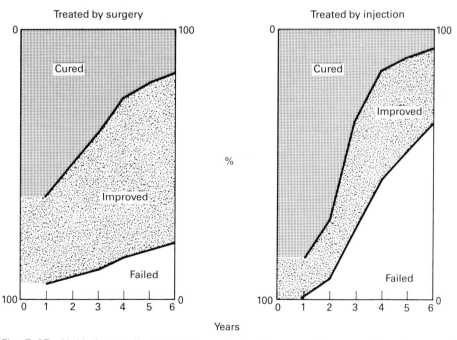

Fig. 7.45 Hobbs' controlled comparison of sclerotherapy with surgery. It can be seen that many more patients were improved or cured 5 years after the initial treatment in the surgical group than in the injection group, but at 2–3 years the results of the two forms of treatment were comparable.
(Modified from Hobbs).[66]

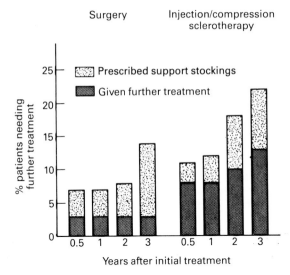

Surgery   Injection/compression
                      sclerotherapy

Fig. 7.46 Chant's comparison between sclerotherapy and surgery. There was no statistical difference in the number of requests for further treatment in either group at 3 years, though in the sclerotherapy group the percentage of patients needing further treatment was greater throughout the trial.

(Modified from Chant *et al.*)[22]

on the savings accruing to the economy if a policy of injection compression was followed by all, but their estimate was based on the 3-year results of Chant's study[22] not on the 5-year results of Hobbs' study.[66]

Comment Two editorials in the *British Medical Journal*[3,4] and one in the *Lancet*[5] presented a rational case for combining surgery and injections in the treatment of varicose veins, surgery being reserved for major long and short saphenous vein incompetence, and sclerotherapy being the treatment of choice for veins of the lower leg and isolated varicosities. The place of surgery versus sclerotherapy in the treatment of incompetent lower leg communicating veins is still debatable. In our opinion, the combined approach is sensible and logical. We continue to find that most of our patients require surgery because they present with advanced disease involving long or short saphenous vein incompetence, and we consider that the only effective treatment for incompetent communicating veins is surgical ligation. If our patients presented earlier, many of them would be treated initially by injection sclerotherapy before their saphenous system became incompetent. If surgery is to be

undertaken, it is obviously reasonable to avulse as many of the varicosities as possible at the same time. Injections may be required to obliterate residual varices after surgery.

We have been unable to find any studies comparing physiological tests of calf pump function in patients treated by surgery with those in patients treated by sclerotherapy (Fig. 7.47). Such studies would be valuable and might help to clarify the role of these forms of treatment. A recent study has shown that appropriate surgery on varicose veins does reduce foot swelling.[137]

Varicose veins of pregnancy and vulval varicosities

These are two sub-groups of varicose veins that deserve special mention.

Pregnancy

The aetiology of these veins has already been discussed (page 159). During pregnancy new varicose veins may appear or existing varicose veins may enlarge. Twenty per cent of mothers develop varicose veins in pregnancy.[36] The treatment is always expectant and should await the completion of the pregnancy. Support stockings may help both symptomatically and prophylactically. Surgery

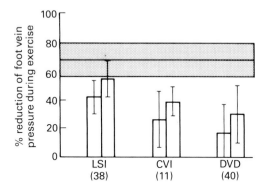

Fig. 7.47 The effect of surgery on calf pump function in three group of patients. The left-hand histogram indicates the reduction of foot vein pressure during exercise before surgery, the right-hand histogram shows the reduction of foot vein pressure during exercise after surgery. It can be seen that surgery almost returns the foot vein pressure to normal limits in patients with long saphenous vein incompetence (LSI), but does not return the pressure to normal in patients with incompetent calf communicating veins (CVI) or in patients with evidence of post-thrombotic damage on phlebography (DVD).

should not be carried out until after breast-feeding has been completed, and even sclero-therapy should be delayed for several months to ensure maximum regression of the veins after parturition. It is better, if possible, to delay definitive treatment until no further pregnancies are envisaged. Compression sclerotherapy may provide a useful interim measure.

Vulval varicosities

Dixon and Mitchell[36] found that 33 per cent of women who developed varicose veins in pregnancy had vulval involvement; Dodd and Payling-Wright[41] found that the incidence was only 2 per cent. Both these studies suggested that vulval varicosities regressed after parturition, but Craig and Hobbs[30] have reported a group of 12 women in whom the veins persisted after childbirth. Contrast radiology of these veins[30,38] has shown that many of them are connected to tributaries of the internal iliac vein (Fig. 7.48). Craig and Hobbs[30] associate the continued presence of vulval varicosities with 'the pelvic congestion syndrome' (dyspareunia, dysmenorrhoea and menorrhagia) but the exact aetiology of this syndrome remains obscure. Dixon and Mitchell[36] advocated that the following measures could be taken to eradicate vulval varicosities.

- Ligation of the internal pudendal vein
- Ligation of the obturator vein
- Ligation of the veins of the round ligament
- Ligation of the upper tributaries of the long saphenous vein

Craig and Hobbs have also suggested that hysterectomy may be helpful![30]

Comment   Treatment of vulval varicosities should be aimed at ligating the sites of communication that are shown on contrast radiology.[80] Hysterectomy is a draconian option for most women with this condition.

Treatment of dilated intradermal venules

The physical findings of dilated intradermal venules have already been described in Chapter 6. A number of descriptive terms have been given to these veins, including: spider veins, tache bleu, brush veins, blue shoots, birch sprigs, spider webs, spider bursts, sunburst veins, angetids, thread veins and hair veins.[50,54]

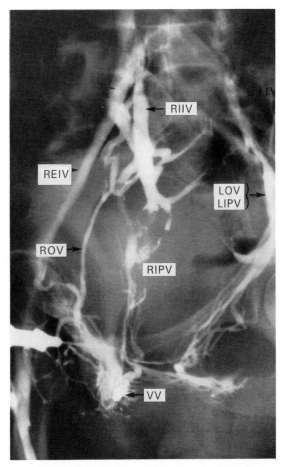

Fig. 7.48   A varicogram showing the connections of vulval varicosities. Vulval varicosities drain to the pudendal veins, the vaginal veins and the internal iliac veins.
RIIV = right internal iliac vein. REIV = right external iliac vein. ROV = right ovarian vein. RIPV = right internal pudendal vein. VV = vulval varices. LOV = left ovarian vein. LIPV = left internal iliac vein.

Dilated intradermal venules may be associated with varicose veins or they may occur independently.[50,54] They are symptomless but patients complain of their unsightliness. They were thought to be more common after pregnancy[50] but this has not been confirmed.[54] They are more common in women and increase with age,[54] and they may be related to occupation and diet.

Treatments for dilated intradermal venules include:

- reassurance
- camouflage creams

- injection of sclerosant through a microneedle
- electrocautery
- surgical intracuticular or subcuticular lancing
- laser photocoagulation

Many of these treatments carry a considerable risk of scarring.

References

1. Albanese AR. New instruments of varicose vein surgery. *J Cardiovasc Surg* 1965; **6**: 65.
2. Albanese AR, Albanese AM. Radical and esthetic surgery for varicose veins of the legs. *Vasc Surg* 1969; **3**: 194.
3. Anon. Economics of varicose veins. *Br Med J* 1973; **2**: 626.
4. Anon. Tailored treatment for varicose veins. *Br Med J* 1975; **1**: 593.
5. Anon. The treatment of varicose veins. *Lancet* 1975; **2**: 311.
6. Babcock WW. A new operation for the extirpation of varicose veins of the leg. *NY Med J* 1907, **86**: 153.
7. Barabas AP. The long saphenous in primary varicose veins. *Br J Surg* 1986; **73**: 320.
8. Batch AJG, Wickremesinghe SS, Gannon ME, Dormandy JA. Randomized trial of bandaging after sclerotherapy for varicose veins. *Br Med J* 1980; **2**: 423.
9. Biegeleisen HI. La cronicidad de las venas varicosas. Un estudio estadistico de cirugia vs escleroterapia. *Medicina* (Mexico) 1953; **33**: 193.
10. Bisgaard H. *Ulcers and Eczema of the leg. Sequels of Phlebitis: Studies on Stasis Diseases of the Lower Limbs and their Treatment.* Copenhagen. Munksgaard 1948.
11. Bishop CCR, Jarrett PEM. Outpatient varicose vein surgery under local anaesthesia. *Br J Surg* 1986; **73**: 821.
12. Bjordal RI. Blood circulation in varicose veins of the lower extremities. *Angiology* 1972; **23**: 163.
13. Bjordal RI. Circulation patterns in incompetent perforating veins in the calf and in the saphenous system in primary varicose veins. *Acta Chir Scand* 1972; **138**: 251.
14. Bjordal RI. Circulation patterns in the saphenous system and the perforating veins of the calf in patients with previous deep venous thrombosis. *Vasa* 1974; Suppl **3**: 1.
15. Bjordal RI. Pressure patterns in the saphenous system in patients with venous leg ulcers. *Acta Chir Scand* 1971; **137**: 495.
16. Bjordal RI. Simultaneous pressure and flow recordings in varicose veins of the lower extremity. *Acta Chir Scand* 1970; **136**: 309.
17. Boyd AM, Robertson DJ. Treatment of varicose veins. Possible dangers of injection of sclerosing fluids. *Br Med J* 1947; **2**: 452.
18. Boyd AM. Discussion on primary treatment of varicose veins. *Proc R Soc Med* 1948; **41**: 633.
19. Burnand KG, O'Donnell TF, Lea Thomas M, Browse NL. Relation between post phlebitic changes in the deep veins and results of surgical treatment of venous ulcers. *Lancet* 1976; **1**: 937.
20. Burnand KG, O'Donnell TF, Lea Thomas M, Browse NL. The relative importance of incompetent communicating veins in the production of varicose veins and venous ulcers. *Surgery* 1977; **82**: 9.
21. Burnand KG. Intérêt de la varicographie dans l'appréciation des varices essentielles des membres inférieurs. *Phlebologie* 1983; **1**: 269.
22. Chant ADB, Jones HO, Weddell JM. Varicose veins: A comparison of surgery and injection/compression sclerotherapy. *Lancet* 1972; **2**: 1188.
23. Chant ADB, Magnussen P, Kershaw C. Support hose and varicose veins. *Br Med J* 1985; **290**: 204.
24. Chassaignac E. *Nouvelle Méthode pour la Traitement des Tumours Haemorhoidales.* Paris. Baillière 1885.
25. Cockett FB. Diagnosis and surgery of high pressure venous leaks in the leg: a new overall concept of the surgery of varicose veins. *Br Med J* 1956; **2**: 399.
26. Cockett FB. The pathology and treatment of venous ulcers of the leg. *Br J Surg* 1955; **43**: 260.
27. Cole DS. 'Save our saphenous veins'. *Medical Tribune International Edition*, Scandinavia 1973; **5**: 3.
28. Corbett CR, McIrvine AJ, Aston NO, Jamieson CW, Lea Thomas M. The use of varicography to identify the sources of incompetence in recurrent varicose veins. *Ann R Coll Surg Engl* 1984; **66**: 412.
29. Cox SJ, Wellwood JM, Martin A. Saphenous nerve injury caused by stripping of the long saphenous vein. *Br Med J* 1974; **1**: 415.
30. Craig O, Hobbs JT. Vulval phlebography in the pelvic congestion syndrome. *Clin Radiol* 1975; **26**: 517.
31. Dale WA. Ligation, stripping, and excision of varicose veins. *Surgery* 1970; **67**: 389.
32. Davy A, Ouvry P. Recurrence of varicose veins. *Phlebology* 1986; **1**: 15.
33. Daseler EH, Anson BJ, Reimann AF, Benton LE. The saphenous venous tributaries and related structures in relation to the technique of high resection. *Surg Gynec Obstet* 1946; **82**: 53.

34. De Palma RG. Surgical therapy for venous stasis. *Surgery* 1974; **76**: 910.

35. Dejode LR. Injection compression treatment of varicose veins. A follow up study. *Br J Surg* 1970; **57**: 285.

36. Dixon JA, Mitchell WA. Phlebographic and surgical observations in vulval varicose veins. *Surg Gynec Obstet* 1970; **130**: 458.

37. Dodd H. The diagnosis and ligation of incompetent perforating veins. *Ann R Coll Surg Engl* 1964; **34**: 186.

38. Dodd H. Varicose veins. *Br J Hosp Med* 1968; 1101.

39. Dodd H, Cockett FB. *The Pathology and Surgery of the Veins of the Lower Limb.* London. Livingstone 1956.

40. Dodd H, Calo AR, Mistry M, Rushford A. Ligation of the ankle communicating veins for the treatment of the venous ulcer syndrome of the leg. *Lancet* 1957; **2**: 1249.

41. Dodd H, Payling-Wright H. Vulval varicose veins in pregnancy. *Br Med J* 1959; **1**: 831.

42. Doran FSA, White M. A clinical trial designed to discover if the primary treatment of varicose veins should be by Fegan's method or by an operation *Br J Surg* 1975; **62**: 72.

43. Edwards JM. Shearing operation for incompetent perforating veins. *Br J Surg* 1976; **63**: 885.

44. Eger M, Goleman L, Torok G, Hirsch M. Inadvertent arterial stripping in the lower limb: Problems of management. *Surgery* 1973; **73**: 23.

45. Fegan WG. Continuous compression technique for injecting varicose veins. *Lancet* 1963; **2**: 109.

46. Fegan WG. Injection, compression treatment of varicose veins. *Br J Hosp Med* **1969**; 1297.

47. Field ES, Kakkar VV, Stephenson G, Nicolaides AN. The value of cinephlebography in detecting incompetent venous valves in the postphlebitic state. *Br J Surg* 1972; **59**: 304.

48. Field P, Van Boxel P. The role of the Linton flap procedure in the management of stasis, dermatitis and ulceration of the lower limb. *Surgery* 1971; **70**: 920.

49. Fletcher EWL, Tibbs DJ. Directional flow in superficial veins as a guide to venous disorders of the lower limbs. *Surgery* 1983; **93**: 758.

50. Foote RR. *Varicose Veins.* London. Butterworths 1954.

51. Fraser IA, Perry EP, Hatton M, Watkin DFL. Prolonged bandaging is not required following sclerotherapy of varicose veins. *Br J Surg* 1985; **72**: 488.

52. Génévrier M. Du traitement des varices par les injections coagulantes concentrées de sels de quinine. *Soc De Med Mil Franc* 1921; **15**: 169.

53. Glass GM. Regrowth of veins in recurrence of varicose veins after surgical treatment. *Br J Surg* 1984; **71**: 991.

54. Gubéran E, Widmer LK, Rougement A, Glaus L. Epidemiology of spider webs. *Vasa* 1974; **4**: 391.

55. Hadfield GJ. In: *The Treatment of Varicose veins by Injection and Compression. (Proceedings of the Stoke Mandeville symposium).* Hereford. Pharmaceutical Research STD Ltd. 1971; 52.

56. Haeger K. Indications for surgery in ankle perforator insufficiency. *Zent Phlebol* 1969; **8**: 158.

57. Haeger K. The surgical anatomy of the saphenofemoral and sapheno-popliteal junctions. *J Cardiovasc Surg* 1962; **6**: 420.

58. Haliday P. Repeat high ligation. *Aust NZ J Surg* 1970; **39**: 354.

59. Hilty H. *Die makroskopiche Gefässvariibilität im Mündungsgebiet der Vena saphena des Menschen.* Basel. Schwabe 1955.

60. Hoare MC, Nicolaides AN, Miles CR, Shull K, Jury RP, Needham T, Dudley HAF. The role of primary varicose veins in venous ulceration. *Surgery* 1983; **82**: 450.

61. Hoare MG, Royle JP. Doppler ultrasound detection of saphenofemoral and saphenopopliteal incompetence and operative venography to ensure precise saphenopopliteal ligation. *Aust NZ J Surg* 1984; **54**: 49.

62. Hobbs JT. Peroperative venography to ensure accurate sapheno-popliteal ligation. *Br Med J* 1980; **2**: 1578.

63. Hobbs JT. In: Negus D, Jantet G (Eds) *Phlebology '85.* London. Libbey 1986; 143.

64. Hobbs JT. Treatment of varicose veins. A random trial of injection compression therapy versus surgery. *Br J Surg* 1968; **55**: 777.

65. Hobbs J. Compression sclerotherapy of varicose veins. In Bergan JJ, Yao JST (Eds) *Venous Problems.* Chicago. Year Book Medical Publishers 1976.

66. Hobbs J. Surgery and sclerotherapy in the treatment of varicose veins. A random trial. *Arch Surg* 1974; **109**: 793.

67. Holm J, Nilsson NJ, Schersten T, Sivertsson R. Elective surgery for varicose veins; A simple method for evaluation of the patients. *J Cardiovasc Surg* 1974; **15**: 565.

68. Homans J. Operative treatment of varicose veins and ulcers. *Surg Gynec Obstet* 1916; **22**: 143.

69. Homans J. The etiology and treatment of varicose ulcers of the leg. *Surg Gynec Obstet* 1917; **24**: 300.

70. Howard Jones N. Origins and early development of hyperdermic medication. *J Hist Med* 1947; **2**: 201.

71. Hurst P A, Kinmonth J B, Rutt D L. A gut and mesentery pedicle for bridging lymphatic obstruction. *J Cardiovasc Surg* 1978; **19**: 589.

72. Kakkar V V, Howe C T, Flank C. Compression sclerotherapy for varicose veins: A phlebographic study. *Br J Surg* 1969; **56**: 620.

73. Kent S J S. Personal communication. 1985.

74. Keith L M, Smead W L. Saphenous vein stripping and its complications. *Surg Clin North Am* 1983; **63**: 1303.

75. King E S J. The genesis of varicose veins. *Aust NZ J Surg* 1950; **20**: 126.

76. Kinmonth J B, Hurst P A, Edwards J M, Rutt D L. Relief of lymph obstruction by use of a bridge of mesentary and ileum. *Br J Surg* 1978; **65**: 829.

77. Kosinski C. The anatomy of the veins of the lower limb. *J Anat* (London) 1926; **60**: 131.

78. Larsson R H, Lofgren E, Myers T T, Lofgren K A. Long term results after vein surgery: Study of 1000 cases after 10 years. *Mayo Clin Proc* 1974; **49**: 114.

79. Lea Thomas M, Bowles J N. Incompetent perforating veins: Comparison of varicography and ascending phlebography. *Radiology* 1985; **154**: 619.

80. Lea Thomas M, Fletcher E W L, Andreas M R, Cockett F B. The venous connections of vulval varices. *Clin Radiol* 1967; **18**: 313.

81. Ledentu A. *Recherches anatomiques a considerations physiologiques sur la circulacion veineuse du pied et de la jambe.* Thesis Paris 1867.

82. Li A K C. A technique for re-exploration of the saphenofemoral junction for recurrent varicose veins. *Br J Surg* 1975; **62**: 745.

83. Linser P. Die Behandlung der Krampfadern mit intravarikösen Kochsalzinjektionen. *Derm Wochenschr* 1925; **81**: 1345.

84. Linser P. Die Behandlung der Varizen mit Künstlicher Thrombosierung. *Derm Z* 1925; **45**: 22.

85. Linser P. Über die konservative Behandlung der Varicen. *Med Klin* 1916; **12**: 847.

86. Linton R R. The communicating veins of the lower leg and the operative technique for their ligation. *Ann Surg* 1938; **107**: 582.

87. Lofgren E P, Coates H L C, O'Brien P C. Clinically suspect pulmonary embolism after vein stripping. *Mayo Clin Proc* 1976; **51**: 77.

88. Lofgren E P, Lofgren K A. Recurrence of varicose veins after the stripping operation. *Arch Surg* 1971; **102**: 111.

89. Lofgren E P, Lofgren K A. Recurrence of varicose veins after the stripping operation. *Arch Surg* 1971; **102**: 111.

90. Lofgren K A. Management of varicose veins: Mayo Clinic experience. In: Bergan J J, Yao J S T (Eds) *Venous Problems.* Chicago. Year Book Medical Publishers 1978.

91. Ludbrook J. Valvular defect in primary varicose veins. Cause or effect? *Lancet* 1963; **2**: 1289.

92. Luke J C, Miller G G. Disasters following the operation of ligation and retrograde injection of varicose veins. *Ann Surg* 1948; **127**: 426.

93. Luke J C. The management of recurrent varicose veins. *Surgery* 1954; **35**: 40.

94. Lumley J S P. Surgical treatment of varicose veins. *Br J Hosp Med* 1977; **508**.

95. MacGowan W A L. Sclerotherapy: Prevention of accidents. A review. *J R Soc Med* 1985; **78**: 136.

96. MacGowan W A L, Holland P D J, Browne H I, Byrnes D P. The local effects of intra-arterial injections of sodium tetradecyl sulphate (S.T.D.) 3 per cent. *Br J Surg* 1972; **59**: 103.

97. Maingot R H, Carlton C H. Injection treatment of varicose veins. *Lancet* 1928; **1**: 806.

98. Marston A. Treatment of varicose veins. *Lancet* 1975; **2**: 453.

99. Massel T B. The problem of adequate therapy for varicose veins: A new procedure. *West J Surg* 1950; **58**: 112.

100. May R, Nissl R. Phlebographic Studien zur Anatomie der Beinvenen. *Fortschr Roentgenstr* 1966; **104**: 171.

101. May R. Varicose veins. In: May R (Ed) *Surgery of the Veins of the Leg and Pelvis.* Stuttgart. Georg Thieme 1979.

102. Mayo C H. Treatment of varicose veins. *Surg Gynec Obstet* 1906; **2**: 385.

103. Mercier R, Fouques P H, Portal N, Vanneuville G. Anatomie chirurgicale de la veine saphene externe. *J Chir* 1967; **93**: 54.

104. Moosman A, Hartwell W. The surgical significance of the subfascial course of the lesser saphenous vein. *Surg Gynec Obstet* 1964; **118**: 761.

105. Munn S R, Morton J B, Macbeth W A G, McLeish A R. To strip or not to strip the long saphenous vein? A varicose veins trial. *Br J Surg* 1981; **68**: 426.

106. Myers T T, Cooley J C. Varicose vein surgery in the management of the post-phlebitic limb. *Surg Gynec Obstet* 1954; **99**: 733.

107. Nabatoff R A. Surgical technique for stripping the long saphenous vein. *Surg Gynec Obstet* 1977; **145**: 81.

108. Nabatoff R A. Three thousand stripping operations for varicose veins on a semi-ambulatory basis. *Surg Gynec Obstet* 1970; **130**: 497.

109. Negus D, Friedgood A. The effective management of venous ulceration. *Br J Surg* 1983; **70**: 623.

110. Negus D. Prevention and treatment of venous ulceration. *Ann R Coll Surg Engl* 1985; **67**: 144.

111. O'Reilly K. A technique of diathermy sclerosis of

varicose veins. *Aust NZ J Surg* 1981; **51**: 379.

112. O'Reilly K. Endovenous diathermy sclerosis of varicose veins. *Aust NZ J Surg* 1977; **47**: 393.

113. Otsu A, Mori N. Therapy of varicose veins. The lower limb spy light calculator. *Angiology* 1971; **22**: 107.

114. Ouvry P A, Davy A. Traitement sclerosant de la saphène externe variqueuse. In Negus D, Jantet G (Eds) *Phlebology '85* London. Libbey 1986; 115.

115. Petrov ML, Pennin BA. Khirurgicheskoe Lechenie pri posttromboflebiticheskom sindrome. *Vestn Khir* 1976; **116**: 48,

116. Piachaud D, Weddell JM. The cost of treating varicose veins. *Lancet* 1972; **2**: 1191.

117. Pulvertaft TB. General practice treatment of symptoms of venous insufficiency with oxerutins. *Vasa* 1983; **12**: 373.

118. Raivió E. Untersuchungen über die Venen der unteren extremitaten mit besonderer berucksichtigung der gegenseit igen verbindungen zwischen den oberflachigen und tiefen Venen. *Ann Med Exp Finn* 1948; **26**: 1.

119. Raj TB, Makin GS. A random controlled trial of two forms of compression bandaging in outpatient sclerotherapy of varicose veins. *J Surg Res* 1981; **31**: 440.

120. Reid RG, Rothnie NG. Treatment of varicose veins by compression sclerotherapy. *Br J Surg* 1968; **55**: 889.

121. Reiner L. Activity of anionic surface compounds in producing vascular obliteration. *Proc Soc Exp Biol Med* 1946; **62**: 49.

122. Rivlin S. The surgical cure of primary varicose veins. *Br J Surg* 1975; **62**: 913.

123. Rogers L, Winchester AH. Intravenous sclerosing solutions. *Br Med J* 1930; **2**: 120.

124. Rose SS, Ahmed A. Some thoughts on the aetiology of varicose veins. *J Cardiovasc Surg* 1986; **27**: 534.

125. Rose SS. Personal communication. 1985.

126. Royle JP. Operative treatment of varicose veins. *Hosp Update* 1984; : 941.

127. Royle JP. In Greenhalgh RM. (Ed) *Vascular Surgical Techniques*. London. Butterworths 1984.

128. Schiassi B. La Cure des varices par l'injection d'une solution d'iode. *Sem Méd Paris* 1908; **28**: 601.

129. Scott A, Dormandy J. Outpatients ligation of varicose veins. *Proc R Soc Med* 1976; **69**: 22.

130. Scurr JH, Coleridge-Smith P, Cutting P. Varicose veins: Optimum compression following sclerotherapy. *Ann R Coll Surg Engl* 1985; **67**: 109.

131. Sedden J. The management of varicose veins. *Br J Surg* 1973; **60**: 345.

132. Sheppard M. A procedure for the prevention of recurrent saphenofemoral incompetence. *Aust NZ J Surg* 1978; **48**: 322.

133. Sherman RS. Varicose veins: Further findings based on anatomic and surgical dissections. *Ann Surg* 1949; **130**: 218.

134. Sicard J A, Gaugier L. *Les Traitment des Varices par les Injections Locals Sclerosantes*. Paris. Masson 1927.

135. Sigg K. Treatment of varicosities and accompanying complications (ambulatory treatment of phlebitis with compression bandage). *Angiology* 1952; **3**: 355.

136. Somerville JF, Brow GO, Byrne PJ, Quill RD, Fegan WG. The effect of elastic stockings on superficial venous pressures in patients with venous insufficiency. *Br J Surg* 1974; **61**: 979.

137. Spearman MJ, Collins J. Are swelling and aching of the legs reduced by operating on varicose veins? *Br Med J* 1986; **293**: 105.

138. Stother IG, Bryson A, Alexander S. Treatment of varicose veins by compression sclerotherapy. *Br J Surg* 1974; **61**: 387.

139. Tavel E. Die Behandlung der varicen durch die künstliche Thrombose. *Dtsch Z Chir* 1912; **116**: 735.

140. Tournay R. Indications et resultats de la methode sclerosantes dans la traitment des varices. *Bull Méd Paris* 1931; **45**: 73.

141. Tournay R. Traitment des varices: Chirurgie ou injections sclerosantes. *Bull Soc Med Pract Lille* 1937.

142. Trendelenburg F. Über die Unterbildung der Vena saphena magna bei unterschenkel Varicen. *Beitr Klin Chir* 1891; **7**: 195.

143. Turner-Warwick W. *The Rational Treatment of Varicose Veins and Varicocele (with notes on the obliterative method of treatment of other conditions)*. London. Faber & Faber 1931.

144. Van Limborgh J. L'anatomie du système veineux de l'extrémité inférieux en relation avec la pathologie variqueuse. *Folia Angiol* 1961; **8**: 3.

145. Watts GT. The treatment of varicose veins. *Lancet* 1973; **1**: 435.

146. Wilkins RW, Mixter G, Stanton JR, Litter J. Elastic stockings in the prevention of pulmonary embolism: a preliminary report. *N Engl J Med* 1952; **246**: 360.

147. Wilkins RW, Stanton JR. Elastic stockings in the prevention of pulmonary embolism. II. A progress report. *N Engl J Med* 1953; **248**: 1087.

148. Williams RA, Wilson SE. Sclerosant treatment of varicose veins in deep vein thrombosis. *Arch Surg* 1984; **119**: 1283.

149. Wilson MG. A method of treatment of varicose veins. *Lancet* 1953; **1**: 1273.

150. Winstone N. In *The Treatment of Varicose Veins by Injection and compression. (Proceedings of the Stoke Mandeville Symposium)*. Hereford. Pharmaceutical Research STD Ltd 1971; 41.

8

Primary (non-thrombotic) deep vein incompetence

The demonstration that the valves in the veins ensured a unidirectional flow of blood was the keystone experiment in Harvey's investigations which proved that the blood circulated from the heart through the arteries and capillaries and returned through the veins.

The valves in the veins of the lower limbs are particularly important because hydrostatic forces encourage retrograde flow in the erect posture.

The valve cusps are extremely delicate but very strong structures (see Chapter 3). Congenital abnormalities of the cusps are rare. Although valvular incompetence is usually the result of a primary vein wall abnormality or the post-thrombotic destruction of normal valves, primary deep vein incompetence is an important abnormality which should always be considered as a possible diagnosis in patients with the clinical features of the calf pump failure syndrome.

The treatment of primary deep vein incompetence is, in many circumstances, similar to the treatment of secondary deep vein incompetence; this chapter and Chapter 12 should therefore be considered together.

Pathology

Retrograde flow in the deep veins may be permitted by one of the following abnormalities.

Absent valves (See Chapter 23, page 606) Congenital absence of the valves of the deep veins is a very rare abnormality;[25,28,29] in 20 years of clinical practice and after viewing more than 3000 phlebograms we have seen only two cases. In these patients no valves were visible in any of the deep veins of the lower limb, and in one patient no valves were present in the deep veins of his arms. No study has examined close relatives of patients without deep vein valves; it is therefore not known

if this is an inherited or a sporadic abnormality.

Vein valve prolapse (floppy valve cusps) The length of the free edge of a valve cusp is critical to its competence. When closed, the edge should be taut and straight and abut against its fellow across the whole width of the vein, with the valve sinus full and tense. If the valve edge is too long, it can evert in an upstream direction and render the valve incompetent. The incompetence, but not the valve eversion, can be demonstrated by descending phlebography. This abnormality has been called 'the floppy valve' by Kistner who has found a series of such cases in different races in Hawaii.[8,19] These patients have no evidence of previous venous thrombosis; it is therefore assumed that this is a congenital abnormality but as the surgical treatment is to repair the valve, none has been removed for histological or bio-mechanical studies to define the nature of the tissue abnormality. It is clear that this is not a valve ring abnormality because the valve commissures are not separated. Since Kistner's description of this abnormality, other surgeons (mainly American) have reported seeing and treating it.[11,33,34] We have searched hard and long for patients with this abnormality but have not yet found a single case. We assume that this is related to either a very low incidence in the population which we treat or a difference in our methods of investigation.

Valve ring dilatation Normal valve cusps will not meet across the lumen of the vein, if the valve ring (the cross-section of the vein at the level of the commissures) dilates. The most common example of this form of incompetence is seen in varicose superficial veins when either an underlying defect in the strength of the vein wall or prolonged high pressure dilates not only the valve ring but the whole vein, making the valves incompetent and the vein large and tortuous (see Chapter 5).

This type of valvular incompetence is rare in the deep veins, perhaps because they are supported by the surrounding muscles and the connective tissues of the neurovascular bundle. The phlebographic diameter of the deep veins is remarkably uniform from patient to patient and is only slightly increased even when there is gross reflux. The deep veins of the authors' two patients with primary avalvular deep veins were of normal size.

A few cases of patients with very large deep veins have been reported in association with arteriomegaly but there is no equivalent condition that can be called 'phlebomegaly'.[22]

There are publications which describe varicose veins of the deep compartment. These veins may have incompetent valves secondary to valve ring dilatation but this abnormality is rare and usually localized to one or two veins in the calf – the other veins being of normal size.[24]

The vein walls relax during pregnancy under the influence of raised hormone levels. This certainly makes the superficial veins dilate and become incompetent and sometimes the deep veins follow suit but the incidence and degree of the deep vein change has not been documented. Most of the vein changes of pregnancy reverse after delivery.

Fixed or thickened valve cusps (possibly post-thrombotic) (see Chapter 11) Thrombosis invariably causes irrecoverable damage to the valve cusps and causes secondary deep vein incompetence. It is such an important cause of deep vein reflux, accounting for 95 per cent or more of cases, that it is mentioned in this chapter to ensure that the reader appreciates the rarity of 'primary' reflux.

If the whole lumen of the vein is occluded by thrombus, the valve cusps become completely fixed within it and can no longer function. Recannalization by the confluence of lytic areas within the thrombus produces an avalvular tube. Retraction of the thrombus to one side of the vein leaves one cusp within the thrombus and the other fixed to the vein wall. Even complete therapeutic or spontaneous thrombolysis usually leaves the valve cusps fixed or thickened and immobile. A delicate functioning valve in a vein that has been thrombosed is very rarely seen, however good the restoration of the lumen. It is not known whether other pathological events can cause thickening and contraction of valve cusps.

Diagnosis

Clinical presentation

Swelling This is the principal complaint and has usually been present for many years. Swelling begins at the ankle and slowly extends to involve the lower leg and sometimes the thigh. It is rarely so great that it impedes the movements of the limb but it does restrict activity because it makes the leg feel tight. Swelling increases as the day passes and goes down a little after a night in bed.

Swelling is caused by the lack of venous hypotension during exercise; its presence therefore implies that there is poor calf pump function. Some patients with severe reflux have no swelling because they are able to reduce their superficial vein pressure by exercise. This makes it likely that the swelling associated with deep vein reflux is not caused by the axial vein reflux alone but by the secondary effects of this reflux on the veins of the calf, particularly the lower leg communicating veins.

Pain Pain is not a common complaint. The leg becomes tight and aches as the day passes but the patient rarely says that the ache is severe enough to merit calling it a pain.

Venous claudication A few patients develop muscle pain on exercise similar to the venous claudication caused by severe outflow tract obstruction. This is difficult to explain when there is no mechanical obstruction to venous outflow from the limb and indicates that the reflux is so great that it is producing the same effect as a severe outflow tract obstruction.

Nightcramps are common.

Skin changes Skin changes such as eczema, pigmentation, lipodermatosclerosis and ulceration rarely appear while the calf pump is efficient, even when there is Grade 4 reflux, but as soon as the communicating veins become incompetent as a result of the prolonged strain on the pump caused by the reflux, the subcutaneous tissues and the skin rapidly deteriorate.

The skin changes in the 'gaiter' area of the leg are identical to those seen following severe calf vein thrombosis.

Clinical examination reveals the swelling and the skin changes and may also detect *superficial varicose* veins. Varicosities are not invariably present but, like the skin changes, they indicate

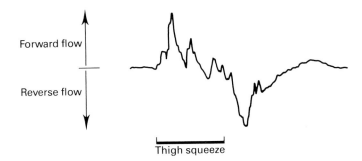

Forward flow

Reverse flow

Thigh squeeze

Fig. 8.1 The Doppler signal from an incompetent superficial femoral vein. Forward blood flow occurs when the lower thigh is squeezed, but the direction of blood flow reverses when the pressure on the lower thigh is released.

calf pump insufficiency and communicating vein incompetence.

Investigations

Doppler insonation (see also Chapter 4, page 83) Retrograde flow in the deep veins can be detected using a bi-directional Doppler flow probe. The transducer is placed over the common or superficial femoral vein to observe the direction of blood flow during and after a Valsalva manoeuvre, and a thigh squeeze. In a normal person venous blood flow stops when the intrathoracic pressure is raised by a Valsalva manoeuvre. If the valves are incompetent, the flow stops and then reverses to flow retrogradely down the vein. A similar biphasic signal (forward and reversed flow) will be heard during and after squeezing the thigh (Fig. 8.1).

The common and superficial femoral veins are easy to insonate with the Doppler probe. It is not easy to find the popliteal vein. When popliteal vein blood flow is being studied it must be done with the short saphenous vein occluded because incompetence of this vein allows retrograde flow in the segment of the popliteal vein above its termination. In fact there are a number of anatomical variations and pathological abnormalities which can allow retrograde flow in a segment of the popliteal vein between competent valves (Fig. 8.2); this vein must therefore be examined very carefully and the results interpreted with caution. The combined use of venous imaging with flow observations will make flow studies much more reliable as the point of flow measurement will be visible on the grey scale image.

When the popliteal vein is examined, the patient must be standing with the knee slightly flexed and the weight on the opposite leg. The transducer is placed over the centre of the pop-

liteal fossa at an angle of 45–60°. The vein usually lies over or to one side of the arterial signal. Blood flow in the vein can be heard if it is accelerated by squeezing the calf. If retrograde flow follows squeezing the calf, the test should be repeated with a finger compressing the short saphenous vein. If the retrograde flow persists, the popliteal vein is incompetent.

Figure 8.3 shows the various situations in which retrograde flow can occur in a segment of popliteal vein, even when its valves are competent, and indicates that this test should be interpreted with caution.

In our laboratory we have not found a good correlation between Doppler detected popliteal vein reflux and descending phlebography but other workers have reported a correlation

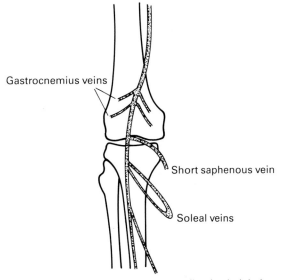

Gastrocnemius veins

Short saphenous vein

Soleal veins

Fig. 8.2 The tributaries of the popliteal vein join it above and below the knee joint. Many of the muscle veins do not have valves so blood can flow retrogradely into them from the main vein.

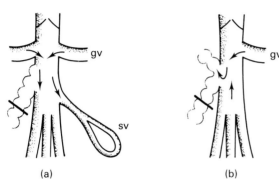

Fig. 8.3 The situations in which retrograde blood flow can occur in the popliteal vein even when the short saphenous vein is occluded. (a) Blood flowing into the popliteal vein from a gastrocnemius vein (gv) and out into a valveless soleal sinusoid (sv).
(b) Blood flowing out into incompetent tributaries deep to the popliteal fascia and above the point of short saphenous vein obstruction. In both these circumstances blood may be flowing forwards in the lower half of the popliteal vein and backwards in the upper half, even when the popliteal vein contains a competent valve.

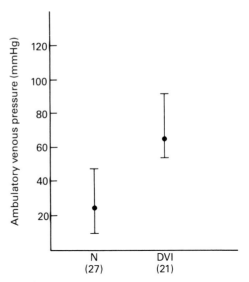

Fig. 8.4 The median and 95 per cent tolerance levels of ambulatory venous pressure (foot vein pressure during exercise) in 27 normal subjects and 21 patients with Doppler-detected popliteal vein reflux. Patients with popliteal reflux were unable to reduce their foot vein pressure; the difference between these patients and normal subjects is statistically significant.
(Redrawn from Schull K.C. *et al. Arch Surg* 1979; **114**: 1304.)

between the presence of popliteal vein reflux and calf pump efficiency assessed by exercising foot vein pressures (Fig. 8.4).

Refilling time All the methods which measure the rate of refilling of the veins of the lower limb (photo, strain-gauge, and isotope plethysmography, foot volumetry and measurement of foot vein pressure) can be used to detect deep vein reflux. All these techniques depend upon the same principle. The veins are emptied by exercise or compression and the rate of refilling is measured with and without superficial vein reflux prevented by a superficial vein occluding tourniquet.

The refilling rate can be expressed in various ways — the complete refilling time, the 90 per cent or the 50 per cent refilling time, or the maximum rate of refilling.

None of these expressions is particularly superior to any other. All are acceptable provided each laboratory establishes its own normal range and adheres to a standardized method.

Normal refilling of the veins of the leg when the superficial veins are occluded is a slow process depending solely upon the arterial inflow. The normal rate of refilling determined by foot volumetry is between 2.0 and 2.5 ml/100 ml of calf/min. When there is gross deep or super-

ficial reflux this rate can increase to 10–15 ml/100 ml/min.[40] When measured with isotope plethysmography[42] the normal refilling rate is 5%/min, deep vein incompetence alone can increase this to 10%/min, and a combination of deep and superficial vein incompetence increases it to 15%/min (Fig. 8.5).

Figure 8.6 shows a foot volume trace of a normal limb and the tracing of a patient with deep vein incompetence, with and without the superficial veins occluded by a tourniquet. The rapid refilling caused by the deep vein reflux is quite obvious.

Phlebography Although the non-invasive tests can detect and quantify deep vein reflux, they do not delineate the state of the deep veins, the extent of the reflux or the presence or absence of normal or abnormal valves. At the moment this can only be done by phlebography[10,23,27] but it may be possible with real-time ultrasound imaging when this method is fully developed.

The technique of descending phlebography is fully described in Chapter 4.

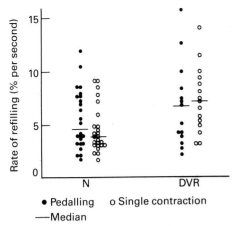

Fig. 8.5 The rate of venous refilling of the calf measured with isotope plethysmography after pedalling (●) and a sustained calf muscle contraction (o) in 25 normal subjects (N) and 15 patients with phlebographically proven deep vein reflux (DVR). The increased rate of refilling in the patients was statistically significant.
(Redrawn from Whitehead *et al.*)[42]

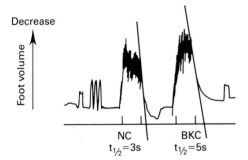

Fig. 8.6 The foot volume trace of a limb with deep vein incompetence. (NC = no superficial vein occluding cuff; BKC = below-knee cuff)

The $t_{1/2}$ (refilling time) without a cuff was 3 s. The $t_{1/2}$ was 5 s when the superficial veins were occluded below the knee.

If the rapid refilling had been caused by superficial vein reflux, the below knee cuff would have restored the refilling time to normal (i.e. 15–25 s).

Provided the position of the patient is kept constant (we prefer the patient to be supine, other investigators favour a 65° head up tilt) and the stimulus to reflux is controlled (a Valsalva manoeuvre at 40 mmHg for 30 seconds), the distance the X-ray contrast medium refluxes down

the leg is reproducible and measurable.[23]
Five grades of reflux are recognized[13] (see Chapter 4 page 112 and Figs. 8.7 and 8.8).

0 — None
1 — Reflux down to the first valve below the site of injection
2 — Reflux down to the upper third of the thigh
3 — Reflux down to, but not below the knee joint
4 — Reflux below the knee joint

An examination of the correlation between the presence of symptoms and signs and the degree of reflux strongly suggests that Grades 0, 1 and 2 reflux are normal, whereas the reflux of Grades 3 and 4 is abnormal and usually, but not always,[3,35] associated with calf pump failure.

Descending phlebography also shows the valve cusps. Stiff fixed cusps are easy to identify. To date we have not seen any floppy prolapsing valve cusps.

As the contrast rarely enters the tributaries of either the main axial vein in the thigh or the stem veins of the calf, descending phlebography gives little information about the state of veins in the calf pump. *Ascending phlebography* is therefore an essential investigation to exclude post-thrombotic changes (recanalization, collaterals, and absent valves) and incompetent communicating veins.

We usually do the ascending before the descending phlebogram because one can be 90 per cent certain that there is little or no reflux if it shows normal valved axial veins, but the presence of a recanalized femoral vein obviously damaged by thrombosis does not necessarily mean that there will be Grade 3 or 4 reflux.

The correlation between the phlebographic state of the veins on ascending phlebography and the degree of reflux is shown in Table 8.1.

An *arm phlebogram* should be performed if a valve transplant is being considered for avalvular or congenitally absent abnormal lower limb valves. In one of our patients valves were absent from both the arms and the legs.

Treatment

All varieties of deep axial vein incompetence should, initially, be treated conservatively. The most important objective is the reduction and

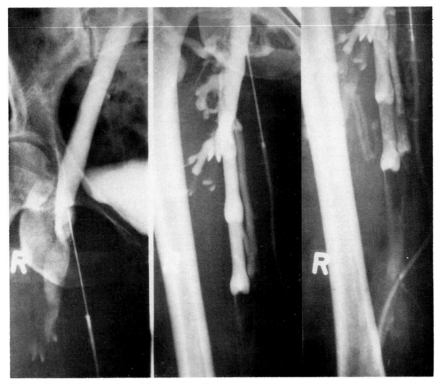

Fig. 8.7 A descending phlebogram showing reflux down to a valve in the mid-thigh during a Valsalva manoeuvre (middle panel) with a small amount of contrast medium trickling through down to a point just above the knee. We would classify the mid-thigh valve as normal and call this Grade 2, not Grade 3, reflux.

control of the swelling with good quality compression stockings and elevation of the leg whenever possible.

Below-knee stockings are usually sufficient as most of the swelling is usually below the knee. Effective stockings should compress the limb with

Table 8.1 Correlation between degree of deep vein damage seen on ascending phlebograms and the degree of deep vein reflux detected by descending phlebography

State of deep veins on ascending phlebography	Grade of Reflux	
	0–2	3–4
Normal deep veins (44 legs)	100%	0
Post-phlebitic deep vein damage (19 legs)	70%	30%
Post-phlebitic deep vein damage and no visible valves (12 legs)	40%	60%

a pressure of 30–40 mmHg at the ankle. The patient must be told to avoid standing still, put their legs up on a leg rest when sitting and, if possible, spend 10–15 minutes each day lying on the floor with their legs propped up vertically against a wall. At night the patient should raise the foot of the bed by 12 inches (30 cm) and elevate the affected limb or limbs still further by resting them upon a wedge of pillows.

Regular support and elevation of the limb, assisted by gentle massage of the whole limb, with special attention to areas of skin or subcutaneous thickening, will often relieve the aching and keep the limb to an acceptable size.

If the swelling or the skin changes deteriorate in spite of good conservative treatment, the veins should be investigated to determine the relative importance of the deep vein incompetence *vis-à-vis* the calf pump insufficiency. If there are no detectable incompetent communicating veins, it is reasonable to consider an operation that will

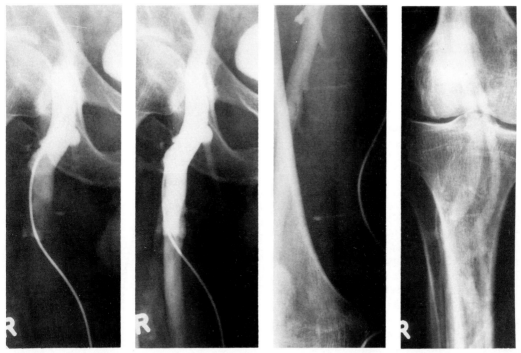

Fig. 8.8 A descending phlebogram showing reflux of radio-opaque contrast medium down to the mid-calf. This is Grade 4 reflux.

restore deep vein competence. If there are many large incompetent communicating veins, we prefer to treat these veins first (by ligation) and wait to see the effect of this procedure before deciding whether the deep vein incompetence requires treatment.

It is not known whether failure to treat the deep vein reflux after treating the communicating vein incompetence will inevitably lead to early recurrence of symptoms. If the calf pump abnormality is secondary to the axial vein incompetence, it is logical to argue that both should be corrected. This has been Kistner's approach[8] because his initial studies suggested that correction of the deep vein reflux without correction of the communicating vein reflux was associated with a high rate of recurrence.

Avalvular incompetence

If avalvular incompetence causes severe symptoms, it may be possible to perform a brachial to popliteal vein valve transplant provided the patient has a brachial valve. This operation is described in the next section.

The only solution for the extremely rare patient without valves in the arm or the leg is a valve allograft. Living vein allografts transplanted for the treatment of arterial ischaemia show the histological changes of rejection and have a high incidence of thrombosis. Valves are likely to behave in the same way but have not been studied clinically.

Denatured tissue does not excite an immune response. We have shown that it is possible to harvest human femoral veins, denature the protein and crosslink the collagen with gluteraldehyde and yet preserve almost normal valve cusp and vein wall mechanical properties.[2] Unfortunately, we found a high incidence of thrombosis when these valves were inserted into dogs veins; the thrombosis was probably caused by residual gluteraldehyde.[1] If the problem of thrombosis can be overcome, it should be possible to create a bank of preserved human vein valves for surgical insertion when the patient's brachial vein is not suitable or when more than one valve is required. The cross linking of the collagen may also stop the dilatation and recurrent incompetence that has been observed in some of the autogenous valve transplants.

Valve cusp prolapse

When Kistner first detected this condition[19] he devised an operation to tighten and repair the valve cusps; he has used this technique to treat most of his patients.[15,16,17,18]

Valve cusp repair

The valve to be repaired, which is usually a valve in the upper part of the superficial femoral vein, is exposed through a longitudinal incision over the course of the vein. The incompetence of the valve vein is confirmed by Harvey's test. A good valve will ballon out and prevent reflux; a prolapsing valve will let blood flow through it. Although the cusps can be seen at the commissures, the prolapse of the edge of the cusp cannot be seen as this is occurring in the middle of the opaque blood.

Kistner believes that it may be necessary to repair valves in more than one vein, for example the superficial femoral and the deep femoral or long saphenous vein, depending upon which of these vessels is the main outflow tract of the leg.

The patient is anticoagulated with heparin and the vein is occluded with soft atraumatic vascular clamps. The vein is then opened through a longitudinal venotomy beginning just below the cusps and passing between them precisely at the commissure so that the cusps are not damaged (Fig. 8.9a). The vein is held open with stay sutures and a stitch of fine non-absorbable monofilament material (usually Prolene) is placed so that it passes through the vein wall, from outside to inside, adjacent to the commissure, through the edge of the cusp 2 mm from the commissure and back through the vein wall. When this stitch is tied on the outside of the vein, it shortens the cusp by 2 mm (Fig. 8.9b). Similar stitches are placed

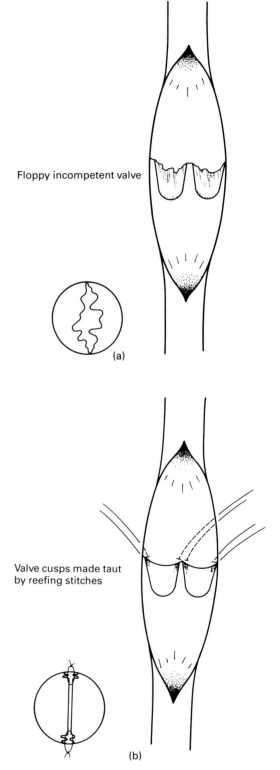

Floppy incompetent valve

(a)

Valve cusps made taut by reefing stitches

(b)

Fig. 8.9 The valve repair operation.

(a) The vein is opened longitudinally, between the valve cusps, to expose the 'floppy valve'.

(b) Stitches are placed through the vein wall, at the commissures and through the edges of the cusps, to shorten their free margins and so make the valve competent when the venotomy is closed.

through the other cusp close to the other edge of the venotomy and through the undivided commissure at the centre of the open vein; this stitch passes through both cusps. Further reefing sutures are inserted until the cusp lies loosely (not tightly) across the surface of the vein. The venotomy is then closed and the competence of the valve is tested.

The patient is given heparin for 3 days and oral anticoagulants for 3 months to maintain anticoagulation.

Results Ferris and Kistner have given a detailed account of their experience with 31 valve repair operations[8] and they have reported that the majority of the valves were made competent by the repair and remained competent for up to 13 years. Their experience is summarized in Fig. 8.10.

Before operation, 5 of the 31 patients refluxed to the upper calf and the other 26 had massive reflux. In 27 patients repeat descending phlebography within 1 year of operation showed no

reflux in 11, reflux to the thigh in 2, reflux to thigh and calf in 10, major reflux to the calf in 3 and massive reflux to the calf in 1. Although Kistner's classification of reflux differs from Herman's classification, which is now in general use, all 31 patients had pathological reflux before operation whereas 13 of the 27 studied soon after the operation had no reflux, 10 were improved and 4 did not improve.

Twenty patients were examined again between 3 and 13 years after operation (Fig. 8.10); 8 patients were unchanged, 7 had improved by one more grade and 5 had deteriorated, but only 2 of these 5 had severe pathological reflux. Seven of the 8 patients who had foot vein pressure studies before and after operation showed an improvement (Fig. 8.11).

These results suggest that the valve repair operation can correct or improve phlebographically detected reflux. It is, however, difficult to assess the clinical value of this operation because in many of these patients the communicating

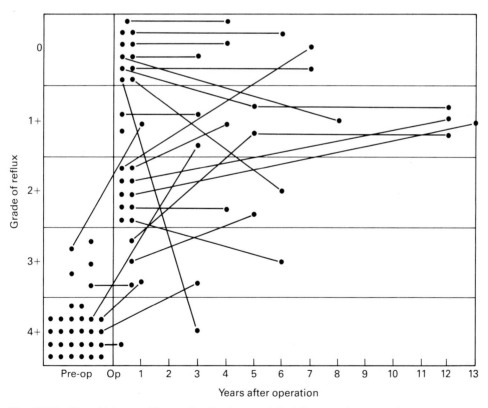

Fig. 8.10 The phlebographic results of valve repair 3–13 years after operation. (Redrawn from Ferris and Kistner.)[8]

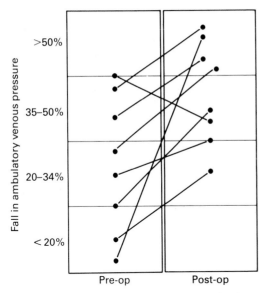

Fig. 8.11 The effect of valve repair on the foot vein pressure during exercise. Seven of the 8 patients studied had improved calf pump function. (Redrawn from Ferris and Kistner.)[8]

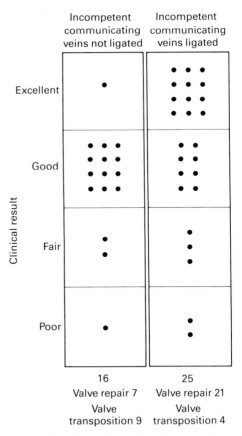

Fig. 8.12 The effect of ligating coincidental incompetent communicating veins at the time of performing valve repair or valve transposition.
Excellent = full relief, no need for elastic stockings.
Good = full relief provided elastic stockings were worn.
Fair = mild to moderate symptoms when elastic stockings worn.
Poor = no improvement or recurrent symptoms.
(Redrawn from Ferris and Kistner.[8] We are grateful to Dr Kistner for additional information included in Figs. 8.11 and 8.12.)

veins had also been ligated. In fact 28 of the 32 patients (90 per cent) who had had a valve repair had communicating vein incompetence and in 21 out of 28 patients (66 per cent) these veins had been ligated before, at the same time, or soon after the valve repair. In only 7 patients had a valve repair been carried out without additional venous surgery, and Kistner states that the best results were seen in those patients in whom both the deep vein valve and the communicating vein abnormality had been corrected.

When the clinical results of both the valve repairs and the valve transpositions are combined (41 patients) but subdivided according to whether or not the communicating veins were ligated, Kistner found that of the 13 patients with an excellent result (full relief of clinical condition *without* elastic compression) only 1 patient had not had a communicating vein ligation, whereas of the 20 patients with a moderate result (good clinical relief provided they wore their elastic stocking) 12 did not have communicating vein ligation (Fig. 8.12).

Our interpretation of these studies is that valve repair is not in itself sufficient to relieve the swelling and skin changes of deep axial vein incompetence. We think that these studies suggest that

symptoms do not appear until the communicating veins become incompetent and that axial vein valve repair will have only a temporary effect if the communicating vein abnormality is not corrected.

These views are in accord with those of Kistner who believes that the whole system should be repaired whenever possible. Repairing one abnormality and leaving another untreated strains the first repair so much that it is likely to fail.

Axial vein valve operations are still in their infancy, and they should only be performed as part of a careful clinical research study. In our opinion communicating vein ligation followed by good elastic compression remains the treatment of choice until more extensive and long-term follow-up studies confirm the value of deep vein valve procedures.

Valve ring plication

Jones *et al.*,[13] have described an alternative procedure to the valve cusp plication. The vein is exposed and the valve ring is reduced in circumference by a longitudinal series of plication stitches, at right angles to the valve ring and midway between the commissures (Fig. 8.13). This does not not shorten the cusps but may prevent them prolapsing. No long-term results of this operation have been published but, as it avoids both opening and stitching through the valves, it should reduce the risk of postoperative thrombosis.

Valve ring dilatation appears to be the main cause of the failure of valve transplants and transpositions, and a method for preventing this is needed. Wrapping the vein with a non-elastic material is the obvious solution but this may cause an inflammatory reaction and thrombosis. Rings placed around the vein to hold it open tend to move or tilt and have not proved successful. Unfortunately, the A–V fistula (the accepted method for keeping venous anastomoses patent) stretches the valve ring and increases the chance of the valve becoming incompetent, particularly if the fistula is not closed within a few months of the repair.

Fixed or irreparable valves

Valve repair operations can only be performed when the valve cusps are pliable and healthy. Some patients with no phlebographic evidence of previous deep vein thrombosis appear to have normal veins with thickened short cusps which cannot be restored to normal. Two operations have been proposed to solve this problem. The

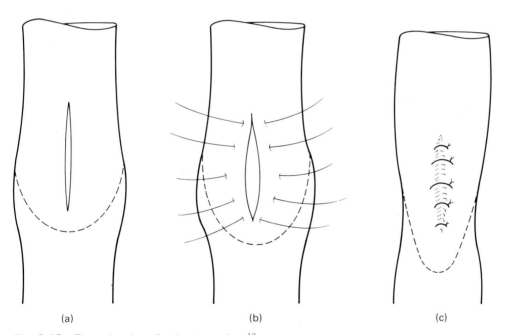

(a) (b) (c)

Fig. 8.13 The valve ring plication operation.[13]

 (a) A longitudinal venotomy is made level with the edge of the valve cusp, midway between the commissures. It is then enlarged towards the centre of the attached border of the cusp.

 (b) A series of sutures are placed to close the venotomy but at an increasing distance from the edge of the venotomy at its centre.

 (c) When the sutures are tied the circumference of the valve ring is reduced.

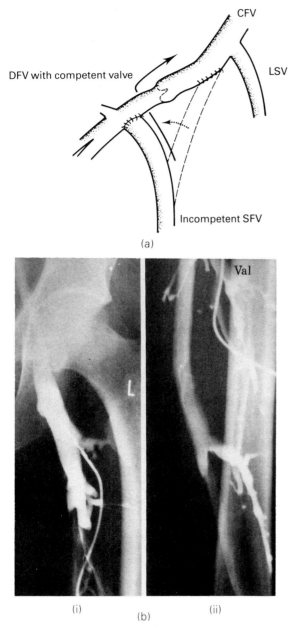

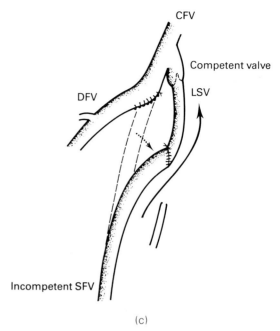

(c) An incompetent superficial femoral vein anastomosed to the long saphenous vein below a competent valve. This operation is rarely performed as the long saphenous vein is usually incompetent in patients with long-standing post-thrombotic deep vein damage.

valve transposition procedure and the valve transplant.

Valve transposition operations

The valves of the three major veins that meet below the inguinal ligament – the superficial and deep femoral veins and the long saphenous vein – are not usually afflicted with the same abnormality. In 1979 Kistner and Sparkuhl[14] suggested that when one of the main veins was incompetent it could be anastomosed to an adjacent vein that contained a competent valve, thus restoring its competence.

Two of the anastomoses which are possible and a phlebogram of a patient in whom one of these procedures might be suitable are shown in Fig. 8.14. The best operation is probably the anastomosis of the superficial femoral vein to a competent deep femoral vein. The saphenous vein is often unsuitable because it is incompetent in most forms of chronic venous insufficiency.

The anastomosis must be made with care using fine monofilament materials. A–V fistulae are not

Fig. 8.14 The valve transposition operation.

(a) An incompetent superficial femoral vein (SFV) anastomosed to the deep femoral vein (DFV) below a competent valve.

CFV = common femoral vein; LSV = long saphenous vein.

(b) A phlebogram showing a competent deep femoral vein (i) and an incompetent superficial femoral vein (ii). This patient could be treated with the operation shown in Fig. 8.14a.

usually employed but the patient should be given anticoagulants for 3–6 months.

Results Kistner has described the results of 14 valve transposition operations followed for 1–6 years (Fig. 8.15).[8] All these patients had reflux to the calf – 2 major, 12 massive. Phlebograms in 10 limbs performed during the first year after operation showed no reflux in 8 and reflux to the thigh and calf in 2. Three years later, further phlebograms on 7 of these 10 patients showed that 3 of the 4 that had been restored to normal were still normal, one that was normal had developed severe reflux, and two patients with reflux to the thigh and calf after operation had deteriorated over the follow-up period and developed severe calf reflux.

The long-term phlebographic results of the valve transpositions were therefore not as good as the valve repairs, though postoperative improvement was seen in 10 of the 11 patients on whom foot vein pressure studies had been carried out before and after operation (Fig. 8.16).

Once again the effect of the valve transposition on the clinical results is difficult to determine because nearly all the patients also had communicating vein ligations. The results suggest that the combination of communicating vein ligation with vein transposition operation produced better results than vein transposition alone.

Queral and his colleagues performed a study of valve transposition alone in 12 patients.[30] All the anastomoses remained patent, and when the patients were assessed 3 months after operation

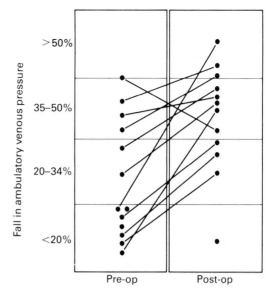

Fig. 8.16 The effect of valve transposition on the foot vein pressure during exercise. Ten of the 11 patients studied had improved calf pump function. (Redrawn from Ferris and Kistner.)[8]

the post-exercise foot vein pressure recovery time had returned to normal limits suggesting that the valves in the new circuit were patent. Twelve months later, however, the mean recovery time had become abnormal again, and 9 patients had developed recurrent ulcers.[12]

These results support the suggestion that correction of axial vein reflux alone will not provide good long-term relief of symptoms. Long-term competence may well depend upon the concomitant and complete correction of any communicating vein abnormality or the prevention of valve dilatation. The latter may be achieved by encircling the vein with a cuff of Dacron.[9]

Autogenous valve transplantation

During the past 20 years a number of surgeons have studied the feasibility of autogenous vein valve transplantation in the experimental animal. They concentrated upon the effect of transplantation on the integrity of the valve[31] and on ancillary methods for maintaining patency,[4,5,6,20,21,28] but they all showed that valve transplantation is a practical possibility.

The presence of irreparably damaged valves in

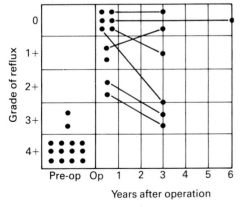

Fig. 8.15 The phlebographic results of valve transposition operations 3 years after operation. (Redrawn from Ferris and Kistner.)[8]

major veins below the groin stimulated Taheri to explore the possibility of transplanting a healthy valve from an arm vein to the leg.[37,38]

The method used by Taheri to assess incompetence was retrograde injection through a catheter introduced via an arm vein. Taheri stated that even when a competent valve was found in the common femoral vein the catheter could be passed through the valve cusps so that valves below this level could be assessed. Taheri therefore advocates valve transplants for patients with segmental valvular incompetence as well as complete axial vein valve incompetence when there is reflux to the knee and below (Grades 3 and 4), and when there has been no response to conservative treatment, providing the phlebographic abnormality is confirmed by foot vein pressure studies and atrophic changes in a calf muscle biopsy.[36]

Technique of valve transplantation

An incision is made on the medial aspect of the thigh centred on the adductor tubercle so that the upper part of the popliteal vein can be exposed. Division of the long head of adductor magnus greatly enhances this exposure. If the popliteal vein wall is healthy, the brachial vein is exposed through a 4 cm incision, beginning just below the axilla. The valves are tested with Harvey's manoeuvre, and 2 cm segment of vein with a healthy valve is removed.

The popliteal vein is divided, approximately 1 cm is excised and the transplant is sewn in, end to end, with fine (7/0) monofilament sutures. An A-V fistula is not fashioned.

Postoperatively, the legs are elevated and intermittent pneumatic compression is applied to the calf until the patient is walking well. Anticoagulants are given for 3–6 months.

Results Taheri has performed 67 transplants on 62 patients over a 4-year period. Sixty-four per cent (43 limbs) have been followed up by a postal or telephone enquiry and some were examined clinically.[36,39] Figure 8.17 shows pre- and postoperative phlebograms of one of these patients demonstrating the restoration of valvular competence.

The patients stated that 32 of the 43 limbs were improved, 10 were no better and one patient had died (Fig. 8.18).

Seventy-five per cent of the limbs examined had

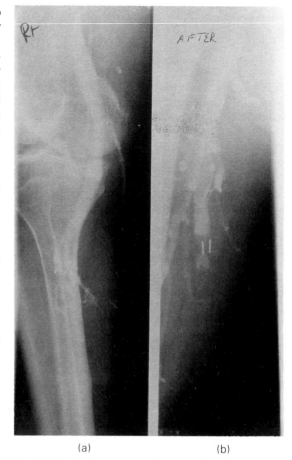

(a)   (b)

Fig. 8.17 Autogenous valve transplantation.
A pre-operative descending phlebogram (a) showing reflux to the calf, and a postoperative phlebogram showing a competent transplanted valve in the middle of the superficial femoral vein (b). The metal clips indicate the level of the upper anastomosis of the transplanted segment of brachial vein.
(Reproduced by kind permission of Dr Syde Taheri.)

a reduction of oedema and 17 of the 18 ulcers had healed.

Foot vein pressures were only measured before and after operation in 18 patients. The pressure during exercise had decreased in 14 patients by an average of 13 per cent, in 2 patients it was worse and in 2 it had not changed. The percentage changes are shown in Fig. 8.19.

Unfortunately, the small objective clinical, as opposed to postal, follow up and the lack of postoperative phlebograms make these results diffi-

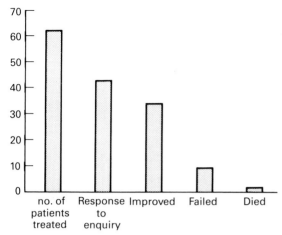

Fig. 8.18 The results of a postal and telephone survey of 67 valve transplants performed on 62 patients.

(Reproduced by kind permission of Dr Syde Taheri.)

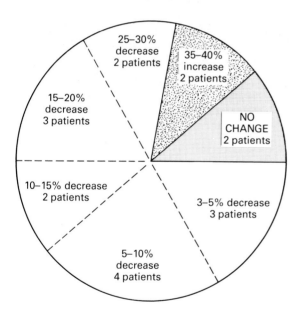

Average change = 13% decrease

Fig. 8.19 The changes in foot vein pressure during exercise 1 month to 4 years after valve transplantation in 18 patients. The average decrease in foot vein pressure was 13%.

(Reproduced by kind permission of Dr Syde Taheri.)

cult to interpret. The fall in foot vein pressure with exercise in patients with Grades 3 and 4 reflux might be expected to be approximately 15–25 mmHg. An improvement of 20 per cent would increase the pressure drop to 18–30 mmHg but still leave the patient with grossly abnormal foot vein pressure profiles. The changes in venous refilling rate have not been published. Figure 8.19 suggests that only 5 of the 18 patients had post-operative pressure profiles approaching the normal range.

Raju[33] has published the results of 22 valve transplants. He does not provide objective evidence of the effect of the operation on deep vein reflux but states that 'axillary vein valve transfers tend to fail with the passage of time'.

We conclude that the efficacy of valve transplantation is not yet proven but that carefully monitored clinical studies should continue.

O'Donnell (personal communication), who has performed nine valve transplants, has observed a discrepancy between the improvement of symptoms (which has been good) and the improvement of calf pump function tests (which has been poor). This raises the question – do tests of refilling truly measure deep vein reflux, and is this reflux the feature of disordered physiology that is responsible for the symptoms? Some of these questions will be answered by making careful physiological studies before and after valve transplant and vein transposition operations.

It would clearly be wrong to embark upon studies of preserved valve transplantation before the results of autogenous valve transplantation are known. If, however, the problem is valve ring dilatation, a preserved valve with a fine Dacron mesh covering might give better long-term results than an autogenous valve; the tanning will strengthen the tissues and prevent immunological reactions.[41]

Commentary

The veins would not have valves if they were unnecessary and yet it is difficult to define the clinical and physiological effect of pure axial vein valve incompetence. Provided the muscle of the calf pump and the valves in the veins within and adjacent to it are competent, it seems that the pump can cope with a considerable degree of reflux down the main outflow tract. In these circumstances the patient has no symptoms. We have seen legs with reflux from the groin to the ankle that have been absolutely normal, without swelling or aching.

Symptoms appear as soon as the pump begins to fail. This is commonly secondary to damage within the pump caused by the same thrombosis that caused the axial vein incompetence, but in the patients described by Kistner and Taheri (with no evidence of previous thrombosis) the pump failure is probably the result of chronic overloading. We suspect that the critical event is failure of the competence of the communicating veins.

The clinical problem is to decide whether to treat the axial vein and the communicating vein incompetence simultaneously, sequentially, or independently. Unfortunately, the available methods of investigation cannot quantify the communicating vein defect. If the relative contribution of the deep and communicating vein abnormalities to superficial venous hypertension during exercise could be measured, at least it would be possible to know which to treat first.

Developments in this field therefore await better quantitative forms of investigation and better methods of valve repair or replacement. Until that time it is wiser for the generalist to rely on the long established and understood procedure of communicating vein ligation and leave the specialist clinical researcher to attack the deep vein valve problem. The published efforts so far are promising but there is a lot to learn before the techniques and indications for deep vein valve surgery are clarified.

References

1. Ackroyd JS, Browse NL. Transplantation of gluteraldehyde preserved venous valves. Unpublished observations.
2. Ackroyd JS, Pattison M, Browse NL. A study of the mechanical properties of fresh and preserved human femoral vein wall and valve cusps. *Br J Surg* 1985; **72**: 117.
3. Ackroyd JS, Thomas ML, Browse NL. Deep vein reflux: an assessment by descending phlebography. *Br J Surg* 1986; **73**: 31.
4. Aschberg S, Hindmarsh T. Distal arteriovenous shunts in autotransplantation of canine venous valves. *Acta Chir Scand* 1971; **137**: 503.
5. Browse NL, Clemenson G. Vein surgery during defibrinogenation. *Br J Surg* 1978; **65**: 452.
6. Bush HL, Nobseth DC. Autogenous venous valve

7. Eriksson I, Almgren B, Norgren L. Late results of venous valve repair. *Int Angiol* 1985; **4**: 413.
8. Ferris EB, Kistner RL. Femoral vein reconstruction in the management of chronic venous insufficiency. *Arch Surg* 1982; **117**: 1571.
9. Hallberg D. A method for repairing incompetent valves in deep veins. *Acta Chir Scand* 1972; **138**: 143.
10. Herman RJ, Neiman JL, Yao JST, Egan TJ, Bergan JJ, Malave SR. Descending venography: a method of evaluating lower extremity venous valvular function. *Radiology* 1980; **137**: 63.
11. Huse JB, Nabseth DC, Bush HL, Widrich WC, Johnson WC. Direct venous surgery for venous valvular insufficiency of the lower extremity. *Arch Surg* 1983; **118**: 719.
12. Johnson ND, Queral LA, Flinn WR, Yao JST, Bergan JJ. Late objective assessment of venous valve surgery. *Arch Surg* 1981; **116**: 1461.
13. Jones JW, Elliot F, Kerstein MD. Triangular venous valvuloplasty. *Arch Surg* 1982; **117**: 1250.
14. Kistner RL, Sparkuhl MD. Surgery in acute and chronic venous disease. *Surgery* 1979; **85**: 31.
15. Kistner RL. Primary venous valve incompetence of the leg. *Am J Surg* 1980; **140**: 218.
16. Kistner RL. Surgical repair of the incompetent femoral vein valve. *Arch Surg* 1975; **110**: 1336.
17. Kistner RL. Transvenous repair of incompetent femoral vein valves. In Bergan JJ, Yao JST (Eds) *Venous Problems.* Chicago, Year Book Medical Publishers 1978.
18. Kistner R. Deep venous reconstruction (1968–1984). *Int Angiol* 1985; **4**: 429.
19. Kistner R. Surgical repair of a venous valve. *Straub Clin Proc* 1968; **34**: 41.
20. Kroener JM, Bernstein EF. Valve competence following experimental venous valve autotransplantation. *Arch Surg* 1981; **116**: 1467.
21. Kunlin J, Lengua F, Richard S, Tregonet T, Mourton A. Grafting of valvulated veins. *J Cardiovasc Surg* 1966; **7**: 520.
22. Lea Thomas M, Andress MR. Phlebographic changes in arteriomegaly. *Acta Radiol (Diagn) (Stockh)* 1970; **10**: 427.
23. Lea Thomas M, Keeling FP, Ackroyd JS. Descending phlebography: A comparison of three methods and an assessment of the normal range of deep vein reflux. *J Cardiovasc Surg* 1986; **27**: 27.
24. Lea Thomas M. *Phlebography of the Lower Limb.* Edinburgh. Churchill Livingstone 1982; 164.
25. Leu HJ. Familial congenital absence of valves in the deep leg veins. *Humangenetik* 1974; **22**: 347.
26. Lodin A, Lindvall N. Congenital absence of valves

transplantation in the dog. *J Surg Res* 1982; **32**: 313.

in the deep veins of the leg. *Acta Derm Venereol (Stockh)* 1961; **41**(Suppl 45): 1.

27. Lundstrom B, Osterman G. Assessment of deep venous insufficiency by descending phlebography. *Acta Radiol (Diag) (Stokh)* 1983; **24**: 375.

28. McLachlin AD, Carroll SE, Meads GE, Amacher AL. Valve replacement in the recanalized incompetent superficial femoral vein in dogs. *Ann Surg* 1965; **162**: 446.

29. Plate G, Brudin L, Eklof B, Jensen R, Ohlin P. Physiologic and therapeutic aspects in congenital vein valve aplasia of the lower limb. *Ann Surg* 1983; **198**: 229.

30. Queral LA, Whitehouse WM, Flinn WR, Neiman HL, Yao JST, Bergan JJ. Surgical correction of chronic deep venous insufficiency by valvular transposition. *Surgery* 1980; **87**: 688.

31. Raju S, Perry JT. The response of venous valvular endothelium to autotransplantation and *in vitro* preservation. *Surgery* 1983; **94**: 770.

32. Raju S. Valvuloplasty and valve transfer. *Int Angiol* 1985; **4**: 419.

33. Raju S. Venous insufficiency of the lower limb and stasis ulceration. *Ann Surg* 1983; **197**: 688.

34. Schanzer H, Pierce EC. A rational approach to surgery of the chronic venous stasis syndrome. *Ann Surg* 1982; **195**: 25.

35. Shumacker HB, Moore TC, Campbell JA. Functional venography of the lower extremities. *Surg Gynec Obstet* 1954; **98**: 257.

36. Taheri SA, Heffner R, Meenaghan MA, Budd T, Albini B, Elias SM, Pollack LH, Pendergast DR, Shores RM. Technique and results of venous valve transplantation. In Bergan JJ, Yao JST (Eds). *Surgery of the Veins*. Orlando, Grune & Stratton 1985.

37. Taheri SA, Lazar L, Elias SM, Marchand P. Vein valve transplant. *Surgery* 1982; **91**: 28.

38. Taheri SA, Lazar L, Elias S, Marchand P, Heffner R. Surgical treatment of post-phlebitic syndrome with vein valve transplant. *Am J Surg* 1982; **144**: 221.

39. Taheri SA, Lazar L, Elias S. Status of vein valve transplant after 12 months. *Arch Surg* 1982; **117**: 1313.

40. Thulesius O, Norgren L, Gjores JE. Foot volumetry a new method for objective assessment of edema and venous function. *Vasa* 1973; **2**: 329.

41. Waddell WG, Vogelfanger IJ, Prudhomme P, Ram JD, Beattie WG, Ewing JB. Venous valve transplantation. *Arch Surg* 1964; **88**: 227.

42. Whitehead S, Clemenson G, Browse NL. The assessment of calf pump function by isotope plethysmography. *Br J Surg* 1983; **70**: 675.

9

Primary (non-thrombotic) deep vein obstruction

Non-thrombotic occlusion of the deep axial veins of the lower limbs is uncommon. Minor degrees of compression by external structures, such as compression of the left common iliac vein by the right common iliac artery, are found in the majority of the population making it difficult to define what is normal and what is abnormal. The ultimate test of an obstruction must be the physiological demonstration of an increased resistance to blood flow, not the demonstration of an anatomical abnormality or even the presence of collateral vessels. It is function, not appearance, that matters. The symptoms and signs of obstruction caused by deep vein thrombosis are discussed in Chapter 17.

Pathology

Non-thrombotic deep vein obstruction may be caused by abnormalities outside, in the wall, or within the lumen of a vein.

External causes

Right common iliac artery compression of the left common iliac vein

The left common iliac vein is crossed by the right common iliac artery in the mid-line, in front of the body of the fifth lumbar vertebra, just before it unites with the right common iliac vein to form the vena cava (Fig. 9.1).

It is not surprising that this part of the vein is always flatter and wider than the vein upstream because it is compressed by the taut pulsating artery in front and the vertebral body behind. This compression is visible on a phlebogram as a segment with reduced opacification or an area of non-filling (Fig. 9.2a–e) and is a normal appear-

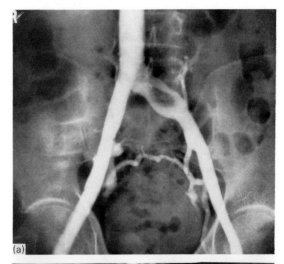

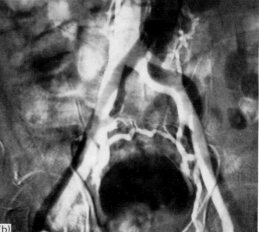

Fig. 9.1 A phlebogram (a) and superimposed arteriogram (b) showing the right common iliac artery crossing and compressing the termination of the left common iliac vein. A kink in the left common iliac artery is causing a filling defect in the left common iliac vein.

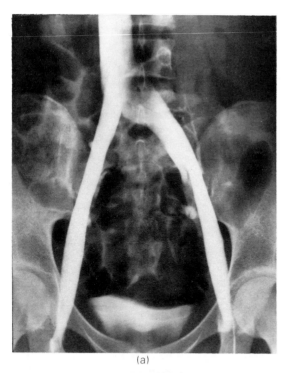

(a)

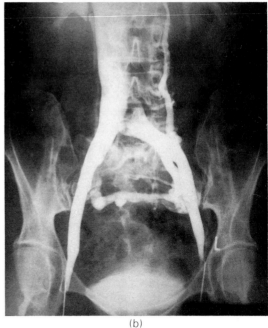

(b)

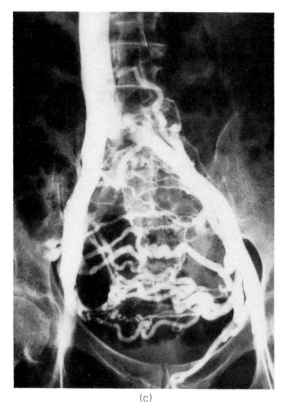

(c)

Fig. 9.2   Five examples of compression of the left common iliac vein by the right common iliac artery varying from minor compression to complete occlusion. None of these patients had any symptoms from his/her abnormality.

(a) A minor degree of arterial compression with no collateral vessels.

(b) Arterial compression occluding half the width of the iliac vein with dilated ascending lumbar and presacral veins.

(c) Arterial compression causing an almost complete band-like occlusion of the iliac vein with many dilated presacral veins.

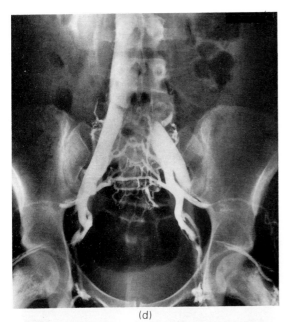

(d)

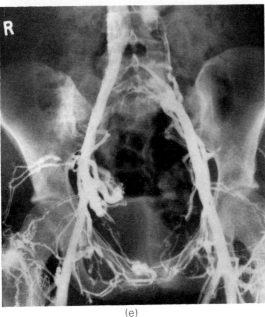

(e)

Fig. 9.2 (d) Arterial compression causing a wide and almost complete occlusion of the whole common iliac vein with a few small presacral collateral veins.

(e) Arterial compression causing a complete occlusion of the common iliac vein with remarkably few collateral veins.

ance. If the lumbar lordosis increases or the intra-abdominal pressure rises (e.g. in pregnancy), the venous compression increases. When this happens blood flow is obstructed and a normal anatomical variant becomes a pathological entity.[1,9,11,57] This is an uncommon event. The clinical significance of iliac vein compression lies in its predisposing effect on deep vein thrombosis.[57] Compression of the vein and any small effect it has on blood flow does not matter under normal circumstances but if the patient is ill or has an operation, events which are thrombogenic, a minor degree of compression may increase the chances of the patient developing a left iliofemoral thrombosis. Compression and webs in the left common iliac vein are thought to be the prime cause of the high incidence of left-sided deep vein thrombosis.

Malignant disease

Malignant disease around the iliac veins can compress and obstruct them. The tumours most likely to do this are carcinoma of the cervix, ovary, colon and rectum all of which may spread directly across the floor of the pelvis and encircle the vein. Secondary thrombosis in a vein constricted by tumour is common (see Fig. 10.3, page 293).

Malignant enlargement of the iliac lymph nodes can also compress or occlude the iliac veins. The secondary tumours which commonly spread to the iliac lymph glands are neoplasms of the uterus, cervix, rectum and the anal canal. Testicular tumours which have spread outside the tunica albuginea and tumours of the leg and scrotal skin (e.g. malignant melanoma and squamous cell carcinoma) also metastasize to the iliac lymph nodes.

Retroperitoneal fibrosis

This condition is mainly found in front of and lateral to the aorta and vena cava, but it can spread across the posterior wall of the true pelvis and involve the iliac veins before it affects the vena cava (see Fig. 10.4, page 294).

Internal iliac artery compression of the external iliac vein

The internal iliac artery crosses the termination of

the external iliac vein on both sides to run down into the pelvis with its companion vein.

It sometimes compresses the external iliac vein in a manner similar to that in which the right common iliac artery compresses the left common iliac vein (Fig. 9.2). This rarely causes symptoms but may increase the risk of an external iliac vein thrombosis.

Tortuous or dilated arteries in any site may cause compression of an adjacent vein.

Compression of the femoral vein (Gullmo's phenomenon)

Phlebograms of the femoral veins sometimes show an indentation on the medial side of the vein at the level of the inguinal ligament. There is much argument about the cause of this compression which can produce a total occlusion.

Gullmo[29] considers that it occurs when a weakness in the region of the femoral canal – a latent femoral hernia – allows the extraperitoneal fat to herniate downwards and laterally to compress the vein when the intra-abdominal pressure rises (Fig. 9.3). Nylander[59] believes that it is the combination of compression of the vein by abdominal pressure and retrograde flow, permitted by incompetent or absent common femoral vein valves, that allows the vein to empty. An indentation which is visible in the absence of a raised intra-abdominal pressure, is probably caused by direct compression by the lacunar part of the inguinal ligament. This appearance is often exacerbated by hyperextension of the hip joint (Fig. 9.4).

Gullmo's phenomenon and inguinal ligament compression are phlebographic abnormalities. They probably never cause symptoms and are therefore of some anatomical interest but are physiologically irrelevant.

Masses in the thigh

Large tumours or aneurysms in the thigh may compress the deep femoral vein and may stretch and compress the common and superficial femoral veins. The tumours are usually liposarcomata and fibrosarcomata, the aneurysms (true or false) in the common, superficial or deep femoral arteries.

The superficial femoral vein may also be com-

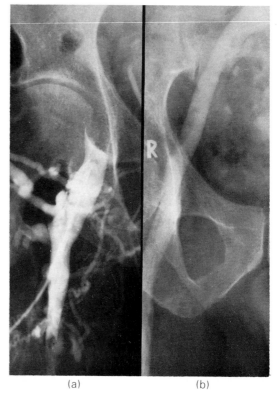

(a) (b)

Fig. 9.3 Gullmo's Phenomenon. (a) During a Valsalva manoeuvre the common femoral vein was completely occluded. (b) When the raised intra-abdominal pressure was released the vein opened out to a normal size.

pressed by the tendon forming the adductor canal (Fig. 9.5).

Popliteal masses

A popliteal aneurysm, a large Baker's cyst or distended bursae can compress the popliteal vein. They may not be discovered until the patient presents with a popliteal or calf vein thrombosis caused by the venous obstruction. An abnormal band of muscle may cause popliteal vein entrapment (see Chapter 23, page 623).

Vein wall abnormalities

Aplasia

Aplasia of the pelvic veins is uncommon. When it occurs it is often part of a congenital venous

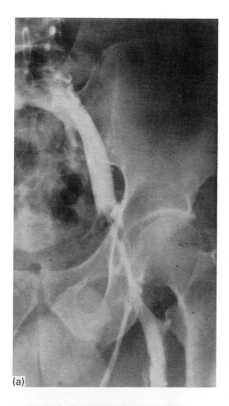

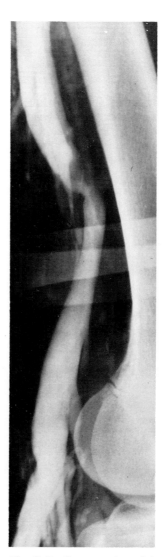

Fig. 9.5 Compression of the superficial femoral vein as it passes through the adductor canal.

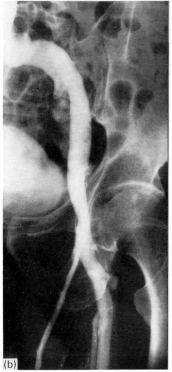

Fig. 9.4 Compression of the common femoral vein by the inguinal ligament (a), which disappeared when the hip joint was slightly flexed (b).

abnormality such as the Klippel–Trenaunay syndrome (see Chapter 23).

Tumours

Primary tumours of the vein wall are rare but are found more often in the lower limb than in the upper limb. They are usually leiomyosarcomata (see Chapter 26). Cystic degeneration producing a lesion which is similar to the common subcutaneous ganglion and the cystic mucoid degeneration of the popliteal artery has been reported as a rare cause of femoral vein obstruction (see Chapter 26).

Intraluminal causes

Spurs/webs

The most important intraluminal cause of venous obstruction is the venous web or septum. Webs (spurs) occur at the termination of the left common iliac vein in 20 per cent of the population at the point where the vein is compressed by the iliac artery.[48,53,63] May has described three varieties, the lateral spur, the central spur and the perforated septum (Fig. 9.6a).[48]

Histological studies have shown these spurs to consist of connective tissue and endothelium but they do not contain elastic tissue, muscle or haemosiderin. These observations suggest that they are not congenital remnants of the vein wall or the remnant of a thrombus. May believes they are caused by the combination of an inflammatory response and endothelial proliferation in response to repeated minor trauma of the two adjacent surfaces of the vein by the overlying compressing iliac artery.[48]

Only when obstruction of the veins is almost complete do these spurs cause symptoms, and then only when the collateral vessels are inadequate. Similar webs have been observed in the femoral vein.[68]

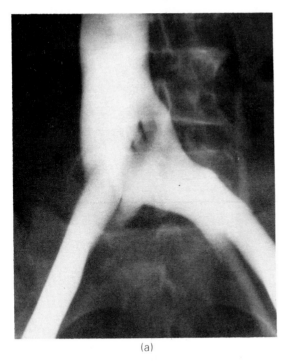
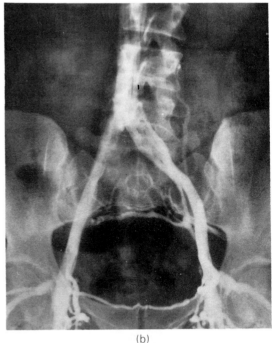

(a) (b)

Fig. 9.6 (a) Two left common iliac vein webs (central spurs). The two filling defects correspond to two bands of connective tissue connecting the anterior to the posterior wall of the iliac vein. Note that they lie within the area of vein compressed by the right common iliac artery but they are not post-thrombotic.

(b) Multiple synaeciae between the anterior and posterior wall of the left common iliac vein. These are the remnants of an iliac vein thrombosis.

There is also a similar synaecium in the inferior vena cava.

Post-thrombosis webs

Although this chapter is concerned with non-thrombotic abnormalities, this condition is mentioned here to remind the reader that post-thrombotic lesions are by far the most common cause of intraluminal obstruction in the deep veins of the lower limbs (Fig. 9.6b).

Clinical presentation

Many of the conditions described above are symptomless and only present when they precipitate a deep vein thrombosis. Their symptoms and treatment in such circumstances are described in Chapters 17 and 18.

The symptoms that occur when a non-thrombotic extraluminal or intraluminal abnormality causes an impediment to blood flow fall into two categories, those of the venous obstruction and those of the underlying abnormality.

Venous obstruction

Distended veins Collateral veins enlarge as the obstruction to blood flow increases. Common iliac vein obstruction is mainly bypassed by collateral veins in the pelvis and posterior abdominal wall, which cannot be seen, and by subcutaneous veins running across the lower abdominal wall just above the pubis and inguinal ligament which may become very large (Fig. 9.7).

If there is some obstruction of the inferior vena cava, the collateral vessels may extend across the abdominal wall towards the axilla. Proof that these veins are collaterals is obtained by confirming the retrograde flow of blood within them by Harvey's test (see Fig. 1.6, page 7)

Oedema Iliac vein obstruction usually causes swelling of the whole leg and sometimes causes swelling of the buttock and lower abdominal wall.

Obstruction of the superficial femoral vein below the termination of the deep femoral vein may cause swelling of the lower leg and ankle but may be symptomless.

Pain If there is only a minor obstruction to blood flow, the patient will complain of an aching pain in the leg that is made worse by standing and is relieved by rest and elevation.

Severe obstruction may cause venous claudication – a deep (muscle) pain within the leg which is induced by the rise in venous and interstitial pressures within the muscle compartments during exercise (see Chapter 12).[64]

Skin changes Prolonged severe obstruction will eventually damage the skin. This damage may be visible as pigmentation 'atrophie blanche', lipodermatosclerosis and ulceration (see Chapter 11). These symptoms are unusual if the obstruction has not been complicated by secondary thrombosis.

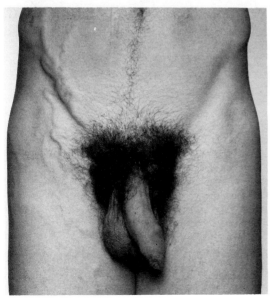

Fig. 9.7 Large tortuous subcutaneous veins crossing the groin carrying blood around an occluded iliac vein.

Evidence of the underlying pathology

Iliac compression and webs only cause the symptoms and signs described above. Patients with obstruction caused by disease outside the veins may have other local or distant evidence of their underlying disease. For example, debility, loss of weight, lower abdominal pain and vaginal bleeding would suggest the presence of pelvic malignancy. Testicular enlargement, palpable inguinal lymph nodes, and lesions on the skin of the leg would suggest the possible presence of iliac lymphadenopathy.

It is absolutely essential to conduct a complete clinical examination to exclude such abnormalities in a patient who presents with recent symptoms or signs of venous obstruction.

Secondary thrombosis

Patients with venous compression or obstruction may develop an acute thrombosis and present with acute pain in the iliac fossa and groin and rapid swelling of the leg. The leg may be white (phlegmasia alba) or blue (phlegmasia cerulea) depending upon the degree of venous obstruction. Although the initial clinical management should be directed towards treating the thrombosis, it is important to remember that there may be an underlying local abnormality, and this must be excluded by a careful clinical assessment. Local or distant malignant disease is the underlying cause of half of the cases of phlegmasia cerulea dolens.

Pulmonary embolism is not a common complication of thrombosis secondary to obstruction because the obstruction prevents the downstream propagation of the thrombus and the upstream thrombosis is 'locked in' by the obstruction.

Investigations

The initial investigations should define the state of the veins and the cause of the obstruction.

Phlebography

Phlebography is an essential, primary, investigation because it will confirm or refute the clinical diagnosis of a venous obstruction. All forms of phlebography may be required but bilateral ascending and percutaneous direct femoral vein phlebograms are sufficient in most patients.

Common iliac compression causes a variety of phlebographic appearances (Fig. 9.2): mildly reduced opacification, a lateral defect, or a full-width complete filling defect. Collateral vessels may be visible across the floor of the pelvis (Fig. 9.8) and the ascending lumbar and ovarian veins may be enlarged. The presence of large collateral veins must not be interpreted as indicating a major degree of obstruction; in fact the larger the collaterals the less the obstruction. Large collaterals indicate that there *has been* a significant obstruction not that it still exists. Obstruction can only be diagnosed by a physiological test (see page 280).

A series of films taken after a femoral vein injection of radio-opaque contrast medium will show the direction of blood flow in the collaterals.

Tumour compression causes irregular filling defects on the vein wall (Fig. 9.9a), usually the

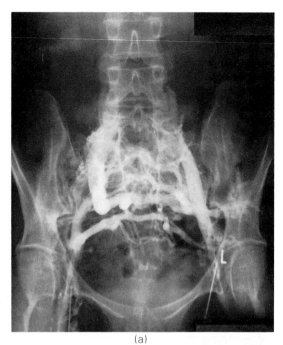

(a)

(b)

Fig. 9.8 The vessels that bypass an iliac vein occlusion.
(a) The presacral veins. (b) The vesical and rectal plexi and the subcutaneous pubic veins.

result of external compression but sometimes caused by mural thrombosis developing in response to tumour infiltrating the vein wall.

When enlarged lymph glands surrounding a vein are irradiated the subsequent fibrosis may

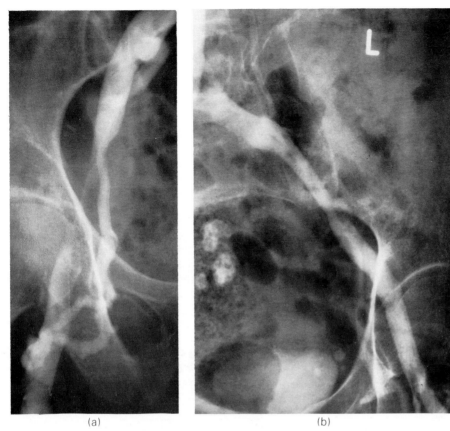

(a)   (b)

Fig. 9.9   (a) A phlebogram showing indentation and compression of the common femoral and external iliac veins by enlarged lymph glands.

(b) A phlebogram showing a long stenosis of the external iliac vein caused by fibrosis and contraction in a mass of iliac lymph glands treated with radiotherapy.

cause a long stricture (Fig. 9.9b).

Arterial impressions are common but can only be confirmed by the superimposition of an arteriogram on a phlebogram (see Fig. 9.1). Indentations of the common and external iliac veins by their accompanying arteries, are common especially as the arteries dilate and elongate with age.

Femoral vein compression is best seen if the patient performs a Valsalva manoeuvre during the phlebogram as this accentuates the size of the impression (see Fig. 9.3).

Primary vein wall tumours produce filling defects which are usually indistinguishable from defects caused by external compression (see Chapter 26).

General investigations

General investigations such as a chest radiograph and blood studies (haematological and biochemical), are important screening tests to exclude distant primary abnormalities.

Coagulation studies may be necessary.

Special techniques such as lymphography, ultrasound imaging and computerized tomography (CT) scanning may help to detect and define masses compressing the veins.

Physiological tests of venous obstruction

Quite major anatomical abnormalities may not obstruct blood flow when the limb is at rest, but will cause obstruction during exercise when the limb blood flow and consequently the deep vein blood flow increases ten- or twenty-fold. The non-invasive techniques for detecting venous outflow obstruction are extremely insensitive because they are usually performed with the leg at rest.

Phleborheography is usually normal in the presence of long standing femoral or popliteal occlusion.

Venous outflow strain-gauge plethysmography may help. It has been claimed[58] that a maximum venous outflow of less than 65 ml/100 ml/min is diagnostic of outflow obstruction and that a decrease in calf volume during exercise of less than 0.75 ml/100 ml indicates calf pump insufficiency secondary to outflow obstruction and communicating vein incompetence. In our own laboratory we find the measurements of maximum venous outflow are extremely variable and no help with diagnosis.

Isotope plethysmography which can measure the amount of blood expelled by both exercise and compression detects only severe obstruction (Fig. 9.10).

Comment We do not find any of the non-invasive tests helpful in the diagnosis of venous outflow obstruction. The few patients who do have grossly abnormal test results usually have venous claudication, a symptom which makes the tests almost superfluous.

Femoral vein pressure Measurement of this pressure before and during exercise will indicate the severity of an iliac vein obstruction.[56] The technique is simple. A fine needle or cannula is inserted into the femoral vein with the patient lying supine. The patient is then asked to forcibly plantarflex the foot against a resistance, once every second.

Under normal circumstances the femoral vein pressure will rise by only 1 or 2 mmHg. When there is an iliac obstruction it will increase by 5–10 mmHg. An increase of more than 5 mmHg is significant but the best test of significance is the comparison of the pressure rise in the abnormal limb with that in the normal limb (Fig. 9.11).

The ability of the clinician to diagnose superficial femoral vein obstruction would be improved if popliteal vein pressure could be measured during exercise. Perhaps the new ultrasound venous imaging techniques will enable us to measure and use changes in popliteal vein diameter as an indication of intraluminal pressure.

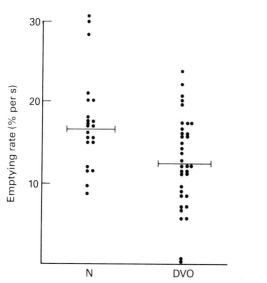

Fig. 9.10 The rate of emptying of the calf veins of 22 normal limbs (N) and 35 limbs with deep vein obstruction (DVO) in response to a single calf contraction, measured with isotope plethysmography. There is no significant difference between the mean rate of emptying of the two groups. Only two patients' calves did not empty at the normal rate. This type of test does not reveal even moderate outflow obstruction.

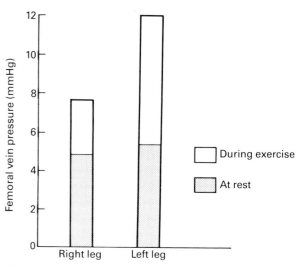

Fig. 9.11 The effect of leg exercise on the femoral vein pressures in a patient with a left iliac vein occlusion.

In the normal leg pressure rose by only 2.2 mmHg. In the abnormal leg the pressure rose by 6.7 mmHg indicating a physiologically significant obstruction. (Modified from May *et al.*)[46]

Treatment

Operations should only be considered when conservative treatment has failed.

Elastic compression

The symptoms of pain and swelling can usually be relieved by the external compression provided by elastic stockings. Below-knee stockings are usually sufficient, but full-length stockings can be used if there are many large veins in the thigh and the thigh is swollen. In most patients the swelling and discomfort are mainly in the calf and a below-knee stocking is adequate.

If the patient wears a stocking regularly the dilatation of the peripheral subcutaneous veins will slow down, and the development of skin changes and ulceration will be delayed.

If lipodermatosclerosis is present, its resolution may be accelerated by the use of drugs which stimulate interstitial fibrinolysis (see Chapter 12).

There are two surgical methods for relieving deep vein obstruction – a bypass operation or a local disobliteration.

Iliac vein bypass operations

Iliac occlusion or compression causing symptoms can be bypassed by the simple, extra-anatomic, extra-abdominal, femoro-femoral saphenous vein bypass operation, described by Palma in 1959 and 1960 (Fig. 9.12a and b).[61,62]

The Palma operation This operation is indicated when there are severe symptoms in the leg which are unrelieved by elastic compression.[13,15,16] The most important symptom is venous claudication. Operations for mild swelling and moderate aching are unlikely to be successful.

The Palma operation should only be considered when there is physiological evidence of venous obstruction during exercise as shown by an *an abnormal rise in femoral vein pressure during exercise* (Fig. 9.11).[46,51] Only under these circumstances can the surgeon be certain of an adequate perfusion pressure to maintain graft patency.

The femoral vein in the groin of the abnormal leg is explored through a vertical incision, and its tributaries are dissected until a healthy patent segment is found, usually in the deep femoral vein. The results are better if the femoral vein does not have post-thrombotic changes.

The long saphenous vein of the normal leg is

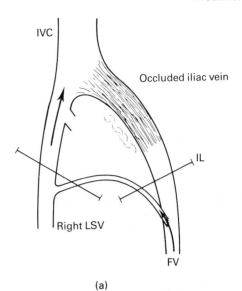

(a)

(b)

Fig. 9.12 The Palma operation

(a) A diagrammatic representation showing the right long saphenous vein (LSV) swung across the pubis and anastomosed to the left femoral vein (FV). (IL = inguinal ligaments.)

(b) The arterial and venous phases of a digital subtraction arteriogram of a patient with a Palma crossover saphenous vein graft and an arteriovenous fistula.

The white arrow indicates the site of the arteriovenous fistula. The lower black arrow indicates the saphenous vein crossover graft and the upper black arrow indicates the right spheno-femoral junction. The right iliac and femoral arteries are opacified because the injection was intra-arterial.

exposed through either a single or multiple incisions. After ligating its tributaries, the vein is divided between ligatures at a point well down the thigh where it will be long enough to stretch, still attached to the femoral vein, across the abdomen to the opposite groin.

A subcutaneous tunnel is made across the lower abdomen by blunt dissection or with a tunneler, above the crest of the pubis to the opposite groin, and the saphenous vein is threaded through it.

An end-to-side anastomosis is made between the saphenous vein and the healthiest segment of femoral vein that can be found, sometimes the common or superficial femoral vein but often the deep femoral vein.

Most surgeons fashion an arteriovenous fistula just below the anastomosis to help maintain patency, using a segment of the saphenous vein or one of its tributaries.[22,24,44]

The patient is given anticoagulants for 3–6 months. If a fistula is fashioned, it should be closed 3 months after operation. This can be a difficult operation, and it is facilitated by leaving a loose non-absorbable suture around the fistula to help to indentify it within the scar tissue.

Results   The results of this operation may be judged by clinical or phlebographic criteria; the clinical results are usually better than the phlebographic results for reasons that are not entirely clear. Clinical improvement in the presence of an occluded graft may be related to an increase in the number of collaterals, or the proper use of better quality elastic stockings, factors which may also be responsible for clinical improvement in patients with patent grafts.

The results of 50 operations performed by Halliday are shown in Fig. 9.13.[32] Unfortunately, pre-operative femoral vein pressure studies had not been carried out on any of these patients. None had arteriovenous fistulae. All had patency judged on clinical grounds (patency = relief of symptoms). Postoperative phlebograms were performed on only 34 patients.

It can be seen that at 5 years when 21 patients were available for assessment, 90 per cent had clinical relief, and 75 per cent had patent grafts. Beyond 5 years the number of patients available for study was too small for detailed analysis but there were clearly a considerable number of patients whose graft was patent 10 years after the operation.

The majority of Halliday's series of Palma

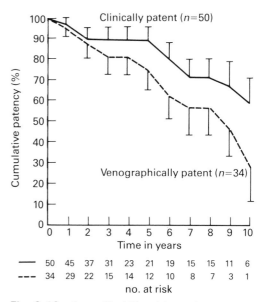

—	50	45	37	31	23	21	19	15	15	11	6
- - -	34	29	22	15	14	12	10	8	7	3	1

no. at risk

Fig. 9.13   A modified life table analysis of the cumulative patency of femoro-femoral vein crossover grafts as determined by clinical examination and phlebography.
(Modified from Halliday *et al.*)[32]

operations were for post-thrombotic occlusion and, consequently, some patients had post-thrombotic changes in the femoral vein at and below the site of the anastomosis. In Fig. 9.14 the results are sub-divided according to the state of the superficial femoral vein. At 5 years those patients with normal femoral veins had better patency rates but this was not the case with the 10 patients studied 6 years after operation.

Other surgeons have reported similar long-term patency rates of 75 per cent.[19,37] Few surgeons have measured femoral vein pressures *after* this operation[46]. It has been suggested that some bypasses thrombose and then recanalize so that the clinical benefit does not appear for 3–6 months.[18]

The development of better vascular prostheses has tempted some surgeons to use these artificial materials for femoro-femoral bypass when the long saphenous vein is inadequate. Only small numbers have been reported[17,72] but the results with prostheses made of PTFE (polytetrafluoroethylene) are encouraging, particularly if the prostheses are strengthened with external ring supports.[8] An arteriovenous fistula is probably

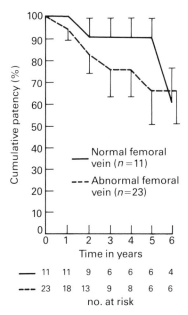

Fig. 9.14 A modified life table analysis of the cumulative phlebographic patency of 34 femoro-femoral vein crossover grafts subdivided according to the pre-operative state of the superficial femoral vein – normal (11), or post-thrombotic damage (23). (Modified from Halliday *et al.*)[32]

essential when using a prosthesis. External support of the anastomosis with rings[41,42] and anticoagulation by defibrinogenation[5,34,39,60] appear to be of value in maintaining the patency of venous anastomoses in experimental animals but there are no clinical studies to confirm the value of these techniques in man.

Other bypass operations Kunlin inserted a saphenous vein between the left external iliac vein and the right common iliac vein to bypass a terminal common iliac vein occlusion.[43] Hardin used the ipsilateral saphenous vein as a bypass between the femoral vein and the vena cava.[33]

These operations have not been widely practised because entering the abdomen adds a morbidity to the procedure which can be avoided by using the Palma operation which is entirely subcutaneous.

Now that better prostheses are available there are some reports of femoral-caval bypasses of iliac blocks using externally supported PTFE.[3,8,12]

Iliac vein disobliteration

A localized obstruction at the termination of the common iliac vein can be treated by a direct operation on this vein.[10]

The vein is best approached through an abdominal incision. The right common iliac artery is mobilized and the underlying common iliac vein is exposed. After the vena cava and both iliac veins have been controlled with soft clamps, the iliac vein can be opened and any spurs or membranes carefully excised. It is sometimes necessary to enlarge the vein with a patch of autogenous superficial vein, as a long-standing occlusion often narrows the vein.

This type of procedure is only applicable to short localized stenoses. The iliac artery should be freed so that it does not compress the site of the operation; if necessary it can be held to one side with a peritoneal sling.

Some authors have suggested placing a plastic bridge beneath the artery to protect the vein.[71] No long-term results of this procedure have been published. We have not used this technique because of the potential risk of arterial erosion and late aneurysm formation.

Iliac vein decompression

If the left common iliac vein is compressed between the fifth lumbar vertebra and the right common iliac artery, the compression can be relieved by dividing and elongating the artery or removing the bony prominence of the vertebra. Both these operations have been proposed by Dick[21] but no long-term results have been published.

Femoral vein bypass operations (Warren-May-Husni operation)[73,50,38]

Non-thrombotic obstruction of the superficial femoral vein is rare. Post-thrombotic obstruction is common, and most of the published series of femoral vein bypass operations have been for post-thrombotic problems.[36]

Popliteal to common femoral vein bypass using the *in situ* long saphenous vein was first described by Warren in 1954,[73] and a few surgeons have used it occasionally since the early 1970s (see Fig. 9.15).

This bypass is indicated when there is severe pain and swelling below the knee caused by a

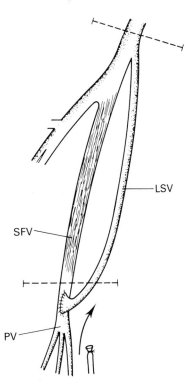

Fig. 9.15 A diagrammatic representation of the Warren popliteal-to-common femoral vein saphenous vein bypass operation.

The long saphenous vein (LSV) has been divided and anastomosed to a patent popliteal vein (PV) to bypass an occluded superficial femoral vein (SFV). The broken lines indicate the level of the hip and knee joints.

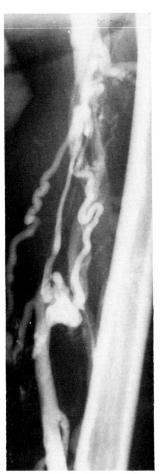

Fig. 9.16 This superficial femoral vein occlusion is suitable for a saphenous vein bypass operation because the popliteal vein is healthy. This patient's symptoms were, however, mild, and surgical interference was not justified.

superficial femoral vein occlusion without adequate collaterals. Although maximum venous outflow rates may be prolonged in this situation, there is no good test of femoral vein obstruction during calf exercise and so the indications for these operations are entirely clinical. The long saphenous vein must be patent, and the popliteal and common femoral veins must be healthy.

The most valuable investigations are phlebography (Fig. 9.16) and a foot vein pressure study confirming a severe degree of obstructive calf pump insufficiency.

The saphenous vein is exposed at the level of the knee, divided and anastomosed end-to-side to the popliteal vein. Provided its valves are competent, its tributaries do not have to be ligated. Gruss[26,28] adds an arteriovenous fistula, not just below the anastomosis, but well down the leg, just above the medial malleolus between the posterior tibial artery and saphenous vein. As the saphenous vein has been divided at the knee level, it is assumed that the additional arterial blood flowing through the fistula travels up the long saphenous vein, into the deep veins via the communicating veins, up the deep veins and then through the venous anastomosis into the bypass. Whether it actually does this is debatable.

Results Gruss[27] has described the results of 12 popliteal to femoral vein bypass operations, 4 without and 8 with arteriovenous fistulae. The late follow-up studies (6–10 years later) revealed that 3 bypasses had occluded, and 8 were patent but the calf pump function (assessed by foot vein pressure measurements) of 4 of the 8 that were patent had deteriorated. Two of the bypasses in the 4 patients whose calf pump function had improved had become dilated and varicose.

May[47] described the initial results in 16 patients and the late results of 7; 4 had improved, 3 had deteriorated. Husni has reported a 60 per cent late patency rate. Frileux[25] has described a series of 20 patients with similar results.

An alternative bypass has been suggested by Annous and Queral.[1] They anastomosed the lower end of a divided femoral vein, at the level of the adductor hiatus end-to-side to the saphenous vein. No long-term results are available.

Comment

It seems that only half of these bypasses remain patent and in a smaller proportion of patients there is worthwhile improvement in calf pump function. The results are not encouraging, and this operation should not be carried out unless it is part of a careful clinical research trial. It may be that functioning valves are required as well as a patent conduit. If the long saphenous vein is already acting as a collateral, there seems little point in dividing and anastomosing it to a deep vein. Perhaps the operation should be restricted to those patients in whom the application of a mid thigh superficial vein occluding tourniquet does *not* adversely affect calf pump function (i.e. those patients in whom the long saphenous vein is not already acting as a collateral vessel).

Other measures

When venous obstruction is caused by an external mass, it may be relieved by removing the mass or reducing its size.

Popliteal aneurysms can be bypassed or resected. Enlarged lymph nodes can be excised or reduced in size by radiotherapy, which may also be used to relieve the effect of infiltrating tumours.

Compression of the femoral vein by the inguinal ligament can be relieved by dividing the ligament.

It is important to relieve any functionally significant persistant compression of a major axial vein to reduce the risk of secondary thrombosis.

Experimental studies

The relatively few clinical reports of vein grafts and vein replacement belie the intense interest in this problem. Over the past 20 years there have been many laboratory studies which have aimed to produce a satisfactory method of replacing occluded veins. Autografts,[20,23,65,74] heterografts,[35] inverted small bowel and many types of prosthesis have been studied.[2,4,6,7,8,14,30,31,40,54,55,66,67,70] The results have been disappointing. The only consistent finding has been the increased patency rate conferred by the use of a temporary arteriovenous fistula.

Direct venous surgery remains in its infancy because of the unsolved technical problems and the small number of patients whose symptoms justify direct surgical interference.

References

1. Annous MO, Queral LA. Venous claudication successfully treated by distal superficial femoral-to-greater saphenous vein bypass. *J Vasc Surg 1 1985;* **2**: 870
2. Baird RJ, Lipton IH, Miyagishima RT. Replacement of the deep veins of the legs. *Arch Surg* 1964; **89**: 797.
3. Bernstein EF, Chan EL, Bardin JA. Externally supported grafts for inferior vena cava bypass. In: Bergan JJ, Yao JST (Eds) *Surgery of the Veins.* New York. Grune & Stratton 1985; 33.
4. Bower R, Fredericci V, Howard JM. Continuing studies of replacement of segments of the venous system. *Surgery* 1960; **47**: 132.
5. Browse NL, Clemenson G. Vein surgery during defibrinogenation. *Br J Surg* 1978; **65**: 452.
6. Bryant MF, Lazenby WD, Howard JM. Experimental replacement of short segments of vein. *Arch Surg* 1958; **76**: 289.
7. Ceriso M, McGraw JY, Luke JC. Autogenous vein graft replacement of thrombosed deep veins. Experimental approach to the treatment of the postphlebitic syndrome. *Surgery* 1964; **55**: 123.
8. Chan EL, Bardin JA, Bernstein EF. Inferior vena cava bypass, Experimental evaluation of externally supported grafts and initial clinical application. *J Vasc Surg* 1984; **1**: 675.
9. Chermet J. Left common iliac vein syndrome. *Anat Clin* 1979; **1**: 347.
10. Cockett FB, Thomas Lea M. The iliac compression syndrome. *Br J Surg* 1965; **52**: 816.
11. Cockett RB, Thomas ML, Negus D. Iliac vein compression, its relation to iliofemoral thrombosis and the post thrombotic syndrome. *Br Med J* 1967; **2**: 14.

12. Dale W A, Harris J, Terry R B. Polytetrafluor-ethylene reconstruction of inferior vena cava. *Surgery* 1984; **95**: 625.

13. Dale W A, Harris J. Crossover vein grafts for iliac and femoral venous occlusion. *J Cardiovasc Surg* 1969; **10**: 458.

14. Dale W A, Scott H W. Grafts of the venous system. *Surgery* 1963; **53**: 52.

15. Dale W A. Crossover grafts for iliofemoral venous occlusion. In: Bergan J J, Yao J S T (Eds) *Venous Problems*. Chicago & London. Year Book Medical Publisher 1978.

16. Dale W A. Crossover vein grafts for relief of ilio-femoral venous block. *Surgery* 1965; **57**: 608.

17. Dale W A. Synthetic grafts in venous reconstruc-tion. In Bergan J J, Yao J S T (Eds) *Surgery of the Veins*. New York. Grune & Stratton 1985; 233.

18. Dale W A. Thrombosis and recanalization of veins used as venous grafts. *Angiology* 1961; **12**: 603.

19. Dale W A. Venous bypass surgery. *Surg Clin North Am* 1982; **62**: 391.

20. De Weese J A, Nignidulie R. The replacement of short segments of veins with functional autogenous venous grafts. *Surg Gynec Obstet* 1960; **110**: 303.

21. Dick W. Klinik und therapie der venensperre am confluens der beiden gemeinsamen iliacalvenen. *Langenbecks Arch Chir* 1962; **301**: 573.

22. Dumanian A V, Santschi D R, Park K, Walker A P, Frahm C J. Cross-over saphenous vein graft combined with a temporary femoral arterio-venous fistula. A case report. *Vasc Surg* 1968; **2**: 116.

23. Eadie D G, de Takats G. The fate of autogenous grafts in the canine femoral vein. *J Cardiovasc Surg* 1966; **7**: 148.

24. Ecklof B, Albrechtson V, Einarsson E, Plate G. The temporary arteriovenous fistula in venous reconstructive surgery. *Int Angiol* 1985; **4**: 455.

25. Frileux C, Pillot-Bienayme P, Gillot C. Bypass of segmental obliterations of ilio-femoral venous axis by transposition of saphenous vein. *J Cardiovasc Surg* 1972; **13**: 409.

26. Gruss J D, Vargas-Mantano H, Bartels D, Hanschke D, Fietze-Fischer B. Direct recons-tructive venous surgery. *Int Angiol* 1985; **4**: 441.

27. Gruss J D. The saphenopopliteal bypass for chronic venous insufficiency (May-Husni Operation). In: Bergan J J, Yao J S T (Eds) *Sur-gery of the Veins*. New York. Grune and Stratton 1985; 255.

28. Gruss J D. Zur Modifikation des Femoral bypass nach May. *Vasa* 1975; **4**: 59.

29. Gullmo A. The strain obstruction syndrome of the femoral vein. *Acta Radiol Scand* 1957; **47**: 119.

30. Haimovici H, Hoffert P W, Zinicola N, Steinman C. An experimental and clinical evaluation of the grafts in the venous system. *Surg Gynec Obstet* 1970; **131**: 1173.

31. Haimovici H, Zinicola N, Noorani M, Hoffert P W. Vein grafts in the venous system. *Arch Surg* 1963; **87**: 542.

32. Halliday P, Harris J, May J. Femoro-femoral crossover grafts (Palma Operation). A long term follow up study. In Bergan J J, Yao J S T (Eds) *Surgery of the Veins*. New York. Grune Stratton 1985; 241.

33. Hardin C. Bypass saphenous grafts for the relief of venous obstruction of the extremity. *Surg Gynec Obstet* 1962; **115**: 709.

34. Hobson R W, Croom R D. Influence of heparin and low molecular weight dextran on the patency of autogenous vein grafts in the venous system. *Ann Surg* 1973; **178**: 773.

35. Horsch S, Pichlmaier H, Walter P, Landes T H. Replacement of the inferior vena cava and iliac veins with heterologous grafts in animal tests. *Surgery* 1978; **84**: 644.

36. Husni E A. Clinical experience with femoro-popliteal venous reconstruction. In Bergan J J, Yao J S T (Eds) *Venous Problems*. Chicago. Year Book Medical Publishers 1978, 485.

37. Husni E A. Reconstruction of veins, the need for objectivity. *J Cardiovasc Surg* 1983; **24**: 525.

38. Husni E A. *In situ* saphenopopliteal bypass graft for incompetence of the femoral and popliteal veins.*Surg Gynec Obstet* 1970; **130**: 279.

39. Ishimaru S, Fujiwara Y, Domeki D, Horiguchi Y, Furukawa K, Takahashi M. Defibrinogenation therapy in venous reconstructive surgery with PTFE Graft. *J Japanese Coll Angiol* 1977; **17**: 515.

40. Katy N M, Spence I J, Wallace R B. Reconstruction of the inferior vena cava with a PTFE tube graft after resection for hypernephroma of the right kidney. *J Thorac Cardiovasc Surg* 1984; **87**: 791.

41. Kunlin J, Benitte A M, Richard S. La suspension de la suture veineuse. Etude experimentale. *Bull Soc Int Chir* 1960; **19**: 336.

42. Kunlin J, Kunlin A, Richard S, Tregovet T. Le remplacement et l'anastomose latéro-latérale des veines par greffon avec suture suspendue à anneau. *J Chir (Paris)* 1963; **85**: 305.

43. Kunlin J. Le rétablissement de la circulation veineuse par greffe en cas d'obliteration trau-matique ou thrombophlétique. Greffe de 18 cm entre la veine saphène interne et la veine iliaque externe. Thrombose après trois semaines de perméabilité. *Mem Acad Chir* 1953; **79**: 109.

44. Levin P M, Rich N M, Hutton J E Jr, Barker W F, Zeller J A. Role of arteriovenous shunts in venous reconstruction. *Am J Surg* 1971;**122**: 183.

45. Matsumoto T, Homes R H, Burdick C O, Herster-

kamp CA, O'Connell TJ. The fate of the inverted segment of small bowel used for the replacement of major veins. *Surgery* 1966; **60**: 739.

46. May R, DeWeese JA. Surgery of the Pelvic Veins. In May R (Ed) *Surgery of the Veins of the Leg and Pelvis*. Stuttgart. Georg Thieme 1974; 171.

47. May R, Nissl R. The post-thrombotic syndrome. In May R (Ed) *Surgery of the Veins of the Leg and Pelvis*. Stuttgart. Georg Thieme 1974; 153.

48. May R, Thurner J. Ein gefasseporn in der V. iliaca comm. sin. als wahrscheinliche Ursache der uberwiegend linksseifigen Beckenvenenthrombose. *Z Kreislaufforsch* 1956; **45**: 912.

49. May R, Thurner J. The cause of the predominantly sinistral occurence of thrombosis of the pelvic vein. *Angiology* 1957; **8**: 419.

50. May R. Femoralis bypass beim posthrombotischen Zustandsbild. *Vasa* 1972; **1**: 267.

51. May R. The femoral bypass. *Int Angiol 1985;* **4**: 435.

52. May R. Veins of the pelvis. In May R (Ed) Surgery of the veins of the leg and pelvis. Stuttgart. Georg Thieme 1974; 25.

53. McMurrich JP. The occurrence of congenital adhesions in the common iliac veins and their relation to the thrombosis of the femoral and iliac veins. *Am J Med Sci* 1908; **135**: 342.

54. Mitsuoka H, Howard JM. Experimental grafting of the vena cava. *J Cardiovasc Surg* 1968; **9**: 190.

55. Moore TC, Young NK. Experimental replacement and bypass of large veins. *Bull Soc Int Chir* 1964; **23**: 274.

56. Negus D, Cockett FB. Femoral vein pressures in postphlebitic iliac vein obstruction. *Br J Surg* 1967; **54**: 522.

57. Negus D, Fletcher EWL, Cockett FB, Lea Thomas M. Compression and band formation at the mouth of the left common iliac vein. *Br J Surg* 1968; **55**: 369.

58. Nicolaides AN, Fernandes JF, Schull K, Miles C. Calf volume plethysmography. In Nicolaides AN, Yao JST (Eds) *Investigation of Vascular Disorders*. New York. Churchill Livingstone 1981; 495.

59. Nylander G. Haemodynamics of the pelvic veins in incompetence of the femoral vein. *Acta Radiol (Stockh)* 1961; **56**: 369.

60. Olsson P, Ljungqvist A, Goransson L. Vein graft surgery in Defibrase defibrinogenated dogs. *Thromb Res*1973; **3**: 161.

61. Palma EC, Esperon R. Tratamiento del sindrome posttrombo-flebitico mediante transplante de safena interna. *Angiologica* 1959; **11**: 87.

62. Palma EC, Esperon R. Vein transplants and grafts in the surgical treatment of the post-phlebitic syndrome. *J Cardiovasc Surg* 1960; **1**: 94.

63. Pinsolle J, Videau J. Anomalies du carrefour ilio-cave. *Chirugie* 1982; **108**: 451.

64. Qvarfordt P, Eklof B, Ohlin P, Plate G, Saltin B. Intramuscular pressure blood flow and skeletal muscle metabolism in patients with venous claudication. *Surgery* 1984; **95**: 191.

65. Scobie AH, Scobie TK, Vogelfeueger LJ. Venous autografts. *Can J Surg* 1962; **5**: 471.

66. Silver D, Anlyan WG. Peripheral vein grafts in dogs. *Surg Forum* 1961; **12**: 259.

67. Sitzmann JV, Imbembo AI, Ricotta JJ, McManama GP, Hutchins GM. Dimethylsulfoxide treated cryopreserved venous allografts in the arterial and venous system. *Surgery* 1984; **95**: 154.

68. Stirling GA, Tsapogas MJ. Extrapulmonary vascular bands and webs. *Ann Surg* 1969; **169**: 308.

69. Sztankasy G, Szabo Z. Ilio-caval dysplasia. Studies on the pathogenesis of venous diseases in the lower extremities. *J Cardiovasc Surg* 1969; **10**: 16.

70. Takaro T, Smith DE, Peasley ED, Kim JS. Experimental vena caval anastomoses and grafts. *Surg Gynec Obstet* 1962; **115**: 49.

71. Trimble C, Bernstein EF, Pomerantz M. A prosthetic bridge device to relieve iliac venous compression. *Surg Forum* 1972; **23**: 249.

72. Vollmar J. Reconstruction of the iliac vein and inferior vena cava. In Hobbs JT (Ed) The Treatment of Venous Disorders. Philadelphia. Lippincott 1977; 308.

73. Warren R, Thayer T. Transplantation of the saphenous vein for postphlebitic stasis. *Surgery* 1954; **35**: 867.

74. Zinicola N, Hoffert PW, Haimovici H. Autogenous vein bypass grafts in the venous system. *Bull Soc Int Chir* 1962; **21**: 265.

10

Acquired obstruction of the inferior vena cava (IVC)

Most of the congenital variations of the inferior vena cava (IVC) do not cause symptoms because they either provide additional pathways for blood flow, as in the double vena cava, or are well compensated by collateral vessels because the abnormality has been present since fetal life. Aplasia and other congenital abnormalities of the IVC are discussed in Chapter 23.

Acquired obstruction of the vena cava is a distinct clinical entity commonly caused by spontaneous thrombosis in a normal vessel, thrombosis secondary to external compression or thrombosis upon pathological changes in the vein wall.

Pathology

The causes of obstruction of the vena cava are as follows.

Thrombosis

Spontaneous thrombosis

Spontaneous thrombosis usually follows a *surgical operation* or major systemic trauma, and is commonly an extension of an ilio-femoral vein thrombosis into the vena cava but may occur in isolation or in association with deep vein thrombosis elsewhere in the lower limbs.

Thombosis secondary to local trauma

Direct trauma, caused by blunt and penetrating injuries, iatrogenic injuries inflicted during arterial operations, and indirect trauma such as tears and bruising from spinal fractures are the injuries that commonly cause secondary thrombosis.

Thrombosis secondary to malignant tumour invasion

(i) Primary and secondary malignant disease in the lymph nodes, and carcinoma of the pancreas, stomach and pelvic organs may infiltrate into the wall of the vena cava and, by damaging the endothelium, initiate thrombosis.

(ii) Renal carcinoma can spread via the lumen of the renal vein into the vena cava where it may cause an occluding thrombosis, or spread along the lumen without blocking it and give rise to tumour emboli.

Thrombosis secondary to external compression (see below)

Iatrogenic

Caval ligation or partitioning with stitches, clips, or filters (all procedures performed to prevent pulmonary embolism) may cause a partial or total obstruction or initiate an occlusive thrombosis.

External compression

External compression may in itself occlude the vena cava but it commonly causes a secondary thrombosis once the compression significantly reduces the rate of blood flow. The common causes of external compression are given below.

Lymph glands

The pre-aortic and para-aortic lymph nodes are often enlarged by lymphomatous change and secondary carcinoma.

Retroperitoneal fibrosis

This begins as a plaque of fibrous tissue across the front of the vena cava and aorta and may totally occlude it as the fibrosis thickens and contracts.

Aortic aneurysms

These commonly stretch and partly compress the IVC but rarely cause a complete occlusion or a thrombosis. Rupture of an aneurysm into the IVC to produce an aorto-caval fistula raises the pressure in the distal IVC and causes symptoms similar to those caused by an IVC block. The increased venous return causes congestive cardiac failure. Inflammatory aneurysms with retroperitoneal fibrosis may occlude the vena cava.

Large abdominal malignant tumours

Tumours such as carcinoma of the kidney and tumours of the ovary may compress the IVC.

Ascites

This may become so tense that it compresses the IVC, obstructs venous return and causes oedema of the legs.

Clinical presentation

The symptoms of occlusion of the vena cava which were first described in 1644[17] may appear suddenly or slowly.[12,14,21] A rapid onset is almost always caused by an acute thrombosis. The gradual development of symptoms may be caused by a slowly increasing compression that causes symptoms as it develops or the slow decompensation of collateral vessels and the slow development of peripheral valve incompetence.

Acute thrombosis

The symptoms of an acute IVC thrombosis may appear spontaneously or following a recent unrelated operation or injury. They may also follow a chronic debilitating illness or as an addition to the symptoms of a chronic IVC obstruction.

The patient often complains of low back or buttock pain which is frequently misdiagnosed as lumbago and treated by putting the patient to bed – an action which exacerbates the thrombotic process. If a renal vein becomes involved, the patient will develop loin pain and haematuria. Abdominal pain is uncommon and the abdomen is rarely tender.

The legs become oedematous within 6–12 hours of the IVC becoming totally blocked. The whole of both limbs, buttocks and sometimes the lower abdominal wall become oedematous. The swelling is soft and pits but is not tender.

The abdomen may become swollen with ascitic fluid or may already be swollen before the onset of the leg swelling, if the caval obstruction is caused by an intra-abdominal abnormality.

The skin of the legs may develop a bluish tinge. If there is extensive thrombosis in the pelvic and femoral veins as well as in the IVC, the skin may turn a deep blue (phlegmasia cerulea dolens) and develop areas of skin blistering and gangrene.

Renal vein thrombosis will cause haematuria, oliguria or anuria and the symptoms of uraemia.[12]

The patient may complain of chest pain and breathlessness if there is an associated pulmonary embolus.

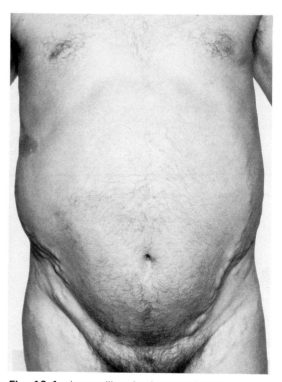

Fig. 10.1 Large dilated veins crossing the anterolateral aspect of the abdominal wall in a patient with occlusion of the inferior vena cava.

There may be other physical signs indicating the cause of the thrombosis, such as a large abdominal mass.

Dilated veins appear on the abdominal wall between the groins and the axillae within days of the thrombosis (Fig. 10.1).

Chronic occlusion (plus thrombosis)

The symptoms and signs of a slowly progressive occlusion are similiar to those of an acute thrombosis but their time course is different.[10]

There may be a history of a serious illness, accident or operation years before, often in the teenage years, which produced no symptoms or minimal leg swelling which regressed rapidly and spontaneously. Some patients will give a history of symptoms relevant to the cause of the IVC compression whilst others will complain of no symptoms other than those caused by the venous obstruction.

A few patients have no symptoms, the IVC occlusion being discovered during a routine examination when collateral veins are found on the abdominal wall.

The principal symptoms of a chronic IVC occlusion are swelling and dull aching pains in the legs and the appearance of varicose veins on the abdomen and the legs. The swelling often becomes gross and may extend into the buttocks and lower abdominal wall.

The large varicosities on the abdominal wall follow the course of the superficial inferior epigastric and superficial external iliac veins (Fig. 10.1). Normally, blood flows down these veins to the sapheno-femoral junction. Compression and stroking the veins (Harvey's test) will reveal that the blood flow is upwards towards the tributaries of the superior vena cava.

The longer the history of leg swelling and varicose veins, the more likely is there to be skin pigmentation, eczema, lipodermatosclerosis and ulceration. If these changes develop, they are invariably extensive often affecting the whole of the lower legs, not just the gaiter areas, with multiple areas of ulceration.

The patient may complain of bursting pain on exercise which is relieved by rest and elevation (venous claudication) and notice that the leg swelling increases with exercise.

General examination may reveal evidence of the cause of the IVC obstruction such as an abdominal mass or generalized lymph node enlargement.[6] Albuminuria in patients with chronic renal vein occlusion is rare.[10]

Investigations

Two questions need to be answered. Is the IVC obstructed? What is the cause of the obstruction?

The state of the IVC is best determined by cavography which was first performed by Dos Santos in 1938.[4]

IVC phlebography[5,7,11,13,20]

Bilateral simultaneous foot injections of a radio-opaque contrast medium, combined with the application of thigh tourniquets during the injection which are suddenly released to allow a bolus of contrast to enter the pelvic veins, usually gives good quality images of the IVC, but they are not as good as those obtained with bilateral femoral vein injections.

Thrombotic IVC occlusion is often associated with iliac and femoral vein thrombosis; it is therefore worthwhile performing bilateral ascending phlebograms first to determine both the state of the veins in the legs and the patency of the femoral veins. A recanalized or fully patent femoral vein can then be punctured for a femoral injection using the ascending phlebogram to identify the position of the patent vein at the groin. Twenty millilitres of contrast medium should be injected into both veins by hand.

On the rare occasion when both femoral veins are occluded, the IVC can be opacified with bilateral intratrochanteric injections,[18] or with a retrograde injection from a catheter passed down into the IVC from an arm vein, or by digital subtraction enhancement of the venous phase of a lumbar aortogram.

The typical appearances of IVC obstruction and the common collaterals (the inferior epigastric, deep external iliac, ascending lumbar and azygos veins) are shown in Fig. 10.2.

If the IVC is not completely blocked, phlebography may reveal external compression by enlarged lymph glands (Fig. 10.3 a and b), retroperitoneal fibrosis (Fig. 10.4), a caval clip (Fig. 10.5) or the intraluminal spread of a tumour (Fig. 10.6). A chest radiograph may reveal an enlarged azygos vein (Fig. 10.7).

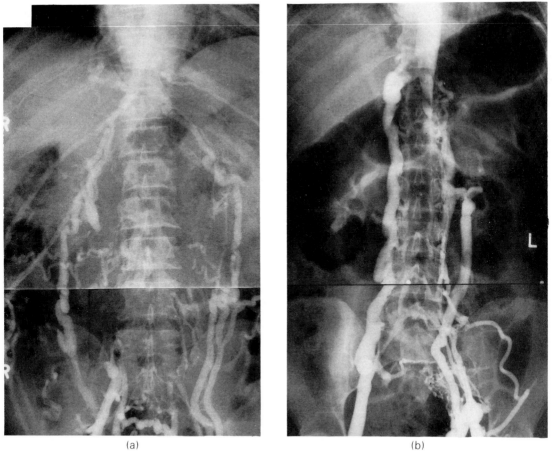

(a)   (b)

Fig. 10.2   The phlebographic appearances of inferior vena cava obstruction.

(a) Total occlusion of the inferior vena cava from its origin to the entry of the renal veins. This phlebogram shows large inferior epigastric, deep circumflex iliac and ascending lumbar veins draining into the lower intercostal and azygos veins just below the diaphragm. This is the pre-operative phlebogram of the patient illustrated in Fig. 10.9.

(b) The phlebogram of a patient with a total occlusion of the inferior vena cava. The two collateral vessels are a large azygos vein on the patient's right and a large ascending lumbar vein on the left.

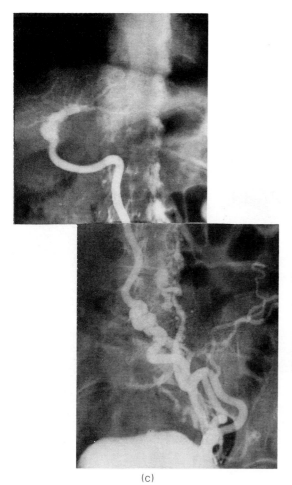

(c)

Fig. 10.2 (c) A montage of the phlebograms of a patient with a total occlusion of the inferior vena cava showing collateral vessels carrying blood from the internal iliac veins into the perirectal venous plexus and from there into the inferior mesenteric vein and the portal vein.[11]

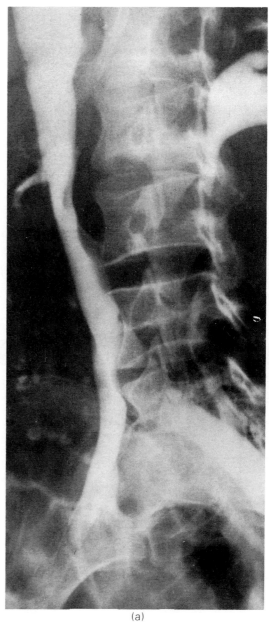

(a)

Fig. 10.3 (a) Compression of the inferior vena cava by a large mass of lymphomatous pre-aortic lymph nodes.

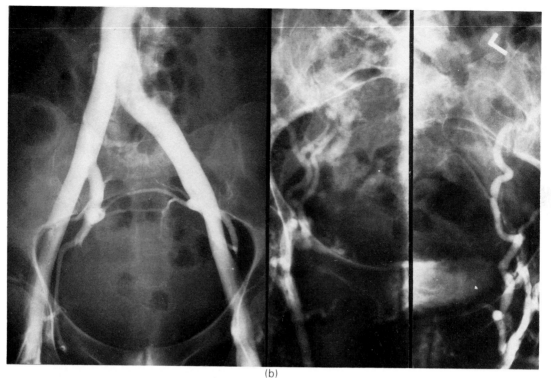

(b)

Fig. 10.3 (b) Two phlebograms taken 2 months apart. The left-hand panel shows an irregular filling defect at the termination of the left common iliac vein and the beginning of the vena cava. This is too lateral and too irregular to be confused with a physiological iliac vein compression. CT scanning confirmed a mass of enlarged lymph nodes in this region. Two months later the patient developed oedema of both legs. A new phlebogram (right-hand panel) showed total occlusion of the vena cava and iliac veins.

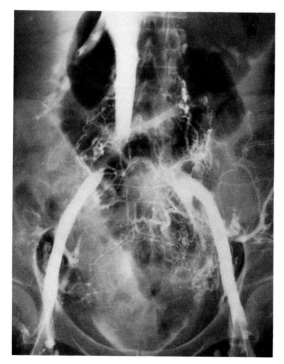

Fig. 10.4 A phlebogram showing stenoses of the iliac vein and the first part of the inferior vena cava caused by retroperitoneal fibrosis.

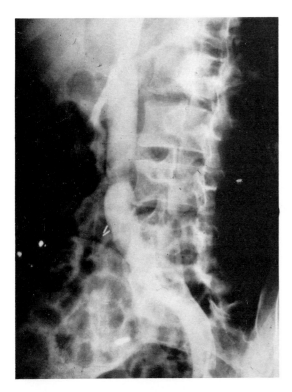

Fig. 10.5   A linear partial transverse filling defect caused by a Miles clip (see Chapter 21, page 586).

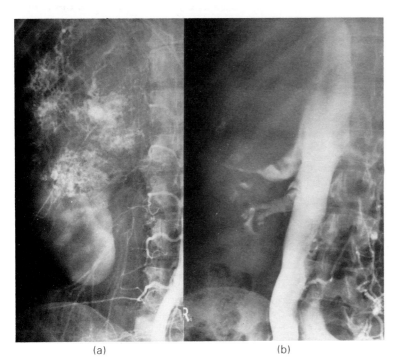

(a)   (b)

Fig. 10.6   A carcinoma of the kidney spreading into the inferior vena cava via the renal vein. (a) An arteriogram showing a large vascular carcinoma of the kidney. (b) A cavagram of the same patient, during a Valsalva manoeuvre, showing tumour in the right renal vein spreading into the vena cava.

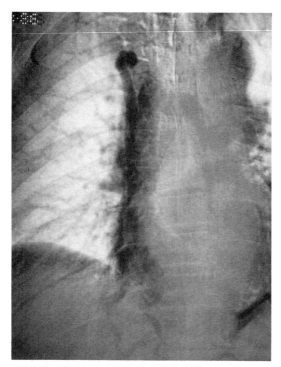

Fig. 10.7 A subtraction film showing a dilated azygos vein carrying blood past an occluded inferior vena cava. The distortion of the mediastinal shadow at the point where the azygos' vein turns forwards to join the superior vena cava may be the first indication that a patient has a vena cava occlusion. Ligation of an azygos vein such as this which is carrying the whole of the visceral and lower limb venous return can cause renal vein thrombosis and death (see Chapter 23, page 609).

The cause of an IVC obstruction can usually be determined by the combination of clinical examination, phlebography and other radiological investigations.

Unless there is a definite history of a previous venous thrombosis, it is wise to exclude all other reasons for a thrombosis before accepting that it is spontaneous.

Physical examination may reveal an abdominal mass, generalized lymphadenopathy or signs of a distant neoplasm.

Blood investigations

These are rarely helpful. A raised erythrocyte sedimentation rate should raise the suspicion of a generalized disease or retroperitoneal fibrosis.

Coagulation factors are usually normal in patients with venous thrombosis, though the rare condition of anti-thrombin III deficiency must not be forgotten. The haemoglobin concentration and white cell count should be measured as they will be abnormal in patients with generalized debilitating disease, infections and retroperitoneal fibrosis. Biochemical tests of renal function may suggest the presence of ureteric obstruction by retroperitoneal fibrosis or renal vein thrombosis.

The CT scan is the most useful investigation for detecting retroperitoneal abdominal masses as it reveals both the lumen of the great abdominal vessels and the anatomy of any masses compressing them.[15] Ultrasound will detect masses but does not give as much information about the vessels as a CT scan.

Retroperitoneal fibrosis is not always visible on a CT scan and may only be diagnosed when an intravenous excretory urogram shows the ureters to be drawn medially and perhaps partially obstructed.

A surgical biopsy of an enlarged peripheral lymph node may be required to define the histology of lymph node disease.

Bipedal lymphangiography is occasionally helpful in defining the extent of an abdominal lymph node mass but has been largely superceded by CT scanning.

Arteriography is rarely required.

The decision to investigate the cause of an IVC occlusion depends upon the degree of suspicion raised by the history and clinical findings that an extravascular abnormality might exist.

Treatment

The treatment of an acute thrombosis of the IVC is similiar to the treatment of any other type of venous thrombosis, fully discussed in Chapter 18. Removal of the thrombus, if possible, and by whatever means, will not, however, result in long lasting patency if the cause of the thrombosis (e.g. external compression) is not corrected.

It is, therefore, essential to decide before beginning treatment whether the thrombosis is spontaneous (idiopathic) or secondary to compression. The investigations required may take some time to carry out and so the immediate treatment, the administration of heparin to prevent further thrombosis, must be based upon a clinical diagnosis. A loading dose of 10,000 units of heparin intravenously should be followed by 40,000 units/24 hours, with the dose controlled and monitored by a laboratory test (the clotting time or the activated partial thromboplastin time) until a definite diagnosis is made and plan of treatment formulated.

Acute 'idiopathic' thrombosis

If no abnormality is detected other than the caval thrombosis, the clinician has three choices – prevent further thrombosis by giving heparin, remove the thrombus surgically or pharmacologically, or confine the thrombus to the vena cava to prevent embolism. The second and third approaches should be considered when the thrombus is fresh and non-adherent or only partially adherent to the vein wall. The first approach is only safe when the whole thrombus is fixed to the vein wall.

Thrombolysis of fresh non-adherent thrombus This may be achieved with urokinase, streptokinase or the newer plasminogen activators which are all described in Chapter 18.

The worry about dissolving a large IVC thrombus is that it might fragment and become a large pulmonary embolus. Emboli do occur during thrombolysis, and the larger the thrombus being lysed the greater this concern. A decision about the use of thrombolysis will depend upon the general state of the patient, evidence of previous emboli and any contraindications to lytic therapy. Our preference is to remove large non-adherent thrombi surgically (Fig. 10.8) and to reserve thrombolysis for relatively small caval thrombus which is usually just an extension of an iliac vein thrombus.

Thrombectomy Thrombectomy of fresh IVC thrombus is performed through a long mid-line abdominal incision. The IVC is exposed by reflecting the caecum, ascending colon and duodenum to the right and controlled with a clamp above the upper limit of the thrombus as displayed by the phlebogram. The thrombus is then extracted with a Fogarty balloon catheter passed directly through a venotomy in the lower half of the IVC. Bleeding from the IVC below the venotomy and the lumbar veins is controlled by direct digital pressure or by a balloon catheter.

Renal vein thrombectomy can be performed but is a considerable surgical 'tour de force'.

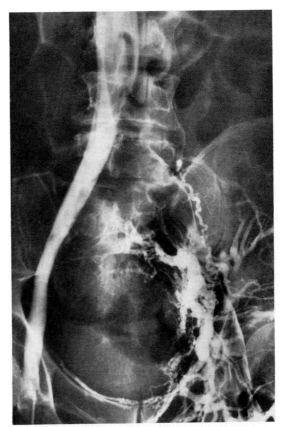

Fig. 10.8 A large loose coiled non-adherent thrombus floating in the inferior vena cava. We prefer to treat such a threat to the patient's life by thrombectomy rather than thrombolysis. The left iliac and common femoral veins also contain fresh partially adherent thrombus. The vena caval thrombus is an extension of the iliac vein thrombus.

There is little point in removing thrombus from the IVC if both iliac veins are irretrievably occluded. If one iliac vein is patent, it is worthwhile clearing the IVC, even if the occluded iliac vein cannot be cleared, because a patent IVC will benefit both the leg with the normal iliac vein and the leg with the blocked iliac vein by increasing the outflow routes of its potential collaterals.

If both iliac veins and the IVC are cleared of thrombus, which implies bilateral groin incisions as well as the abdominal incision, then patency should be maintained with bilateral A-V fistulae fashioned between the femoral arteries and veins.

Caval blockade Patients who are not fit enough to withstand a major abdominal operation and who have contraindications to thrombolysis should be considered for caval blockade (see Chapter 21). It is not possible to predict whether a fresh thrombus will fragment and embolize; it must therefore be assumed that it will. A history of chest pain, haemoptysis or a positive lung scan suggests that the risk of further embolism is high.

Caval blockade can be performed under local anaesthesia by inserting a filter into the upper part of the IVC, usually below the entry of the renal veins, through a venotomy in the right internal jugular vein.

Most forms of filter or external clip effectively prevent further emboli, and in these circumstances we are not concerned with IVC patency. Indeed if there is a large fresh thrombus in the IVC, it is highly likely that the IVC will become totally occluded after inserting a filter. Heparin must be given to reduce further thrombosis, and placing the filter below but as close to the entry of the renal veins as possible will also reduce the chances of thrombosis above the filter.

Heparin Patients who have a complete vena caval occlusion by the time they present, with no propagating tail of thrombus and no symptoms or signs of embolism, should be treated with a 7-day course of heparin followed by oral anticoagulation for at least 6 months. Thrombectomy or thrombolysis when the phlebogram shows a completely occluded IVC and well-developed collateral channels usually fails because the thrombus is frequently more than 6 days old.

Acute secondary thrombosis

Most of the conditions that compress the vena cava and precipitate thrombosis are unsuitable for surgical treatment. In such cases anticoagulants to prevent further thrombosis and caval blockade to prevent embolism are the main forms of treatment.

Even surgically correctable conditions such as aortic aneurysms are not easy to treat at the same time as IVC thrombectomy, though a combined operation is technically feasible. It is safer to allow the acute thrombosis to settle before treating the aneurysm, or opt for embolus prevention by inserting a caval filter before proceeding to repair the aneurysm.

Thrombus in a compressed or infiltrated IVC is usually adherent and without a propagating tail so controllable with anticoagulants. Direct venous surgery is rarely indicated.

Chronic occlusion

When the initial cause of the IVC occlusion is compression the compression should if possible be treated first. Many of the patients in this group have advanced malignant disease. The cause of their IVC obstruction is often beyond treatment and their symptoms are often clinically insignificant.

The symptoms of the patients with a long-standing IVC occlusion following thrombosis fall into two groups: swelling and post-thrombotic changes in the skin of the legs, and venous claudication.

Swelling and skin changes can usually be controlled by conservative measures. Venous claudication is uncommon and can only be relieved by some form of direct vascular surgery.

Conservative treatment Conservative treatment of the leg swelling, varicose veins and skin changes caused by a long-standing IVC obstruction aims to reverse the effect of the high peripheral venous pressure by counteracting it with external compression.

Patients must wear high quality, high compression (40 mm Hg), full-length, bilateral, elastic compression stockings at all times (see Chapter 12, page 339). Patients should elevate their legs whenever possible. At night the feet of their beds should be raised 12 inches (30 cm). During the day they should avoid standing and sitting. When sitting they should raise their legs on a foot stool so the legs are horizontal. Patients should lie on the floor and raise their legs vertically against a wall for 15 minutes at least once each day. If the swelling is severe, they may have to spend 1 or 2 days in bed each week.

Once lipodermatosclerosis and ulceration have developed, elastic compression alone has little effect. Long periods of bed rest are required to heal chronic ulcers, and areas of severe tissue damage may have to be excised and replaced with skin grafts. Patients who have reached this state and those with venous claudication can only be helped by bypass surgery.

Vena cava bypass operations Venous bypass operations have not been widely practised because of their high failure rate.[19,22] Recently, a number of animal studies have shown that prostheses made of expanded polytetrafluoroethylene (PTFE) will stay patent in the venous system if venous blood flow is enhanced by a distal A-V fistula.[2,3,8]

Some isolated clinical reports of bypasses of the iliac veins remaining patent for 2 years are encouraging.[1,2]

For the bypass procedure to be successful there must be a relatively healthy vein at both ends of the bypass for the anastomoses. Unfortunately, many patients with an IVC occlusion have extensive post-thrombotic damage of the iliac and femoral veins as well as of the IVC, and a bypass is therefore not possible.

If, however, a patient has disabling symptoms of claudication or extensive skin damage in the lower limb and patent, moderately healthy femoral veins, it is worthwhile attempting a bi-femoral caval bypass with an externally supported PTFE prothesis with A-V fistulae below the lower anastomoses (Fig. 10.9).

The patient who is to have a bypass operation must be well past the thrombotic state of his original illness and have severe symptoms. Anti-coagulants must be given postoperatively, and the fistulae must be closed 3–6 months later.

While the fistulae are open swelling of the patient's leg may increase because the venous pressure in the legs will be increased.

When a Budd–Chiari syndrome is associated with a vena caval thrombosis a cavo-atrial bypass may relieve the symptoms in the legs.[9]

Much careful clinical experimentation needs to be done before these procedures become generally adopted. Venous claudication should improve following a bypass operation but improvement in the state of the skin of the lower leg depends mainly on the degree of post-thrombotic damage in the calf. Additional surgery may be needed to ablate secondarily incompetent communicating veins.

Excisional operations

When the vena caval occlusion is caused by tumour infiltration, or intraluminal spread of the tumour, a wide excision of the tumour and the vena cava may produce worthwhile palliation of symptoms and an occasional cure.[16]

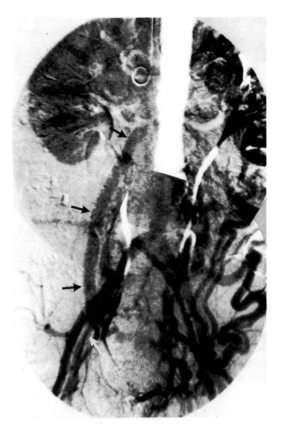

Fig. 10.9 A montage of two films from a digital subtraction angiogram showing an externally supported PTFE graft between the right external iliac vein and the inferior vena cava, just below the entry of the right renal vein.

In the upper part the aorta is white but in the lower part arteries are black. In the lower part the ureters are white. The black arrows indicate the bypass. The white arrow indicates the external iliac vein just below the anastomosis. This is the patient illustrated in Fig. 10.2a.

Prognosis

The prognosis for patients with IVC obstruction depends upon their ability to form collateral channels, the likelihood of further episodes of thrombosis, and the presence of post-thrombotic damage in the deep veins of lower limb.

The younger the patient the better the collaterals. Many of the cases of spontaneous IVC thrombosis seen in our clinic occurred during the teenage years but did not present until the patient was 30 or 40 years old, presentation being related to the slow progression of symptoms or to a new episode of thrombosis. Once symptoms have appeared their progression is inexorable unless the patient is exceptionally diligent with the use of their elastic stockings. Direct venous surgery will be applicable to only a small proportion of these patients, even when the techniques are fully developed; the clinical emphasis must therefore be on the prevention of thrombosis or its effective treatment when it first occurs. Progressive destruction of the skin of the lower leg following bilateral femoral and iliac thrombosis plus an IVC thrombosis sometimes ends with the patient requesting an amputation.

References

1. Chan EL, Bardin JA, Bernstein EF. Inferior vena cava bypass. Experimental evaluation of externally supported grafts and initial clinical experience. *J Vasc Surg* 1984; **1**: 675.
2. Dale WA, Harris J, Terry RB. Polytetrafluorethylene reconstruction of the inferior vena cava. *Surgery* 1984; **95**: 625.
3. Dale WA. Synthetic grafts for venous reconstruction. In Bergan JJ, Yao JST (Eds) *Surgery of the Veins.* New York. Grune & Stratton 1985; 233.
4. Dos Santos JC. La phlebographie directe. *J Int Chir* 1938; **3**: 625.
5. Filler RM, Edwards EA. Collaterals of the lower inferior vena cava in man as revealed by venography. *Arch Surg* 1962; **84**: 10.
6. Filler RM, Harris SH, Edwards EA. Characteristics of inferior vena cava venogram in retroperitoneal cancer. *N Engl J Med* 1962; **266**: 1194.
7. Fletcher EWL, Lea Thomas M. Chronic post thrombotic obstruction of the inferior vena cava investigated by cavography. *Am J Roentgenol* 1968; **102**: 363.
8. Gloviczki P, Hollier LH, Dewanjee MK, Trastek VF, Hoffman EA, Kaye MP. Experimental replacment of the inferior vena cava. Factors affecting patency. *Surgery* 1984; **95**: 657.
9. Huguet C, Deliere T, Ollivier JM, Levy VG. Budd Chiari syndrome with thrombosis of the inferior vena cava: long term patency of meso-caval and cavo-atrial prosthetic bypass. *Surgery* 1984; **95**: 108.
10. Jackson BT, Thomas ML. Post thrombotic inferior vena caval obstruction. A review of 24 patients. *Br Med J* 1970; **1**: 18.
11. Kendall B. Collateral flow to portal system in obstruction of iliac veins and inferior vena cava. *Br J Radiol* 1965; **38**: 798.
12. Missal ME, Robinson JA, Tatum RW. Inferior vena cava obstruction. Clinical manifestations, diagnostic methods and related problems. *Ann Intern Med* 1965; **62**: 133.
13. O'Loughlin BJ. Roentgen visualisation of inferior vena cava. *Am J Roentgenol* 1947; **58**: 617.
14. Pleasants JH. Obstruction of the inferior vena cava with a report of eighteen cases. *Johns Hopkins Hosp Rep* 1911; **15**: 363.
15. Schechter DC, Vogel JM. The challenge of venous extension in malignant renal neoplasms. *N Y State J Med* 1983; **83**: 55.
16. Schechter DC. Cardiovascular Surgery in the management of exogenous tumours involving the vena cava. In Bergan JJ, Yao JST (Eds) *Venous Surgery.* New York. Grune & Stratton 1985; 393.
17. Schenk. *Observationum Medicarum Rariorum.* Lugduni 1644; 339.
18. Schobinger RA. *Intra-osseus Phlebography.* New York. Grune & Stratton 1960.
19. Stansel HC. Synthetic inferior vena cava grafts. *Arch Surg* 1964; **89**: 1096.
20. Stein S, Blumsohn D. Clinical and radiological observations of inferior vena caval obstruction. *Br J Radiol* 1962; **35**: 159
21. Welch WH. In Allbutt TC, Rollerton HD (Ed). *A System of Medicine.* Vol 6. London. Macmillan 1899; 217.
22. Wilson SE, Jabour H, Stone R, Stanley TM. Patency of biological and prosthetic inferior vena cava grafts with distal limb fistula. *Arch Surg* 1978; **113**: 1174.

11

The calf pump failure syndrome: pathology

The changes in the veins, subcutaneous tissues and skin of the lower limb that follow a deep vein thrombosis have for many years been called the post-phlebitic syndrome. The terms thrombophlebitis and phlebothrombosis are misleading[20,27,37] because they imply a dominance of one form of pathological change and furthermore suggest that it is possible to identify the dominant abnormality, namely, the thrombosis or the vein wall inflammation.

Most clinicians and pathologists now prefer to use the all embracing and non-committal term 'deep vein thrombosis' for all forms of venous thrombosis except for the variety in the superficial veins which is called 'superficial thrombophlebitis' (see Chapter 22) because it is obviously associated with an inflammation of the vein wall.

As the principal cause of the late sequelae of deep vein thrombosis is the thrombosis rather than the vein wall inflammation, it is preferable to use the term 'post-thrombotic syndrome' rather than post-phlebitic syndrome. This chapter is, however, entitled 'The calf pump failure syndrome', not the post-thrombotic syndrome because the clinical features of this condition can develop in the absence of any evidence of a previous deep vein thrombosis. Patients with the calf pump failure syndrome fall into three distinct groups: those with a definite history of proven deep vein thrombosis, those with no history of thrombosis but phlebographic evidence of a previous thrombosis, and those with no history of a thrombosis and a normal phlebogram. The syndrome in the latter group is not post-thrombotic. Its ultimate cause is failure of the calf pump hence the name 'calf pump failure syndrome' which can be preceded by the adjective post-thrombotic if there is definite evidence of thrombosis.

Aetiopathology

The starting point of the post-thrombotic syndrome is presumed to be the first episode of deep vein thrombosis. The severity of the syndrome is, however, only loosely linked to the severity of the initial thrombosis. This discrepancy is usually attributed to the remarkable ability of the peripheral veins and the calf pump to compensate for a considerable degree of obstruction and reflux on the one hand, and on the other hand the susceptibility of calf pump function to serious derangement following a minor degree of thrombosis in a critical part of the pump (e.g. the communicating veins). However, as a considerable number of patients with the post-thrombotic syndrome have no demonstrable evidence of a previous thrombosis, we believe that a less specific description such as 'calf pump failure syndrome' is more suitable for this condition until our knowledge and understanding of its aetiology improves.

The role of deep vein thrombosis in the development of calf pump failure

The aetiology and pathology of deep vein thrombosis is discussed in detail in Chapter 16. The initiating factor is usually trauma (e.g. an accident or a surgical operation), a severe medical illness, or pregnancy and childbirth.

The risk of a thrombosis complicating these conditions is exacerbated by increasing age, a previous episode of deep vein thrombosis, the presence of malignant disease, the presence of varicose veins, obesity, and abnormalities in the blood such as polycythaemia, thrombocytosis, abnormal coagulation factors, a raised plasma fibrinogen or defective fibrinolysis.

In many patients these risk factors play a very small part; the ultimate trigger of the coagulation cascade is the undefined 'hypercoagulability' induced by the operation or injury, in association with the reduced venous blood flow that accompanies the prohibition of exercise enforced by the initial trauma or illness. Nevertheless, all the conditions which predispose to thrombosis must be considered as risk factors of the post-thrombotic syndrome.

The post-thrombotic syndrome is a clinical syndrome which many clinicians are prepared to diagnose even in the absence of clinical evidence of a previous thrombosis. Clinicians justify this approach with the argument that at least 50 per cent of episodes of deep vein thrombosis are symptomless. There are, however, two important facts which belie this approach.

First, 30 per cent of general surgical patients over the age of 40 years have a deep vein thrombosis but only a small proportion subsequently develop the post-thrombotic syndrome.

Secondly, in the Basle survey of patients with varicose veins and the skin changes of chronic venous insufficiency, which would be called by many clinicians 'post-thrombotic' only 6 per cent of men and 14 per cent of women had any knowledge of a predisposing venous thrombosis (see Chapter 5).

Nevertheless, there is no doubt that a major deep vein thrombosis will cause the post-thrombotic syndrome. Bauer[2], reviewed a series of patients with phlebographic evidence of thrombosis and found a 20 per cent incidence of venous ulceration at 5 years and a 52 per cent incidence at 10 years but these patients had actually had a post-thrombotic syndrome for many years before their ulcer appeared because 40 per cent and 72 per cent had skin and subcutaneous tissue induration at 5 and 10 years respectively.

Two questions therefore need to be answered. Is the severity of the syndrome related to the site of the thrombosis? Is the syndrome always, and only caused by thrombosis?

The effect of the site of thrombosis

The calf   The most minor form of deep vein thrombosis is the asymptomatic calf vein thrombosis that occurs in 20–30 per cent of patients after a major operation.[38,66] However, one-third of all patients who have had a major operation do not develop a post-thrombotic syndrome; the significance of these minor postoperative thrombi is therefore not clear.

Calf thrombosis alone may or may not alter calf pump function depending upon its effect on the communicating veins. It is almost impossible for a deep vein thrombosis to obliterate all the deep veins of the calf. Many thrombosed veins recanalize, collaterals always develop and the pump may return to normal if the outflow tract is undamaged and the communicating veins remain competent.

In 1974 we reviewed 44 patients, between 3 and 4 years after they had had a positive postoperative Fibrinogen Uptake Test.[13] Their mean age was 60 years. Three and a half years after operation one-fifth of the limbs that had contained a thrombus still ached, one-fifth were slightly swollen and one-half had varicose veins.

Of particular interest was the finding that one-tenth of the legs *without* thrombus (negative Fibrinogen Uptake Tests) ached, one-tenth had some ankle swelling, and half had visible varicose veins. If the combination of aching, swelling and varicose veins is thought to be the beginning of the post-thrombotic syndrome, 20 per cent of the legs that had a post-operative thrombosis and 10 per cent of legs that did not have a thrombosis were developing the syndrome 3 years after an operation. However, 50 per cent of the legs studied had mild varicose veins before the operation. Only 10 per cent of the legs without varicose veins before operation developed new varicose veins. When the legs without pre-operative venous abnormalities were analysed we found that 6 of the 34 legs known to have a thrombosis had developed an ankle flare and 2 of these had developed pigmentation and mild lipodermatosclerosis. At the same time 2 of the 15 legs without a pre-existing venous abnormality that did not develop a thrombosis (negative Fibrinogen Uptake Test) had developed an ankle flare and one of these had developed lipodermatosclerosis. We cannot be absolutely certain that a thrombosis did not develop in these limbs as a late event, after the fibrinogen scanning, but this is unlikely.

Thus in the 49 legs without any evidence of pre-operative venous abnormality, 8 (16 per cent) had developed signs suggestive of calf pump failure and the incidence of this change was similar in those legs with, and in those legs without thrombosis (18 per cent and 14 per cent respectively).

A similar study was performed by Mudge and Hudges in 1978[64] on patients who 3 years previously had entered a trial of postoperative Dextran prophylaxis. They found that 26 patients (out of 564) had clinical evidence of the post-thrombotic syndrome. This was present before the operation (3 years earlier) in 14 patients but was a new event in 12 patients, all of whom had had a postoperative deep vein thrombosis. This result (24 per cent) is similar to ours (18 per cent). Three-quarters of these patients developed their skin changes within 1 year of operation. The incidence of the post-thrombotic syndrome in the patients who did not develop a postoperative thrombosis was not studied as not all patients had a fibrinogen uptake test.

Widmer studied the incidence of the post-thrombotic syndrome 5 years after the initial thrombosis in 37 patients who had had localized calf thrombosis.[89] Although some patients had minor symptoms none had developed a post-thrombotic syndrome. These results are difficult to interpret as some patients had been treated with streptokinase and others with heparin. Also Widmer's symptom score differs from ours in placing far more weight on ulceration; for example, in Widmer's study a patient with an ankle flare, oedema and skin changes would not be classified as having a post-thrombotic syndrome, whereas in both the other studies they would. Such differences highlight the problems of definition and comparibility in long-term follow-up studies.

Lindhagen *et al.*,[61] found no difference in the incidence of the post-thrombotic syndrome between patients who had a positive or negative postoperative fibrinogen uptake test (23 per cent and 21 per cent respectively) but found a foot vein pressure fall during exercise of less than 30 mmHg more often in those who had had a positive test (18 per cent compared with 7 per cent).

The outflow tract A thrombosis that affects the venous outflow tract of the limb alone will obstruct the blood flow from the calf pump until the thrombosed vessels recanalize and collaterals develop. The obstruction will then become less but the valves in the recanalized segment will invariably be incompetent making reflux an additional burden on the pump. At first the pump may be able to deal with the combined stress of outflow obstruction and reflux but it will become inefficient if progressive dilatation of the veins in the pump causes communicating vein incompetence. A thrombosis which is localized to the superficial femoral or the iliac vein will cause less of an obstruction than a thrombosis involving both these veins because, though both have potentially good collateral circulations, two sets of collaterals in series are rarely adequate. Thrombosis involving the whole of the deep venous system, from the calf veins to the vena cava has a much greater chance of causing a post-thrombotic syndrome.

There is little point in classifying these different distributions of thrombosis for two reasons. First, there are many possible combinations, but considering them all together oversimplifies the problem. Secondly, the available methods of diagnosis are not sufficiently accurate to allow the clinician to say with certainty, for example, that a patient has thrombus in the iliac vein but no thrombus in the calf. Such a patient is highly likely to have small undetectable calf thrombi which combined with a proximal outflow obstruction might cause a severe post-thrombotic syndrome.

We examined 130 legs of 67 patients, 5–10 years after they had suffered a thrombosis to see if there was any relationship between the site of the initial thrombosis and the subsequent development of the post-thrombotic syndrome.[12] All the patients had been treated with anticoagulants. Forty-seven of the legs were clinically and phlebographically normal and therefore acted as controls. The site and severity of the thrombosis was graded from the phlebogram and the current signs and symptoms assigned a symptom score. There was a higher incidence of post-thrombotic sequelae in the patients who had had a severe thrombosis when compared with those who had had a minor thrombosis (Fig. 11.1).

Thirteen per cent of the legs with no thrombosis, 20 per cent of the legs with small localized thrombosis (regardless of site), and 40 per cent of the legs with an extensive thrombosis had developed the post-thrombotic syndrome. Many of these patients wore elastic stockings which may have retarded the development of the syndrome but the incidence of 40 per cent with post-thrombotic symptoms 6 years after an extensive thrombosis is close to Bauer's finding of an incidence of 45 per cent with induration 5 years after a thrombosis.

It is important to note that 13 per cent of limbs

No or minor initial thrombosis (87 legs)

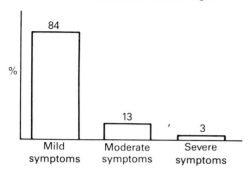

Severe initial thrombosis (15 legs)

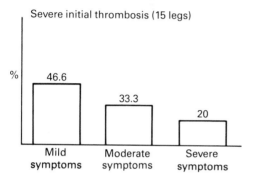

Fig. 11.1 The leg symptom scores of patients with minor and major degrees of deep vein thrombosis (phlebographically determined) 5–10 years after the thrombosis. Only 16% of patients with a minor thrombosis had moderate or severe symptoms compared to a 53% incidence of moderate or severe symptoms amongst those who had a severe thrombosis.

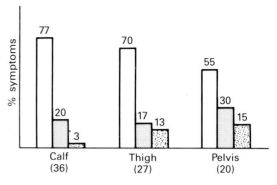

Upper limit of thrombosis

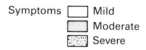

Fig. 11.2 The leg symptom scores of patients 5–10 years after a deep vein thrombosis related to the site of the thrombosis. The symptom score was higher the more extensive the thrombosis but the differences were not statistically significant.

developed symptoms in the absence of evidence of a thrombosis. As there was no evidence to suggest that these patients had had a late thrombosis, 6 months or more after the initial episode when their anticoagulants were stopped, we assume that their calf pump failure was not post-thrombotic.

An analysis of the effect of the site of the thrombosis was unexpectedly inconclusive (Fig. 11.2). Legs with an axial vein thrombosis did not have a significantly higher incidence of problems (calf thrombus – 20 per cent, thigh thrombus – 30 per cent, and pelvic thrombus – 45 per cent), though there was a definite trend which might have reached significance in a larger study. Almost half (42 per cent) of the 12 legs with a total calf-femoral-iliac thrombosis had no symptoms at 6½ years.

Widmer's 5-year follow-up of 415 patients with deep vein thrombosis,[89] some of whom had been treated with streptokinase, found a 21 per cent incidence of post-thrombotic syndrome and a 6.5 per cent incidence of ulceration. When the limbs were subdivided according to the extent of the initial thrombosis, the incidence of the post-thrombotic syndrome following calf and popliteal vein thrombosis was 17 per cent (5 per cent with ulcers) for calf, popliteal, and superficial femoral vein thrombosis It was 23 per cent (7 per cent with ulcers), and for calf, popliteal, femoral and iliac vein thrombosis it was 34 per cent (8 per cent with ulcers) (Fig. 11.3). There may be two reasons for the lower incidence of post-thrombotic syndrome found by Widmer. First, his definition of the post-thrombotic syndrome placed more weight on ulceration and less on pre-ulcer skin changes. Secondly, the selection for treatment and the method of treatment was different. Despite these differences the results of all the studies quoted follow the same trend and emphasize the high chance of late sequelae after a deep vein thrombosis.

We also found a positive correlation between the age of the thrombus – assessed radiographically at the time of presentation – and subsequent symptoms.[12] Fresh thrombi (which were also an indication of earlier diagnosis and subsequent treatment with anticoagulants) were associated

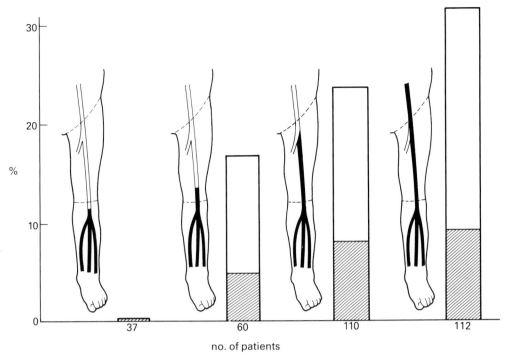

Fig. 11.3 The incidence of the post-thrombotic syndrome and ulceration (hatched area) related to the site of thrombosis (black shading) in 341 patients 5 years after the thrombosis. This study showed a close correlation between the extent of the thrombosis and the incidence of symptoms.
(Modified from Widmer.)[89]

with a 9 per cent incidence of symptoms, whereas thrombi more than 7 days old at presentation (which was usually an indication of occluding thrombi and late treatment) had a 46 per cent incidence of symptoms (Fig. 11.4). Perhaps some of the differences between the results of our study and those of Bauer are related to the time of diagnosis and the early use of heparin.

It can be deduced from these studies that a patient with a thrombosis that extends into the popliteal vein or above has a 35 per cent chance of getting a mild post-thrombotic syndrome and a 40 per cent chance of getting a severe post-thrombotic syndrome within 6 years. Without doubt 75 per cent of these patients will get some symptoms.[30]

It must also be remembered that 20 per cent of patients with minor calf or small non-adherent axial vein thrombi and 13 per cent of patients with no evidence of postoperative thrombosis will get symptoms. This later figure is almost identical to the 14 per cent incidence of post-thrombotic syndrome that we found in patients who had had a

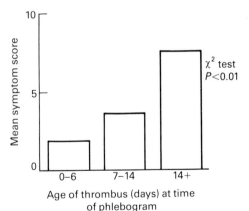

Fig. 11.4 The relationship between the incidence of post-thrombotic symptoms 5–10 years after the thrombosis and the age of the thrombosis (judged phlebographically) at the time of clinical presentation.

The older the thrombosis at presentation the greater the severity of the symptoms 5 years later.

negative Fibrinogen Uptake Test after operation, a fact not detected by Bauer because he only studied legs with thrombosis.

The role of varicose veins

Many of the patients in the studies discussed above had varicose veins, and this raises the question of the role of simple primary varicose veins in the aetiology of the post-thrombotic syndrome.[85,91]

Mudge and Hudges[64] observed that 24 per cent of their patients had varicose veins pre-operatively but that new varicose veins had appeared 1 year later in 16 per cent of the patients who did not have a postoperative thrombosis, and in 35 per cent of the patients who had had a thrombosis. We found a similar incidence of new varicose veins in previously normal legs (14 per cent) but a lower incidence (18 per cent) in the legs that had had a thrombosis.[12]

Varicose veins reduce calf pump efficiency by allowing superficial vein reflux during pump diastole; it is therefore possible that the calf pump failure symptoms that developed in the patients without evidence of thrombosis were related to the development of varicose veins and their effect on the calf pump.

Phlebographic studies of the deep veins of patients with venous ulceration show that a significant proportion have normal looking deep veins.[68,75] Unless it is postulated that these veins, or the communicating veins, have been the site of minor thrombosis not detectable by phlebography, it is difficult to postulate that the ulceration, and the pre-ulcer calf pump failure was caused by a thrombosis.

The arguments set out above do not explain how an operation can induce the appearance of varicose veins if it is not through the mechanism of thrombotic valve destruction. We have no alternative hypothesis to advance.

Superficial varicose veins can produce skin changes and ulceration[47,77] but we suspect that this only happens when the communicating veins are involved in the varicose process and dilate, thus making the valves incompetent. This is normally a very slow process. We would not expect it to occur in 1 year and so can see no mechanism that would rapidly affect the veins except minor thrombosis that is undetectable and confined to the communicating veins and destroys their valves.

The argument therefore turns full circle. The 'post-thrombotic syndrome' occurs in patients with varicose veins and in patients with no firm evidence of a past thrombosis, yet we know of no mechanism by which an operation can cause the development of varicose veins other than valve destruction by deep vein thrombosis. There is still much to investigate and unravel.

The role of tissue fibrinolysis

One of the predisposing causes of deep vein thrombosis is a deficiency of fibrinolysis.[46,72] A number of studies have suggested that patients who have had a thrombosis have a reduced level of blood fibrinolytic activity. Of all the haematological factors that have been studied before and after surgical operation,[51] the level of plasma fibrinogen and tests of blood fibrinolytic activity are the most reliable predictors of the likelihood of thrombosis.[23,41,52,73]

Varicose veins also have a reduced tissue fibrinolytic activity. This is mentioned here because if tissue fibrinolytic activity mirrors blood fibrinolytic activity, this may be the reason why varicose veins are a risk factor for thrombosis, and a major risk in the development of the post-thrombotic syndrome. The relationship between blood and vein wall fibrinolytic activator levels and the development of the post-thrombotic syndrome requires further study.

Comment

The interaction of factors such as interstitial fibrosis, valve ring dilatation and fibrinolysis may explain why a simple correlation between the degree of thrombosis and the post-thrombotic syndrome has not yet been found. Until an incontrovertible connection between thrombosis and all cases of the post-thrombotic syndrome can be established we shall continue to use the term 'calf pump failure syndrome'.

The effect of thrombosis on the vein

Most venous thrombi seem to begin within valve cusps and muscle sinusoids[20,29,39,45,71,78,80,82,84] (see Chapter 16).

As the thrombus grows it gets thicker changing from a thin non-adherent non-obstructing thrombus to one that completely obstructs the vein. The obstruction becomes haemodynamically significant when the thrombus occupies more than 75 per cent of the cross-sectional area of the vein. When this occurs collateral vessels begin to open, the main stimulus to collateral vein dilatation being the pressure gradient between the occluded vein's tributaries on either side of the obstruction.

Venous collaterals can become large and effective within a few hours and their development is helped by the presence of many small veins throughout all tissues. The best example of a pre-existing potential collateral vein is the common connection between the upper part of the popliteal vein and the deep femoral vein which immediately dilates and becomes a collateral pathway when the superficial femoral vein occludes.

The effect of thrombosis on the valves

As the thrombus grows it either surrounds the valve cusps or pushes them flat against the wall of the vein. These are the most serious effects of thrombosis because they destroy the valves. At first the valves become stiffened by a covering of fibrin and thrombus, soon they adhere to the vein wall and eventually they fragment. These changes destroy the valve's ability to function and leave the vein incompetent if it recanalizes.[32] Valves can only be saved from destruction by thrombosis if the thrombus is dissolved or removed during the first few hours of its life, before it has engulfed the valve (see Fig. 18.4, page 508). The period of time which is necessary for a valve to be completely destroyed has not been established.

The natural history of a thrombus

This may follow one of three courses.

Retraction As a thrombus ages, its fibrin matures and contracts causing the whole thrombus to shrink.[4,53,58] This is a slow process which takes many months to complete. As the thrombus gets smaller it usually becomes adherent to the vein wall, fixing and destroying any remaining valves which were not incorporated within it when it first formed. Sometimes the thrombus adheres to opposite sides of the vein and then, as it retracts, turns the vein into a double channelled vessel (see Fig. 16.12, page 461).[62,74]

Adhesion Most thrombi grow steadily until they fill the whole vein and engulf the valves. They then adhere to the vein wall and stimulate an inflammatory process in the wall.[32] The thrombus may then retract but more often it totally occludes the vein which either remains permanently occluded or recanalizes.

The inflammatory response in the vein wall is the first step in the organization of the thrombus. The thrombus is infiltrated by chronic inflammatory cells and new capillary loops. The whole process leads to the conversion of the thrombus into an organized scar consisting of fibrin, fibrous tissue, and a few capillaries. The end result is a solid cord of tissue consisting of the original vein containing a thin totally organized thrombus.

Recanalization The term recanalization is often used loosely to describe the new channels that can be seen to replace the original vein on a phlebogram. The reopening of most veins results from the retraction and adhesion of the thrombus to one side of the vein leaving part of the *original* lumen open. True recanalization is rare.

True recanalization is the development of a new channel through the thrombus.[79] As time passes, areas within the thrombus soften and liquify, just as a haematoma liquifies, by spontaneous proteolysis. The role of the venous endothelium and the fibrinolytic activator it produces in this process of recanalization is not known.[22,55] Cystic spaces develop throughout the thrombus and if they join together and reach to both ends of the thrombus a new channel is formed (Fig. 11.5). The chances of this process producing a good-sized channel are few, and the new channel is valveless.

The development of large patent channels at the site of a previously thrombosed major vein should not be called recanalization. If the channel is large and in direct continuity with anatomically recognizable vessels above and below, it is probably the original vein which has *reopened* as a result of thrombus *retraction* (Fig. 11.5). If there are one or two large vessels, almost but not precisely in the anatomical course of the thrombosed vein, they are probably *dilated vena venorum acting as collaterals* (Fig. 11.6). If there is a narrow and irregular channel bridging the gap between two anatomically definable veins, the thrombus may have recanalized.

Whatever the form of channel that develops it will probably be valveless, certainly incompetent, but not necessarily an obstruction to blood flow. The lumen of a reopened iliac or femoral vein can be as large as the normal vein if the thrombus retracts down to a thin cord on one side of the vein

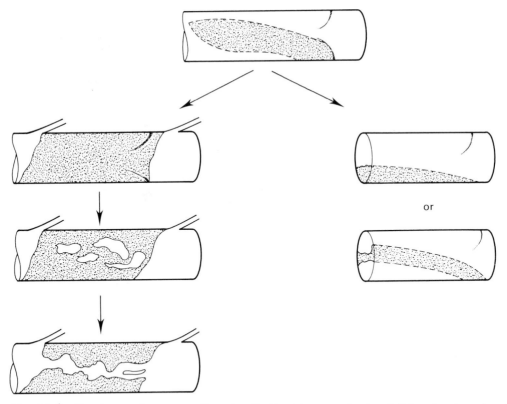

Fig. 11.5   The changes in a venous thrombus that lead to recanalization (left-hand pathway) and reopening (right-hand pathway). The former is true recanalization (i.e. intrinsic thrombolysis producing a channel through the thrombus). The latter is simply retraction and adherence of the thrombus to one or both sides of the vessel wall.

but this is unusual (Fig. 11.7). Collateral vessels and truly recanalized veins are rarely as big as the orginal vessel and usually cause some obstruction to blood flow.

Collateral vessel formation

Collateral vessels bypassing an occluded vein can develop very quickly. They are often visible on a phlebogram within 24 hours of an acute occlusion.

The peripheral veins are multiple, variable and frequently interconnect. Potential collateral channels are therefore immediately available. New vessels do not have to grow as they do in the arterial circulation.

The main sites for collateral vessel development are discussed in Chapter 2. The deep femoral vein provides an escape route for blood from the calf to the outflow tract at the root of the limb. The gluteal veins and their tributaries deep in the thigh help bypass an ilio-femoral occlusion by conducting blood into the internal iliac system, across the floor of the pelvis, to the contralateral internal iliac vein. The epigastric veins can conduct blood up the abdominal wall in cases of iliac and vena caval obstruction. Within the abdomen, vena caval obstruction is bypassed by the ascending lumbar, ovarian and azygos veins.

Collateral vessels on a phlebogram often appear to have a larger total cross-sectional area than the original blocked vessel. Collateral vessels, however, nearly always obstruct blood flow and contribute to calf pump dysfunction because their valves are incompetent as a result of valve ring dilatation.

It must always be remembered that the superficial subcutaneous veins of the lower limb may also act as collateral vessels when the deep veins are blocked but in order to drain blood from the

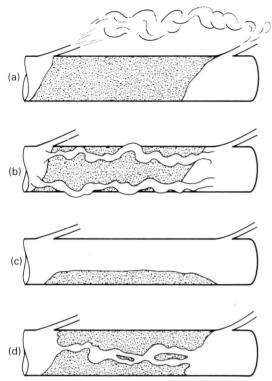

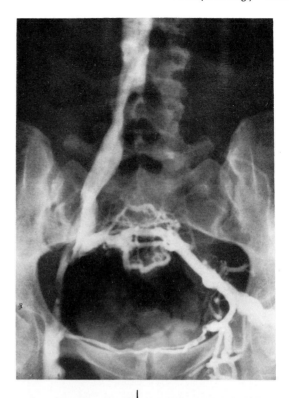

Fig. 11.6 The four ways in which blood can bypass or pass through an obstruction caused by thrombosis.
- (a) Via true collateral vessels.
- (b) Via dilated vena venora.
- (c) Alongside retracted thrombus.
- (d) Through true recanalization.

calf pump they must receive blood via the communicating veins. They can only do this if the communicating vein valves are incompetent. Communicating vein incompetence is a common sequel to the high pressure that develops within the calf when there is pump outflow obstruction. This can occur with isolated pelvic vein obstruction but more often follows combined popliteal and femoral vein obstruction. Under these circumstances the communicating veins are acting more as a safety valve to reduce the intrapump

Fig. 11.7 An example of complete reopening of a major vein probably caused by retraction of the thrombus rather than true recanalization. The lower phlebogram was obtained 2 years after the upper film.

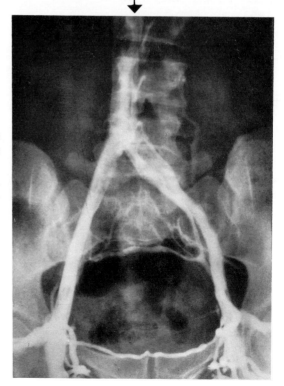

pressure than as vessels conducting a significant volume of blood flow, but the effect remains the same whether they are safety vents or blood conductors – superficial venous hypertension – which leads to the tissue damage we recognize as the calf pump failure syndrome.

The effect of thrombosis on calf pump function

Chapter 3 describes the function of a normal calf pump by dividing it into two compartments: the *deep (pump) compartment* (the veins within the deep fascia lying within and between the muscles) and the *superficial (pump) compartment* (all the veins in the subcutaneous tissues and skin). In addition there are *the communicating veins* connecting the two compartments and the *out-flow tract* from the pump (the popliteal, femoral and iliac veins).

Thrombosis can occur in one, or any, combination of the four parts of this system with varying effects.

Superficial vein thrombosis

This is mentioned first because superficial thrombophlebitis in superficial varicose veins is probably the most common form of thrombosis. In the Basle study[90] 16 per cent of women with varicose veins claimed to have had an episode of 'thrombosis'.

Thrombosis in a varicose vein can be beneficial because it occludes the vein in a manner similar to sclerotherapy, though this benefit is often short-lived because the vein usually recanalizes. Thrombosis of a large superficial varix may stop the reflux, improve the appearance of the leg and reduce the symptoms.

Superficial thrombophlebitis does not cause the 'post-thrombotic syndrome' unless it extends into the communicating veins (Fig. 11.8) It is not known how often this happens but phlebographic evidence suggests that it occurs in 20–40 per cent of patients without varicose veins but in only 2–4 per cent of patients with varicose veins.[3]

It is unusual to see the radiological features of recanalization in either the superficial veins or the communicating veins. Nevertheless, some authorities consider that it must be the cause of all

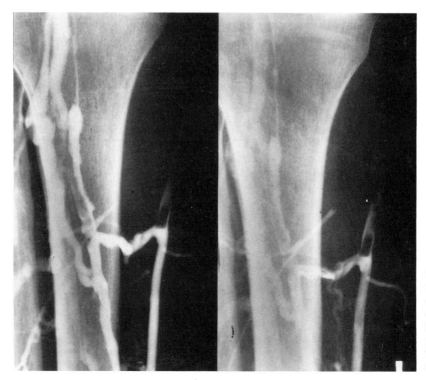

Fig. 11.8 Thrombosis in the posterior tibial vein extending into a communicating vein (seen best in the right-hand panel) associated with a fresh thrombus in a superficial vein.

communicating vein incompetence even when there is no evidence of deep vein thrombosis.[25] Extension of thrombosis into the communicating veins certainly occurs if an intravenous infusion is given into the long saphenous vein at the ankle. This site of superficial thrombophlebitis has long been recognized as a cause of the post-thrombotic syndrome and ulceration, and is the reason why intravenous infusions should always be given into arm veins. In most cases superficial thrombophlebitis in varicose veins does little harm to calf pump function and may improve it if it occludes a major pathway of superficial reflux.

Calf and communicating vein thrombosis

Thrombosis of the communicating veins is usually an extension of deep vein thrombosis. The important medial communicating veins drain directly into the posterior tibial veins, veins which are a common site of deep vein thrombosis. Other (indirect) communicating veins drain via the intramuscular veins of the gastrocnemius and soleus muscles which are also common sites of venous thrombosis. Autopsy studies have shown thrombus in the deep veins extending into the communicating veins.

If the thrombosis destroys the valves, the veins will be incompetent when they reopen or recanalize, and the high pressure developed during muscle contractions within the deep fascia will be transmitted directly into the superficial system.[54]

Communicating vein incompetence makes the pump 'leaky'[28,36,56] but the volume of blood that flows retrogradely through these veins is probably not the important factor. If the patient is upright, the superficial veins are full and at the top their stress – strain curve (see Fig. 3.3, page 55). The veins cannot dilate further and so the addition of even a small amount of blood from the contracting calf pump produces a significant increase in pressure, and it is this increase in pressure rather than the volume of retrograde blood flow that causes the microvascular damage.[39,78]

It is unusual for all the communicating veins to be incompetent; the superficial vein pressure during exercise therefore depends upon the balance between those communications that are working normally and helping to decompress the superficial veins and those which are incompetent and allow blood to reflux and distend the superficial system. The blood may literally be going round in circles – in through one communicating vein and out through another. It is not the blood flow or its disordered direction that matters, it is the failure of the pump to produce superficial venous hypotension during exercise (i.e. the venous hypertension) that leads to the tissue changes described later.

The communicating veins have a relatively small cross-sectional area when compared with the large axial and muscle veins of the calf which combine to form the popliteal vein. A normal outflow tract presents less resistance to flow than three or four incompetent communicating veins.

It is therefore not surprising that the pump still works quite well when the only abnormality is communicating vein incompetence with the superficial venous pressure falling during exercise to a moderate level (40–50 mmHg).[17,57] Communicating vein incompetence alone therefore takes a long time to cause the microcirculatory changes of the calf pump failure syndrome; this explains why the majority of patients have forgotten the symptoms of their initiating thrombosis (if they ever had any) by the time their skin changes develop. Isolated thrombosis within the calf veins that does not involve the communicating veins has little effect on the calf pump. Two long-term follow-up studies have failed to find an increased incidence of post-thrombotic symptoms in patients with minor calf vein thrombosis detected with radioactive fibrinogen.[13,64]

Calf vein thrombosis that propagates into the popliteal vein often leads to a severe post-thrombotic syndrome because it invariably causes a severe obstruction to the outflow of blood from the calf[89] or severe reflux if it recanalizes.[81] The muscle and stem veins of the calf all drain into the popliteal vein and are not connected with other veins which can become collaterals. If the communicating veins were involved in the initial thrombosis, the pump rapidly becomes inadequate. If the communicating veins were not involved in the initial thrombosis, they gradually dilate, become incompetent and act as collateral outflow channels from the pump. In these circumstances superficial venous pressure falls by only 10 or 20 mmHg during exercise and the calf pump failure syndrome quickly develops.

Outflow tract thrombosis (normal calf)

Thrombosis in the outflow tract usually follows

one of four common patterns: ilio-femoral vein thrombosis, superficial femoral vein thrombosis, superficial femoral and popliteal vein thrombosis, and ilio-femoro-popliteal vein thrombosis (i.e. thrombosis of the upper third, the middle third, the lower two thirds or the whole tract) (Fig. 11.9). Solitary popliteal vein thrombosis is uncommon.

Isolated iliac vein thrombosis   This increases the resistance to the outflow of blood from the whole leg but is sufficiently distant from the calf pump and often so well compensated by collateral pathways that it may cause little or no symptoms. The veins below the obstruction dilate and connect with many vessels on the floor of the pelvis and posterior abdominal wall which act as collateral pathways.[26,63] Provided the valves in the superficial femoral vein remain competent the calf pump can function normally, even though it has an increased load; the skin of the lower leg remains normal. In some patients the pump cannot push enough blood past the obstruction during exercise and the veins become distended and painful – a symptom called venous claudication.[67,87]

If the veins upstream to the obstruction (i.e. in the femoral and popliteal veins) dilate, two complications may develop.

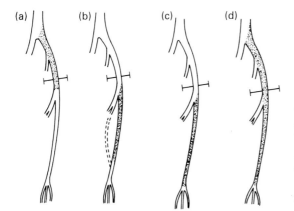

Fig. 11.9   The four common varieties of calf pump outflow tract thrombosis.
  (a) Ilio-femoral thrombosis.
  (b) Superficial femoral vein thrombosis.
  (c) Superficial femoral and popliteal vein thrombosis.
  (d) Complete popliteal, femoral and iliac vein thrombosis.

At first, the valves of the outflow tract become progressively incompetent down to, and including, those in the popliteal vein[81] so the pump becomes overloaded with blood refluxing into it during diastole. The response of the calf pump is similar to that of the heart. The capacity of the pump and the ejection fraction increases but usually neither change is sufficient and so pump efficiency falls and less blood is drawn from the superficial into the deep compartment during diastole. Although the superficial vein pressure during exercise does not fall to the normal range, the resulting venous hypertension is often not sufficient to cause post-thrombotic changes in the skin. In other words – minimal outflow tract obstruction plus secondary outflow tract reflux, in the presence of a good pump with normal calf and communicating vein valves, rarely causes severe symptoms or serious skin changes.

Eventually, the higher pressures and volumes within the pump caused by the minimal outflow tract obstruction and reflux may cause communicating vein incompetence. As soon as this occurs the calf pump failure syndrome rapidly appears because the combination of outflow obstruction and reflux with a leaky pump makes the pump extremely inefficient. Superficial venous pressure is reduced during exercise by only 10–20 mmHg and the persistent venous hypertension quickly causes the microcirculatory changes that lead to eczema, pigmentation, lipodermatosclerosis and ulceration.

Isolated superficial femoral vein thrombosis   This can cause the same sequence of events but in many patients the collateral circulation from the upper popliteal vein to the deep femoral vein becomes an adequate and competent outflow tract and the patient has no symptoms. If, however, the collateral veins are inadequate, the pump begins to fail, the soleal sinusoids and the communicating veins dilate and a calf pump failure syndrome appears.

The superficial femoral vein often partially reopens but usually remains an obstruction to pump outflow. It is also incompetent and the pump therefore has to cope with obstruction during systole and reflux during diastole. This combination overloads the pump much more than obstruction alone and leads to communicating vein incompetence. Patients affected in this way may occasionally complain of venous claudication as well as the calf pump failure syndrome but this is uncommon if the popliteal vein in patent.

Isolated popliteal vein thrombosis This is extremely rare. It is usually the result of extension of thrombus from a calf vein tributary. When it results from retrograde spread of a low superficial femoral vein thrombosis and the calf veins are normal the symptoms are similar to those describe above but appear sooner and are more severe.

Combined iliac and superficial femoral vein thrombosis This causes a rapid onset of the symptoms and disturbance of the calf pump physiology similar to those described above, because the collateral channels are seldom adequate.[93] Reopening and recanalization does occûr but is rarely sufficient to relieve the outflow obstruction. It is uncommon for extensive axial vein thrombosis to occur without the calf veins being involved. Even when the calf veins are spared, however, the obstruction and reflux rapidly overload the pump and cause communicating vein incompetence and the appearance of pump failure changes in the skin.

Once this occurs the superficial veins become incompetent and superficial vein reflux is added to the load of the pump. These patients often present with a combination of venous claudication and skin changes.

Combined calf and outflow tract thrombosis

The post-thrombotic syndrome develops in 80–90 per cent of patients with extensive thrombosis but it is quite extraordinary that some patients can have an extensive continuous thrombosis of their calf, popliteal, femoral, and iliac veins and yet be free of symptoms 10 years later. We were surprised to find that half of our patients who had this degree of thrombosis were without symptoms 5 years after their thrombosis.[12] These results may, however, have been influenced by the length of follow-up and the relatively small numbers that we were able to study.[2,40,89]

When both the outflow tract and the communicating veins are damaged, pump failure is almost inevitable. As the calf muscles contract the blood flow meets a massive resistance. The principal communicating veins cannot act as collaterals because they are occluded by thrombus, every other small unnamed vein therefore dilates to fill this role. Later the communicating veins reopen or recanalize and act as collateral outflows to the pump during exercise and at rest. By this stage some of the axial veins may have reopened but they are usually narrow and incompetent. There is no way in which such a damaged system can propel sufficient blood towards the heart to reduce the superficial venous pressure during exercise. There is constant superficial venous hypertension which is often exacerbated by exercise. The leg swells, becomes painful and the skin steadily deteriorates. Venous claudication and venous ulceration often appear within 2–3 years of a severe thrombosis.

The above descriptions of the haemodynamic effects of deep vein thrombosis explain why the pathophysiological sequelae are unpredictable and variable.

The damaged outflow tract may obstruct blood flow or permit reflux; in many patients it does both. As a result of these abnormalities the communicating veins become incompetent. It is impossible with our current methods of investigation to isolate and quantify each of these abnormalities, and so we are usually unable to determine which of them is the cause of a patient's symptoms.

Obstruction, even with a healthy pump, may cause venous claudication, but it is debatable whether reflux alone can do the same. Skin changes appear once the valves in the communicating veins fail, and when this occurs the skin problems tend to overshadow the claudication. It is not known whether outflow obstruction or reflux is more likely to lead to communicating vein failure. Consequently, when a patient has a combination of outflow tract obstruction and incompetence we do not know which to correct. The problem is not academic because surgical repair of secondarily incompetent communicating veins will provide only a temporary improvement if the primary problem is not corrected. We will not be able to answer these questions and treat our patients rationally until we can measure the size of each abnormality individually and accurately.

The effect of an inefficient calf pump on the skin and subcutaneous tissues

Inefficiency of the calf pump whether it be the result of overloading from superficial venous incompetence, communicating vein leakage or outflow tract obstruction or incompetence or, as is most often the case, combinations of all these abnormalities, causes a persistent rise in the mean superficial venous pressure throughout the patient's daily life. The first effect of this venous hypertension appears in the subcutaneous veins and skin capillaries.

Subcutaneous veins

The raised venous pressure eventually causes the subcutaneous veins to dilate and their valves to become incompetent. The resulting retrograde blood flow exacerbates the venous hypertension and the veins become varicose. Very large dilated veins may appear over the point where incompetent communicating veins pierce the deep fascia. These localized varicosities have been called 'blow-out' veins by Cockett[25] and 'blow-down' veins by Gottlob.[42] We prefer the term 'blow-out' because it reminds us of the underlying and more important abnormality.

Capillaries

The venules and venular capillaries also dilate and become tortuous. A cross-section of dermis from an area of the leg showing the skin changes of the calf pump failure syndrome reveals many more capillaries cut in cross-section than a cross-section of normal skin (Fig. 11.10).[18,88]

We have called this 'capillary proliferation' but it is probably mainly elongation and tortuosity of the capillaries rather than an increase in the number of capillaries.[34]

The number of venular capillaries seen in histological preparations of the skin is directly related to the efficiency of the calf pump as assessed by the reduction of foot vein pressure during exercise (Fig. 11.11).[18]

This change can be seen clinically as the leash of small intradermal venules that appears over the medial aspect of the ankle in patients with calf pump failure, known as the *ankle flare* or the

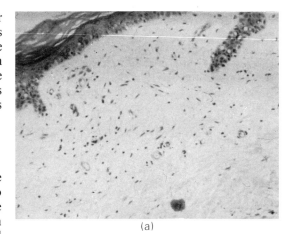

(a)

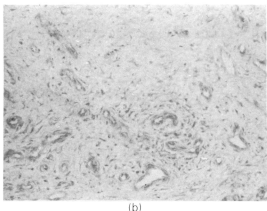

(b)

Fig. 11.10 Photomicrographs of (a) normal skin and (b) skin showing the changes of lipodermatosclerosis. The magnification is slightly different but the increased number of capillaries seen in the abnormal skin is clearly apparent.

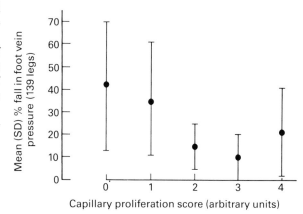

Fig. 11.11 The relationship between the percentage reduction of foot vein pressure during exercise and the number of skin capillaries (capillary proliferation in arbitrary units). The less efficient the calf pump the greater the number of capillaries seen in the skin.

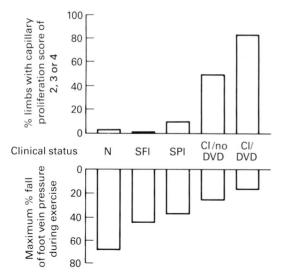

Fig. 11.12 The relationship between the clinical state of the limb and the proliferation of the capillaries in skin biopsies removed from an area 7 cm above the medial malleolus.

N = Normal. SFI = Sapheno-femoral incompetence. SPI = Sapheno-popliteal incompetence. CI/no DVD = Communicating vein incompetence with phlebographically normal deep veins. CI/DVD = Communicating vein incompetence with phlebographic evidence of post-thrombotic deep vein damage.

corona phlebectatica (see Chapter 6 and Colour plate 4). The degree of capillary proliferation is closely related to the clinical severity of the calf pump failure (Fig. 11.12).

Capillary permeability

The dilated elongated dermal capillaries have an increased permeability to large molecules because the raised venous pressure enlarges the inter-epithelial pores, the pathway through which large molecules leave the capillaries. We sought proof of this by measuring the accumulation of radio-actively labelled sodium chloride, albumin and fibrinogen in the fluid that collects in the centre of a Guyton capsule implanted into the subcutaneous tissues of a dog's hind limb with venous hypertension produced by fashioning an A–V fistula at the groin.[16] These experiments showed that the accumulation of fibrinogen in the capsule fluid was significantly greater in the limbs which had a high venous pressure (Fig. 11.13). A similar

increase in extravascular fluid can be seen in man, using skin capillaroscopy, when a halo is seen around the capillaries.[33,35]

Venous hypertension, both acute and long-term, also increases the concentration of fibrinogen in the lymph leaving the limb. An increase in the venous pressure from 2 mmHg to 20 mmHg trebles the lymph flow and doubles the lymph fibrinogen concentration (Table 11.1). As the only source of fibrinogen in lymph is the plasma fibrinogen, the venous hypertension must have made the capillaries more permeable.[7,8,9]

The interstitial spaces

The raised venous pressure and increased capillary permeability increase the flow of capillary transudate through the interstitial spaces. Most of this transudate is cleared by the lymphatics but some remains and is clinically apparent as oedema. Venous hypertension increases the amount of fibrinogen crossing the interstitial spaces by 600 per cent (Table 11.1). Accompanying the fibrinogen are all the other components of plasma including clotting factors, fibrinolytic activators and inhibitors. Our measurements of lymph composition in dogs' legs with venous hypertension showed only a slight reduction of fibrinolytic activator activity but revealed the appearance of an inhibitor of fibrinolysis, α_2-antiplasmin. Thus not only is the amount of fibrinogen passing through the interstitial spaces increased[59,60] but the interstitial fluid also contains

Table 11.1 The effect of venous hypertension on canine hind limb lymph flow and lymph fibrinogen concentration[59]

Acute venous hypertension

Venous pressure (mmHg)	Lymph flow (μl/min)	Lymph fibrinogen (g/l)
2.4	14.0	0.07
18.0	40.5	0.14

(An increased interstitial fluid transport of fibrinogen of 623%)

Chronic venous hypertension

Venous pressure (mmHg)	Lymph flow (μl/min)	Lymph fibrinogen (g/l)
1.0	11.6	0.11
25.0	38.6	0.20

(An increased interstitial fluid transport of fibrinogen of 602%)

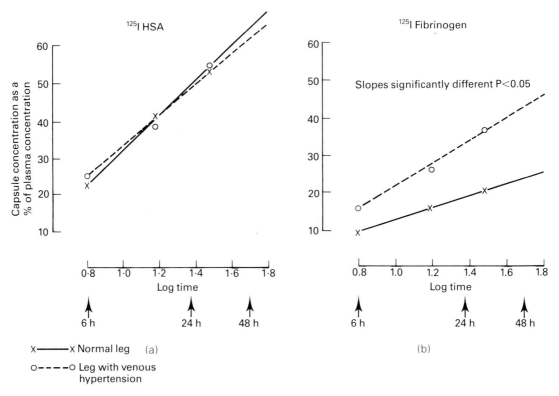

Fig. 11.13 The rate of accumulation of (a) albumin and (b) fibrinogen in Guyton capsules in the subcutaneous tissues of six canine hind limbs with and six limbs without venous hypertension produced by an arteriovenous fistula. The accumulation of fibrinogen in the capsules in the limbs with venous hypertension was significantly increased.

a fibrinolytic inhibitor and less fibrinolytic activator. It may be that these changes explain the deposition of fibrinogen/fibrin around the capillaries.

Careful staining with specific dyes and fluorescent antibodies has revealed layers of fibrinogen/fibrin around the dermal capillaries of lipodermatosclerotic skin.[19] The presence of pericapillary fibrin is associated with calf pump inefficiency. The mean reduction in foot vein pressure during exercise in 26 legs with pericapillary fibrin in their skin biopsies was 18 mmHg, whereas the mean reduction in foot vein pressure during exercise in 15 legs without pericapillary fibrin was 55 mmHg.[15,19] The presence of fibrin also correlates well with the degree of capillary 'proliferation', fibrin only being seen in limbs with an excessive number of dermal capillaries.

The presence of interstitial fibrin may be the result of an increased deposition of fibrin but

could also be caused by a decreased rate of clearance.

Vein wall fibrinolytic activator activity

The amount of fibrinolytic activator produced by the vein wall can be measured by incubating thin slices of vein wall on a fibrin plate and measuring the areas of fibrinolysis (see Fig. 16.3, page 450).[86] Veins taken from limbs with the calf pump failure syndrome have a reduced level of tissue activator activity (Fig. 11.14). Veins from the hands of these patients also have a reduced activity (Fig. 11.15).[15] Furthermore, the plasma fibrinogen is raised, the dilute blood clot lysis time is prolonged and the fibrin plate lysis area is reduced.[14,52] This implies that these patients have a *systemic* reduction of blood and tissue fibrinolytic activity. Whether this is a primary abnormality or is secondary to exhaustion of the activator stores in the

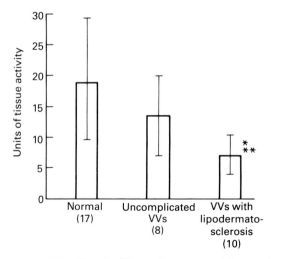

*Significantly different from normal (P=0.001)

**Significantly different from uncomplicated VVs
(P=0.01)

Fig. 11.14 The tissue fibrinolytic activity of veins removed from the feet of normal subjects, limbs with uncomplicated varicose veins and limbs with lipodermatosclerosis. The mean fibrinolytic activity of the veins from the limbs with skin changes was significantly less than the normal (means and standard deviations).

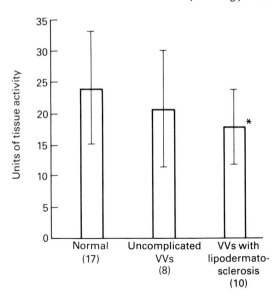

*Significantly different from normal (P=0.05)

Fig. 11.15 The tissue fibrinolytic activity of veins removed from the dorsum of the *hands* of normal subjects and patients with uncomplicated varicose veins and varicose veins (VVs) with lipodermatosclerosis. The mean fibrinolytic activity of the veins from the patients with lipodermatosclerosis was significantly less than the normal (means and standard deviations.)

legs caused by the chronic venous hypertension is not known. In favour of a primary systemic defect is the observation that patients with a history of deep vein thrombosis have a reduced blood fibrinolytic activity.[15] It may be this abnormality which triggers the initial thrombosis and later exacerbates the interstitial changes caused by the damaged calf pump. This hypothesis would explain why only a proportion of a group of patients with similar calf pump dysfunction develop post-thrombotic syndrome skin changes.

Whatever the cause of the fibrinolytic deficiency, it definitely reduces the clearance of subcutaneous fibrin clots in limbs with lipodermatosclerosis (Table 11.2).

Tissue anoxia

Although most venous ulcers are started by an injury, none of the other changes of the calf pump failure syndrome is related to trauma. Skin and subcutaneous tissue fibrosis – which we have called 'lipodermatosclerosis' – and 'atrophie blanche' are the visible evidence of slow tissue death and replacement by scar tissue. The tissue death must be caused by anoxia if there is no trauma and no other detectable chemical or physical cause.

If a sheet of fibrin is studied in a diffusion chamber, it can be shown that it acts as a barrier to oxygen diffusion.[19] Oxygen must leave the capillaries and pass through the interstitial spaces to reach the cells. We have postulated that the layer of fibrin that appears around the capillaries when the calf pump fails acts as a barrier to the passage of oxygen from the blood to the cells so rendering them fatally anoxic (Fig. 11.16).[63]

There is a considerable amount of circumstantial evidence to support this 'fibrin barrier/physiological shunt' hypothesis. A number of workers have shown that the oxygen content of the blood in the veins draining a limb with the post-thrombotic syndrome is increased.[5,6] This could only be caused by physiological shunting or the development of patho-

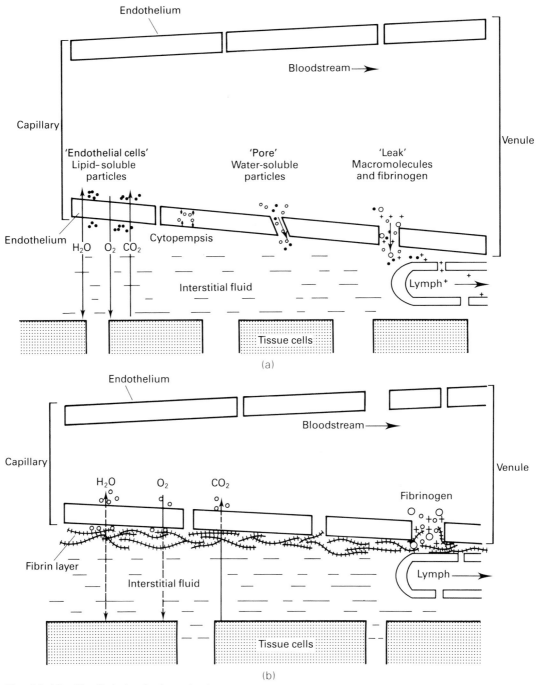

Fig. 11.16 The fibrin barrier hypothesis.

(a) *Normal microcirculation* Under normal circumstances lipid-soluble substances diffuse through the capillary wall and water-soluble substances pass through interendothelial pores to reach the cells.

Excess water and protein are removed by the lymphatics.

(b) *Microcirculation in the calf pump failure syndrome* When there is venular capillary hypertension and a reduced tissue fibrinolysis, fibrin becomes deposited around the capillaries (see Colour plates 25, 26 and 27). This blocks the passage of oxygen and nutrients to the cells and causes cellular anoxia.

Lipodermatosclerosis, which is the slow replacement of the skin and subcutaneous tissues by scar tissue in response to anoxia, is therefore primarily caused by the combination of the increased capillary permeability caused by the venous hypertension and the reduced fibrin/fibrinogen interstitial fluid clearance caused by the reduced plasma and interstitial fluid fibrinolytic activity.

(Modified from Browse and Burnand.)[11]

Table 11.2 The clearance of radioactive fibrin clots from the subcutaneous tissues of normal legs and legs with lipodermatosclerosis[60]
(Subcutaneous clot = 0.05 ml ^{125}I-fibrinogen + 0.05 ml human thrombin)

	Count rate (% of initial injection)			
	24 hr	48 hr	72 hr	5 days
Normal legs	9 ± 1.8	4 ± 0.9	1 ± 0.5	0
Liposclerotic legs	17 ± 2.1*	12 ± 1.6*	8 ± 1.8*	9 ± 2.7*

* $P < 0.001$

logical arteriovenous shunts.[1] Slow flow (stasis) would reduce the oxygen content.

Attempts to detect arteriovenous shunts by physiological methods have failed, though some workers claim, on the basis of arteriography and anatomical dissections, that they do exist.[43,44,76] If arteriovenous fistulae were present, there would be an increased blood flow, a high venous oxygen concentration and a normal or increased tissue oxygen utilization. Studies with Positron Emission Tomography[50] have shown that areas of lipodermatosclerosis have an increased blood flow but a *reduced* oxygen utilization; this finding is consistent with the fibrin barrier/physiological shunt hypothesis.

The permeability of the capillaries in the granulation tissue in the base of venous ulcers has also been shown to be directly related to the mean venous pressure; permeability reverts to normal when the patient is put to bed.[48] If A-V shunts were present, the venous pressure would remain high and the permeability would not fall during bedrest.

Further support for the physiological shunt hypothesis comes from measurements of transcutaneous oxygen tension which have shown that areas of lipodermatosclerosis have significantly lower oxygen diffusion than normal skin,[24] and the observation that the venous hypertension seen in the hand after the formation of an A-V shunt at the wrist causes lesions in the fingers which are similar to those seen in lipodermatosclerosis.[92] In addition to all this evidence we have been unable to develop a hypothesis which would explain how a deep vein thrombosis could cause the development of A-V fistulae in a previously normal limb.

Nevertheless, it must be stressed that the fibrin diffusion barrier explanation for the cause of the tissue changes of the calf pump failure syndrome is a *hypothesis* not a proven fact. The physiological and pathological evidence available to date

supports the fibrin barrier hypothesis, and does not support the stasis or the A–V fistulae hypotheses but only time will tell which is correct.[49]

The lymphatics

The main lymphatic trunks of the limb are normal in patients with primary and post-thrombotic venous disease[69] but the small collecting lymphatics in the skin and subpapillary dermal plexus are abnormal in areas of lipodermatosclerosis. Bollinger has described a lymphatic microangiopathy causing an increase of permeability to fluorescent dextrans,[7,8,9] and Fagrell has described a reduced lymphatic clearance from tissues showing post-thrombotic changes.[35]

A limb which has a chronically raised venous pressure has an increased lymph flow which can be shown by isotope lymphography to be two or three times higher than normal.[83]

Our assessment of the available evidence is that the lymphatics play no part in the initiation of the post-thrombotic syndrome but are affected by the changes in the capillaries and interstitial fluid and thereafter contribute as a secondary factor to the deterioration of the skin and subcutaneous tissues.

Prevalence

It is extremely difficult to determine the prevalence of the calf pump failure (post-thrombotic) syndrome. It certainly does not occur in every patient who has had a venous thrombosis. Indeed, if clinical history, Fibrinogen Uptake Tests and phlebographic studies are accepted, it would appear to affect some patients who have never had a thrombosis. Most workers, however, believe that it is always caused by a thrombosis and refuse to entertain other possibilities.

We think that 'calf pump failure syndrome'

would be a better name than post-thrombotic syndrome as this would encompass pump failure associated hereditary varicose veins or a fibrinolytic deficiency without evidence of an initiating thrombosis.

As there is no clear definition of the post-thrombotic syndrome, estimation of its incidence is extremely difficult. The symptoms and signs may vary from mild pain to severe venous claudication and from an ankle flare with a little pigmentation to a large ulcer.

Estimates of the prevalence of venous ulcers lie between 0.1 per cent and 0.25 per cent (see Chapter 13). If we knew the proportion of patients with the post-thrombotic syndrome that had ulcers, we could deduce the prevalence of the post-thrombotic syndrome.

The incidence of varicose veins, chronic venous insufficiency and ulcers in the 4529 people (3744 men, 785 women) examined in the Basle survey was 45 per cent, 15 per cent and 1 per cent respectively.[31,89] 'Chronic venous insufficiency' occurred in 16 per cent of the men and 13 per cent of the women. 'Chronic venous insufficiency without ulceration' was also divided into mild, medium and severe, medium being hyperpigmentation or hypopigmentation with or without a 'corona phlebectatica'. If it is accepted that these changes are the early signs of calf pump failure, the Basle study suggests that calf pump failure was present in 6 per cent of men and 5 per cent of women.

This means that the prevalence of calf pump failure is five times that of ulceration. If we accept a figure of 0.1–0.2 per cent as the prevalence of ulceration in the Western Hemisphere (one-tenth of that of the Basle III study), between 5 and 10 of every 1000 adults over the age of 25 years have an inadequate calf pump.

All the epidemiological studies have shown an increasing incidence with age, approximately tenfold in men and twenty-fold in women between the ages of 25 years and 65 years. As many as 100–200 of every 1000 women (10–20 per cent) over the age of 65 years have some signs of chronic venous insufficiency which are compatible with a diagnosis of calf pump failure syndrome.[10] The prevalence in men is half this figure.[21]

The obvious difference in a woman's life compared to a man's life is pregnancy and childbirth. Both events are known to be complicated by venous dilatation and deep vein thrombosis. This supports the belief that thrombosis, even though small and unnoticed, is the main cause of calf pump failure and helps to justify the continued use of the term post-thrombotic syndrome.

Mudge and Hughes[64] reviewed the limbs that developed a deep vein thrombosis during a study of Dextran prophylaxis, 5 and 10 years later. They found 26 out of 564 (4.5 per cent) patients had a post-thrombotic syndrome but this was present before the operation in 14 (2.5 per cent). Their pre-operative incidence matches the prevelance figures discussed above, and the post-operative incidence of 4.5 per cent suggests that a major traumatic event in a person's life such as a surgical operation doubles the chances of developing a post-thrombotic syndrome.

The problem is massive. In a country with a population of 50 million, between 250,000 and 500,000 people will have a post-thrombotic syndrome. This figure will increase steadily as the mean age of the population rises. There are 8.0 million people over 65 years old in the United Kingdom – 3.2 million men and 4.8 million women. At least 0.65 million (160 000 men and 480 000 women) probably have clinical evidence of the calf pump failure – post-thrombotic syndrome.

References

1. Arnoldi CC, Linderholm H. On the pathogenesis of venous leg ulcer. *Acta Chir Scand* 1968; **134**: 427.
2. Bauer G. A roentgenological and clinical study of the sequels of thrombosis. *Acta Chir Scand* 1942; **86** (supply 74): 1.
3. Bergqvist D, Jaroszewski H. Deep vein thrombosis in patients with superficial thrombophlebitis of the leg. *Br Med J* 1986; **292**: 658.
4. Bergvall U, Hjelmstedt A. Recanalization of deep venous thrombosis of the lower leg and thigh. A phlebographic study of fracture cases. *Acta Chir Scand* 1968; **134**: 219.
5. Blalock A. Oxygen content of blood in patients with varicose veins. *Arch Surg* 1929; **19**: 898.
6. Blumoff RL, Johnson G. Saphenous vein pO_2 in patients with varicose veins. *J Surg Res* 1977; **23**: 35.
7. Bollinger A, Jäger K, Geser A, Sgier F, Seglias J. Transcapillary and interstitial diffusion of Na-fluorescein in chronic venous insufficiency with white atrophy. *Int J Microcirc Clin Exp* 1982; **1**: 5.

8. Bollinger A, Jäger K, Roten A, Timeus C, Mahler F. Diffusion, pericapillary distribution and clearance of Na-fluorescein in the human nailfold. *Pflügers Arch Ges Physiol* 1979; **382**: 137.

9. Bollinger A, Jäger K. Trans and pericapillary diffusion of Na-fluorescein in scleroderma and venous insufficiency. *Bibl Anat* 1981; **20**: 679.

10. Borschberg E. *The Prevalence of Varicose Veins in the Lower Extremities*. Karger 1967.

11. Browse NL, Burnand KG. The cause of venous ulceration. *Lancet* 1982; **2**: 243.

12. Browse NL, Clemenson G, Lea Thomas M. Is the postphlebitic leg always postphlebitic? Relation between phlebographic appearance of deep vein thrombosis and late sequelae. *Br Med J* 1980; **282**: 1167.

13. Browse NL, Clemenson G. Sequelae of an[125] I-fibrinogen detected thrombosis. *Br Med J* 1974; **2**: 468.

14. Browse NL, Gray L, Jarrett PEM. Blood and vein wall fibrinolytic activity in health and vascular disease. *Br Med J* 1977; **1**: 478.

15. Burnand KG, Browse NL. The post-phlebitic leg and venous ulceration. In: Russell RCG (Ed) *Recent Advances in Surgery II*. Edinburgh. Churchill Livingstone 1982.

16. Burnand KG, Clemenson G, Whimster I, Gaunt J, Browse NL. The effect of sustained venous hypertension on the skin capillaries of the canine hind limb. *Br J Surg* 1982; **69**: 41.

17. Burnand KG, O'Donnell TF, Lea Thomas M, Browse NL. The relative importance of incompetent communicating veins in the production of varicose veins and venous ulcers. *Surgery* 1977; **82**: 9.

18. Burnand KG, Whimster I, Clemenson G, Lea Thomas M, Browse NL. The relationship between the number of capillaries in the skin of the venous ulcer bearing area of the lower leg and the fall in foot vein pressure during exercise. *Br J Surg* 1981; **68**: 297.

19. Burnand KG, Whimster I, Naidoo A, Browse NL. Pericapillary fibrin in the ulcer bearing skin of the leg. *Br Med J* 1982; **285**: 1071.

20. Byrne JJ. Phlebitis. A study of 748 cases at the Boston City Hospital. *N Engl J Med* 1955; **253**: 579.

21. Callam MJ, Ruckley CV, Harper DR, Dale JJ. Chronic ulceration of the leg: extent of the problem and provision of care. *Br Med J* 1985; **290**: 1855.

22. Chakrabarti R, Birks PM, Fearnley GR. Origin of blood fibrinolytic activity from veins and its bearing on the fate of venous thrombi. *Lancet* 1963; **1**: 1288.

23. Clayton JK, Anderson JA, McNicol GP. Preoperative prediction of post operative deep vein thrombosis. *Br Med J* 1976; **2**: 910.

24. Clyne CAC, Ramsden WH, Chant ADB, Webster JHH. Oxygen tension in the skin of the gaiter area of limbs with venous disease. *Br J Surg* 1985; **72**; 644.

25. Cockett FB, Elgan Jones DE. The ankle blow-out syndrome. *Lancet* 1953; **1**: 17.

26. Cockett FB, Thomas ML. The iliac compression syndrome. *Br J Surg* 1965; **52**: 816.

27. Coon WW. Problems in thromboembolism. *Surg Clin North Am* 1961; **41**: 1343.

28. Corrigan TP, Kakkar VV. Early changes in the postphlebitic limb: their clinical significance. *Br J Surg* 1973; 60: 808.

29. Cotton LT, Clark C. Anatomical localization of venous thrombosis. *Ann R Coll Surg Engl* 1965; **36**: 214.

30. Cranley JJ, Krause RJ, Strasser ES. Chronic venous insufficiency of the lower extremity. *Surgery* 1961; **49**: 48.

31. Da Silva A, Widmer LK, Martin H, Mall TH, Claus L, Schneider M. Varicose veins and chronic venous insufficiency. *Vasa* 1974; **3**: 118.

32. Edwards EA, Edwards JE. Effects of thrombophlebitis on venous valves. *Surg Gynec Obstet* 1937; **65**: 310.

33. Fagrell B. Local microcirculation in chronic venous incompetence and leg ulcers. *Vasc Surg* 1979; **13**: 217.

34. Fagrell B. Microcirculatory changes of the skin in venous disorders of the leg; studied by vital capillaroscopy. In: Schneider KW (Ed) *Die Venose Insuffizienz*. Baden-Baden. Witztrock 1972; 202.

35. Fagrell B. Microcirculatory disturbances – the final cause for venous ulcers. *Vasa* 1982; **11**: 101.

36. Fell SC, McIntosh HD, Hornsby AT, Horton CE, Warren JV, Pickrell K. The syndrome of the chronic leg ulcer. The phlebodynamics of the lower extremity: physiology of the venous valves. *Surgery* 1955; **38**: 771.

37. Fine J, Starr A. The surgical therapy of thrombosis of the deep veins of the lower extremity. *Surgery* 1945; **17**: 232.

38. Flanc C, Kakkar VV, Clarke MB. The detection of venous thrombosis of the legs using[125] I-labelled fibrinogen. *Br J Surg* 1968; **55**: 742.

39. Gibbs NM. Venous thrombosis of the lower limbs with particular reference to bed rest. *Br J Surg* 1957; **45**: 209.

40. Gjöres JF. The incidence of venous thrombosis and its sequelae in certain districts of Sweden. *Acta Chir Scand* 1956; Suppl **206**.

41. Gordon-Smith IC, Hickman JA, LeQuesne LP. Postoperative fibrinolytic activity and deep vein thrombosis. *Br J Surg* 1974; **61**: 213.

42. Gottleb R. The clinical insignificance of the rami perforantes or communicantes in primary vari-

coses. In: May R, Partsch H, Staubesand J (Eds) *Perforating Veins*. Munich Urban & Scharzenberg 1981.

43. Guis J A. Arteriovenous anastomoses and varicose veins. *Arch Surg* 1960; **81**: 299.

44. Haimovici H. Arteriovenous shunting in varicose veins. *J Vasc Surg* 1985; **2**: 684.

45. Hamer J D, Malone P C, Silver I A. The pO$_2$ in venous valve pockets. Its possible bearing on thrombogenesis. *Br J Surg* 1981; **68**: 166.

46. Hedner U, Nilsson I M, Isaacson S. Effect of ethyl-oestranol on fibrinolysis in the vessel wall. *Br Med J* 1976; **2**: 729.

47. Hoare M C, Nicolaides A N, Miles C R, Shull K, Jury R P, Needham T N, Dudley H A F. The role of primary varicose veins in venous ulceration. *Br J Radiol* 1971; **44**: 653.

48. Hopkins N F G, Jamieson C W. Antibiotic concentration in the exudate of venous ulcers. A measure of local arterial insufficiency. *Br J Surg* 1982; **69** (Suppl): 676.

49. Hopkins N F G, Jamieson C W. Diffusion barriers in venous ulceration. *J R Soc Med* 1985; **78**: 355.

50. Hopkins N F G, Spinks T J, Rhodes C G, Ranicar A S O, Jamieson C W. Positron emission tomography in venous ulceration and liposclerosis, study of regional tissue function. *Br Med J* 1983; **286**: 333.

51. Hume M, Chan Y K. Examination of the blood in the presence of venous thrombosis. *JAMA* 1967; **200**: 747.

52. Isaacson S, Nilson I M. Defective fibrinolysis in blood and vein walls in recurrent idopathic venous thrombosis. *Acta Chir Scand* 1972; **138**: 313.

53. Kakkar V V, Howe C T, Flanc C, Clarke M B. Natural history of postoperative deep vein thrombosis. *Lancet* 1969; **2**: 230.

54. Killewich L A, Martin R, Cramer M, Beach K W, Strandness D E. An objective assessment of the physiologic changes in the post thrombotic syndrome. *Arch Surg* 1985; **120**: 424.

55. Kwaan H C, Astrup T. Fibrinolytic activity in thrombosed veins. *Circ Res* 1965; **17**: 477.

56. Lawrence D, Kakkar V V. Post phlebitic syndrome – a functional assessment. *Br J Surg* 1980; **67**: 686.

57. Lawrence D. *Haemodynamic Studies Relating to the Postphlebitic Syndrome*. MS Thesis. London University 1982.

58. Lea Thomas M, McAllister V. The radiological progression of deep vein thrombosis. *Radiology* 1971; **99**: 37.

59. Leach R D, Browse N L. Effects of venous hypertension on canine hind limb lymph. *Br J Surg* 1985; **72**: 275.

60. Leach R D. Venous ulceration, fibrinogen and

fibrinolysis. *Ann R Coll Surg Engl* 1984; **66**; 258.

61. Lindhagen A, Bergqvist D, Hallbook T. Deep venous insufficiency after post operative thrombosis diagnosed with ^{125}I labelled fibrinogen uptake test. *Br J Surg* 1984; **71**: 511.

62. Luke J C. The deep vein valves: a venographic study in normal and post-phlebitic limbs. *Surgery* 1951; **29**: 381.

63. May R, Thurner J. Ein Gefässsporn in der V. iliaca communis sinistra als Ursache der vorwiegend linksseitigen Beckenvenenthrombosen. *Z Kreislaufforsch* 1956; **45**: 912.

64. Mudge M, Hudges L E. The long term sequelae of deep vein thrombosis. *Br J Surg* 1978; **65**: 692.

65. Negus D, Cockett F B. Femoral vein pressures in postphlebitic iliac vein obstruction. *Br J Surg* 1967; **54**: 522.

66. Negus D, Pinto D J, Le Quesne L P, Brown N, Chapman M. ^{125}I-labelled fibrinogen in the diagnosis of deep vein thrombosis and its correlation with phlebography. *Br J Surg* 1968; **55**: 835.

67. Negus D. Calf pain in the post thrombotic syndrome. *Br Med J* 1968; **2**: 156.

68. Negus D. Prevention and treatment of venous ulceration. *Ann R Coll Surg Engl* 1985; **17**: 144.

69. Negus D. The iliac veins in relation to lymph-oedema. *Br J Surg* 1969; **56**: 481.

70. Nicolaides A N, Clark C T, Thomas R D, Lewis J D. Soleal veins and local fibrinolytic activity. *Br J Surg* 1972; **59**: 914.

71. Nicolaides A N, Kakkar V V, Field E S, Renney J T G. The origin of deep vein thrombosis. *Br J Radiol* 1971; **44**: 653.

72. Nilsson I M, Isacson S. New aspects of the pathogenesis of thrombo-embolism. In: Allgower M, Bergentz S E (Eds) *Progress in Surgery*. Basel. Karker 1973.

73. Pandolfi M, Isacson S and Nilsson I M. Low fibrinolytic activity in the walls of veins of patients with thrombosis. *Acta Med Scand* 1969; **186**: 1.

74. Phillips R S. Prognosis in deep vein thrombosis. *Arch Surg* 1963; **87**: 44.

75. Recek E. A critical appraisal of the role of the ankle perforators for the genesis of venous ulcers in the lower leg. *J Cardiovasc Surg* 1971; **12**: 45.

76. Schalin L. Arteriovenous communications to varicose veins in the lower extremities studied by dynamic angiography. *Acta Chir Scand* 1980; **146**: 397.

77. Sethia K K, Darke S G. Long saphenous incompetence as a cause of venous ulceration. *Br J Surg* 1984; **71**: 754.

78. Sevitt S, Gallagher N G. Venous thrombosis and pulmonary embolism. A clinico pathological study in injured and burned patients. *Br J Surg* 1961; **48**: 475.

79. Sevitt S. The mechanism of canalization of deep vein thrombosis. *J Pathol* 1973; **110**: 153.

80. Sevitt S. The structure and growth of valve-pocket thrombi in femoral veins. *J Clin Pathol* 1974; **27**: 517.

81. Shull KC, Nicolaides AN, Fernandes E Fernandes J, Miles C, Horner J, Needham T, Cooke ED, Eastcott FH. Significance of popliteal reflux in relationship to ambulatory venous pressure and ulceration. *Arch Surg* 1979; **114**: 1304.

82. Stamatakis JD, Kakkar VV, Lawrence D, Bentley PG. The origin of thrombi in the deep veins of the lower limb: a venographic study. *Br J Surg* 1978; **65**: 449.

83. Stewart G, Gaunt J, Croft DN, Browse NL. Isotope lymphography, a new method of investigating the role of the lymphatics in chronic limb oedema. *Br J Surg* 1985; **72**: 906.

84. Thomas ML, O'Dwyer JA. Site of origin of deep vein thrombosis in the calf. *Acta Radiol (Diagn) (Stockh)* 1977; **4**: 418.

85. Thuleseius O, Gjöres JE, Eriksson O, Berlin E. Mechanische und biochemische Voraussetzungen der chronisch-venosen insuffizienz. *Vasa* 1984; **13**: 195.

86. Todd AS. The histological localization of fibrinolysis activator. *J Path Bacteriol* 1959; **78**: 281.

87. Tripolitis AJ, Milligan EB, Bodily KC, Strandness DE Jr. The physiology of venous claudication. *Am J Surg* 1980; **139**: 447.

88. Whimster I. In Dodd H, Cockett FB (Eds) *The Pathology and Surgery of Veins of the Lower Limb*. Edinburgh. Churchill Livingstone 1953.

89. Widmer LK, Zemp E, Widmer MTh, Schmitt HE, Brandenberg E, Voelin R, Biland L, da Silva A, Maggs M. Late results in deep vein thrombois of the lower extremity. *Vasa* 1985; **14**: 264.

90. Widmer LK. *Peripheral Venous Disorders*. Bern. Hans Huber 1978.

91. Wolfe JHN, Morland M, Browse NL. The fibrinolytic activity of varicose veins. *Br J Surg* 1979; **66**: 185.

92. Wood ML, Reilly GD, Smith GT. Ulceration of the hand secondary to a radial arteriovenous fistula, a model for varicose ulceration. *Br Med J* 1983; **287**: 1167.

93. Young AE, Thomas ML, Browse NL. Comparison between sequelae of surgical and medical treatment of venous thromboembolism. *Br Med J* 1974; **4**: 127.

12

The calf pump failure syndrome: diagnosis and treatment

The development of symptoms after a deep vein thrombosis is not entirely predictable. Nevertheless a considerable proportion of patients will get problems in their legs after a deep vein thrombosis which are sufficiently distinctive to be recognizable as the clinical syndrome known as the post-thrombotic syndrome, but more easily understood as 'the calf pump failure syndrome'.

Diagnosis

Clinical presentation

History

Not every patient with the post-thrombotic syndrome gives a history of a deep vein thrombosis. Some patients have never been seriously ill, undergone surgery or had any previous leg symptoms. The phlebograms of many of these patients are normal which makes one question whether their symptoms are truly post-thrombotic (see Chapter 11). In our experience less than one-third of patients with a post-thrombotic syndrome give a definite history of a previous deep vein thrombosis. It is easy for patients to forget past events and they may not have been told their diagnosis; when taking a history it is therefore important to ask directly about episodes of leg swelling or pain in relation to pregnancy, to the puerperium, to previous operations, or to accidents. A number of women will deny a history of 'thrombosis' but then inform you that they had a 'white leg' after the birth of a child! Thromboembolic events are sometimes familial; it is therefore important to ask about a family history of varicose veins, venous thrombosis or pulmonary embolism.

Symptoms and signs

Pain and tenderness The most common complaint is of *an aching pain* in the leg that is exacerbated by standing. The pain is felt in the muscles of the calf or thigh and is relieved by rest and elevation of the leg. The muscles are not particularly tender.

Localized *throbbing pain* may be felt over areas of acute lipodermatosclerosis and superficial thrombophlebitis.

Ischaemic skin about to break down and form into an ulcer often causes *persistent pain* which is not relieved by rest and is similar to the rest pain of arterial ischaemia. The surrounding skin is often very tender but the centre may be numb.

Venous claudication is a *bursting pain* experienced during exercise. It occurs when there is severe outflow obstruction and venous hypertension during exercise. The bursting sensation is felt deep inside the leg, mainly below the knee, though a few patients complain that the thigh becomes painful before the calf. The amount of exercise needed to produce the pain is not so constant and reproducible as that needed to cause the pain of arterial claudication. When the muscles are tense and 'bursting' they are usually tender. The acute pain subsides quickly with rest and elevation but a residual dull ache and mild tenderness often persists for some time.

Swelling Oedema caused by venous obstruction may vary from mild ankle swelling to gross oedema of the whole leg from the foot to the groin. If the inferior vena cava (IVC) has been thrombosed, the oedema may extend into the lower abdominal wall and over the buttocks. The oedema of venous obstruction varies from day to day, is soft, pits easily and is not tender. It subsides rapidly with bedrest and limb elevation.

Localized oedema occurs in areas of lipodermatosclerosis and thrombophlebitis. An oedematous patch of acute lipodermatosclerosis, found commonly in the gaiter area of the leg, is usually hot, red and tender with an easily palpable edge.

Varicose veins The subcutaneous veins become dilated after a deep vein thrombosis for two reasons. First, they are distended by the high venous pressures in the leg that follow the outflow obstruction and the valvular incompetence of the communicating veins. Secondly, they enlarge to carry more blood as they become collateral channels bypassing the occluded deep veins.

Some patients with the post-thrombotic syndrome have no visible varicose veins, and it was their absence in some patients with venous ulcers that confused the early physicians and stopped them recognizing the 'venous' nature of many ulcers.

When varicose veins do appear they may be situated anywhere but are often most prominent on the lower medial third of the leg, close to the important communicating veins. A very large dilated vein over the site of an incompetent communicating vein is often called a *blow-out*.[19]

The long and short saphenous veins and their tributaries may also be dilated and incompetent, particularly when they are acting as collateral veins. Dilatation is more common in patients who had varicose veins before their thrombosis or who have a family history of varicose veins.

Post-thrombotic communicating vein incompetence often causes lower leg varicosities but may take many years to make the whole subcutaneous venous system dilated and incompetent. Once incompetent, the communicating veins may act as *collateral vessels*, but the direction in which blood flows in lower leg varicose veins during exercise cannot be deduced from their size or site.

Varicose veins which appear in the upper thigh, groin and lower abdomen following an iliofemoral thrombosis are usually acting as collaterals. Large dilated veins at the root of the limb and crossing the groin are diagnostic of an iliac vein obstruction.

Varicose veins that appear as a sequel to deep vein damage cause the same symptoms as primary varicose veins, namely aching pains, night-cramps, mild oedema and cosmetic disfigurement. They are often the patient's *presenting complaint*, especially if the patient is unaware of the initial thrombotic episode.

It is important to remember the patient's principal symptoms and their cause when phlebograms and other minor symptoms are tempting you to perform deep vein surgery.

Intradermal venules Chronic venous hypertension dilates the veins, the venules and the venular capillaries (see Chapter 11). This is manifest clinically by the appearance of fine dilated veins in the skin. They bulge up under the epidermis making the skin bosselated and irregular. They are prone to localized thrombosis. This turns them into small black nodules which eventually peel off and may bleed profusely after minor trauma. Intradermal venules are commonly seen in a triangular area, whose apex begins just above the medial malleolus and whose base is at the edge of the sole of the foot. This patch of dilated venules has been called the *ankle flare*,[19] or the corona phlebectactica[84] (see Colour plate 4). This is an apt description and its presence indicates long-standing calf pump failure, usually caused by communicating vein incompetence.

Venous 'stars' The valves begin in venules which are 1 mm in diameter. If the first few valves of a venule become incompetent, the fine venular capillaries become distended and are visible on the skin as fine thread-like red–purple vessels. Their draining vein is situated either at their centre – the vessels radiating from it like the spokes of a wheel (hence the name 'stars')–,or at one corner with the vessels radiating out in a triangle. Extensive venous stars can give the skin of the whole leg an unsightly blue colour. Venous stars can occur in normal limbs without varicose veins and their aetiology and significance is therefore far from clear. They cause distress solely because of the cosmetic disfigurement. They do not cause pain or bleeding and are clinically and prognostically insignificant when compared with the intradermal venules discussed above.

Pigmentation Prolonged venous hypertension causes venular dilatation and the extrusion of red blood cells through the interendothelial pores. The red cells are broken down and absorbed but the *haemosiderin* remains as a brown pigment staining the skin.

Pigmentation occurs mainly on the lower

medial third of the lower leg but may slowly spread around the leg to involve the whole of the 'gaiter' area. (see Colour plate 6).

As the years pass the pigmentation may get darker and eventually look almost black. The epidermis over such pigmented skin tends to become hypertrophic and scaly, probably as a result of the venous hypertension rather than as a response to the pigment.

Pigmentation may also occur in a linear form over the course of a subcutaneous vein and commonly occurs over a segment of superficial thrombophlebitis. The more vigorous the inflammatory response, the more likely it is that the inflammatory exudate will contain red cells.

Dermatitis Dermatitis appears over prominent subcutaneous varicose veins and in areas of skin which have been subjected to chronic venous hypertension – usually the lower medial third of the leg. These changes are presumably a response to venous congestion, fibrin, and haemosiderin deposition and local oedema but the exact mechanism is not known.

Venous dermatitis (or 'varicose eczema') may be dry and scaly or vesicular, 'ulcerated' and weeping. Once the epidermis is lost there is a serious risk that a venous ulcer may develop but as this is not an invariable sequence of events it is likely that the disorders of the microcirculation that cause the dermatitis are not always the same as those that cause ulcers. Ulcers are invariably started by minor local trauma, dermatitis is not. The difference between ulceration and dermatitis is particularly apparent in the patient with a linear patch of dermatitis over a large vein on the lateral aspect of the thigh, a site at which venous ulcers are never found.

The skin of patients with chronic venous disease appears to be more sensitive than normal. *Contact dermatitis* in response to any or all of the medicaments placed on ulcers, to the rubber in elastic bandages, and to the creams in impregnated bandages is extremely common. This may be induced sensitization from repeated dressings but it is so common that it is conceivable that chronic venous hypertension, in some unknown way, increases skin sensitivity to chemical agents.

Lipodermatosclerosis This is a rather unwieldy term which we coined to describe the progressive fibrosis of the skin and subcutaneous tissues induced by chronic venous hypertension.[13] Other investigators have called it fat necrosis, panniculitis and chronic cellulitis but none of these names indicates the true pathology.

It appears in two forms – acute or chronic. It is usually found on the lower medial third of the leg but sometimes spreads around the whole of the lower third of the limb (the gaiter area) and occasionally higher up the calf. The acute variety eventually becomes chronic, but the chronic variety can develop without passing through an acute stage.

Acute lipodermatosclerosis is a painful disabling condition. It begins as a thickened, sometimes slightly raised red–brown, tender area in the skin of the lower leg (see Colour plate 7). The patient's main complaint is of pain and tenderness and a constant sensation of heat. The area gradually enlarges and has a distinct edge. The edge is not elevated like that of erysipelas but there is a palpable change between the hot red tense skin and subcutaneous tissue and the soft normal tissue. The redness, heat and tenderness frequently lead to a mistaken diagnosis of cellulitis or thrombophlebitis. The afflicted area may increase in size or the centre may suddenly break down and ulcerate.

The inguinal lymph nodes are not enlarged and the patient does not have a pyrexia or a leucocytosis. Acute lipodermatosclerosis occasionally resolves spontaneously but usually progresses to the chronic form, if an ulcer does not supervene.

Chronic lipodermatosclerosis may develop spontaneously or from burnt-out acute lipodermatosclerosis. The skin is stiff and shiny and fixed to the hard indurated contracting subcutaneous tissues. It has a palpable edge, and the dilated veins within it feel like deep pits. The skin is not red and hot but brown and shiny.

The progressive contraction of the skin and subcutaneous tissues make the gaiter area shrink and, with slight oedema of the calf above, gives the leg an inverted 'champagne bottle' shape (see Colour plate 8).

The pigmented skin is often scarred from previous ulceration and the subcutaneous fat may become calcified, and feel rock hard.

Atrophie blanche Skin can die and be replaced by scar tissue without ulcerating or sloughing. Atrophie blanche is the name given to small areas of skin scarring caused by chronic venous hypertension (and in other circumstances by arteritis).

The patches are grey–white and usually only a few millimetres in diameter. They form a slight depression on the skin surface and are covered with a thin transparent-looking epithelium which may be surrounded by a halo of fine dilated venules (see Colour plate 9).

Sometimes multiple small areas of atrophie blanche coalesce to form a large scar. These larger scars are fragile and may break down spontaneously or following minimal trauma to become an ulcer.

Stiffness of the ankle joint   The progressive subcutaneous thickening and scarring of lipodermatosclerosis may also extend into the subcutaneous tissue around the ankle joint. This restricts ankle movements, reduces calf pump efficiency and exacerbates the venous hypertension. The ankle joint may become completely fixed by scar tissue – *a fibrous ankylosis.*

Fixed plantar flexion   Chronic pain from lipodermatosclerosis or an ulcer makes patients avoid bearing weight on the sole of the foot. The patient limps on the toes of the affected leg to reduce ankle movements and gradually the ankle stiffens in plantar flexion and the Achilles tendon shortens. The calf muscles do not contract as the patient limps and calf pump efficiency diminishes. Painful callosities form on the ball of the foot and toes which also impede walking.

Walking with a plantar flexed ankle disturbs the whole leg, the knee, hip, and back, and can exacerbate any pre-existing symptoms of osteoarthritis.

Periostitis   Long-standing inflammation in the subcutaneous tissues may induce a hyperaemia in the underlying periosteum which then produces new subperiosteal bone. This can sometimes be felt as patchy thickening and roughening of the subcutaneous surface of the lower third of the tibia but is more often a coincidental finding observed on a plain radiograph (Fig. 12.1).

Ulceration   All the conditions described above and collectively called the post-thrombotic syndrome are pre-ulcer changes. They are the signs of impaired tissue oxygenation and slow tissue death which can be exacerbated in minutes by an injury and then progress rapidly to ulceration, Venous ulceration is discussed in detail in Chapters 13, 14 and 15.

Investigations

There are two main objectives in investigating a patient with symptoms and signs suggestive of the

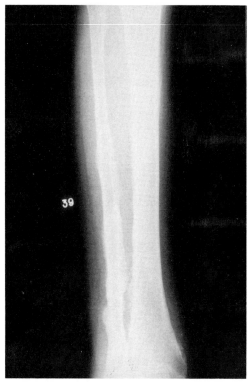

Fig. 12.1   A plain radiograph showing periosteal new bone formation on the surface of the fibula underneath an area of chronic lipodermatosclerosis and recurrent ulceration.

post-thrombotic syndrome. The first is to confirm the diagnosis, the second is to assess the severity of the venous disease and the possible forms of treatment. The investigations comprise a general physical examination, blood studies and special radiological tests.

Investigations to exclude other diagnoses

Other conditions which cause symptoms and signs which can be confused with the calf pump failure syndrome are given below.

Peripheral arterial disease

Arterial insufficiency can cause muscle pain on exercise, pain in the leg when at rest and skin ulceration. In each of these circumstances there will be some detectable abnormality of the arterial circulation such as pallor of the limb, absent peripheral pulses or arterial bruits. Many elderly patients have both peripheral arterial and venous disease, and it is sometimes difficult to decide which system is the cause of the symptoms. Special tests such as ankle arterial pressure measurements using Doppler ultrasound after treadmill exercise may be needed before arterial insufficiency can be excluded as a cause of symptoms.

Myositis and arteritis

These both cause muscle pains which are exacerbated by exercise and relieved by rest. Clinical examination may reveal persistent tenderness in the muscles after exercise and tenderness of the upper limb muscles. The erythrocyte sedimentation rate (ESR) is usually raised and there may be abnormal levels of immunoglobulins in the blood. A biopsy of the muscles or arteries may be needed to confirm the diagnosis.

Deep vein thrombosis

An acute thrombosis will not cause skin changes but may occur in a limb which is already the site of post-thrombotic damage and exacerbate the existing pain and swelling. Sudden onset of pain, calf tenderness and mild oedema should arouse suspicion of this diagnosis. Phlebography is the quickest and most accurate method for excluding fresh thrombus.

Arteriovenous fistulae

These can cause pain, varicose veins and skin ulceration – which are all symptoms of the post-thrombotic syndrome. This diagnosis should be suspected if the patient is young, the limb is hot and enlarged and if there are flow murmurs over the main limb arteries. Arteriography and measurements of peripheral blood flow will confirm or exclude this diagnosis.

Lymphoedema

Lymphoedema is a possible diagnosis if the swelling is marked, the skin healthy and the varicose veins sparse. Lymphoedema can be distinguished from venous oedema by isotope lymphangiography. Venous oedema causes an increase of lymph flow, while in lymphoedema the lymph flow is reduced.

Other causes of pigmentation and dermatitis

The whole of the patient's skin should be carefully examined. Abnormalities in skin not subjected to chronic venous hypertension should raise the possibility of a primary skin disease. Biopsy of lesions on the legs and elsewhere may be necessary to determine whether pigmentation or dermatitis is venous in orgin.

Locally applied medicaments may make the skin pigmented. A careful history should be taken of all previous local and systemic treatment.

Atrophie blanche

This can be caused by cutaneous vasculitis. The clue is often found in the site of the scarring. If the white patches are on the toes or feet and the other signs of venous insufficiency are unconvincing, the efficiency of the calf pump should be measured and, if it is normal, the blood should be examined for evidence of abnormal immunoglobulins and rheumatoid factors. These tests are often unhelpful, and non-venous atrophie blanche is often diagnosed by exclusion after finding that the calf pump function tests and the phlebograms are normal.

Rheumatoid arthritis

This may present with acute pain and redness of the subcutaneous tissues. Joint pain and immobility is usually severe. Serological tests and radiographs will help confirm this diagnosis.

Cellulitis

Acute lipodermatosclerosis is red, hot and tender, as is cellulitis, but the former has a long history and does not cause a pyrexia, lymphangitis, a leucocytosis or inguinal lymphadenopathy. A diagnostic course of antibiotics may, however, be the only way to prove that an area of lipodermatosclerosis is not a subcutaneous infection.

Superfical thrombophlebitis

If the inflammation in the vein is severe and spreads into the surrounding tissues, it may be difficult to confirm the diagnosis of superficial thrombophlebitis by feeling the underlying 'cord-like' thrombosed vein. Superficial thrombophlebitis is rarely confined to the lower third of the leg and settles quickly with bedrest. Phlebography is not helpful unless it shows thrombus in other veins.

Neurological disease

Peripheral neuropathy, ankle deformities, ulcers and oedema can all complicate neurological disease. A full neurological examination of the limb is essential.

Periostitis

This may be noticed by chance on a radiograph. Other causes of periostitis (e.g. ulcerative colitis) must be excluded.

Comment The differential diagnoses of the post-thrombotic calf pump failure syndrome can be excluded in most patients by a careful clinical history and examination. Simple blood tests, the occasional skin biopsy, phlebograms and arteriograms will help sort out the confusing clinical situation where the patient has post-thrombotic type symptoms and signs but normal calf pump function test results. The differential diagnoses of leg ulcers are discussed in Chapter 14.

Investigations to confirm and assess the severity of the venous disease

Clinical examination

The severity of the pain and the extent of the swelling, pigmentation and lipodermatosclerosis indicate the severity of the damage to the micro-circulation but are poorly related to the crude measurements of calf pump function that are available and often have little correlation with the phlebographic abnormalities. It is therefore important to remember while performing special investigations on the veins that the main object is to treat the symptoms not just the anatomical or physiological abnormalities demonstrated by the investigations; this objective can often be achieved with an elastic stocking. Surgery should be the last form of treatment.

Whatever treatment is prescribed it is important to know which aspect of calf pump physiology is abnormal. The *tourniquet tests* should be used during clinical examination to see if the long or short saphenous systems or the communicating veins are incompetent. The latter assessment is difficult if the veins are not prominent and the tissues are thickened. Laboratory tests are more informative.

Tests of calf pump efficiency

The simple methods of assessing calf pump function are useful for confirming the presence of a venous abnormality and obtaining an estimate of its severity.

The best assessment of pump function is to measure venous emptying during exercise. This can be qualitatively assessed with *photoplethysmography*, which can be crudely calibrated to make it semi-quantitative. We find, however, that the simplest quantitative method is *foot volumetry*. This method gives a measure of venous emptying and refilling in absolute terms and in relation to the initial foot volume. The normal values of these measurements are remarkably similar in different laboratories and so can be used to diagnose the presence or absence of pump inefficiency with confidence (see Chapter 4, page 97).

We have found similar measurements based on calf strain gauge plethysmography to be unreliable but *isotope plethysmography* gives an excellent measure of the percentage of the calf blood volume expelled in response to either a sustained or repeated calf contraction (see Chapter 4, page 96).

It is essential to watch the patient performing these tests. A painful stiff ankle will reduce movements and the strength of the calf contractions and show that correction of the joint problem might have a greater effect on the calf pump than correction of the venous abnormality.

Saphenous reflux

Superficial vein reflux can add a large burden to the work of the calf pump. Reflux can be detected with the clinical tourniquet tests and heard with the Doppler flow detector but its contribution to the calf pump failure syndrome can only be measured by combining the tourniquet tests with plethysmography (see Chapter 4).

The simplest test is to combine the *tourniquet tests with photoplethysmography*. This only gives a qualitative answer but if the refilling rate becomes normal when a tourniquet is applied, the superficial vein reflux probably needs to be corrected surgically.

We prefer to measure the superficial reflux with the *foot volumeter* because it gives a quantitative measure of reflux. Isotope plethysmography is more accurate but too complicated and too expensive for routine use (see Chapter 4).

Descending phlebography will often show the presence of long saphenous reflux but is not indicated for this purpose alone because the simpler methods such as Doppler flow detection and the tourniquet tests are probably just as accurate (see Chapter 4).

Communicating vein reflux

There is no way of measuring the amount of blood that refluxes through the communicating veins. If a tourniquet is placed just below the knee, it will prevent reflux down the saphenous veins but not through the communicating veins. An abnormally fast refilling with a below-knee tourniquet in place implies that the communicating veins are incompetent. A tourniquet at the ankle will only restore refilling to normal if it is below the lowest incompetent communicating vein, compresses all the subcutaneous veins and does not interfere with ankle movements. As the lowest communicating vein is behind and just below the medial malleolus, and the subcutaneous tissues are often hard and incompressible, an ankle tourniquet is frequently ineffective.

Only 50–60 per cent of incompetence communicating veins can be detected with a *Doppler flow detector* (see page 84). This test also produces a high rate of false-positives. We find that the most reliable technique for the detection of incompetent communicating veins is *ascending phlebography* (see Chapter 6, page 187) but accept that, though its positive test accuracy is high, it also has a high false-negative rate. Phlebography does not measure the amount of reflux, and so it has to be assumed that any detectable incompetence is clinically significant.

By a complex series of manoeuvres involving multiple cuffs, passive squeezing of the calf, and the use of isotope plethysmography it is possible to detect the reflux of blood into the superficial compartment and measure the resulting increase in superficial venous volume. The volume of the reflux is very small; this explains why it is so difficult to measure.

A decision that the communicating veins are playing a significant role in the symptomatology of a patient's post-thrombotic syndrome is based primarily on finding that these veins are incompetent by clinical or radiological means, and from the site and distribution of the skin changes. The non-invasive tests are not very helpful.

The role of the deep veins

The deep veins may be contributing to calf pump inefficiency by obstructing forward blood flow or allowing blood to reflux. Maximum venous outflow measured with a plethysmograph around the calf gives a crude measure of femoral vein obstruction but is not very accurate. Wheeler[84] has devised a measurement called the 'venous diameter index' derived from an impedance plethysmograph tracing but the accuracy and significance of this measurement is still being assessed (see Chapter 4).

Iliac vein obstruction can be assessed from *femoral vein pressures* measured during exercise.

The presence of deep vein reflux can be detected and estimated using the *photoplethysmograph* or the foot volumeter if an increased rate of refilling persists after all the superficial reflux has been prevented with tourniquets, but the extent of the reflux can only be assessed by *descending phlebography*.

Ultrasound imaging may offer new ways of detecting and quantifying deep vein blood flow (see Chapter 4).

The anatomy of the venous abnormalities

None of the tests of function indicates the precise site of the post-thrombotic abnormalities; this can only be done with ascending and femoral phlebography. Phlebography reveals calf, axial and communicating vein damage. Prefemoral or intraosseus phlebography may be needed to show abnormalities in the ilio-femoral segment (see Chapter 4).

Biopsy

It may be necessary to take a biopsy of an area of

post-thrombotic lipodermatosclerotic change to assess the effect of the venous hypertension on the skin and confirm the diagnosis.

Blood studies

Part of the post-thrombotic syndrome is related to a deficiency of fibrinolysis. The fibrinolytic system of a patient with surgically incurable or recurrent post-thrombotic disease should be studied by measuring the *plasma fibrinogen* and *euglobulin clot lysis time*, and *vein wall fibrinolytic activator production* should be assessed from a vein biopsy from the dorsum of the foot. The new techniques for measuring tissue plasminogen activator and its inhibitors await further assessment.

Comment

Whereas most patients with simple varicose veins can be treated on the basis of clinical examination alone, patients with post-thrombotic calf pump failure need careful evaluation before advising treatment.

In our opinion the minimum investigations should be the following.

- A careful clinical examination supplemented with tourniquet tests and a Doppler flow detector analysis of saphenous reflux.
- A foot volumetric or photoplethysmographic assessment, with and without tourniquets, of overall calf pump function, saphenous and deep vein reflux.
- Ascending phlebography to detect incompetent communicating veins, post-thrombotic calf vein damage, axial vein obstruction and collaterals.
- Descending phlebography to define the extent of any deep vein reflux if indicated.
- Measurements of blood and vein wall fibrinolytic activity when surgical correction of the calf pump is not possible.

Natural history

What happens once the symptoms and signs of calf pump failure have appeared?

Although collectively and individually the skin changes of the calf pump failure syndrome can be called pre-ulcer changes, not every patient develops an ulcer. It is not known whether the rate of progression of tissue damage is related to:

- a critical level of calf pump inefficiency,
- a deteriorating efficiency,
- the effect of the circulatory changes on tissue fibrinolysis,
- the presence of a pre-existing deficiency of fibrinolysis,
- age and repeated trauma.

Probably all these factors are involved, but much more information is needed about the day-to-day and year-to-year fluctuations of lower limb superficial vein pressures, blood and tissue fluid fibrinolysis, and their relation to the development of symptoms.

When a patient with a history of venous thrombosis with a few varicose veins and early skin pigmentation asks if he/she will develop a venous ulcer, we normally answer in the affirmative in order to stimulate the patient to take preventative measures and wear an elastic stocking. In truth, we do not know the answer. The calf pump function tests of a patient with mild symptoms are usually not grossly abnormal, and yet one such patient may develop an ulcer 1 year later whereas another patient will have no new changes in the leg 10 or 20 years later, partly because the cause of an ulcer is often an unrelated event such as a minor injury.

When symptoms get worse the results of the function tests are usually found to have deteriorated. It has been suggested that patients with exercising foot vein pressures which are lower than 45 mmHg never develop ulcers.[64] This may be close to the truth but the converse is not true. Not all, or even the majority, of patients with high exercising foot vein pressures develop ulcers. The lack of a close correlation between the onset of symptoms and the degree of calf pump inefficiency suggests that the clinical natural history is significantly affected by another factor. Whereas skin deterioration, once the skin changes are present, coincides with the deterioration of the calf pump, the initiation of skin changes may depend upon local factors such as tissue fibrinolysis.

What makes the pump deteriorate? This is another unanswered question. Valves not destroyed by the initial thrombosis probably become incompetent because of valve ring dilatation. Dilatation is caused by the raised venous pressures, but must also be related to vein wall strength. Is it the patient with a familial tendency to varicose veins who gets a thrombosis because of the varicose veins,[3] which in turn causes further incompetence because of vein wall weakness? Is this another vicious circle like the thrombolytic deficiency/thrombosis/fibrin cuff circle?

There is much to be discovered about the factors which effect the progression of the symptoms of the post-thrombotic syndrome. In general it can be said that pigmentation and dry eczema are early mild signs that may remain static. Lipodermatosclerosis indicates serious tissue damage which will advance either to overt skin necrosis, an ulcer, or to a latent fibrous replacement of the skin and subcutaneous tissue–clinically visible as atrophie blanche and the 'champagne bottle' leg. Lipodermatosclerosis rarely regresses if the abnormalities of the calf pump and tissue fibrinolysis are not treated. Its rate of progression is variable but usually inevitable.

The clinician has a problem. Mild disease causes few symptoms but is easier to investigate and treat than advanced disease which is complex and difficult to investigate and treat. If we knew that early treatment with external support, fibrinolysis or surgery would definitely stop the progression of skin changes, we would not hesitate to advise treatment at an early stage, but there is no scientifically acceptable evidence to support such an approach. As we are considering a pathological process that may progress over 30 years, or even longer, a good experimental study would outlast a surgeon's working life making its conduct a considerable challenge. Short-term studies based on the results of non-invasive investigations may be possible if we can improve the quality, reproducibility, and sensitivity of the tests and define their significance and relationship to the clinical problems.[77]

Treatment

The common presenting symptom – aching pain – is often relieved by wearing a good quality elastic stocking.[30,47,68] Stockings can be prescribed after the patient's first consultation and worn while the investigations are being arranged. Relief of pain by a stocking is not only gratifying to the patient but is also a good diagnostic test confirming the clinical impression that the symptoms are caused by venous hypertension.

Once the diagnosis has been made and the severity and type of the venous abnormality defined, treatment falls into · two distinct categories.[1]

- Curative treatment = surgical correction of the calf pump abnormality
- Palliation of symptoms = principally, reducing the venous transmural pressure

The term 'cure' when applied to venous disease is an optimistic overstatement; it might be loosely applied to the treatment of some types of primary varicose vein but should never be used to describe the treatment of the post-thrombotic syndrome. All forms of surgical treatment throw added stress on the remaining veins unless the treatment restores every part of the pump to normal, which is usually impossible. When one incompetent communicating vein is ligated another has to take over its function as a collateral vessel and in time becomes incompetent. At best surgery improves calf pump function for a limited time, it rarely restores it permanently to normal – which is what most patients would consider to be a 'cure'.

Surgical correction of calf pump abnormalities

The two abnormalities of the veins of the lower limb that can be corrected surgically are valvular incompetence and obstruction to blood flow. The former is corrected by restoring valve function or ligating the incompetent vessel, the latter is corrected by bypassing the obstruction.

All patients admitted to hospital for the investigation and treatment of the post-thrombotic syndrome should be given 5000 units of heparin subcutaneously 12-hourly from the day of their admission until discharge to prevent further deep vein thrombosis (see Chapter 19).

Prevention of reflux

The veins which become incompetent and strain the pump are those in the saphenous system, the communicating veins and the deep outflow tract. All these veins will become incompetent if the thrombosis has been extensive. It is usually impractical to correct all three systems at once and so most surgeons prefer to correct the superficial and communicating vein incompetence first, and leave the deep vein incompetence to be treated, if necessary and if technically possible, at a later date.

Saphenous vein reflux

Saphenous vein reflux is treated by *ligation* of the saphenous vein at the sapheno-femoral junction. This operation is described in detail in Chapter 7 (page 205). The long saphenous vein above the level of the knee often connects with the superficial femoral vein in the middle of the thigh through the Hunter's canal communicating vein and so the saphenous vein should be *stripped* out from the knee to the groin to abolish this site of deep-to-superficial reflux and so prevent an early or late recurrence.

The saphenous vein should not be ligated or stripped if it is acting as a major collateral around a superficial femoral vein block. It is difficult to be certain from a clinical examination when this situation is present. If phlebography shows no filling of the superficial and deep femoral veins with all the contrast medium ascending from the mid calf to the groin in the saphenous vein, the wisdom of removing the long saphenous vein should be questioned. But phlebography is an anatomical not a physiological test. The only physiological way to assess the role of the long saphenous vein is to measure the change of foot volume, or the foot vein pressure during exercise before and after occluding the superficial veins in the thigh with a tourniquet. If the long saphenous vein is acting as a significant collateral, calf pump function will deteriorate when the tourniquet is inflated (i.e. the venous volume and pressure during exercise will increase when the cuff is inflated) (Fig. 12.2a). The pressure may even increase above the resting level.

Much more commonly, occlusion of a large incompetent saphenous vein that is allowing gross reflux to overload the pump will improve calf pump function (Fig. 12.b). In these circumstances an incompetent long saphenous vein can safely be ligated and stripped. The long saphenous vein functions as a significant collateral channel in only 5–10 per cent of patients but this small group must be identified because ligation of their long saphenous veins will make their symptoms worse.

Communicating vein reflux

The presence of skin and subcutaneous tissue changes in the lower leg are usually sufficient to justify a diagnosis of communicating vein incompetence but an attempt should always be made to

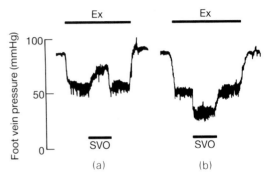

Fig. 12.2 The effect of superficial vein occlusion (SVO) at mid thigh level on the foot vein pressure during exercise (Ex).

(a) If superficial vein occlusion causes an increase in foot vein pressure during exercise, the superficial veins must be acting as collateral outflow channels.

(b) If superficial vein occlusion reduces foot vein pressure during exercise, the superficial veins must be incompetent and the reflux impeding calf pump function.

confirm the presence of the reflux with tourniquet and Doppler flow detection tests and the sites of reflux should be determined by ascending phlebography.[16,67,77]

Whereas ligation of an incompetent long saphenous vein acting as a major collateral channel will do harm, ligation of communicating veins acting as collaterals does not appear to cause problems. The volume of blood that these veins conduct is small when compared to the deleterious effect of their incompetence on the superficial venous pressure, and it is this pressure abnormality that must be abolished to stop the progression of the calf pump failure syndrome.

Unfortunately, the patient's symptoms will only be relieved until new incompetent communicating veins develop. It is not possible to predict how long this process will take but it is clearly related to the degree of deep vein damage. The rapid re-appearance of new, dilated, incompetent communicating veins usually indicates a severe degree of outflow tract obstruction; this process often takes 1–3 years. The usual phlebographic indication that this will occur is severe post-thrombotic changes in the calf veins and a totally occluded or very poorly recanalized popliteal vein.

Although the ligation of communicating veins which are acting as collaterals does no harm clinically because it reduces the superficial venous hypertension and so helps the subcutaneous tissues and skin to recover, it must harm the pump. Ligating these veins when the outflow tract is obstructed is the equivalent of introducing mitral stenosis in place of mitral incompetence in a patient with severe aortic stenosis. The incompetent communicating veins are the 'blow out' safety vents for the pump. Ligating them increases the end systolic volume and the work that the pump must do during systole. If we could measure intrapump volumes and pressures, with and without the incompetent communicating veins occluded, we could decide how their ligation would affect pump function in a way similar to the assessment of the role of an incompetent long saphenous vein that might be acting as a collateral or as a source of regurgitation. At present we cannot do this because we can neither pin-point and occlude every incompetent communicator, nor measure the pressure – volume relationships within the pump.

The only means we have of predicting the long-term effect of communicating vein ligation is by examining the phlebogram for evidence of severe deep vein damage. In a series of our patients whose communicating veins were ligated following conservative treatment to heal a venous ulcer, the ulcer recurred within 5 years in all those with extensive deep vein damage. The ulcer did not recur in those patients with healthy deep veins. Neither group was provided with elastic stockings.[15]

How is deep vein damage assessed phlebographically? Occlusion, recanalization and stenosis of the main outflow tract is easy to see (see Fig. 16.13, page 461). Post-thrombotic changes in the stem and muscle veins of the calf are much more difficult to describe and are not easy to quantify. The deep vein changes that predict a poor result from communicating vein ligation (i.e. an early chance of recurrence) are narrowing and irregularity of clusters of veins, tortuous collateral vessels within the calf, occluded calf axial veins (there should always be three pairs of axial veins in the calf – posterior tibial, peroneal, and anterior tibial) and the absence of valves (Fig. 12.3).

These abnormalities are rarely present in isolation, they are commonly all present. We try to avoid ligating the communicating veins when these changes are present because the results are often no better than those obtained with elastic compression but some patients prefer to have an operation even though they will experience a relapse in 3–5 years time. It is important to discuss the prognosis in detail with the patient before proceeding to surgery.

Communicating vein ligation This is described in detail in Chapter 7. If the deep veins are healthy, it is possible to cut through thick pigmented skin and obtain primary healing provided maximum care is taken to avoid skin damage, undercutting, and skin ischaemia as a result of tight stitches. If there is an ulcer, the incision can be moved posteriorly to avoid cutting through unhealthy skin.[25,26,57,58]

When there are post-thrombotic skin changes exploration to find the communicating veins should *always be subfascial*. Undercutting the skin in the subcutaneous layer is likely to cause skin necrosis or delayed healing. The last thing a surgeon wants is to cause an ulcer when he is doing an operation to prevent ulceration. The skin should be closed with the minimum of stitches. It is often possible to hold the incision together with surface adhesive strips and thus avoid skin stitches altogether (Colour plate 28).

The leg should be firmly bandaged. If the patient has had an ulcer and is used to an impregnated bandage (e.g. Viscopaste or Calaband) this can be applied at the end of the operation and left in place for 2–3 weeks.

The patient should be kept in bed with the leg elevated for 2 or 3 days before being allowed to walk because ankle movements disturb the edges of the lower part of the incision, Patients are normally encouraged to walk as soon as possible after varicose vein operations but in these patients the main objective is to obtain healing by first intention and this requires a period of rest to give the wound a chance to knit together before being disturbed by weightbearing and walking.

A delayed healing rate of 10–15 per cent is inevitable when operating through unhealthy tissues. If the wound is very painful, it must be inspected. Skin necrosis and haematomata are the common causes of postoperative pain and should be treated by excision and evacuation respectively, the resulting defect may have to be closed with a skin graft.

Prophylaxis with subcutaneous heparin is essential in these patients, throughout their stay in hospital, as they are at risk of getting a further thrombosis – an event which could make their leg

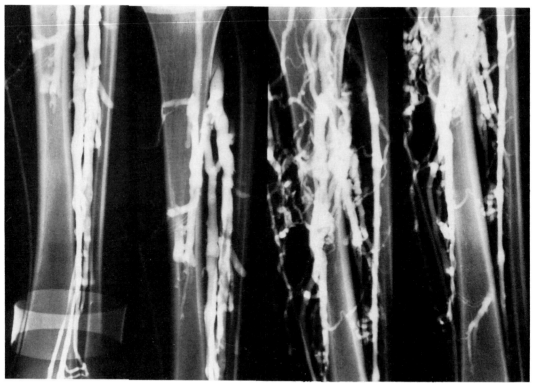

Fig. 12.3   Phlebograms showing normal (left-hand panels) and damaged (right-hand panels) deep calf veins. The deep vein thrombosis has caused a mixture of partial and complete occlusion, tortuous collaterals and many thin irregular valveless vessels meandering in all directions.

much worse. The heparin should not increase the incidence of wound haematomata if care is taken with haemostasis during the operation and the limb is firmly bandaged and elevated afterwards.

The effect of communicating vein ligation on the pre-ulcer calf pump failure syndrome skin changes has not been evaluated. The majority of surgeons have studied ulcer recurrence and claim a 5-year ulcer-free rate of 85 per cent but few have assessed the state of the deep veins with phlebography pre-operatively.[4,10,32,38,45,46,50,53,63,65,78] It is our experience that those legs that develop recurrent ulcers or show progression of their lipodermatosclerosis are those with extensive deep vein damage.

Patients with incompetent communicating veins and scarred unhealthy skin often do better if the damaged skin is excised and replaced by a split skin graft. A few patients with extensive circumferential skin damage do best when all the skin of the lower leg is excised, from the ankle to the mid calf, in a way similar to the Charles' operation

(reducing operation) for lymphoedema. When there is extensive deep vein damage this may be the only treatment that can be offered. It should reduce the incidence of recurrence because the excision of all the communicating veins with the skin and subcutaneous fat leaves none to become incompetent. We have only performed this operation on four patients.

Communicating vein shearing   To avoid cutting through the unhealthy skin some surgeons push a blunt-ended shearing knife up and down the leg beneath the deep fascia to divide all the communicating veins.[27] This method can cause haematomata, bruising of the skin, and occasionally, skin necrosis. Until it has been shown that this technique divides all the incompetent communicating veins, it cannot be recommended.

Another method of ligating communicating veins is to perform the subfascial exploration through a small incision and use long retractors and malleable lights. The simplest apparatus to use for this procedure is the Magill laryngoscope;

it can be used to elevate the fascia, and illuminate the wound and it has a lumen which is large enough to accommodate a metal clip applicator.[9] No results of this approach to communicating vein ligation have been published.

Deep vein reflux

The treatment of non-thrombotic deep vein reflux has been discussed in Chapter 8. When reflux follows deep vein thrombosis the valves are totally destroyed making attempts at valve repair inappropriate. The only two methods by which a valve can be inserted to prevent reflux in a previously thrombosed vein are valve transplantation[81] and valve segment transposition.[55] *Valve transplantation* had been described on pages 265–268. It only works when a healthy valve can be transferred into a relatively healthy vein. In reflux without evidence of post-thrombotic damage (for which valve transplantation has been used by Taheri)[82] the popliteal or superficial femoral veins of the recipient legs have been healthy.[82] After popliteal or femoral vein thrombosis the segment of vein that recanalizes least well is the portion above and below the adductor canal – perhaps this is because of the stiff surrounding structures. Consequently, it is rarely possible to transplant a valve to this position after a thrombosis because of the poor quality of the recipient vein. It is unwise to sew a valve into a vein that is fibrosed, thickened and stenosed with endothelialized mural thrombus. Such a vein can be guaranteed to thrombose in spite of anticoagulants and the use of an adjuvant arteriovenous fistula.

Valve transplantation has little place in the treatment of the post-thrombotic syndrome and, because suitable patients are extremely hard to find, no large series describing its use has been published. For the same reasons the insertion of a preserved allograft valve will rarely be feasible.

Valve transposition Deep vein thrombosis often affects the superficial femoral vein and spares the deep femoral vein. In such circumstances it may be possible to perform a transposition of the upper end of an incompetent superficial femoral vein into the side of a competent deep femoral vein, below a healthy valve (see Fig. 8.14, page 264).[55]

A number of the valve transpositions described in the recent Chicago study were performed for post-thrombotic incompetence. Although the patients in this study had a significant prolongation of deep vein refilling 3 months after operation, refilling became abnormal again 9 months later, indicating that this simple and logical operation has not stood the test of time.[52,72] This does not mean that it should be abandoned but that it should be studied when combined with additional procedures that might prevent valve ring dilatation and recurrent reflux.

During the time that an obstructed segment of vein takes to recanalize to allow sufficient reflux to cause symptoms, the original obstruction will have stimulated other veins to dilate and thus made them incompetent. We do not know whether the restoration of deep vein competence will encourage superficial incompetent veins, which have dilated to act as collaterals, to constrict and become competent. Fegan has claimed that this phenomenon can occur in the long saphenous vein following occlusion of incompetent calf communicating veins,[29,73] but whether a similar change follows a successful valve transplant or transposition is not known. The evidence from Kistner's valve repair studies[31] suggest that the communicating veins do not recover as the majority of his patients still needed communicating vein surgery after a successful valve repair. This is not surprising because the pump still generates the same systolic pressure so that blood will continue to flow retrogradely in the communicating veins even after the axial veins have been rendered competent. This means that incompetent communicating veins must be ligated at the same time as deep vein valve competence is restored.

A number of other anti-reflux procedures on the deep veins have been advocated over the years; none has stood the test of time.

Femoral vein and popliteal vein ligation These methods have been tried and found to be unsatisfactory. The theories of Homans, Bauer and Linton[5,6,7] that femoral vein ligation would improve calf pump function were based on the belief that reflux down the recanalized femoral or popliteal vein was the main cause of the post-thrombotic syndrome and venous ulceration. Deep vein reflux cannot, however, be the only or even the main cause of post-thrombotic symptoms because many patients with incompetent communicating veins have normal popliteal and femoral veins.

Other investigators[21,76] have tried both these

operations and have not found them to be of clinical benefit. Sometimes the bursting pain on walking is relieved for a few months but it soon returns. Oedema is unaffected, and the measurements of calf pump function deteriorate. The only explanation that can be advanced for Bauer's claim that two-thirds of his 136 patients were improved by deep vein ligation must lie in his simultaneous prescription of proper conservative treatment, particularly the use of elastic compression. Linton[57] frequently stated that femoral vein ligation must be followed by permanent elastic support otherwise the operation will fail. *Deep vein ligation should not be practised for the post-thrombotic syndrome.*

In 1964 Psathakis[71] devised an operation in which the tendon of the gracilis muscle was rerouted deep to the popliteal vein so that the vein was occluded when the muscle contracted, making it in effect an *external compression valve*. Recently[70] Psathakis has suggested using a plastic cord attached to the muscle in place of the tendon. This operation has not been widely practised as other investigators have reported poor results (e.g. 4 successes in 46 cases).[40,60] Unless the gracilis contracts and occludes the popliteal vein immediately the calf contraction stops – the time when the reflux begins – the operation cannot work. Such a course of events is most unlikely. Psathakis states that superficial vein and communicating vein incompetence should be treated at the same time as the sling operation. It seems likely that these additional procedures produce the clinical improvement.

The preceding paragraphs reveal the importance of communicating vein incompetence even in the presence of extensive deep vein reflux. Far more benefit is achieved by preventing communicating vein reflux than by preventing deep vein reflux. If it is thought, however, that concomitant repair of the deep reflux will prevent the recurrence of communicating vein reflux, it should always be considered.

Deep vein obstruction

Any combination of lower limb venous outflow tract thrombosis can occur but there are four common varieties, ilio-femoral, superficial femoral, combined superficial femoral and popliteal and total ilio-femoro-popliteal thrombosis (see Fig. 11.9, page 312).

If the diagram of these types of thrombosis is examined it is apparent that the lesion most suited to treatment by a bypass operation is isolated iliac or ilio-femoral occlusion. Superficial femoral vein obstruction may be bypassed if the popliteal vein has been spared or has recanalized well. Total occlusion of the outflow tract is not amenable to surgical cure.

Iliac vein obstruction

This can be treated by femoral-caval bypass or by an extra anatomic femoro-femoral bypass (the Palma operation). These operations are described on pages 281–283.

When an isolated ilio-femoral thrombosis occurs, the inferior vena cava and the opposite iliac vein are not affected. The femoral vein below the block is usually healthy but may contain some organized thrombus. Provided the contralateral long saphenous vein is healthy and of good calibre and there is a patent major vein in the groin of the affected side, a Palma operation is possible.[22] The operation should not, however, be performed without first showing that there is a significant rise in femoral vein pressure in response to leg exercise.

When the femoral vein below the obstruction at the site of the anastomosis is abnormal, it is wise to add an arterio-venous fistula because post-thrombotic damage at the site of anastomosis increases the risk of thrombosis. Some surgeons advocate the use of an arteriovenous fistula in all cases.

The long-term (5-year) patency rates for the Palma operation are approximately 75 per cent, with a lower patency when there are post-thrombotic changes in the femoral vein (see Figs. 9.13 and 9.14, pages 282 and 283).[44] If the graft remains patent, the patient can expect the symptoms of venous claudication to disappear and oedema to decrease. Skin changes in the leg should also improve but this will depend upon the degree of pre-existing damage in the other deep veins and the communicating veins. The main indication for a Palma operation is venous claudication. The addition of communicating vein ligation depends upon the symptoms, the state of the skin of the lower leg and the phlebographic appearance of the calf veins.

In a busy venous disease clinic the number of patients that might be seen who are suitable for this operation is small. Halliday[44] performed 50 operations between 1965 and 1984, less than three each year. Gruss[36] calculated that less than 2 per cent of patients with the post-thrombotic syndrome are suitable for any type of bypass. Careful selection of patients is critically important, and the surgeon must be certain that it is the iliac obstruction that is the principal cause of the symptoms. The Palma operation is so simple that bypasses between the femoral vein and the vena cava with heterologous vein or prosthetic materials should only be considered when the long saphenous vein of the other leg is unsuitable or there is obstruction in the iliac veins of both legs.

Superficial femoral vein obstruction

This can be treated with a popliteal to femoral vein saphenous vein bypass provided the popliteal vein is healthy and draining most of the blood from the calf.[49,83]

All the published series of this operation have been done for post-thrombotic occlusions and the results have been poor; they are summarized on page 00. May performed 16 of these operations;[61] in 3 patients immediate graft thrombosis occurred, but in 13 patients an improvement in calf pump function was seen when assessed by foot vein pressure studies. Gruss has performed 12 operations (5 patients had a simultaneous Palma operation).[36] Three of the popliteal–femoral bypasses thrombosed; in 4 patients the results of calf function tests deteriorated but in 5 patients they improved and the symptoms decreased. The combination of these two studies shows that some improvement occured in 18 out of 28 patients.

When an operation is performed so rarely by experts in the field one must suspect that they doubt its value or find it difficult to decide when to do it. We are sure that both reasons are valid and consider that the difficulty in deciding about the suitability of a patient for this operation lies in the inability of our pre-operative tests either to distinguish the relative importance of deep vein obstruction from calf pump inefficiency and communicating vein reflux or to indicate whether the long saphenous vein is already acting as an important collateral channel.

The deterioration of the calf pump function tests in four of the patients operated on by Gruss suggests that the popliteal vein had thrombosed.

Such an event might cause a severe deterioration of symptoms and is the risk that has deterred us from using this procedure.

As in all cases of post-thrombotic damage, ligation of incompetent communicating veins is likely to produce the most clinical improvement, even though the deep vein damage restricts the duration of the improvement.

Palliative treatment of the post-thrombotic calf pump failure syndrome

The pressure that affects the state and function of the wall of a hollow tube is not solely the pressure within it but the difference between the pressure inside and the pressure outside – the transmural pressure. A high transmural pressure will dilate a vein, venule, or venular capillary, open the interendothelial pores, and make the small vessels more permeable.

A high transmural pressure can be reduced by lowering the intraluminal pressure or increasing the extraluminal pressure. All of the reconstructive surgical techniques described above are designed to lower the intraluminal venous pressure, which *pari passu* reduces the transmural pressure. When surgical methods cannot reduce intraluminal pressure, an alternative method of reducing transmural pressure is to increase the extraluminal pressure. This can be done by bandaging, elastic hosiery or pneumatic leggings. As so many patients have post-thrombotic damage which cannot be cured by surgery, external compression is the mainstay of their treatment.

Many of the effects of venous hypertension on the tissues will not regress when the transluminal pressure is reduced but further deterioration can be prevented.

The palliative treatment of the post-thrombotic syndrome therefore has two objectives:

(a) to reduce the transmural pressure;
(b) to reverse the tissue changes.

Elastic compression

The transmural pressure in the veins of the foot when standing is 90–100 mmHg; at the knee it is 60–70 mmHg and at the groin it is 30–40 mmHg. The pressure applied by an elastic stocking should take account of this gradual reduction of pressure along the limb to avoid overcompressing the veins in the thigh and prevent the stocking acting as a tourniquet.[48,54,59] Modern elastic stockings are designed to apply a known pressure at the ankle which gradually reduces along the length of the leg; this is known as *graduated compression*. The pressure exerted by a stocking varies according to the tension and content of the elastic material in the stocking and the size and fitting of the stocking.

The pressure in the arteriolar capillaries – when the leg is horizontal – is 40 mmHg; when standing it is 130 mmHg at the ankle but proportionally less higher up the leg.[8] Skin blood flow, when measured with xenon clearance, is reduced by external compression greater than 40 mmHg when the leg is horizontal but is not affected when the leg is vertical until the compression reaches 80 mmHg.[56]

In a normal limb the foot vein pressure falls from 90 to 30 mmHg during exercise. This is the effect that we wish stockings to mimic. A stocking pressure of 40 mmHg at the ankle reduces the transmural pressure in the lower leg, when standing, to 50 mmHg. This has little effect on the arterial inflow but helps an inefficient calf pump to reduce foot vein pressure to 20–30 mmHg during exercise instead of 60–70 mmHg. The stocking must therefore exert a pressure which has a worthwhile effect on the venous system when the patient is standing or walking without having a deleterious effect on tissue perfusion.[34,66,79] This is difficult to achieve because each patient's requirement is different. A stocking pressure at the ankle of 40 mmHg seems to be the best compromise in patients with the calf pump failure syndrome. A lower pressure may be adequate when the calf pump abnormality is confined to the superficial veins.

At the first consultation graduated elastic compression stockings which give a pressure of at least 30 mmHg at the ankle should be prescribed for all patients with the post-thrombotic syndrome.[80] There is no evidence that stockings that stretch above the knee are required unless there is marked thigh swelling. Stockings are known to help the calf pump, their effect on the thigh pump has not been studied.

Stockings should be put on before the patient gets out of bed and not removed until bedtime. Two pairs should be prescribed to allow for washing, and they must be replaced every 6 months as frequent washing and wearing causes a loss of elasticity.[74] Most manufacturers make a wide range of garments which will fit most sizes and shapes of leg; a leg which is an unusual shape needs a 'made-to-measure' stocking.

Stockings can be worn over dressings but a bulky mass beneath the stocking disturbs its contour and alters its compressive effect (see Chapter 15, page 433). The legs of patients who have ulcers which need frequent dressings are best supported with some form of bandage because ulcer exudate can damage the fibres of a stocking.

Elastic stockings reduce oedema, improve calf pump function and increase the clearance of subcutaneous fibrin (Fig. 12.4.).[14] The patient usually notices an immediate reduction of the ache and discomfort in the leg.[2,20] This provides a good diagnostic test that the veins are the source of the symptoms. Swelling takes longer to disperse and rarely goes completely. Varicose veins often become a little smaller but revert to their original size within 24 hours of removing the stocking. It is possible, but unlikely, that some of the valves of incompetent veins become competent while they are compressed.

Elderly and fat people often have difficulty in reaching their feet and pulling on a tight stocking and may need to be helped by a friend or nurse. Some people prefer elastic or impregnated bandages.

Some patients develop allergies to the elastic material be it rubber, latex or polymer. They first notice an itching and then develop a dermatitis. They should stop using the stocking immediately. An attempt should then be made to discover the cause of the allergy so that stockings without the allergen can be prescribed.

Bandages

A multitude of ribbon-like and tubular bandages are used on patients with post-thrombotic changes. Only those bandages with an intrinsic elasticity capable of exerting compression are worth using.

A heavy elastic bandage is often easier to apply to legs of an unusual shape or a leg with an ulcer than a stocking but it must be applied carefully in a way that will exert an even and, if possible, a graduated compression. Studies of the skill of nurses and doctors at bandaging reveal that this is

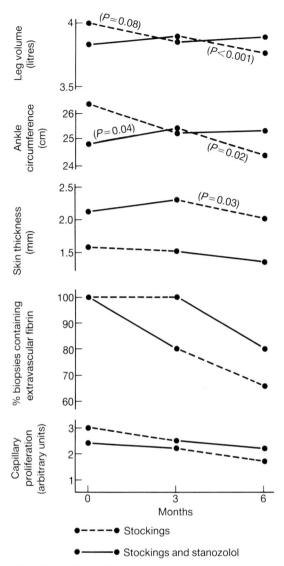

Fig. 12.4 The effect of below-knee elastic stockings (with and without stanozolol) on the leg volume, ankle circumference, skin thickness, extravascular fibrin and capillary proliferation of limbs with lipodermatosclerosis (calf pump failure syndrome). The stockings alone produced significant effects on leg volume, ankle circumference and skin thickness.

not such a simple task as it first may seem (see Chapter 15).

Impregnated bandages are designed for use when the patient has an ulcer (Chapter 15, page 418). It is not advisable to use them when the skin is intact (even when there is severe lipodermatosclerosis) except for the occasional elderly patient who cannot put on a stocking or apply a bandage and who may be more comfortable and active when wearing an impregnated bandage renewed every 2 or 3 weeks; the skin must, however, be tolerant of the medicament in the bandage.

The routine for the use of bandages should be the same as that for the use of stockings; they must be worn whenever the patient is out of bed.

Elevation

Standing still for prolonged periods is the worst thing that a patient with venous disease of the lower limbs can do, as it is the position in which the venous pressure in the lower part of the leg is at its highest. If patients have to stand for long periods, they must exercise their calf muscles by walking, tiptoeing or bracing the knees in order to reduce the venous pressure.

When the legs are above heart level the venous pressure falls to zero and tissue fluid is absorbed. This relieves the aching pains and reduces the swelling. Patients should raise the foot of their bed on 12-inch (30 cm) blocks and sleep with no more than two pillows so that their legs are above the level of their heart throughout the night. This discipline can produce a marked improvement in symptoms.[42]

During the day the legs should be kept 'up' as much as possible – elevated on a stool when sitting, or on pillows when lying down. If the patient can spend 15–30 minutes in the middle of the day resting with the legs elevated at 90° (legs propped up against a wall with the patient lying on the floor), they will notice a reduction of pain and tightness in the legs during the afternoon. We have had one patient who kept his legs in excellent condition by doing 'bicycling exercises', while standing on his head, assisted by a padded head and shoulder support! Exercise with the legs above heart level is the best physiological way of reducing oedema.[24] Unfortunately, the whole of life cannot be conducted in this position, and the amount of time spent like this depends on the patient's occupation and hobbies!

Massage and passive movements

Gentle but firm massage of the skin and subcutaneous tissues with the fingers and a little bland oil in a centripetal direction together with passive movements of the ankle joint has five effects.

1. It disperses the oedema through the tissues, moving it up the leg to areas where it is more likely to be absorbed.
2. It softens the subcutaneous tissues which makes them respond to the compression of the elastic stocking.
3. It breaks up some of the fibrin deposited in the tissue; this softens the tissues and helps to reduce the fibrous reaction.
4. The oil keeps the skin soft and reduces hyperkeratosis, but the patient must be careful not to make the skin so soft that it is more susceptible to trauma.
5. Moving the ankle reduces the chance of ankle stiffness and ensures that reduced ankle movements do not add to the inefficiency of the calf pump.

Diuretics

Diuretics do not help the oedema of chronic venous hypertension. The patient may notice a slight reduction in swelling after the first course of diuretics but the effect is short-lived.[37,41] Diuretics affect the whole body not just the swollen limb and may increase the chance of a deep vein thrombosis or superficial thrombophlebitis if they cause haemoconcentration.[41]

Antibiotics

In the mistaken belief that the redness, heat and tenderness of acute lipodermatosclerosis indicate infection, some practitioners prescribe antibiotics. There is no infection present and antibiotics have no value. The role of antibiotics in the treatment of venous ulceration is discussed in Chapter 15.

Sympathectomy

Venous insufficiency is *not* associated with a reduced skin blood flow, and sympathectomy has no place in the treatment of its symptoms.

Rutosides

A number of publications[12,33,39,43,69,75,86] have claimed that the oral administration of rutosides, which alter capillary permeability in the experimental animal, relieve the symptoms of chronic venous insufficiency. The clinical evidence for this effect is weak, and much of the improvement claimed is probably a 'placebo effect'. More controlled scientifically acceptable evidence is required before these drugs can be recommended.

Stimulation of fibrinolysis

If the fibrin barrier/physiological shunt hypothesis (Chapter 11) is correct, removal of the fibrin should improve tissue oxygenation.[11,18] We have performed two studies to test this thesis, a pilot study[12] and a double blind crossover trial.[14] In the pilot study, 14 patients with active lipodermatosclerosis secondary to venous insufficiency were given stanozolol for 3 months. These patients had failed to respond to elastic compression and surgical treatment of their varicose veins.

The blood fibrinolytic activity increased and the plasma fibrinogen fell significantly during treatment. The mean area of lipodermatosclerosis, which had been unaltered for many months before treatment began, fell from 219 cm^2 to 58 cm^2. These results encouraged us to undertake a controlled clinical trial. Thirty-four legs of 23 patients with active lipodermatosclerosis were studied. Half were given elastic stockings and a placebo for 3 months followed by stockings and stanozolol 5 mg b.d. for another 3 months. The other half were treated in reverse order (i.e. the active drug was given after the placebo). Leg circumference, leg volume, skin thickness, skin biopsies stained for fibrin, foot vein pressures, routine haematology and liver function tests, plasma fibrinogen, and dilute blood clot lysis time were measured at intervals throughout the study.

The mean area of lipodermatosclerosis reduced in response to both the elastic compression and placebo and the elastic compression and stanozolol but the improvement in the group who received the active drug was twice that of the group who took placebo (Fig. 12.5). The probability value of this difference was 0.08. It is conventional to consider any *P* value greater than 0.05 as insignificant but in view of the consistency of these results in all patients, the difficulties of measurement and the pilot study results we considered that the additional improvement caused by the stanozolol was clinically significant.

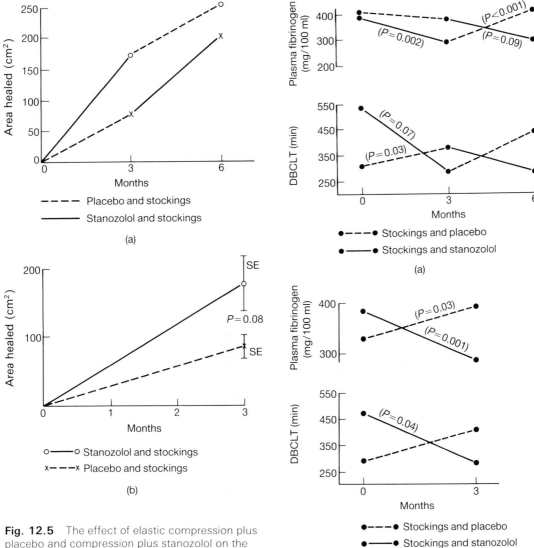

Fig. 12.5 The effect of elastic compression plus placebo and compression plus stanozolol on the healing of lipodermatosclerosis.

(a) The areas of lipodermatosclerosis healed in the two groups of our double blind crossover study.[14]

(b) The results of the two crossover groups combined. The healing rate of the patients given stanozolol was twice that of those given placebo, a difference that was significant at the 8% level.

Fig. 12.6 The effect of elastic compression plus placebo and compression plus stanozolol on the dilute blood clot lysis time (DBCLT) and plasma fibrinogen.

(a) The changes in the blood in the two groups of our double blind crossover study.[14]

(b) The changes in the blood of the two crossover groups combined. The stanozolol caused a significant fall in dilute blood clot lysis time (DBCLT) and plasma fibrinogen. The levels reverted to pretreatment values within 3 months of stopping the stanozolol (a).

The difference in the improvement between the two groups over the first 3 months of treatment was statistically significant $P = 0.03$.

The leg volume and the ankle circumference were significantly reduced by the elastic stockings in the placebo group (Fig. 12.4). Stanozolol causes mild water retention which abolished the effect of the stockings on the leg swelling during treatment with the active drug (Fig. 12.4).

Stanozolol produced the expected 50 per cent reduction of dilute blood clot lysis time and 25 per cent reduction of plasma fibrinogen (Fig. 12.6)[23] and the amount of perivascular fibrin was less in the post-treatment biopsies (Fig. 12.4). Stanozolol caused no serious side-effects.

No other fully controlled trial of stanozolol in the treatment of lipodermatosclerosis has been reported but many clinicians have used stanozolol and confirmed its clinical effectiveness. For example, Gröenewald[35] found that the induration of lipodermatosclerosis improved in 17 of 22 patients given stanozolol compared with 9 of 22 patients given placebo, and discoloration improved in 16 of 22 patients given the active drug compared to 8 of 22 patients given a placebo.

The pain settles in 2–5 weeks. After 3 months the redness, heat and induration begin to go, and in many of our patients a 9-month course of treatment (including good quality stockings) caused the skin to return to normal including a reduction of skin pigmentation.

Stanozolol has three effects; it is mildly androgenic, it stimulates fibrinolysis and reduces plasma fibrinogen, and is a weak steroid. It is possible that the latter property, which might be mildly anti-inflammatory might be responsible for the reduction of pain but, as there are few inflammatory cells in lipodermatosclerotic tissues, this is unlikely. It is difficult to perceive how the androgenic properties would help the skin and so we are left with the conclusion that the beneficial effect of stanozolol comes from the stimulation of defective fibrinolysis. This would fit and support our hypothesis but the problem needs to be studied further; more investigations of the treatment of active lipodermatosclerosis and studies on the chronic, non-painful, 'burnt out' variety are required.

We must stress that we only recommend stanozolol for those patients with acute lipodermatosclerosis (painful, hot and tender) in whom standard treatment with elastic stockings and previous saphenous and communicating vein surgery has failed to prevent the progression of the skin changes. Treatment should be continued for 6 months. The patient should be warned not to expect much change, except for pain reduction, in the first 3 months. We prefer not to continue treatment for more than 12 months but if the lipodermatosclerosis recurs, a further course of treatment can be given with similar clinical benefit.

Twenty of the patients in our 1976 trial were assessed in 1982, 6 years after treatment;[17] 13 of these patients had had frequent recurrent ulceration before entering the trial. All patients but one were still using elastic compression. Nineteen patients thought that their skin was better than it was in 1976. Two patients had had recurrent episodes of ulceration throughout the 5 years. Four of the patients who said that their skin had improved had had one short period of ulceration lasting less than 3 months..One patient had died. Thirteen patients had had no further ulceration. These long-term results suggest that the incidence of recurrent ulceration was reduced, but this needs further clinical evaluation.

If a patient is resistant to stanozolol, a similar effect on fibrinolysis may be obtained with ethyloestranol and phenformin.[28,51]

Surgical excision of damaged skin

It is sometimes worthwhile excising skin which has become scarred, hyperpigmented and hyperkeratotic and replacing it with split skin grafts. This operation also divides and ligates *all* the communicating veins. It is rarely indicated when there has not been recurrent ulceration but sometimes non-ulcerated skin and subcutaneous tissues become so painful and tender that the patient begs for something to be done and excision may be the only answer. The surgeon's natural inclination to preserve adjacent moderately good looking skin should be resisted; if not, the patient will complain of similar problems in the skin surrounding the graft 2 to 3 years later.

An alternative to split skin grafting is a cross leg flap or a vascularized free skin flap with arterial and venous microanastomoses. These operations should be reserved for intractable problems in young adults, usually the result of the combination of compound fractures of the tibia and deep vein thrombosis.

Achilles tendon lengthening

Pain in and around the ankle may cause permanent joint stiffness and a secondary shortening of the Achilles tendon producing a fixed plantar flexion deformity.

If the joint is not completely fixed, the pain can be relieved and the condition of the skin improved by lengthening the Achilles tendon. It is not always easy to find a patch of healthy skin for the operative incision, and the operation should be preceded by a joint consultation between the vascular and the orthopaedic surgeon.

References

1. Ackroyd JS, Browse NL. The investigation and surgery of the post thrombotic syndrome. *J Cardiovasc Surg* 1986; **27**: 5.
2. Allen S. The treatment of chronic venous disorders of the leg. *Practitioner* 1970; **205**: 221.
3. Arnoldi CC. The heredity of venous insufficiency. *Dan Med Bull* 1958; **5**: 169.
4. Arnoldi CC, Haeger K. Ulcus cruris venosum-crux medicorum. *Lakartidningen* 1967; **64**: 149.
5. Bauer G. Division of the popliteal vein in the treatment of so-called varicose ulceration. *Br Med J* 1950; **2**: 318.
6. Bauer G. Indications for popliteal vein ligation. *J Cardiovasc Surg* 1963; **4**: 18.
7. Bauer G. The aetiology of leg ulcers and their treatment by resection of the popliteal vein. *J Int Chir* 1948; **8**: 937.
8. Beaconsfield P, Ginsberg J. Effect of changes in limb posture on peripheral blood flow. *Circ Res* 1955; **3**: 478.
9. Bentley RJ. The obliteration of perforating veins of the leg. *Br J Surg* 1972; **59**: 199.
10. Bertelsen S, Gammelgaard A. Surgical treatment of post-thrombotic leg ulcers. *J Cardiovasc Surg* 1965; **6**: 452.
11. Browse NL, Burnand KG. The cause of venous ulceration. *Lancet* 1982; **2**: 243.
12. Browse NL, Jarrett PEM, Morland M, Burnand KG. The treatment of liposclerosis of the leg by fibrinolytic enhancement: a preliminary report. *Br Med J* 1977; **7**: 434.
13. Browse NL. Venous ulceration. *Br Med J* 1983; **286**: 1920.
14. Burnand KG, Clemenson G, Morland M, Jarrett PEM, Browse NL. Venous lipodermatosclerosis, treatment by fibrinolytic enhancement and elastic compression. *Br Med J* 1980; **280**: 7.
15. Burnand KG, Lea Thomas M, O'Donnell T, Browse NL. Relationship between post-phlebitic changes in the deep veins and results of surgical treatment of venous ulcers. *Lancet* 1976; **2**: 936.
16. Burnand KG, O'Donnell TF, Lea Thomas M, Browse NL. The relative importance of incompetent communicating veins in the production of varicose veins and venous ulcers. *Surgery* 1977; **82**: 9.
17. Burnand KG, Pattison M, Browse NL. The results of a course of Stromba treatment on lipodermatosclerosis of skin of the lower leg. A five year follow up. In *Progress in Fibrinolysis* Vol VI. Edinburgh. Churchill Livingstone 1983; 526.
18. Chilvers AS. A *Study of the Effect of Long Term Stimulation of Fibrinolysis by a Biguanide and an Anabolic Steroid on the Deposition of Fibrin in Arteries.* MCh Thesis, Cambridge University 1971.
19. Cockett FB, Elgan Jones DE. The ankle blow out syndrome. *Lancet* 1953; **1**: 17.
20. Cockett FB. Management of the postphlebitic leg. *Br J Hosp Med* 1971; **6**: 767.
21. Cristian V. Resection of the superficial femoral vein in the treatment of post-phlebitic syndrome. Renewal of therapeutic interest. *Phlebologie* 1974; **27**: 103.
22. Dale WA. Crossover vein grafts for relief of ilio-femoral venous block. *Surgery* 1965; **57**: 608.
23. Davidson JF, Lockhead M, McDonald GA, McNichol GP. Fibrinolytic enhancement by stanozolol: a double blind trial. *Br J Haematol* 1972; **22**: 543.
24. de Takats G. The management of acute thrombophlebitic oedema. JAMA 1933; **100**: 34.
25. Dodd H, Cockett FB. In *The Pathology and Surgery of the Veins of the lower Limb.* Edinburgh. Churchill Livingstone 1956.
26. Dodd H. The diagnosis and ligation of incompetent perforating veins. *Ann R Coll Surg Engl* 1964; **34**: 186.
27. Edwards JM. Shearing operation for incompetent perforating veins. *Br J Surg* 1976; **63**: 885.
28. Fearnley GR, Chakrabarti R, Evans JF. Mode of action of phenformin plus ethyloestranol on fibrinolysis. *Lancet* 1971; **1**: 723.
29. Fegan WG. Treatment of varicose veins by injection compression. In: Hobbs JE (Ed). *Treatment of Venous Disorders.* Philadelphia. JB Lippincott 1977.
30. Fentem PH, Goddard M, Gooden BA, Yeung CK. Control of distension of varicose veins achieved by leg bandages as used after sclerotherapy. *Br Med J* 1976; **2**: 725.
31. Ferris EB, Kistner RL. Femoral vein reconstruction in the management of chronic venous insufficiency. *Arch Surg* 1982; **117**: 1571.
32. Field P, Van Boxall P. The role of the Linton flap procedure in the management of stasis

dermatitis and ulceration of the lower limb. *Surgery* 1971; **70**: 920.

33. Fitzgerald D. A clinical trial of Froxerutin in venous insufficiency of the lower limb. *Practitioner* 1967; **198**: 406.

34. Gjöres JE, Thülesius O. Compression treatment in venous insufficiency evaluated with foot volumetry, *Vasa* 1977; **6**: 364.

35. Gröenewald J. *Communication to the International Vascular Symposium*. London. Sept 1981.

36. Gruss JD. The sapheno-popliteal bypass for chronic venous insufficiency. In Bergan JJ, Yao JST (Eds) *Surgery of the Veins*. Orlando. Grune & Stratton 1985.

37. Haeger K. Hypostatic oedema. *Zbl Phlebol* 1971; **10**: 192.

38. Haeger K. Indications for surgery in ankle perforator insufficiency. *Zbl Phlebol* 1969; **8**: 158.

39. Haeger K. The debatable value of flavinoids in venous insufficiency. *Zbl Phlebol* 1967; **6**: 526.

40. Haeger K. The treatment of the severe post-thrombotic state. *Angiology* 1968; **19**: 439.

41. Haeger K. The treatment of venous hypostatic oedema and its complications. *Zbl Phlebol* 1970; **9**: 23.

42. Haeger K. Treatment of the post thrombotic state in elderly patients. *Zbl Phlebol* 1971; **10**: 178.

43. Halborg-Sorenson A, Hansen H. Chronic venous insufficiency treated with hydroxyethylruto-sides. *Angiologica* 1970; **7**: 192.

44. Halliday P, Harris J, May J. Femoro-femoral crossover grafts. A long term follow-up study. In: Bergan JJ, Yao JST (Eds) *Surgery of the Veins*. Orlando. Grune & Stratton 1985.

45. Halliday P. The place of subfascial ligation of perforating veins in the treatment of the post-phlebitic syndrome. *Br J Surg* 1971; **58**: 104.

46. Hansson LO. Venous ulcers of the lower limb. *Acta Chir Scand* 1964; **128**: 269.

47. Horner J, Fernandes E Fernandes J, Nicolaides AN. Value of graduated compression stockings in deep venous insufficiency. *Br Med J* 1980; **1**: 820.

48. Horner J, Lowth LC, Nicolaides AN. A pressure profile for elastic stockings. *Br Med J* 1980; **1**: 818.

49. Husni EA. *In situ* sapheno-popliteal bypass graft for incompetence of the femoral and popliteal veins. *Surg Gynec Obstet* 1970; **130**: 279.

50. Hyde GL, Hull DA. Long term results of subfascial vein ligation for venous stasis disease.*Surg Gynec Obstet* 1981; **153**: 683.

51. Isacson S, Nilsson I M. Effect of treatment with combined phenformin and ethyloestranol on the coagulation and fibrinolytic systems. *Scand J Haematol* 1970; **7**: 404.

52. Johnson ND, Queral LA, Flinn WR, Yao JST, Bergan JJ. Late objective assessment of venous valve surgery. *Arch Surg* 1981; **116**: 1461.

53. Johnson WC, O'Hara ET, Corey C, Widrich WC, Nabseth DC. Venous stasis ulceration. Effectiveness of subfascial ligation. *Arch Surg* 1985; **120**: 797.

54. Jones NAG, Webb PJ, Rees RI, Kakkar VV. A physiological study of elastic compression stockings in venous disorders of the leg. *Br J Surg* 1980; **67**: 569.

55. Kistner R. Deep venous reconstruction. *Int Angiol* 1985; **4**: 429.

56. Lawrence D, Kakkar VV. Graduated, static, external compression of the lower limb: A physiological assessment. *Br J Surg* 1980; **67**: 119.

57. Linton RR. The communicating veins of the lower limb and the operating technique for their ligation. *Ann Surg* 1983; **107**: 582.

58. Linton RR. The post thrombotic ulceration of the lower extremity: its aetiology and surgical treatment. *Ann Surg* 1953; **138**: 415.

59. Lipmann HI, Briere J-P. Physical basis of external supports in chronic venous insufficiency. *Arch Phys Med Rehabil* 1971; **52**: 555.

60. May R, Nissl R. The post thrombotic syndrome. In May R (Ed) *Surgery of the Veins of the Leg and Pelvis*. Stuttgart. Georg Thieme 1979.

61. May R. Der Femoralis bypass bein postthrombo-tischen Zustandsbild. *Vasa* 1972; **1**: 267.

62. McEwan AJ, McArdle C S. Effect of hydro-xyethylrutosides on blood oxygen levels and venous insufficiency symptoms in varicose veins. *Br Med J* 1971; **1**: 138.

63. Negus D, Friedgood A. The effective management of venous ulceration *Br J Surg* 1983; **70**: 623.

64. Nicolaides AN, Schull K, Fernandes JF, Niles C. Ambulatory venous pressures. New information. In: Nicolaides AN, Yao JST (Eds) *Investigation of Vascular Disorders*. New York. Churchill Livingstone 1981.

65. Nielubowicz J, Szostek M, Staszkiewicz W. Late results of Linton flap operation. *J. Cardiovasc Surg* 1977; **18**: 561.

66. O'Donnell TFJr, Rosenthal DA, Callow AD, Ledig BL. Effect of elastic compression on venous hemodynamics in postphlebitic limbs. *JAMA* 1979; **242**: 2766.

67. O'Donnell TF, Burnand KG, Clemenson G, Lea Thomas M, Browse NL. Doppler examination vs clinical and phlebographic detection of the location of incompetent perforation veins. *Arch Surg* 1977; **112**: 31.

68. Pierson S, Pierson D, Swallow R, Johnson G Jr. Efficacy of graded elastic compression in the lower leg. *JAMA* 1983; **249**: 242.

69. Prerovsky I, Roztocil K, Hlavova A, Koleilat A, Razgova L, Oliva I. The effect of hydroxy-ethylrutosides after acute and chronic oral administration in patients with venous diseases. *Angiological* 1972; **9**: 408.

70. Psathakis ND, Psathakis DN. Rationale of the substitute valve operation by technique II in the treatment of chronic venous insufficiency *Int Angiol* 1985; **4**: 397.

71. Psathakis N. Ein neues operatives verfahren sur rationallen Behandlung des Insuffizien-syndroms der tiefen Beinvenen. *Chirurg* 1964; **35**: 79.

72. Queral N, Whitehouse WM, Flinn WR, Neiman HL, Yao JST, Bergan JJ. Surgical correction of chronic deep venous insufficiency by valvular transposition. *Surgery* 1980; **87**: 688.

73. Quill RD, Fegan WG. Reversibility of femoro-saphenous reflux. *Br J Surg* 1971; **58**: 388.

74. Raj TB, Goddard M, Makin GS. How long do compression bandages maintain their pressure during ambulatory treatment of varicose veins. *Br J Surg* 1980; **67**: 122.

75. Rose SS. A report on the use of hydroxyethylruto-sides in symptoms due to venous back pressure and allied conditions of the lower limb. *Br J Clin Pract* 1970; **24**: 4.

76. Sanberg I, Haeger K. The value of deep venous resection (Bauer's popliteal resection) for deep venous insufficiency. *Acta Chir Scand* 1966; **131**: 50.

77. Schanzer H, Peirce EC II. A rational approach to surgery of the chronic venous stasis syndrome. *Ann Surg* 1982; **195**: 25.

78. Silver D, Gleysteen JJ, Rhodes GR. Surgical treat-ment of the refactory post phlebitic ulcer. *Arch Surg* 1971; **103**: 554.

79. Somerville JJF, Brow GO, Byrne PJ, Quill RD, Fegan WG. The effect of elastic stockings on superficial venous pressures in patients with venous insufficiency. *Br J Surg* 1974; **61**: 979.

80. Stemmer R. Ambulatory elastocompressive treat-ment of the lower extremities particularly with elastic stockings. *Z Arztl Fortbild (Jena)* 1969; **63**: 1.

81. Taheri SA, Heffner R, Meenaghan MA, Budd T, Pollack LH. Vein valve transplantation. *Int Angiol* 1985; **4**: 425.

82. Taheri SA, Lasar L, Elias SM. Surgical treatment of post phlebitic syndrome. *Br J Surg* 1982; **69**(Suppl): 59.

83. Warren R, Thayer TR. Transplantation of the saphenous vein for post-phlebitic stasis. *Surgery* 1954; **35**: 867.

84. Wheeler HB, Anderson FA. The diagnosis of venous thrombosis by impedance plethysmo-graphy. In Bernstein EF (Ed) *Non Invasive Diagnostic Techniques in Vascular Disease.* St Louis. CV Mosby 1985.

85. Widmer LK. In: *Peripheral Venous Disorders.* Bern. Hans Huber 1978.

86. Wismer R. The actions of tri-hydroxyethylrutoside on the permeability of the capillaries in man. *Praxis* 1963; **52**: 1412.

13

Venous ulceration: pathology

Definition

A venous ulcer is a solution of the continuity of the skin of the lower limb caused by an abnormality of the veins draining the limb. There is no single venous abnormality that is always associated with ulceration, and most of the pathological changes in the skin and ulcer base are non-specific.[112] A venous ulcer is usually situated in the gaiter region of the leg and is invariably surrounded by thickened, pigmented and fibrotic skin which we have called lipodermatosclerosis (Colour plates 7 and 8).[22,23,28]

'Varicose ulcer', 'gravitational ulcer', 'stasis ulcer' and 'hypostatic ulcer' have been used in the past as alternative names for venous ulcers. All these terms are semantically incorrect and should be abandoned.

Prevalence and incidence of venous ulceration

It is difficult to obtain an up-to-date and accurate figure of the prevalence of venous leg ulcers because the diagnosis is so imprecise. Various estimates have been made but these are almost certainly inaccurate and rely heavily on extrapolation and guesswork.

In 1931 Dickson Wright[48] suggested that a quarter of a million patients in the United Kingdom had leg ulcers (a prevalence of 0.5 per cent), but the means by which this figure was obtained were not given. Linton[91] took Dickson Wright's figures and extrapolated them to the United States, to produce an estimate of between 300,000–400,000 patients with venous ulcers in North America.

Lockhart Mummery and Smitham[93] used Bauer's figures from Denmark[6] (which, incidentally, he derived from Roholm and it is not known how Roholm obtained his data) to estimate that there were at any one time between 100,000 and 200,000 patients with 'varicose ulcers' in England and Wales, a prevalence of 0.25–0.5 per cent.

Boyd et al.,[20] from their experience of patients with leg ulcers referred to hospitals in the Manchester region, estimated that 5/1000 of the population were affected, this is an identical figure to that of Dickson Wright. Hellgren[69] in Sweden found, however, that only approximately 3000 men and 15,000 women have obvious ulceration of the leg in a population of 7.5 million (a prevalence of less than 0.1 per cent). Bobek et al.,[17] found a much higher incidence of approximately 1 per cent, but they were studying subjects with evidence of venous disease.

Widmer and his co-workers[131,132] investigated the prevalence of venous and arterial disease in 4376 workers in the Basle chemical industry. They found that 1.3 per cent of this cohort of the population had suffered or currently suffered from leg ulceration – 1.1 per cent of the men and 1.4 per cent of the women.

Ruckley's recent survey[31,32,111] on leg ulceration in the West Lothian and Forth Valley regions of Scotland, based on patients located through a postal survey of district nurses, physiotherapists, general practitioners, long-stay hospitals and hospital outpatients during a defined period, found just under 1500 patients with ulcers in a population of approximately 1 million (an incidence of 0.15 per cent). Even in this well conducted study, however, the numbers of true venous ulcers are difficult to obtain, as it was only possible to investigate and confirm the diagnosis in a cohort of the affected patients, and patients with ulcers not under the care of nurses or doctors were undetected. The investigations that were performed on the sample population were clinical tests and Doppler ultrasound arterial ankle pressure measurements. The patients did not have any tests of venous calf pump function, and they were not investigated by phlebography. The diagnosis of venous ulceration was therefore based on 'typical clinical appearances' and an absence of another cause for the ulceration.

A similar study on a defined population in north-west London by Lewis and Cornwall,[39] also based on patients obtained through general practitioners, district nurses and residential homes, detected 357 patients with 424 leg ulcers in a population of approximately 200,000 (giving an incidence of 0.18 per cent). In this survey an attempt was made to differentiate the patients with venous disease and ulcers by the use of non-invasive techniques of venous investigation on a sample of 100 patients with 117 ulcerated limbs. Venous disease was assessed by continuous wave ultrasound and by photoplethysmography (see Chapter 4).

Sixty-three of the 117 ulcerated limbs had evidence of venous disease alone, 36 had signs of superficial venous incompetence and 27 had superficial and deep vein incompetence. Another 132 limbs had an abnormal calf pump function and Doppler evidence of venous reflux, but they also had evidence of ischaemia, as shown by a reduced arterial ankle pressure index (less than 0.9). Fourteen of these 32 'ischaemic' limbs had evidence of superficial venous incompetence and 18 had signs of coexisting deep vein incompetence. Twelve of the ulcerated limbs had no evidence of any venous abnormality but had a reduced ankle pressure index indicative of arterial ischaemia, and in 10 limbs with ulcers all the tests proved normal.

This study suggests that 80 per cent of all leg ulcers have some evidence of venous disease within the affected limb but this is combined with arterial disease in nearly a third.

Comment   As no venous or arterial abnormality could be found in 10 of the ulcerated limbs investigated by Cornwall and Lewis (all tests were normal), it is reasonable to maintain a sceptical attitude to all the published figures of the incidence of 'venous ulceration'.

Nevertheless, on the basis of these two recent major British surveys,[32,39] it is sensible to conclude that approximately 1 per cent of the population have, or have had leg ulceration, with perhaps a quarter of this figure (0.25 per cent) having active ulceration at any one time. About 75 per cent of

all leg ulcers are associated with venous disease. This figure increases with age[32,39] and is higher in the female population (nearly 3:1, women:men). It also increases if arterial disease or rheumatoid arthritis develops.[31] Venous ulceration appears to be common in all countries and does not appear to have any definite racial predilection.

Incidence of superficial vein incompetence, deep vein incompetence and calf communicating vein incompetence in the genesis of venous ulceration

This has been discussed already in Chapter 11, but those studies which have specifically attempted to evaluate the role of these three main sites of valvular incompetence in the genesis of venous ulceration are discussed again here.

Estimates of the incidence of post-thrombotic damage and superficial venous incompetence as a cause of venous ulceration vary considerably between hospitals and between countries.[8,25,92,105,124] These estimates also depend upon the method used to assess deep vein damage (see Chapters 4 and 12) and upon the skill of the clinician examining the superficial veins. The methods that have been used to assess incompetence of the calf communicating veins (which have already been discussed in Chapters 4 and 6) are known to be inaccurate and open to individual interpretation.

Table 13.1 shows the incidence of past deep vein thrombosis or evidence of a deep vein abnormality (valvular incompetence or post-thrombotic changes) which have been reported in patients with venous ulcers. The methods used to make the diagnosis of post-thrombotic limb are also shown.

A past history of thrombosis can be obtained from at least 20 per cent of all patients with venous ulcers, and 'objective tests' of deep vein function or anatomy double this figure. Approximately 40 per cent of the patients with venous ulcers therefore have objective evidence of post-thrombotic damage, though this figure obviously varies considerably in different studies.[25,105,124]

Table 13.2 shows the incidence of incompetence of the calf communicating veins in patients with venous ulceration. These figures must be viewed with some scepticism because of the inaccuracy of the methods used to assess incompetence of the calf communicating veins. They do suggest, however, that incompetence of

Table 13.1 Incidence of post-thrombotic ulceration

Authors	Method of diagnosis	No. ulcerated limbs	No. post-thrombotic limbs	% of post-thrombotic limbs
Birger[9]	History	432	173	40
Bauer[6]	Asc.Phleb.*	38	34	87
DeTakats and Graupner[46]	History			
	Asc.Phleb.*	100	46	46
Anning[3]	History	1026	738	75
Cockett[37]	History			
	Clinical signs	182	38	20
Arnoldi and Haegar[4]	Asc.Phleb.*	1092	486	45
Burnand et al.[25]	Asc.Phleb.*	41	23	55
Negus and Friedgood[105]	Asc.Phleb.*			
	Doppler ultrasound			
	Photoplethysmography	109	44	40
Sethia and Darke[118]	Asc. and Des.Phleb.†	60	20	33
Cornwall and Lewis[39]	Photoplethysmography			
	Ultrasound	99	45	46

*Asc.Phleb. = ascending phlebography.
†Des.Phleb. = descending phlebography.

Table 13.2 Incidence of lower leg communicating vein incompetence in limbs with venous ulcers

	Techniques	Limbs	Incompetent Communicating veins No.	%
Dodd and Cockett[50]	Operative exploration	135	96	71
Thomas et al.[124]	Operative exploration	44	43	99
Sethia and Darke[118]	Operative exploration	60	59	99
Hoare et al.[72]	Ultrasound	80	71	88
Negus[106]	Operative exploration	109	108	99
Haeger[61]	Operative exploration	54	54	100
Arnoldi and Haeger[4]	Operative exploration	509	509	100

these veins is almost always present in limbs with venous ulceration.

Comment Haegar[61] has stated that the calf communicating veins are *always* incompetent in limbs with venous ulceration, and saphenous vein incompetence on its own can *never* cause venous ulceration. We do not believe that this dogma is correct, as the words 'never' and 'always' rarely apply to biological phenomena; in general, however, venous ulceration is rare in limbs with pure saphenous vein incompetence.

It is therefore true that incompetence of the calf communicating veins is found in 'most' limbs with venous ulcers, but it is equally true that this abnormality invariably coexists with superficial (saphenous) vein incompetence and often with post-thrombotic damage of the deep veins and saphenous vein incompetence is the abnormality responsible for the major part of the derangement of calf pump function that our simple tests measure.

Aetiology of venous ulceration

Calf pump dysfunction

The first appreciation of the association between varicose veins and venous ulceration is attributed to Hippocrates (460–377 BC). In Adam's translation of the ancient Greek book *De Ulceribus*,[71] Hippocrates (or members of his School) states

'when the points adjoining to an ulcer are inflamed, the ulcer is not disposed to heal until the inflammation subside, nor when the surrounding parts are blackened by mortification, nor when a varix occasioned an overflow of blood in the part, is the ulcer disposed to heal, unless you bring the surrounding parts into a healthy condition.'

The association between varicose veins and venous ulcers became clearly established in the 16th and 17th centuries[66,133] and a number of authors in the early 19th century[21,38,42,70,73,76,80] stressed the importance of varicose veins in the aetiology of leg ulceration.

In 1867 John Gay[50] gave two Lettsomian lectures entitled *On varicose discolouration, induration and ulcer*. In these lectures he recorded the findings of the dissections he had made in 24 cadavers with clinical evidence of venous disease of the leg. He stated that the relatively small number of observations make his conclusions of 'doubtful validity' and regarded his work as a 'pioneering party'; presumably what we would call a 'pilot study'.

In nine of the limbs he found simple external varicosities around normal skin, but in 10 limbs the varicosities were associated with discoloration of the skin and ulceration, and in one limb there were varicosities, ulceration and skin induration but no discoloration (i.e. nine legs had simple uncomplicated varicose veins and in 11 legs varicose veins were complicated by lipodermatosclerosis). He noted that the worst varicosities were often not associated with skin changes and, conversely, some of the worse skin changes were found in limbs with the least varicosities. These findings caused him to question the accepted association between varicose veins and ulceration. He went on to show that coagula (new and old thrombi) were present in the short saphenous veins of three patients and in the deep veins of six of the nine patients with the cutaneous changes of lipodermatosclerosis (bronzing and induration of the skin with or without ulcers). Some arterial disease was present in six of the limbs.

Gay states 'ulceration is not a direct consequence of varicosity but of other conditions of the venous system with which varicosity is not infrequently a complication, but without which neither of the allied skin conditions is met with.'

The presence of communicating veins between the deep and superficial compartments of the calf was probably first described by Verneuil[127] who stated that 'deep varices are more common than subcutaneous varices'. He drew the following inferences from 21 dissections

'the primitive seat of phlebectasy resides in the deep veins. These first suffer dilatation for reasons which anatomy and physiology render imperative; and from there it passes to the subcutaneous veins. The extension takes place by various anatomical channels which exist between the superficial and deep veins. I affirm that if you find in any part of the limb, a spot ever so limited in which the superficial veins are serpentine, if you trace them with care you will find that they communicate by large tracts with the deep or intramuscular branches'.

Gay[59] confirmed the findings of Verneuil[127] in his cadaver dissections and drew particular attention to the communicating veins of the medial calf which he called 'perforating veins'. These are well shown in a number of illustrations which accompany the text (see Figs. 1.11, 1.12, 1.13, 1.14). He also reported a series of experiments to look at the venous return in cadavers, and in a dog model after the femoral vein had been ligated. He concluded that 'obstruction of the femoral vein is followed by saphenous repletion, repletion of the intercommunicating veins, and capillary cutaneous injection.' He regarded the communicating veins as an alternative means for venous return.

A specific role for incompetence of the valves in the communicating veins of the calf (the perforating veins of Gay) in the genesis of ulceration was first suggested by John Homans in 1918[75] who, apparently ignorant of Gay's work, recognized two varieties of ulcer – the first associated with surface varices and the second associated with surface varices complicated by varicosity of the ankle communicating veins including postthrombotic varices. He suggested that the location of ulceration in the gaiter region was the result of the location of the medial calf communicating veins in the gaiter region of the leg. He then subdivided the incompetence of the communicating veins into those associated with and presumably caused by the varicose process, and those secondary to a thrombosis. He believed that the latter 'develop as an overflow or safety vent from the deep veins'.

In his conclusions based on a series of illustrated cases he states the following.

> '1. Varicose ulcers take origin in profound nutritional disturbances attributable to varicose veins (influenced by trauma, infection and surface stasis).
>
> 2. Varicose ulcers arising from surface varicosities are generally healed by adequate removal of varicose veins.
>
> 3. Varicose ulcers dependant upon a postphlebitic varix are always intractable to palliative treatment, generally incurable by the removal of varicose veins alone and must be excised to be cured.'

Homan's hypothesis of two causes of incompetence of the communicating veins has never been disproved. Phlebographic studies have confirmed that there are certainly two groups of patients with incompetence of the communicating veins – those who have no phlebographic evidence of past deep vein thrombosis and those with post-thrombotic damage (Fig. 12.3).[4,6,25,45,61]

Calf pump function in limbs with incompetent calf communicating veins with phlebographically normal deep veins is often just as poor as in those limbs with unequivocal evidence of deep vein damage.[26] Furthermore, the function of the calf pump cannot be restored to normal by ligating the communicating veins even in limbs with apparently normal deep veins which suggests, if our tests are accurate, that there is subtle damage to the deep veins which is undetectable by phlebography. It is conceivable that post-thrombotic damage may be responsible for all the valvular changes within the communicating veins but this is unlikely and a dual aetiology, from varicose veins or deep vein thrombosis remains a teleologically more attractive hypothesis. Further evidence is, however, required before this hypothesis can be fully accepted.

The role of incompetence of the calf communicating veins in the genesis of ulceration has been amplified by Turner-Warwick,[125] Linton[90,91,92] and Cockett.[35,36,37] These authors have all observed that saphenous vein incompetence, incompetence of the calf communicating veins and post-thrombotic damage commonly coexist,

and it has proved difficult to unravel which of these mechanisms is dominant in ulcer development. The Linton and Cockett schools have argued[4,5,41,55,105,106,124] that incompetence of the calf communicating veins must be present before ulceration can occur.

The pressure flow studies of Bjordal[10,11,12,13,14] have cast doubt on the importance of the communicating veins in affecting calf pump function, but unfortunately have never been repeated or confirmed. Bjordal showed that reflux through the ankle communicating veins has only a minor adverse effect on calf pump function compared with the effect of saphenous vein incompetence. We also found that ligation of the medial calf communicating veins produced a relatively small improvement in the function of the calf pump, whereas the surgical abolition of saphenous reflux almost returns the calf pump function to normal.[26] The fact that correcting the superficial reflux has the greatest effect on our measurement of calf pump function does not, however, mean that superficial reflux is the cause of the ulceration.[117] The reduction in the local superficial venous pressure produced by abolishing reflux through the calf communicating veins may be more important than producing an overall improvement in calf pump function, and rates of pressure change may be more important than absolute or mean levels. The effects of incompetence in the superficial and lower leg communicating veins are probably complementary.

Comment By definition a venous ulcer cannot exist in the presence of normal calf pump function but confusion (fuelled by inadequate methods of investigation) still exists, as to which of the three main venous abnormalities is responsible for, or is the most important cause of a venous ulcer. All three lesions (deep vein damage, lower leg communicating vein incompetence and saphenous incompetence) can and, in many limbs, do coexist. At the same time there are certainly some limbs with ulcers in which the calf communicating veins are not incompetent.

Several recent papers have shown that the diagnosis of simple long saphenous vein incompetence is often inaccurate;[30,101] this makes the crude intraoperative assessment of lower leg communicating vein incompetence even more suspect. If we cannot diagnose the physiological abnormality correctly, we will never be able to assess its importance.

In view of these difficulties it is, at present, impossible to determine which site of incompetence is of major or sole importance. There is some evidence that the role of communicating vein incompetence in the genesis of ulceration has been overstressed. This has partly stemmed from general dissatisfaction with the results of lower leg communicating vein ligation in preventing recurrent ulceration in the post-thrombotic limb,[25,90,92] even though there are many studies which show that this operation is very effective in limbs without post-thrombotic damage.[25,105,124] In recent years a greater emphasis has been attached to deep vein obstruction and reflux in the genesis of ulceration, and this has lead to the development of surgical techniques to reconstruct, repair, or transplant valves into incompetent veins,[82,83,110,128] or techniques to bypass occluded segments,[44,99,129] but there is little evidence that this type of surgery is any more effective than ligation of the communicating veins in preventing the recurrence of post-thrombotic ulceration (see Chapters 8, 9 and 12).

Most patients with uncomplicated and isolated long saphenous vein incompetence do not develop venous ulceration but there is little doubt that there exists a small group of patients without evidence of lower leg communicating vein incompetence who do get ulcers. Nevertheless, the majority of patients with venous ulcers do have incompetent communicating veins.

The relative importance of each site of valvular incompetence will only be discovered when random cohorts of patients with healed ulcers are treated by ligation of the communicating veins in isolation and the results compared with those of other groups treated by saphenous vein surgery alone and deep vein repair alone. These studies have yet to be carried out.

A defective calf pump is essential to the development of ulceration, but it is not known if there is a critical level of increased pressure that will always lead to ulceration, or if the development of lipodermatosclerosis is related to a certain time span of abnormal pressure. Will a pressure in the superficial veins that is always above 50 mmHg inevitably lead to ulceration, unless elastic compression is worn? We do not know the answer to this question and never will unless large scale prospective physiologically monitored clinical studies are undertaken.

It may be that the genesis of lipodermatosclerosis and ulceration is a product of the level of venous pressure and the time that the tissues are exposed to this high pressure. Perhaps skin changes and ulceration develop rapidly in tissues exposed to high pressures, while lower absolute pressures only produce damage after prolonged exposure. We do not know if a constant high pressure is more harmful or less harmful than short episodes of very high pressure. We do not even know whether the absolute amount, type or persistence of the pressure matter at all! Perhaps it is the tissue reaction to the pressure that matters – sensitive tissues responding to minor changes, insensitive tissues withstanding gross changes. All these questions remain to be answered by properly planned prospective human surgical research.

Changes in the microcirculation and tissue anoxia

The mechanism by which calf pump failure causes lipodermatosclerosis and ulceration is just as poorly understood as the type of venous lesion which is responsible for pump failure. Three main theories have been proposed to explain how a disordered calf pump causes tissue death (Fig. 13.1).

- Stasis within the cutaneous microcirculation
- The opening of arteriovenous shunts
- An interstitial barrier

All these theories assume that these changes are secondary to the calf pump failure but even that assumption is debatable.

Capillary and venular stasis

Homans[75] was the first person to suggest that defective venous return from the lower limb caused by post-thrombotic deep vein damage or varicose veins, might result in 'venous stasis'. He thought that the resulting stagnant anoxia was responsible for the tissue death seen as cutaneous ulceration. This theory has been repeated and accepted in countless publications on venous ulceration, though the concept of 'stasis' has been discredited by measurements of the oxygen content of the venous and capillary blood and in the tissues of ulcerated limbs.

The first study which described the oxygen

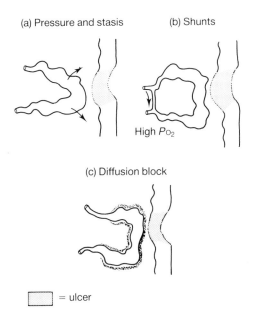

(a) Pressure and stasis   (b) Shunts

High P_{O_2}

(c) Diffusion block

☐ = ulcer

Fig. 13.1 A diagrammatic representation of the three 'theories' of ulcer development.

(a) Pressure and stasis. This theory postulates that the high venous pressure and slow venous blood flow of calf pump failure cause stagnant anoxia and/or pressure necrosis of the overlying skin.

(b) Arteriovenous shunts. This theory postulates that arteriovenous shunts open up in the dermal capillary bed as a result of a persistently high venous pressure. These shunts, by diverting oxygenated blood away from the over-lying skin, cause skin ischaemia and ulceration.

(c) The fibrin diffusion block. This theory postulates that the high venous pressure present during exercise in the calf pump failure syndrome is transmitted back to the capillary bed which distends and elongates. The interendothelial pores enlarge allowing large molecules, including fibrinogen, to escape into the tissues where an associated reduction in fibrinolytic capacity is thought to enable polymerization of fibrin to occur unimpeded. The pericapillary fibrin then acts as a diffusion barrier or interferes with local tissue metabolism. The eventual cause of ulceration is the reduced skin oxygenation caused by the diffusion barrier.

content of venous blood[47] reported that the venous blood oxygen content was lower in blood sampled from a varicose vein than in samples taken from the anticubital vein of the same patient. One year later, however, Blalock[15] repeated these studies and found conflicting results. He showed that the oxygen content of

femoral venous blood was highest during recumbency and declined rapidly when the patient stood. He considered that differences in posture at the time of sampling could account for the conflicting results of these two studies. He also showed that the oxygen content of the femoral venous blood was higher in a limb with varicose veins than its normal counterpart and that this difference was accentuated when ulceration was present. Blalock concluded that his findings suggested that the total blood flow through limbs with venous ulceration was increased.

A number of subsequent studies have confirmed Blalock's findings,[16,54,74,109] and only one study[100] has been contradictory. There is therefore little doubt that the venous blood leaving an ulcerated limb has a high oxygen content.

The blood flow in ulcerated limbs has also been measured. Dye injected into the femoral artery appears more rapidly in the veins of the patients with ulcerated limbs than in normal 'controls'[64,65,109,128] and plethysmographic studies have also shown an increased blood flow in ulcerated limbs.[1]

The development of transcutaneous oxygen electrodes, which measure oxygen diffusion across the skin, has enabled the tissue oxygen in lipodermatosclerotic skin to be measured and compared with that in control sites. Using a probe heated to 45°C, it has been shown that the tissue oxygen concentration is reduced in areas of lipodermatosclerosis.[34,96,121]

Recently, Dodd et al.,[49] using an unheated probe over the anterior tibial compartment, found higher oxygen tensions in patients with active or past venous ulceration. The strange siting of the electrode and the small number of patients included in this study make it difficult to assess.

Hopkins et al.,[78] used positron emission tomography to measure blood flow and oxygen utilization in the skin of a group of 11 patients with venous ulceration and 5 patients with lipodermatosclerosis. They found that there was an increased blood flow with a reduced tissue extraction of oxygen in areas of lipodermatosclerosis and in the abnormal skin around open ulcers. These results indicate that there is no venous stasis but a local functional shunting of blood through an abnormal microcirculation.

All these findings refute the concept of 'stasis' as an important factor in the genesis of venous ulceration, but it is conceivable that there is local slowing of blood flow through the cutaneous capillary bed of the peri-ulcer skin while there is rapid blood flow through other areas of the limb.[113,114,115] Videomicroscopy[18] has provided some support for this concept, though such a change could be an effect of the ulceration rather than its cause. The case for 'venous stasis' as a cause of venous ulceration is not entirely discredited.

Arteriovenous shunting

Holling *et al.*,[74] stated that it was possible that 'a shunt of blood directly from the arterioles to the venules, largely avoiding the capillary bed' might explain their findings of high oxygen levels in the venous blood of ulcerated limbs. This idea was extended by Piulachs and Vidal-Barraquer,[109] who suggested that arteriovenous communications opened up in response to venous obstruction or other causes of defective venous return. Fontaine[57] provided further support for this hypothesis when he reported higher oxygen tensions in the venous blood samples from the limbs of 95 patients with varicose veins than in samples taken from healthy control subjects.

Gius[60] said that he had seen histological evidence of abnormal arteriovenous communications in the skin of the calves of patients undergoing varicose vein surgery whilst using an operating microscope. He conceded, however, that the vessels that he had seen were indistinguishable from thick-walled capillaries. His work has never been confirmed. Schalin[116] has also suggested that all varicose veins are caused by arteriovenous fistulae.

Ryan and Copeman[113] postulated that the normal temperature-regulating arteriovenous fistulae present within the dermis might open up as a result of raised venous pressure, and that these fistulae might be responsible for the arteriovenous shunting that appeared to exist in patients with ulceration.

The reduction in the time taken for radio-opaque contrast medium to traverse arteries and reach the veins in patients with ulcers,[64,65,128] together with an increase in the cutaneous temperature which has been recorded in post-thrombotic limbs[62] all lent additional support to the concept of abnormal 'shunts' opening up in limbs with severe venous dysfunction. The concept of functional arteriovenous shunting was, however, strongly challenged by the work of Partsch and his colleagues.[89,94] They used isotopically labelled macroaggregates of albumin to assess the size of the functional arteriovenous shunt that was present in limbs with venous ulceration and compared this with similar measurements made in normal healthy limbs. No evidence of physiological shunting was found in the vicinity of an ulcer, though the authors did find some evidence of an increased blood flow in the feet of ulcerated limbs. In fact, their gamma camera scans of ulcerated limbs demonstrated an increased trapping of the aggregates in the ulcer-bearing skin – a finding which contradicts the hypothesis that there are arteriovenous shunts. These findings were confirmed by Hehne *et al.*,[67] who, using a similar technique, also failed to demonstrate evidence of shunting in patients with venous ulceration.

An interstitial diffusion barrier caused by increased capillary permeability and a deficiency of tissue fibrinolysis (see Chapter 11)

Whimster originally observed that patients with severe chronic venous disease in their lower limbs appeared to have an increased number of capillaries in biopsies taken from the 'gaiter skin' (Colour plate 25).[130] He suggested that the capillary bed had proliferated in response to the persistently elevated venous pressure.

Other investigators,[55,88] have suggested that dermal capillary loops elongate and become tortuous rather than increase in actual number, and Ryan[114] has suggested that a rise in venous pressure causes dilatation of the horizontal subpapillary venous plexus (Fig. 13.2), with grossly 'coiled' elongated papillary (dermal) capillaries, and a reduction in the number of capillaries supplying the epidermis. Corrigan and Kakkar[40] observed that the endothelial cells of capillaries within the ankle skin of patients with the post-thrombotic syndrome were often swollen and contained large vacuoles. They also reported that the basement membrane of these capillaries was often irregular and thickened.

All these studies suggest that lipodermato-sclerosis and ulceration might be caused by an alteration in the local capillary bed in response to calf pump failure. We confirmed this when we

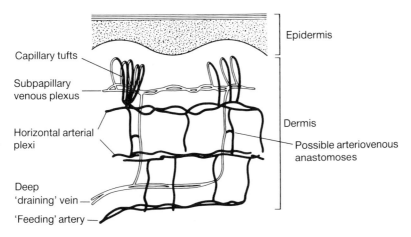

Fig. 13.2 A diagram to show the normal arrangement of the vessels in the dermis. The possible sites of arteriovenous fistulae are shown. The 'elongation' or 'proliferation' that is found in patients with chronic venous hypertension occurs in the capillary tufts that drain into the subpapillary venous plexus. The perivascular fibrin cuff is found around these capillaries.

found a significant correlation between the number of capillaries seen on histological sections of the 'gaiter area' skin and the extent of the venous pressure fall found during exercise (Fig. 13.3).[28] We then showed, in an animal model, that venous hypertension increased capillary permeability and the concentration of fibrinogen in lymph.[7,29,86] Fibrinogen, a large molecule, was found to escape significantly faster from the capillary bed of the skin and subcutaneous tissues in limbs with a high venous pressure.[29,53]

This led us to re-examine the ulcer-bearing skin of patients with severe venous disease and cutaneous complications to see if there was any evidence of fibrinogen or fibrin deposition within the tissues. Biopsies of skin were taken from patients with severe lipodermatosclerosis and were stained for fibrinogen/fibrin with phosphotungstic acid haemotoxylin (PTAH) (Colour plate 25) and also treated with rabbit raised antihuman fibrin/fibrinogen antibodies and then examined with fluorescent labelled markers. Both techniques showed the presence of pericapillary fibrin/fibrinogen (Colour plates 26 and 27).

A controlled study showed that these changes were only present in limbs with lipodermatosclerosis and were associated with a significantly larger dermal capillary bed and a significantly reduced venous pressure fall on exercise (Fig. 13.4).[28]

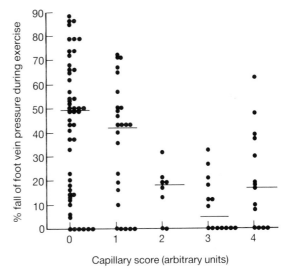

Fig. 13.3 This graph shows the relationship between the capillary 'proliferation' seen in biopsies taken from the ulcer-bearing skin of legs with varying degrees of calf pump failure and the maximal fall in foot vein pressure during exercise. It can be seen that limbs with mild or absent capillary 'proliferation' (scores 0 and 1) had much more efficient calf pumps than limbs with moderate or severe capillary 'proliferation' (scores 2, 3 and 4). This difference was highly significant ($P < 0.001$).[28]

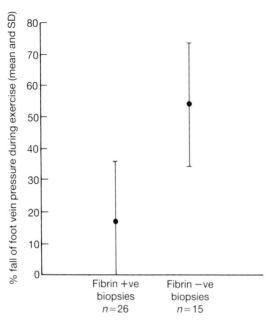

Fig. 13.4 This figure shows the mean maximum fall of foot pressure during exercise in 26 limbs in which the skin biopsies had evidence of pericapillary fibrin (fibrin-positive biopsies) and in 15 limbs in which no fibrin was seen (fibrin-negative biopsies). The limbs with evidence of pericapillary fibrin in the ulcer-bearing skin had significantly worse calf pump function than those whose skin contained no pericapillary fibrin.[29]

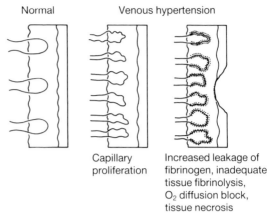

Fig. 13.5 A diagrammatic representation of the development of the pericapillary fibrin cuff. The permanently elevated venous pressure (which is not reduced by the calf pump) distends and enlarges the capillary bed (capillary 'proliferation'). The distended interendothelial pores allow the normally 'pore-bound' fibrinogen to escape and this polymerizes and becomes fixed around the capillaries. The inadequate fibrinolytic capacity of these patients interferes with the removal of the fibrin and the subsequent reduction in the metabolism and oxygenation of the tissues nurtured by these capillaries leads to necrosis and ulceration.[22]

The deposition of fibrin within the tissues is normally prevented by the interstitial fibrinolytic system. We found, however, that patients with lipodermatosclerosis had a significant reduction in both systemic and tissue fibrinolytic activity.[24]

We felt that the pericapillary fibrin/fibrinogen deposition that we had seen in the ulcer-bearing skin might be the result of a persistently elevated venous pressure which distended the capillary bed and dilated the inter-endothelial pores (Fig. 13.5).[108,119] These changes could be expected to increase the concentration of fibrinogen and other large plasma molecules in the intestitial fluid where the fibrinogen/fibrin might become fixed within the tissues around the capillaries because of the defective tissue fibrinolytic activity capacity of these patients. This pericapillary 'cuff' might then act as a diffusion barrier (Fig. 13.5).

The presence of pericapillary fibrils which stain with PTAH has also been reported in the abnormal skin of patients with arteriovenous fistulae formed for renal dialysis access in the upper limb.[134] This is the human equivalent of our animal model.

The presence of pericapillary fibrin/fibrinogen deposition in the skin of more than 90 per cent of patients with lipodermatosclerosis has been confirmed by Marks,[97] Partsch,[107] and Eaglestein.[52] Immunofluorescent pericapillary fibrin has been found in the lipodermatosclerotic skin around venous ulcers but not in the skin adjacent to ulcers of different aetiology.[52]

Electronmicroscopic analysis (Fig. 13.6) and monoclonal antibodies against cross-linked fibrin have shown that the pericapillary material is not necessarily pure cross-linked fibrin. The concept of a mechanical 'fibrin' block may not be correct. There is no doubt that there is a pericapillary cuff of fibrin/fibrinogen but it may be behaving as a tissue metabolic block of indeterminate origin and not simply as a mechanical obstruction to diffusion.

Comment The mechanism by which the cutaneous changes of lipodermatosclerosis and

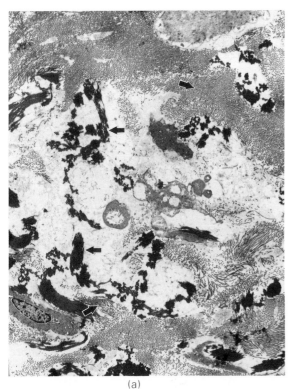

(a)

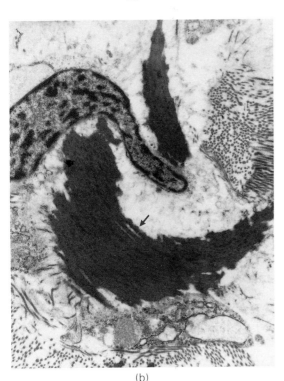

(b)

ulceration develop in response to prolonged venous hypertension remains open to speculation (see Chapter 11 and above).

There is no satisfactory animal model of the venous ulcer. Marks *et al.* have produced slowly healing 'sores' in experimental animals by injecting sodium tetra decyl sulphate subcutaneously,[98] but this does not exactly mimic the human venous ulcer. Other investigators[126] have found that frogs' legs subjected to intensive external compression develop oedema, capillary dilatation, haemorrhage and, eventually, small areas of cutaneous ulceration. It is not clear how long these ulcers take to heal. Until we have a satisfactory 'ulcer model' further progress in understanding both the aetiology and pathology of venous ulceration will be delayed.

We have proposed a hypothesis which fits the known facts better than the 'stasis' and 'arteriovenous shunt' hypotheses but which will certainly have to be modified as our understanding of the changes that occur in the microcirculation improves. We await further studies on the cause of venous ulceration with interest.

The cause of skin breakdown

Injury

It is not known if localized tissue anoxia can in itself cause the skin to ulcerate. Minor trauma, possibly as little as rubbing an itchy patch of skin, is probably necessary for ulceration to begin. It is impossible to prove or disprove the concept that local injury is always the final initiating factor in the genesis of a venous ulcer. Certainly, many of our patients describe an episode of trauma before their ulcers developed, and we advise all patients

---

Fig. 13.6 Two electron micrographs of the tissue in the edge of a chronic venous ulcer.

(a) Many normal collagen fibrils are visible (white edged arrows) but there is also some electron dense material which appears to be coarsely fibrillary (black arrows).

(b) A higher power magnification shows this fibrillary material more clearly. This is probably the material described by Adair, which he thought was degenerating collagen, (see page 363).

These figures were kindly supplied by Gillian Bullock and Paul Sibson of Ciba Geigy.

to protect their legs from injury when their ulcers have healed.

Tissue anoxia may cause the death of skin and its replacement with scar tissue without ulceration. The white scars of 'atrophie blanche' are commonly seen in areas of chronic lipodermatosclerosis. This observation suggests that something else is required to change the slow death with simultaneous repair (atrophie blanche) into the rapid skin death of ulceration.

Oedema

Local tissue oedema has, for some time, been thought to play a part in the development of ulcers,[19,45,63,103,112] however, Myers *et al.* have shown that the presence of oedema does not delay ulcer healing,[104] and that its elimination does not ensure healing. Very few of our patients with lymphoedema develop ulceration of the skin, but we have shown that the combination of lymphoedema and lipodermatosclerosis is usually associated with evidence of defective fibrinolysis.[122] Many of our patients with venous ulceration have no signs of oedema. There is therefore no clear evidence that oedema of the tissues is an important factor in ulceration.

Infection

The role of infection in the genesis of a venous ulcer is still confused. There is little doubt that venous ulcers all become secondarily infected[115] but it is much more difficult to know if bacteria play any part in promoting or perpetuating the ulcer. Some studies have suggested that the numbers of organisms may perpetuate ulceration; high colony counts represent significant infection and low counts represent simple commensal colonization.[115]

Our current ulcer study suggests that the role of anaerobic infection may have been underestimated, because we have found pathogenic anaerobic organisms in nearly half of the ulcers we have examined but it is doubtful if infection ever acts as a primary cause of venous ulceration.

Ischaemia

Ischaemia is, like trauma, a potent cause of ulceration in its own right, and it will be discussed further in Chapter 14 on the differential diagnosis of venous ulcers. It was, however, pointed out by Dodd and Cockett[50] that the skin of the anteriomedial aspect of the lower leg has an extremely poor blood supply, which increases the risk of skin breakdown if an additional noxious stimulus is present. Ischaemia and venous skin damage may therefore combine to cause necrosis and ulceration, and in some patients it may be difficult to distinguish the relative importance of calf pump failure from that of arterial ischaemia in the development of ulceration;[111] Doppler ultrasound ankle pressure measurements and arteriography may be required to define the role of ischaemia in ulcers of mixed aetiology.[39,111]

Obesity

This is reported to be an important predisposing factor in the development of ulceration[115] but it does not appear to be an initiating factor. It does, of course, make ulcer healing more difficult. Many patients with ulcers may become obese because of the reduced activity caused by their ulcer, and perhaps very obese subjects are more likely to develop varicose veins and deep vein thrombosis (see Chapter 5 and Chapter 17).

Malfunction of the calf muscles

Nerve damage, local muscle damage or joint abnormalities all cause malfunction of the calf muscle pump.[95] This is seen in patients with poliomyelitis, after severe soft tissue and bony injury and in association with osteoarthritis of the knee or ankle. Although these conditions may predispose to ulceration, we are not aware of any evidence that they cause ulceration in their own right. However, the fixed equinuus deformity of the ankle that develops in some patients with severe long-standing ulceration around the ankle, certainly impedes healing and predisposes to further ulceration by preventing normal calf pump function.

Erect stance and height

Ulcers do not develop in other members of the animal kingdom, and the assumption of the erect posture by man is obviously important in the development of ulceration.[58] The resting hydrostatic foot vein pressure increases with the height of the individual but, though it is a clinical impression that tall people develop ulcers, there is a low incidence of both varicose veins and ulcers in the Bantu[51] who are an exceptionally tall race.

Intersex states

There is an unexplained relationship between varicose veins, venous ulceration and Klinefelter's syndrome (XXY).[33,79,81] We have seen three patients with an XYY chromosomal pattern who have resistant ulceration of the leg with normal venous physiology and anatomy (Fig. 13.7). It is possible that defective fibrinolysis may play a part in the development of these ulcers.

General health, cleanliness and personal hygiene

Poor general health does not cause venous ulceration, but may be the result of long-standing ulceration with its associated anaemia and protein depletion.[117] Lack of cleanliness and personal hygiene may be associated with poor compliance to treatment, but is unlikely to be an important cause of venous ulceration.

Psychological factors

Some patients appear to need a focus around which to live their lives, and an ulcer together with the medical and nursing care required for its management may provide just such a focus. The role of psychological factors in the development of venous ulceration and its persistence has not been proved.

In mediaeval times ulcers were thought to be necessary to allow the escape of 'evil humours', and healing was actively prevented.[3] This belief is not entirely extinct, and some patients believe that their ulcer serves a useful purpose and that their general health will deteriorate if it heals.

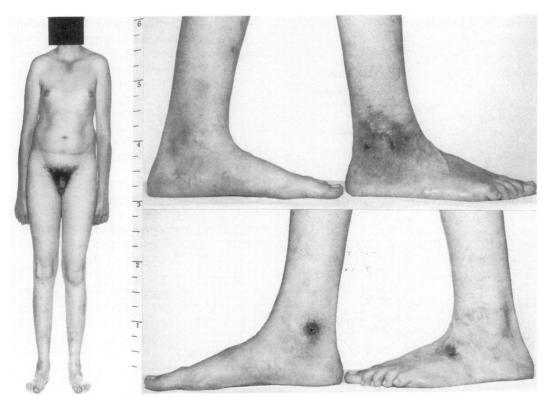

Fig. 13.7 A patient with Klinefelter's syndrome (XXY) (left-hand panel) associated with ulceration around the ankle (right-hand panels). This relationship is well recognized, but the aetiology of the ulceration remains obscure. The low level of male sex hormones in these patients may be associated with defective fibrinolysis.

The cause of associated skin changes

'Atrophie blanche' is an area of white stellate scarring (Colour plate 9) which often accompanies chronic lipodermatosclerosis and may precede venous ulceration. In an area of atrophie blanche the skin becomes shrivelled and scarred rather than thick and hard as in lipodermatosclerosis. The reason for this difference is open to speculation. Is atrophie blanche the result of cutaneous ischaemia, perhaps from capillary thrombosis, or is it just an extreme example of the effect of chronic hypoxia caused by the diffusion barrier? The two apparently dissimilar conditions – lipodermatosclerosis and atrophie blanche – may be the result of different levels of venous hypertension and tissue fibrinolysis. We do not know how the same mechanism, calf pump failure, can produce such different skin reactions.

The relevance of the gaiter region to the aetiology of ulceration

Most venous ulcers occur in the gaiter region of the leg, between the malleoli and the level of the lower edge of the gastrocnemius muscle. Venous ulcers have been described in the upper calf[3] (but we have never seen them) and they can also occasionally occur on the foot, though these are very rare. Ulcers on the foot are more often caused by different mechanisms.

Why then are venous ulcers confined to the 'gaiter skin'? The answer must lie in the relationship between this skin and the large medial calf communicating veins of the calf pump.[75] The calf pump generates pressures of up to 200 mmHg within the fascia,[95] and the high pressure developed within the soleal sinusoids and venae comitantes of the calf is transmitted directly into the surface veins and local capillary bed if the valves within the calf communicating veins are incompetent. Waves of high pressure may reach the superficial veins during calf pump systole, especially if there is obstruction to the pump outflow tract. Although there are foot pumps and thigh pumps, these do not usually generate the same amount of pressure[95] and, consequently, skin changes seldom occur in the skin of the thigh or foot. We have seen lipodermatosclerosis of the sole of the foot in two patients who had total congenital valvular agenesis in their deep veins, and we have seen one case of true lipodermato-sclerosis of the thigh in a patient with severe post-thrombotic disease.

All the evidence indicates that the site of the incompetent communicating veins determines the site of development of lipodermatosclerosis and venous ulceration. The poor arterial blood supply of the skin of the lower leg may increase skin ischaemia, but local venous hypertension is the root cause of the ulcer.

Comment In Chapter 11 we discussed the pathology of the post-thrombotic limb or 'calf pump failure syndrome' in detail. Some of this detail has necessarily been re-examined in this chapter but here we have laid particular emphasis on its relationship to the development of ulceration. We have also discussed again the type of venous abnormality that can lead to ulceration and other factors which may influence ulcer development. We have analysed the evidence for and against the three main theories of ulcer development.

The final pathway to ulceration seems to be through the transmission of high venous pressures (developed within the calf pump during exercise) to the subcutaneous veins and dermal capillaries. This appears to produce tissue anoxia, perhaps as the result of a pericapillary diffusion block, which leads directly to tissue necrosis and sometimes to cutaneous ulceration.

Progressive fibrosis and scarring leads to irreversible skin damage which may be responsible for permanent or recurrent ulceration.

Our own studies of the effect of chronic venous hypertension on the microcirculation of the lower limb was presaged by Arnoldi and Linderholm[5] who in 1968 concluded a study on venous pressure measurements with the following statement:

> 'Dilatation of capillaries causes an increase permeability of capillary walls. Proteins escape easily into the interstitial fluid[85] and after prolonged anoxaemia even blood corpuscles may penetrate the capillary wall.[135] These observations may explain the high protein content of interstitial fluid observed in patients with leg ulcers[67] and the discolouration of the skin of the ankle by haemosiderin which is an almost constant finding in these patients'.

The pathology of a venous ulcer

Ulcer development

The pathological changes of lipodermatosclerosis have already been discussed (see Chapter 11). When ulceration begins there is partial skin loss in an already abnormal area of skin. If this does not heal rapidly, the remaining layers of skin usually necrose to produce full-thickness skin loss. There is invariably some attempt at healing by the underlying tissues, and granulation tissue consisting of capillary loops and fibrous tissue starts to develop from the dermal vascular plexus, if this is still present (Fig. 13.2), or from vessels in the subcutaneous fat.[3,112]

Tissue necrosis with cellular death can occasionally extend into the subcutaneous fat and even down to the deep fascia, muscles and the periosteum of the tibia or fibula. If the ulcer is rapidly extending, the granulation tissue is scanty and the local inflammatory reaction is variable.

Ulcer repair

Once the ulcer has stopped enlarging (i.e. skin necrosis has stopped) and the dead tissue has separated, granulation tissue begins to develop. The natural history of the ulcer is initially determined by the balance between the development of granulation tissue formation and continuing necrosis, and then by the rate of epithelial growth over the granulation tissue. Fibrin, polymorphonuclear leucocytes and phagocytes all appear around the newly formed capillaries and, providing that healing progresses, the granulation tissue extends upwards to 'fill in' the defect left by the necrosis. The fibrin exudate stimulates collagen deposition[84] and the white blood cells attack microorganisms and digest dead tissue.

Re-epithelialization

The edges of the ulcer cicatrize, thus reducing the size of the skin defect, and epidermal cells are stimulated to migrate across the granulation tissue.[2] There is no evidence that epithelial cell mitosis and migration is reduced in the edges of poorly healing venous ulcers but Adair[2] has suggested that the failure of ulcers to heal may be associated with an increased loss or reduced adhesion of epithelial cells as they attempt to migrate across the granulation tissue. Adair also found less collagen in the dermis beneath ulcers than in normal skin and an increase in the number of fibroblasts. Some new capillaries were always present, usually in large numbers. In the region of the epithelial migration in poorly healing ulcers, Adair found coarse extravascular fibrillary material (Fig. 13.6) which had the high electron density usually associated with structurally normal collagen fibrils. He suggested that this material was a degenerating form of collagen.

Adair also noted cytoplasmic vacuolation in the epidermal cells of non-healing ulcers. These vacuoles were found in the granular layers of the epidermis and were associated with a lack of collagen fibrils in the papillary dermis which were replaced by a fine fibrillary material. He did not draw any inferences from these observations but suggested that though local hypoxia does not influence epidermal division and migration[102] it may well effect epidermal survival and be responsible for the changes that he had observed. It is possible that the fine fibrillary material which he saw within the papillary dermis was fibrin.

The ulcer 'base'

In rapidly extending ulcers the necrotic epidermis and dermis may remain as a thick slough lying on top of the granulation tissue in the ulcer base. There may be a considerable volume of moist exudate comprised of oedema fluid and dead polymorphonuclear leucocytes. The bacteria contaminating the surface of the ulcer rarely invade the subcutaneous fat.

Peripheral nerve endings may be directly involved in the inflammatory process and give rise to considerable local pain, but it is surprising how seldom pain is a major symptom in some of the largest and most infected ulcers. It is impossible to equate the pathological features of the ulcer with the presence or absence of pain, though small sloughing young ulcers are often very painful. Perhaps pain is more related to the local release of kinins and other chemical stimuli than to the direct extension of the ulcer into the local nerve endings.

Once an ulcer is clean, its base becomes covered with bright red velvety granulation tissue (Colour plate 12), provided the base is not fibrous and ischaemic. Ulcers which develop in areas of chronic lipodermatosclerosis often have a white fibrous base with scanty granulation tissue; this is an indication that the ulcer will be slow to heal (Colour plate 11).

Development and control of re-epithelialization

Ulcers usually heal by cicatrization and epithelial migration over the granulation tissue from the skin edge. Occasionally, epithelialization develops from multiple islands of epithelium that appear over the whole surface of the granulation tissue (Fig. 13.8). It is not known whether these islands of epithelium originate from deep remnants of the skin and its appendages which were not destroyed when the ulcer developed, or from cells which have migrated from the ulcer edge before becoming fixed. A third possibility is that fibroblasts and other totipotent cells may undergo squamous metaplasia but this seems unlikely. We have no idea what factors control epithelial mitosis, migration and repair, but these factors must be determined before we can fully understand the process of ulcer healing. Local hormones, fibrin, fibronectin, and epithelial growth factor may all be relevant and require further study.

Inspection of the ulcer edge usually gives a good indication of its propensity for healing. If the edge is shallow and sloping with thin purple–pink new epithelial cells extending onto the granulation tissue, healing will proceed (Colour plate 12). If the skin is overhanging the base of the ulcer and there is no evidence that new epithelium is appearing, the ulcer will be slow to heal, especially if the granulation tissue in the base is sparse or fibrotic (Colour plate 13). This type of ulcer may need to be excised before satisfactory granulation tissue will develop and epithelialization can follow.

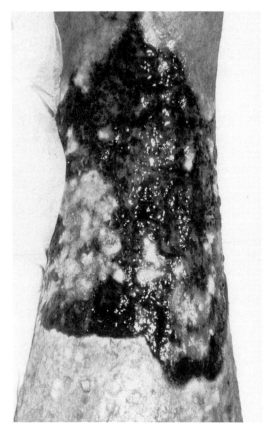

Fig. 13.8 An ulcer which is healing from multiple islands of epithelium developing within the granulation tissue. Although this healing pattern is rare, this photograph demonstrates that not all ulcers heal in from the edge.

Microorganisms in venous ulcers

This subject is discussed in detail in Chapters 14 and 15. Most of the microorganisms found in ulcers are commensals taking the opportunity of growing on an ideal culture medium.[115] Hopkins and Jamieson[77] have shown that antibiotics can permeate ulcer exudate and that their concentration in the exudate varies with both posture and the state of the ulcer. More studies are needed on the relationship between ulcer exudate and microbial flora and on the influence of these factors on ulcer healing. It may be important to relate events such as ulcer healing and extension to the type of microorganism that is growing on the ulcer at the time; as far as we know this has not been done; it would, however, help to establish the role of infection in the natural history of ulceration. It has been repeatedly observed that though venous ulcers are always covered in microorganisms, spreading infection, cellulitis, lymphangitis or septicaemia is extremely rare. Perhaps the fibrinous exudate prevents the access of organisms to the lymphatics or bloodstream.

Organisms presumably reach the ulcer from the general environment and from other areas of the patient's skin that harbour bacteria. Staphylococci and streptococci may be transferred from the upper respiratory tract and nasal passages while Gram-negative bacteria and anaerobes may pass to the ulcer from the perineal area.

Cross contamination can occur when the ulcer is dressed by medical attendants, doctors, nurses and physiotherapists. Despite this possibility, cross-infection does not appear to be of clinical importance in ulcer clinics or hospital wards provided the normal precautions of hand washing and the use of fresh sterile instruments and dressings for each patient are taken. The relevance of high concentrations of organisms and combinations of different types of organisms in the pathology of ulceration remains to be clarified.

The scar (the healed ulcer)

When epithelium finally covers all the granulation tissue in the ulcer base, the ulcer is healed. The new pink epithelium is fragile and unstable. Until it matures and becomes more stable, it easily breaks down or becomes detached if it is not protected from inadvertent injury. As the new skin matures it becomes paler and thicker and the granulation tissue beneath the epithelium contracts and becomes less vascular and more fibrous as the collagen matures. Sometimes the keratin in the skin over the healed surface of the ulcer increases in thickness. The mechanism of this 'hyperkeratinization' is obscure (Fig. 13.9). The depth and extent of the scar tissue beneath the endothelium depends upon the inital size and depth of the ulcer.

The general effects of ulceration

These are discussed in more detail in the section on the natural history of ulceration at the beginning of Chapter 15 (page 412) but they are summarized here.

- Venous ulcers are rarely life threatening, as systemic septicaemia almost never occurs.
- Ulcers may cause much morbidity from pain, discomfort and discharge.
- Ulcers never appear to cause secondary amyloid disease but can cause chronic anaemia and hypoproteinaemia.
- Very occasionally, ulcers may undergo

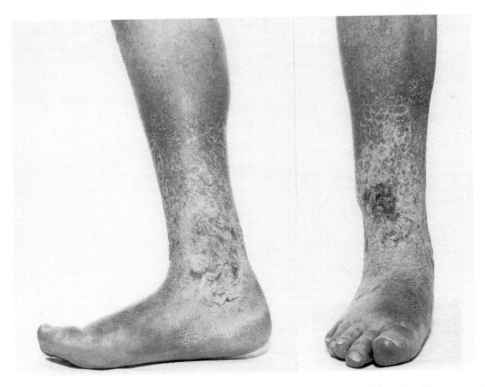

Fig. 13.9 A healed venous ulcer with marked hyperkeratinization of the skin. The cause of this abnormality is obscure.

malignant change (Marjolin's ulcer, see Chapter 14, page 383).

- Ulcers may● have serious economic and psychological effects (see Chapter 15, page 412).
- Ulcers are a considerable drain on medical resources – their treatment requires considerable amounts of medical time and revenue.

References

1. Abramson DI, Fierst SM. Arterial blood flow in extremities with varicose veins. *Arch Surg* 1942; **45**: 964.
2. Adair HM. Epidermal repair in chronic venous ulcers. *Br J Surg* 1977; **64**: 800.
3. Anning ST. *Leg Ulcers: their Causes and Treatment*. London. Churchill. 1954.
4. Arnoldi CC, Haegar K. Ulcus cruris venosum – Crux medicorum. *Läkartidningen* 1967; **64**: 2149.
5. Arnoldi CC, Linderholm H. On the pathogenesis of the venous leg ulcer. *Acta Chir Scand* 1968; **134**: 427.
6. Bauer G. A roentgenologic and clinical study of the sequels of thrombosis. *Acta Chir Scand* (Suppl) 1942; **86**: 74.
7. Beard RC. *Factors Affecting the Composition of Renal Lymph*. Cambridge University. MCh Thesis. 1982.
8. Berquist D. *Post-operative Thromboembolism*. Berlin. Springer Verlag. 1983.
9. Birger I. Ulcus cruris. *Nord Med* 1941; **12**: 3542.
10. Bjordal RI. Blood circulation in varicose veins of the lower extremities. *Angiology* 1972; **23**: 163.
11. Bjordal RI. Circulation patterns in incompetent perforating veins in the calf and in the saphenous system in primary varicose veins. *Acta Chir Scand* 1972; **138**: 251.
12. Bjordal RI. Circulation patterns in the saphenous system and the perforating veins in the calf in patients with previous deep venous thrombosis. *Vasa* 1974; Suppl **3**: 3.
13. Bjordal RI. Pressure patterns in the saphenous system in patients with venous leg ulcers. *Acta Chir Scand* 1971; **137**: 495.
14. Bjordal RI. Simultaneous pressure and flow readings in varicose veins of the lower extremity. *Acta Chir Scand* 1970; **136**: 309.
15. Blalock A. Oxygen content of blood in patients with varicose veins. *Arch Surg* 1929; **19**:898.
16. Blumoff RL, Johnson G. Saphenous vein pO$_2$ in patients with varicose veins. *J Surg Res* 1977; **23**: 35.

17. Bobek K, Cajzl L, Cepelák V, Slaisova V, Opatzny K, Barcal R. Etude de la frequence des maladies phlebologiques ét de l'influence de quelques facteurs etiologiques. *Phlebologie* 1966; **19**: 217.
18. Bollinger A, Jäger K, Geser A, Sgier F, Seglias J. Transcapillary and interstitial diffusion of Na fluorescein in chronic venous insufficiency with white atrophy. *Int J Microcirc Clin Exp* 1982; **5**: 17.
19. Bourne IHJ. Vertical leg drainage of oedema in treatment of leg ulcers. *Br Med J* 1974; **2**: 581.
20. Boyd AM, Jepson RP, Ratcliffe RH, Rose SS. The logical management of ulcers of the legs. *Angiology* 1952; **3**: 207.
21. Brodie BC. Observations on the treatment of varicose veins of legs. *Med Chir Trans* 1816; **7**: 195.
22. Browse NL, Burnand KG. The cause of venous ulceration. *Lancet* 1982; **2**: 243.
23. Browse NL. Venous ulceration. *Br Med J* 1983; **286**: 1920.
24. Browse NL, Gray L, Morland M, Jarrett PEM. Blood and vein wall fibrinolytic activity in health and vascular disease. *Br Med J* 1977; **1**: 478.
25. Burnand KG, O'Donnell TF Jr, Lea Thomas M, Browse NL. The relationship between post-phlebitic changes in the deep veins and results of the surgical treatment of venous ulcers. *Lancet* 1976; **1**: 936.
26. Burnand KG, O'Donnell TF Jr, Lea Thomas M, Browse NL. The relative importance of incompetent communicating veins in the production of varicose veins and venous ulcers. *Surgery* 1977; **82**: 9.
27. Burnand KG, Clemenson G, Whimster I, Gaunt J, Browse NL. The effect of sustained venous hypertension on the skin capillaries of the canine hind limb. *Br J Surg* 1982; **69**: 41.
28. Burnand KG, Whimster I, Clemenson G, Lea Thomas M, Browse NL. The relationship between the number of capillaries in the skin of the venous ulcer-bearing area of the lower leg and the fall in foot vein pressure during exercise. *Br J Surg* 1981; **68**: 297.
29. Burnand KG, Whimster I, Naidoo A, Browse NL. Pericapillary fibrin in the ulcer-bearing skin of the leg: the cause of lipodermatosclerosis and venous ulceration. *Br Med J* 1982; **285**: 1071.
30. Burnand KG, Pattison M, Powell S, Lea Thomas M, Browse NL. Can we diagnose long saphenous incompetence correctly? In Negus D, Jantet G (Eds) *Fibrinolysis '85*. London. Libbey. 1986.
31. Callam MJ, Ruckley CV, Dale JJ, Harper DR. Chronic leg ulcer. The incidence of associated

non-venous disorders. In Negus D, Jantet G (Eds) *Phlebology '85.* London. Libbey. 1986.

32. Callam MJ, Ruckley CV, Harper DR, Dale JJ. Chronic ulceration of the leg: extent of the problem and provision of care. *Br Med J* 1985; **290**: 1855.

33. Campbell WA, Newton NS, Price WH. Hypostatic leg ulceration and klinefelter's syndrome. *J Ment Defic Res* 1980; **24,** 2: 115.

34. Clyne CAC, Ramsden WH, Chant ADB, Webster JH. Oxygen tension on the skin of the gaiter area of limbs with venous disease. *Br J Surg* 1985; **72**: 644.

35. Cockett FB, Jones DE. The ankle blow-out syndrome. A new approach to the varicose ulcer problem. *Lancet* 1953; **1**: 17.

36. Cockett FB. Diagnosis and surgery of high pressure venous leaks in the leg: a new overall concept of surgery of varicose veins and venous ulcers. *Br Med J* 1956; **2**: 1399.

37. Cockett FB. The pathology and treatment of venous ulcers of the leg. *Br J Surg* 1955; **43**: 260.

38. Cooper AP. *Lectures on the Principles and Practice of Surgery.* London. Cox & Portwine. 1835.

39. Cornwall JV, Lewis JD. Leg ulcer revisited. *Br J Surg* 1983; **70**: 681.

40. Corrigan TP, Kakkar VV. Early changes in the postphlebitic limb: their clinical significance. *Br J Surg* 1973; **60**: 808.

41. Cranley JJ, Krause RJ, Strasser ES. Chronic venous insufficiency of the lower extremity. *Surgery* 1961; **49**: 48.

42. Critchett G. *Lectures on the Causes and Treatment of Ulcers of the Lower Extremity.* London. Churchill. 1849.

43. Dale JJ, Callam MJ, Ruckley CV, Harper DR, Berry PN. Chronic ulcers of the leg: A study of prevalence in a Scottish community. *Health Bull* 1983; 41/6: 310.

44. Dale WA. Venous bypass surgery. *Surg Clin North Am* 1982; **62**: 391.

45. Dale WH, Foster JH. Leg ulcers. *Trans South Surg Assoc* 1963; **775**: 399.

46. de Takats G, Graupner GW. Division of the popliteal vein in deep venous insufficiency of the lower extremities. *Surgery* 1951; **29**: 342.

47. de Takats G, Quint H, Tillotsen BI, Crittenden PJ. The impairment of the circulation in the varicose extremity. *Arch Surg* 1929; **18**: 671.

48. Dickson Wright A. The treatment of indolent ulcer of the leg. *Lancet* 1931; **1**: 457.

49. Dodd HJ, Gaylarde PM, Sakarny I. Skin oxygen tensions in venous insufficiency of the lower leg. *J R Soc Med* 1985; **78**: 373.

50. Dodd H, Cockett FB. *The Pathology and Surgery of the Veins of the Lower Limb.* Edinburgh. Livingstone. 1956.

51. Dodd HJ. The cause, prevention and arrest of varicose veins. *Lancet* 1964; **2**: 809.

52. Eaglestein WH. Personal Communication. 1985.

53. Ersek RA, Jones MH, Tilak SP, Howard JM. Studies of peripheral lymphatics following femoral vein occlusion in the dog. *Surgery* 1965; **57**: 269.

54. Fagrell B. Local microcirculation in chronic venous incompetence and leg ulcers. *Vasc Surg* 1979; **13**: 217.

55. Fagrell B. Vital capillary microscopy. *Scand J Clin Lab Invest* 1973; Suppl **133**.

56. Field P, Van Boxel PV. The role of the Linton flap procedure in the management of stasis dermatitis and ulceration in the lower limb. *Surgery* 1971; **70**: 920.

57. Fontaine R. Remarks concerning venous thrombosis and its sequelae. John Homans memorial lecture. *Surgery* 1957; **41**: 6.

58. Foote RR. *Varicose Veins.* London. Butterworths. 1954.

59. Gay J. *Varicose Disease of the Lower Extremities and its Allied Disorders: Skin Discoloration, Induration and Ulcer.* London. Churchill. 1868.

60. Gius JA. Arteriovenous anastomoses and varicose veins. *Arch Surg* 1960; **81**: 299.

61. Haeger K. Three to six year results with standardized surgical therapy of venous ulcers. *Vasc Dis* 1966; **3**: 106.

62. Haeger KMH, Berglan L. Skin temperature in normal and varicose legs and some reflections on the etiology of varicose veins. *Angiology* 1963; **14**: 473.

63. Haeger K. Diuretic treatment of postthrombotic and varicose oedema in the lower extremities. *J Cardiovasc Surg* 1961; **2**: 367.

64. Haimovici H, Steinman C, Caplan LH. Role of arteriovenous anastomosis in vascular diseases of the lower extremity. *Ann Surg* 1966; **164**: 990.

65. Haimovici H. Abnormal arteriovenous shunts associated with chronic venous insufficiency. *J Cardiovasc Surg* 1976; **17**: 473.

66. Harvey W. *Exercitatio Anatomica de Motu Cordis et Sanguinis in Animalibus.* Frankfurt. W Fitzer. 1628.

67. Haxthausen H. Om pathogensen af ulcus cruris varicosum. *Novd Med Tidskv* 1936; **12**: 1665.

68. Hehne HJ, Locher J Th, Waibel PP, Fridrich R. Zur Bedeutung arteriovenösen Anastomosen bei der primären Varicosis und der chronischvenösen Insuffizienz. *Vasa* 1974; **3**: 396.

69. Hellgren L. *An Epidemiological Survey of Skin Diseases, Tattooing and Rheumatic Diseases.* Uppsala. Slinquist Wiksell. 1967.

70. Hilton J. A course of lectures on pain and the therapeutic influence of mechanical and physiological rest in accidents and surgical disease. *Lancet* 1861; **2**: 245.

71. Hippocrates (460 BC). Adams F (Trans, Ed) *The Genuine Works of Hippocrates. De Ulceribus.* London. Sydenham Society.

72. Hoare MC, Nicolaides AN, Miles CR, Shull K, Jury RP, Needham T, Dudley HAF. The role of primary varicose veins in venous ulceration. *Surgery* 1982; **92**: 450.

73. Hodgson J. *A Treatise on Diseases of the Arteries and Veins.* London. Underwood. 1815.

74. Holling HE, Beecher HK, Linton RR. Study of the tendency to oedema formation associated with incompetence of the valves of the communicating veins of the leg. Oxygen tension of the blood contained in varicose veins. *J Clin Invest.* 1938; **17**: 555.

75. Homans J. The etiology and treatment of varicose ulcer of the leg. *Surg Gynec Obstet* 1917; **24**: 300.

76. Home E. *Practical Observations on the Treatment of Ulcers of the Leg, Considered as a Branch of Military Surgery.* 2nd edition. London. Bulmer. 1801.

77. Hopkins NFG, Jamieson CW. Antibiotic concentration in the exudate of venous ulcers. A measure of local arterial insufficiency. *Br J Surg* 1982; **69**: 676.

78. Hopkins NFG, Spinks TJ, Rhodes CG, Ranicar ASO, Jamieson CW. Positron emission tomography in venous ulceration and liposclerosis: a study of regional tissue function. *Br Med J* 1983; **286**: 333.

79. Howell R. Hypostatic ulceration and Klinefelter's Syndrome. *Br Med J* 1978; **2**: 95.

80. Hunt T. *A Guide to the Treatment of Diseases of the Skin: with Suggestions for Their Prevention.* 4th edition. London. Richards. 1859.

81. Jancar J. Hypostatic ulceration and male sex chromosomal abnormalities. *Br Med J* 1971; **1**: 434.

82. Johnson ND, Queral LA, Flinn WR, Yao JST, Bergan JJ. Late objective assessment of venous valve surgery. *Arch Surg* 1981; **116**: 1461.

83. Kistner R. Primary venous valve incompetence of the leg. *Am J Surg* 1980; **140**: 218.

84. Knighton DR, Hunt TK, Thakral KK, Goodson WH. The role of platelets and fibrin in the healing sequence: an *in vivo* study of angiogenesis and collagen synthesis. *Ann Surg* 1982; **196**: 379.

85. Landis EM. Capillary pressure and capillary permeability. *Physiol Rev* 1934; **14**: 404.

86. Leach RD, Browse NL. Effect of venous hypertension on canine hind limb lymph. *Br J Surg*

87. Leach RD. Venous ulceration, fibrinogen and fibrinolysis. *Ann R Coll Surg Engl* 1984; **66**: 258.

88. Leu HJ. The prognostic significance of cutaneous and microvascular changes in venous leg ulcers. *Vasc Dis* 1965; **2**: 77.

89. Lindemayr W, Löfferer O, Mostbeck A, Partsch H. Arteriovenous shunts in primary varicosis? A critical essay. *Vasc Surg* 1972; **6**: 9.

90. Linton RR, Hardy IB. Post-thrombotic syndrome of the lower extremity. Treatment by interruption of the superficial femoral vein and ligation and stripping of the long and short saphenous veins. *Surgery* 1948; **24**: 452.

91. Linton RR. The communicating veins of the lower leg and the operating technics for their ligation. *Ann Surg* 1938; **107**: 582.

92. Linton RR. The post-thrombotic ulceration of the lower extremity: its etiology and surgical treatment. *Ann Surg* 1953; **138**: 415.

93. Lockhart-Mummery HE, Smitham JH. Varicose ulcer: A study of the deep veins with special reference to retrograde venography. *Br J Surg* 1951; **38**: 284.

94. Löfferer O, Mostbeck A, Partsch H. Arteriovenöse Kurzseblüsse der Extremitäten nuclearmedizinische untersuchungen mit besonderer Berücksichtigung des postthrombotischen Unterschenkelgeschwüs. *Zbl Phlebol* 1969; **8**: 2.

95. Ludbrook J. *Aspects of Venous Function in the Lower Limbs.* Springfield. Thomas. 1966.

96. Mani R, Gorman FW, White JE. Transcutaneous measurements of oxygen tension at the edges of leg ulcers: preliminary communication. *J R Soc Med* 1986; **79**: 650.

97. Marks R. Personal Communication. 1981.

98. Marks R, Williams D, Pearse AD. Models to study function and disease of the skin. In Plewig G, Marks R (Eds) *Skin Models.* Berlin. Springer Verlag. 1985.

99. May R. Der Femoralis bypass bein postthrombotischen zustandsbild. *Vasa* 1972; **1**: 267.

100. McEwan AJ, McArdle CS. Effect of hydroxyethylrutosides on blood oxygen levels and venous insufficiency symptoms in varicose veins. *Br Med J* 1971; **2**: 138.

101. McIrvine AJ, Corbett CRR, Aston NO, Sherriff EA, Wiseman PA, Jamieson CW. The demonstration of sapheno-femoral incompetence: doppler ultrasound compared with standard clinical tests. *Br J Surg* 1984; **71**: 510.

102. Medawar PB. The behaviour of mammalian skin epithelium under strictly anaerobic conditions. *Q J Microsc Sci* 1947; **88**: 27.

103. Myers MB, Cherry G. Pathophysiology and treat-

ment of stasis ulcers of the leg. *Am Surg* 1971; 37: 167.

104. Myers MB, Richter M, Cherry G. Relationship between edema and the healing rate of stasis ulcers of the leg. *Am J Surg* 1972; **124**: 666.

105. Negus D, Friedgood A. The effective management of venous ulceration. *Br J Surg* 1983; **70**: 623.

106. Negus D. Prevention and treatment of venous ulceration. *Ann R Coll Surg Engl* 1985; **67**: 144.

107. Partsch H. Personal communication. 1985.

108. Pietra GG, Szidon JP, Leventhal MM, Fishman AP. Haemoglobin as a tracer in haemodynamic pulmonary oedema. *Science* 1969; **166**: 1643.

109. Piulachs P, Vidal-Barraquer F. Pathogenic study of varicose veins. *Angiology* 1953; **4**: 59.

110. Queral LA, Whitehouse WM, Flinn WR, Nieman HL, Yao JST, Bergan JJ. Surgical correction of chronic deep venous insufficiency by valvular transposition. *Surgery* 1980; **87**: 688.

111. Ruckley CV, Callam MJ, Harper DR, Dale JJ. The Lothian and Forth Valley survey. Part 4. Arterial disease. In Negus D, Jantet G (Eds) *Phlebology '85* London. Libbey. 1986.

112. Rutter AG. Chronic ulcer of the leg in young subjects. *Surg Gynec Obstet* 1954; **98**: 291.

113. Ryan TJ, Copeman PMW. Microvascular patterns and blood stasis in skin diseases. *Br J Dermatol* 1970; **8**: 563.

114. Ryan TJ. The epidermis and its blood supply in venous disorders of the leg. *Trans St John's Hosp Derm Soc* 1969; **55**: 51.

115. Ryan TJ. *The Management of Leg Ulcers*. Oxford. Oxford Medical Publications. 1983.

116. Schalin L. Arteriovenous communications localized by thermography and identified by operative microscopy. *Acta Chir Scand* 1981; **147**: 409.

117. Schraibman I, Stratton FJ. Nutritional status of patients with leg ulcers. *J R Soc Med* 1985; **78**: 39.

118. Sethia KK, Darke SG. Long saphenous incompetence as a cause of venous ulceration. *Br J Surg* 1984; **71**: 754.

119. Shirley HH, Wolfram CG, Wasserman K, Mayerson HS. Capillary permiability to macromolecules: stretched pore phenomenon. *Am J Physiol* 1957; **190**: 198.

120. Smirk FH. Observations on the cause of oedema in congestive cardiac failure. *Clin Sci* 1936; **2**: 317.

121. Stacey MC, Burnand KG, Layer GT, Pattison M. Transcutaneous oxygen tension (tcPO$_2$) as a prognostic indicator and measure of treatment of recurrent venous ulceration. *Br J Surg* 1987; in press.

122. Stewart GJ, Pattison M, Burnand KG. Abnormal fibrinolysis: the cause of lipodermatosclerosis or "chronic cellulitis" in patients with primary lymphoedema. *Lymphology* 1984; **17**: 23.

123. Taheri SA, Lazar L, Elias S. Status of vein valve transport after twelve months. *Arch Surg* 1982; **117**: 1313.

124. Thomas AMC, Tomlinson PJ, Boggon RP. Incompetent perforating vein ligation in the treatment of venous ulceration. *Ann R Coll Surg Engl* 1986; **68**: 214.

125. Turner-Warwick W. *The Rational Treatment of Varicose Veins and Varicocele (with notes on the application of the obliterative method of treatment to other conditions)*. London. Faber & Faber. 1931.

126. Van Limborgh J, Boersma W, Van der Lugt L. Experimental production of *ulcus cruris venosum* conditions in frogs. *Zent Phlebol* 1966; **5**: 66.

127. Verneuil A. Du siége réel et primitif des varices des membres inferieurs. *Gaz Méd Paris* 1855; **10**: 524.

128. Vogler E. Angiographische Beiträge zur Eusterhung von Gefässerkrankungen unter besonderer Berücksichtigung der terminalen Strombahn. *Fortschr Roentgenstr* 1954; **81**: 479.

129. Warren R, Thayer TR. Transplantation of the saphenous vein for postphlebitic stasis. *Surgery* 1954; **35**: 867.

130. Whimster I. Cited in: Dodd H, Cockett FB. *The Pathology and Surgery of the Veins of the Lower Limb*. Edinburgh. Livingstone. 1956.

131. Widmer LK, Plechl SCH, Lea HJ, Boner H. Venenerkrankungen bei 1800 Berugstatigen, Basle Studie II. *Schweiz Med Wochenschr* 1967; **97**: 4.

132. Widmer LK. *Peripheral Venous Disorders. Basle Study III*. Bern. Hans Huber. 1978.

133. Wiseman R. *Eight Chirurgical Treaties*. London. Tooke & Meredith. 1705.

134. Wood ML, Reilly GD, Smith GT. Ulceration of the hand secondary to a radial arteriovenous fistula: a model for varicose ulceration. *Br Med J* 1983; **297**: 1167.

135. Zwiefach BW. The structural basis of permiability and other functions of blood capillaries. *Cold Spring Harbor Symp Quant Biol* 1940; **8** 216.

14

Venous ulceration: diagnosis

The clinical features of venous ulceration

History

Leg ulcers may develop slowly or suddenly. The patient will often remember that an area of skin became thickened and discoloured and then, for no apparent reason, began to blister or weep before rapidly breaking into an open sore. If the onset of ulceration is sudden, trauma is often the precipitating factor. The supermarket trolley, an inadvertant hard knock or kick, or an insignificant scratch or scrape may all cause a break in the continuity of the skin which becomes an ulcer.

The patient will often report that varicose veins were present before the ulcer developed, and may recollect a prior episode of deep vein thrombosis.

The association of pain and ulceration is well recognized, but this does not help to differentiate the cause of the ulcer unless there is a clear history of persistent ischaemic rest pain. Some small ulcers are very painful while some large ulcers are painless. A complete absence of pain should suggest the possibility of a gumma or a neuropathic ulcer.

A new untreated ulcer of the leg is a relative rarity in a hospital leg ulcer clinic. When a patient is seen with a first-time ulcer a detailed history must be taken of its onset and development. A history of trauma must be sought and enquiry must be made into any possible venous abnormality or skin changes noticed by the patient before the ulcer appeared.

Direct questions should be asked about the presence of varicose veins, and previous investigations or treatment for any venous problems, especially deep vein thrombosis. Patients must be specifically asked whether leg swelling occurred after an operation or pregnancy, an event which can easily slip from the patient's memory. A complicated or difficult operation or a fracture of the lower limb treated by a plaster cast or prolonged bed-rest may have been the cause of a silent deep vein thrombosis and may subsequently result in a post-thrombotic limb (see Chapter 16). Patients must be questioned about episodes of chest pain, haemoptysis or a known history of pulmonary embolism. Whenever possible, the objective evidence that supported the diagnosis of deep vein thrombosis or pulmonary embolism should be obtained. Treatment with antiocoagulants is only indirect evidence of a thrombosis or embolism and is not completely reliable,[42,44] whereas a phlebogram showing thrombus or an isotope lung scan showing a perfusion ventilation mismatch are positive proof.

Many patients with ulcers give a history of previous ulceration.[12] The number of episodes of ulceration, the time taken for each ulcer to heal, the period that the patient has been free from ulceration, the methods of treatment and any means used to prevent recurrence must all be recorded. Particular attention must be paid to previous operations or sclerotherapy to obliterate varicosities, and the use of elastic stockings. Very rarely, deep vein reconstruction may have been carried out in an attempt to prevent recurrence, but this may become more common in the future.

A list of the common causes of leg ulcers and their approximate incidence is shown in Table 14.1. Many of the causes of leg ulcer are rare, and direct questions designed to elucidate the precise aetiology of the ulcer are usually unhelpful. Arterial, rheumatoid, diabetic and traumatic ulcers are, however, common, and specific questions should be put to confirm or refute these diagnoses.

A history of intermittent claudication, rest

Table 14.1 The common causes of leg ulcer

Cause of ulcer	Incidence (%)
Venous insufficiency	70–90
Arterial insufficiency	5–20
Rheumatoid arthritis	5
Trauma	2
Neoplastic change	1
Others	2–0.05

pain, transient ischaemic attacks or cerebral infarction, supports a diagnosis of underlying arterial disease as does a history of angina pectoris or myocardial infarction. A history of diabetes, treated by oral hypoglycaemic drugs or insulin injections, should raise the suspicion of infective or neuropathic ulceration. Heavy smokers and diabetics are particularly prone to develop ischaemic ulceration.

Joint pain, swelling and restricted movement suggest a diagnosis of rheumatoid ulcer. Any anti-inflammatory drugs taken by the patient for rheumatoid arthritis should be recorded.

A clear history of injury in the absence of any preceding skin changes favours a diagnosis of traumatic ulceration but does not exclude other causes of ulceration.

In addition to obtaining a careful history of the ulcer and these specific enquiries, a full general inquiry must be made into all systems, including past medical conditions, drugs, allergies and the patient's social circumstances.

Physical signs

Examination should be carried out with the patient fully undressed, except for underpants in a man, and brassier and pants in a woman. There is no place for simply examining a patient's leg by rolling up a trouser leg or lifting a skirt while the patient remains seated with all their other clothes left in place, prohibiting examination of the groins, the abdomen and the rest of the body.

The examination should commence with the undressed patient lying comfortably on a couch in a warm well lit room. Blankets should be provided for additional warmth and modesty.

General examination

The general examination is designed to detect evidence of generalized disease. Anaemia,

polycythaemia, cyanosis, jaundice, myxoedema, scleroderma, rheumatoid arthritis and Klein-felter's syndrome are some of the many conditions that can be found on systemic examination that may be relevant to the ulcer. Inspection of the hands can be especially valuable, revealing clubbing of the nails, koilonychia, rheumatoid changes, or the spindle-shaped fingers of scleroderma. Palpation of the pulse may reveal atrial fibrillation, and hypertension may be diagnosed when the blood pressure is measured. Abdominal examination and rectal examination should be performed on all patients. Even simple inspection of the abdomen may reveal distended superficial veins indicative of an ilio-caval obstruction. It is not appropriate to describe the full general examination of a patient in this book, but it is necessary to stress that leg ulcers are so often a manifestation of distant disease that *a complete medical examination is essential in all patients.*

Local examination

Both lower limbs should be examined with the patient lying and standing. It is easier to begin with the leg horizontal and then ask the patient to stand.

The ulcer The site and the number of ulcers should be recorded. It is helpful to draw the areas of ulceration on an outline plan of the leg together with their maximum dimensions. An instant polaroid photograph of the ulcer with a centimetre rule attached to the leg allows later measurement of its surface area and comparison with future appearances,[39] but this may not be possible on the grounds of expense.

Many other techniques have been used for estimating ulcer size. The outline of the ulcer can be traced on plastic sheeting or tracing paper with an indelible pen,[27] a mould can be made to fill in the area of the ulcer and, recently, direct computerized measurements of the surface area using a light pen and a sonic digitizer[15] or complex stereo photographs (stereo-photogrammetry) have been advocated.[6] Whether the introduction of these expensive techniques into the science of ulcer measurement is of value remains to be seen. The simplest and cheapest way of assessing the area of an ulcer and its response to treatment is to calculate the product of accurate measurements of the maximum width and breath (Fig. 14.1). This has been shown to correlate well with more

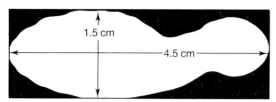

Calculated ulcer area = 1.5 × 4.5 = 6.75 cm²

Fig. 14.1 A diagram to show why the product of the greatest width and the greatest length over-estimates the surface area of an ulcer. Fortunately, most ulcers are oval in shape and this makes the over-estimate (the black area) quite small (10–20% on average).

complex forms of measurement (Fig. 14.2).[50]

Site The site of an ulcer gives an indication of its cause. Venous ulcers typically occur in the gaiter region (Fig. 14.3a). They can occur on the foot or higher up the calf but other causes should be excluded before attributing ulceration in these areas to venous disease (Fig. 14.3b). Venous ulcers tend to be situated on the medial or lateral surfaces of the leg; solitary ulcers on the front or the back of the leg, even though they are in the 'gaiter' area, may not be venous.

Size The size of the ulcer gives little indication of its aetiology but does, of course, have consi-

derable bearing on treatment and must therefore be carefully recorded.

Shape Venous ulcers can appear in many different shapes, but they are mostly oval, circular or irregular.

Edge An established venous ulcer with a granulating base which is trying to heal has a pale pink sloping edge of new epithelium (Fig. 14.4) but a young actively extending ulcer often has a punched-out edge and a slough covered base (Fig. 14.5). *Any elevation of the ulcer edge should arouse suspicions of malignant change.* Tuberculosis should be considered if the ulcer edge is undermined.

Surface (Base) The appearances of the surface of a venous ulcer depend more upon the state of development of the ulcer than on its cause. An extending, infected ulcer is usually covered with slough and has a copious exudate hiding any granulation tissue from view (Fig. 14.5). A chronic ulcer of many years standing often has a pale pink-white fibrous base with little or no granulation tissue, indicating extensive fibrosis and a poor blood supply (Fig. 14.6). A surface of bright red, velvety granulation tissue that bleeds when touched or wiped, indicates a good blood supply and good healing potential (Fig. 14.7). If there is a thin layer of pink epithelium growing over the granulation tissue at the

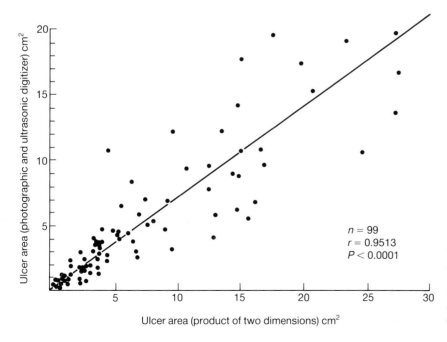

n = 99
r = 0.9513
P < 0.0001

Fig. 14.2 This graph compares the areas of 99 ulcers, estimated by the product of the two greatest diameters, with their areas, measured with an ultrasonic digitizer from scaled polaroid photographs. The correlation is very good but the simple product method invariably over-estimates the true area of the ulcer.

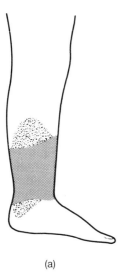

(a)

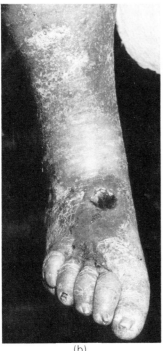

(b)

Fig. 14.3 (a) The ulcer-bearing area of the lower leg is often called the 'gaiter' area. The hatched area is the 'gaiter area' but ulcers may also occur in the stippled area.

(b) This ulcer on the foot looked like a venous ulcer because there was also eczema and pigmentation but the patient had normal veins and polycythaemia rubra vera. Even if an ulcer on the foot appears 'venous' other causes must be excluded.

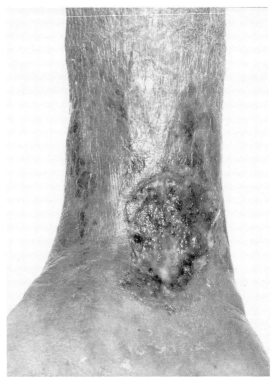

Fig. 14.4 This venous ulcer is in the process of healing. The healthy looking granulation tissue in the base is being rapidly covered by a thin layer of new 'pink' epithelium.

edge of the ulcer, healing is occurring (Fig. 14.7). Very occasionally, the granulation tissue proliferates and rises above the level of the surrounding skin.

The tissues beneath the surface of the ulcer (the base) can only be seen when the surface slough or granulations have been removed; they consist of a mixture of granulation tissue and fibrous tissue. The more chronic the ulcer, the more fibrous is the base. The fibrosis, and sometimes the ulcer itself, can extend into the fascia, periosteum and even into the underlying muscle or tendon but venous ulcers never extend into bone. If there is evidence of cortical bone involvement as opposed to periostitis then osteomyelitis, ischaemia, neoplasia or trauma must be responsible.

Surrounding tissue

Venous ulcers usually arise in an area of

Plate section

Plates 1–40

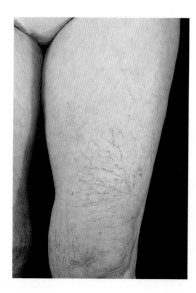

Plate 1. *Venous Telangiectases.* These fine intradermal venules are also called venous stars and spider veins. They are commonly associated with varicose veins. They can be treated by injection sclerotherapy but almost always recur. Treatment is rarely indicated because they are usually symptomless.

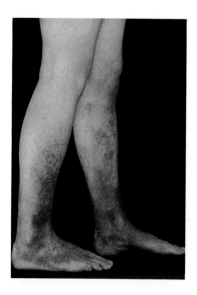

Plate 2. *Progressive arborizing telangiectases.* Sometimes venous telangiectases increase steadily in number and extent giving the skin of the whole lower leg a deep purple colour. This often occurs in young and middle-aged women in the absence of any subcutaneous varicose veins. The cause of this condition is unknown.

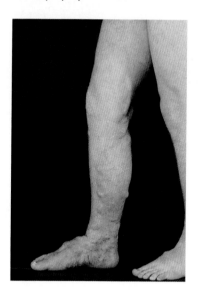

Plate 3. *Varicose veins.* Varicose veins are, by definition, dilated, tortuous veins with incompetent valves. This patient has many large varicose veins below the knee. The large vein just above the knee is not the long saphenous vein but a dilated tributary lying superficial to the long saphenous vein.

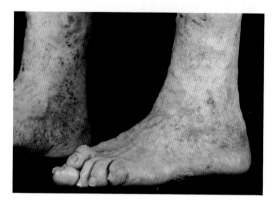

Plate 4. *The 'ankle flare'.* Chronic venous hypertension causes dilatation of the intradermal and subdermal venules around the ankle. This is usually seen as a triangle of dilated venules below the medial malleolus. This patient has medial and lateral ankle 'flares' on both legs.

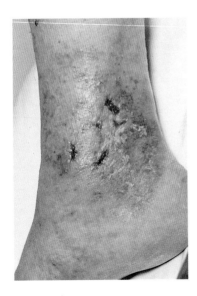

Plate 5. *Venous eczema/dermatitis.* Chronic venous hypertension often causes erythema and a chronic eczema of the skin of the lower leg. Sometimes the eczema overlies prominent varices. This patient has a red weeping rash above the medial malleolus.

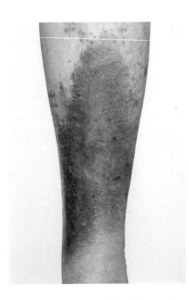

Plate 6. *Pigmentation.* Chronic venous hypertension causes the extravasation of red blood cells into the tissues. The unabsorbed haemosiderin gives the skin a deep brown colour.

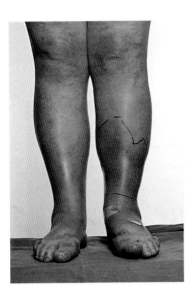

Plate 7. *Acute lipodermatosclerosis.* Chronic venous hypertension slowly destroys the skin and subcutaneous tissues so that they become replaced with scar tissue. The tissues become hot, red, thickened, painful and tender as they become anoxic. We have called this condition acute lipodermatosclerosis. It is often misdiagnosed as cellulitis, thrombophlebitis or panniculitis.

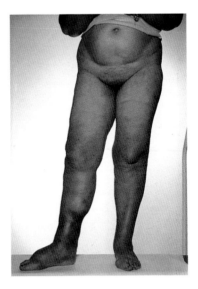

Plate 8. *Chronic lipodermatosclerosis.* Acute lipodermatosclerosis ultimately subsides to leave a hard pigmented constricted cylinder of skin just above the ankle (the 'gaiter area') giving the leg an inverted 'Champagne bottle' shape. This patient shows the typical tight constriction and pigmentation of the gaiter skin caused by longstanding lipodermatosclerosis. The fibrosis and pain has also caused a fixed planter flexion deformity of the ankle.

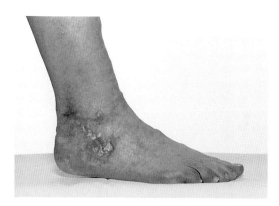

Plate 9. *Atrophie blanche.* When skin has been completely replaced with scar tissue it has a white shiny appearance. This is known as atrophie blanche. It frequently appears without passing through a stage of ulceration but a healed ulcer may present a similar appearance.

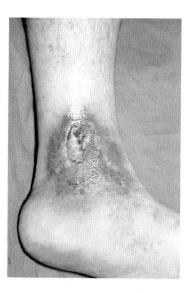

Plate 10. *A young venous ulcer.* This ulcer is only 2 weeks old. It was exuding purulent serum and was extremely painful. The acute lipodermatosclerosis which preceded it can be seen in the surrounding skin.

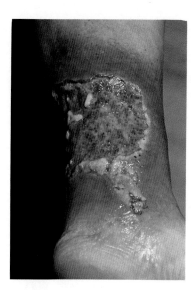

Plate 11. *A chronic venous ulcer.* This large ulcer had been present for 2 years. It was not painful but showed no signs of healing. The base is a mixture of fibrous tissue and small nodules of granulation tissue covered with exudate and slough. The edge is 'punched-out' and the surrounding skin is pigmented and sclerotic.

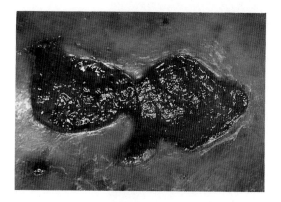

Plate 12. *A clean healing venous ulcer.* This ulcer is healing because it has a base of healthy granulation tissue and a sloping edge of new epithelium growing over the granulation tissue. The surrounding skin also looks healthy.

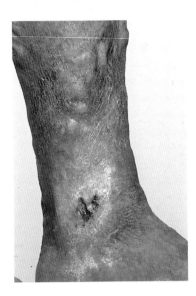

Plate 13. *A 'permanent' venous ulcer.* This ulcer had healed and broken down many times and finally become an unstable layer of epithelium over a plaque of fibrous tissue. The blood supply is insufficient to maintain a healthy epidermis. The only effective treatment is excision of all the diseased skin and subcutaneous tissue and replacement with split skin grafts followed by correction of the underlying venous abnormality (in this case an extensive communicating vein ligation and a sapheno-femoral ligation).

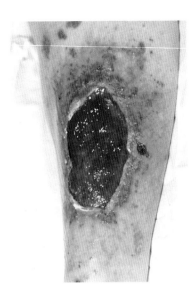

Plate 14. *A 'rheumatoid' ulcer.* This patient had had rheumatoid arthritis for many years before this ulcer appeared on the anterio-medial aspect of the middle third of her left leg. The base is healthy but the edge shows no sign of healing, even though the surrounding skin looks normal.

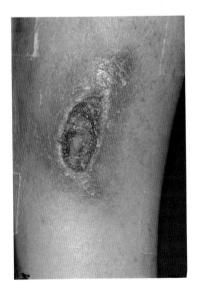

Plate 15. *A traumatic ulcer.* This area of full thickness skin necrosis followed a direct blow. Separation of the necrotic skin and healing by second intention took many months.

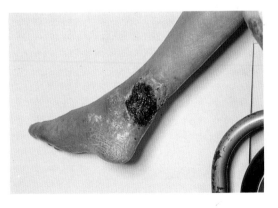

Plate 16. *An 'ischaemic' ulcer.* This patch of gangrenous skin was caused by a minor injury to a leg whose arterial blood supply was diminished. Combined arterial and venous insufficiency is common in the elderly. Treatment of a venous ulcer will fail if coexisting arterial insufficiency is not recognized and corrected.

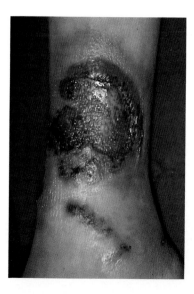

Plate 17. *Pyoderma gangrenosum.* Spontaneous gangrene of the skin is often associated with ulcerative colitis. (We are indebted to Dr D McGibbon for this illustration.)

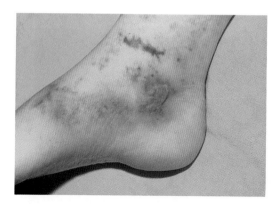

Plate 18. *Acute livedo vasculitis.* This patch of grey necrotic skin was caused by a non-specific vasculitis. When the necrotic skin had separated and the surrounding red skin had turned a blue–brown colour, some weeks later, the overall appearance was indistinguishable from that of a venous ulcer. (We are indebted to Dr D McGibbon for this illustration.)

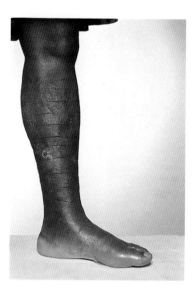

Plate 19. *A sickle cell ulcer.* Leg ulcers are common in patients with sickle cell disease. Some ulcers are secondary to post-thrombotic deep vein damage; other ulcers are caused by arteriolar occlusion and thromboses.

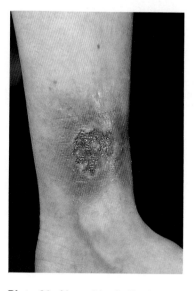

Plate 20. *Necrobiosis lipoidica.* This rare condition, commonly associated with diabetes, looks very like a venous ulcer, especially when it occurs on the lower third of the leg.

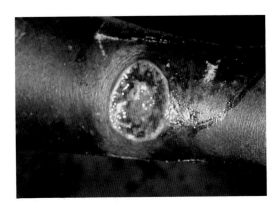

Plate 21. *A 'Tropical ulcer'.* Well defined circular, often multiple, ulcers that appear on the legs and sometimes arms of children and young adults in tropical countries (particularly in West Africa and Papua New Guinea) are a distinct clinical entity justifying the descriptive term 'tropical ulcer', even though their aetiology is unkown. (We are indebted to Dr R Hay for this illustration.)

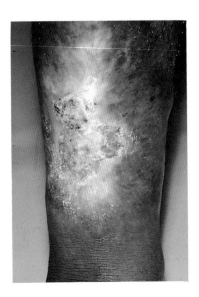

Plate 22. *Yaws.* Yaws, a spirochaetal infection, often causes skin papules which break down and become superficial ulcers. (We are indebted to Dr D McGibbon for this illustration.)

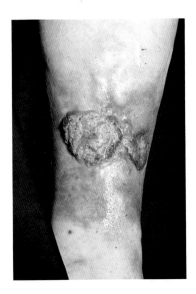

Plate 23. *A 'Marjolin's' ulcer.* This patient developed an ulcerating squamous carcinoma in the edge of a chronic venous ulcer. Malignant change in a chronic ulcer is commonly called a Marjolin's ulcer, even though Marjolin's original description was of malignant change in the scars of burns.

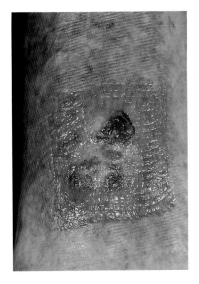

Plate 24. *A 'Marjolin's' ulcer.* This chronic venous ulcer was painful and slightly raised above the surrounding skin. Any atypical or changing area in a chronic ulcer should be biopsed. In this case the biopsy revealed the presence of a basal cell carcinoma.

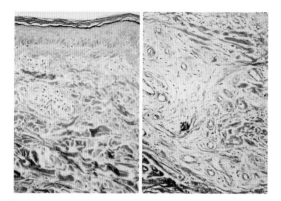

Plate 25. *Capillary 'proliferation'.* These two photomicrographs stained with phosphotungstic acid haematoxylin (PTAH) show the difference between the number of capillaries in the skin of a normal leg (left-hand panel) and the skin of a leg subjected to chronic venous hypertension (right-hand panel). There are very few capillaries in the dermis of the normal skin but many in the abnormal skin. This is mainly caused by elongation and tortuosity of existing capillaries not by growth of new capillaries. Fibrin/fibrinogen stains blue with PTAH. The capillaries in the right-hand panel are surrounded by a 'blue' fibrillary material.

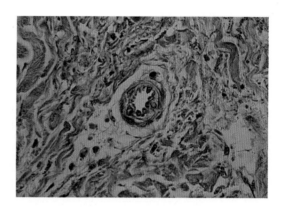

Plate 26. *Pericapillary fibrin/fibrinogen.* A high powered photomicrograph of a venular capillary, taken from skin subjected to chronic venous hypertension, has been stained with phosphotungstic acid haematoxylin (PTAH). The 'blue' fibrillary material seen in and around the wall of the capillary is fibrin/fibrinogen.

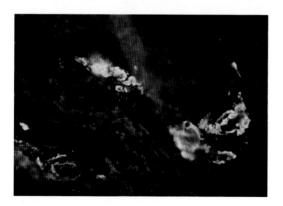

Plate 27. *Pericapillary fibrin/fibrinogen.* This section of skin, taken from an area of lipodermatosclerosis, has been stained with flourescent antibodies to fibrin/fibrinogen. The areas of yellow–green flourescence around the capillaries are deposits of fibrin/fibrinogen. (We are indebted to Dr W Eaglestein for this illustration.)

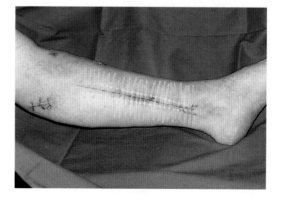

Plate 28. *Communicating vein exploration.* A long incision is required to expose all the medial lower leg communicating veins. The wound should be closed with the minimum of sutures, combined with adhesive skin tapes.

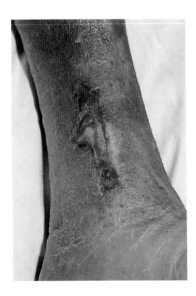

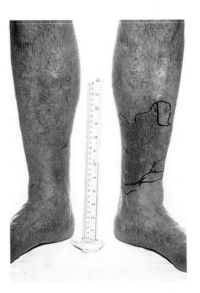

Plate 29. *Wound edge necrosis.* Exploration of the medial lower leg communicating veins through unhealthy damaged tissue occasionally results in incision edge necrosis. During the operation the skin must be handled with great care and not undermined. Incision edge necrosis can usually be treated with bedrest and external compression but sometimes it has to be excised and replaced with split skin grafts.

Plates 30, 31, 32 *Effect of stanozolol on lipodermatosclerosis.*
Plate 30. Before treatment. The area of tenderness and thickening has been outlined and measured.

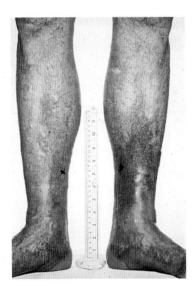

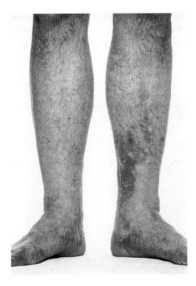

Plate 31. After 3 months of treatment with stanozolol (5 mg b.d.) the tenderness has gone and the area of lipodermatosclerosis has decreased.

Plate 32. After 6 months, the skin is not red or tender and the pigmentation is significantly less.

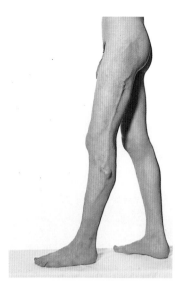

Plate 33. *The lateral vein of the Klippel–Trenaunay syndrome.* This vein is a persistent vestigial lateral limb bud vein. In this patient this large lateral vein drained into the internal iliac vein but also connected with the calf veins beneath the large 'blow out' bulge just below the knee.

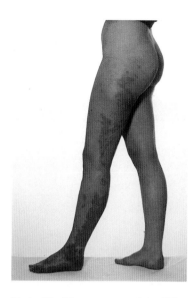

Plate 34. *The naevus of the Klippel–Trenaunay syndrome.* This naevus is pale purple in colour and often metameric in distribution. Its colour tends to fade in adult life.

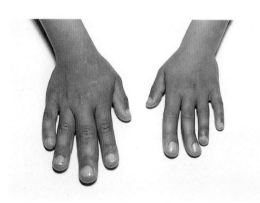

Plate 35. *Gigantism and the Klippel–Trenaunay syndrome.* This young girl had the Klippel-Trenaunay syndrome in all four limbs. Her right hand was very much bigger than her left hand. The left hand was of normal size but the index finger was enlarged. These discrepancies in size were caused by overgrowth of all the tissues (skin and bone) and are best described as localized gigantism.

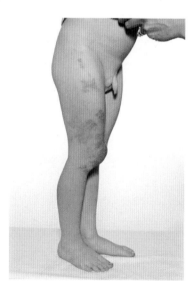

Plate 36. *Multiple venous angiomata.* Venous angioma are often multiple and are usually found in the subcutaneous tissues and the underlying muscles. The anterior aspect of the thigh is commonly affected.

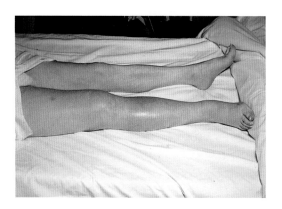

Plate 37. *Deep vein thrombosis.* This patient has a right ilio-femoral thrombosis causing swelling, pain, tenderness, and discoloration of the whole leg.

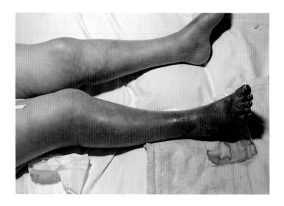

Plate 38. *Venous gangrene.* The blistering and death of the skin of the toes of this patient has been caused by an extensive venous thrombosis. Gangrene is a rare complication of venous thrombosis.

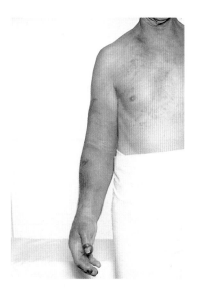

Plate 39. *Venous gangrene.* Venous gangrene can occur in the upper limb. Venous gangrene is frequently associated with advanced malignant disease. This patient had carcinomatosis from carcinoma of the bronchus.

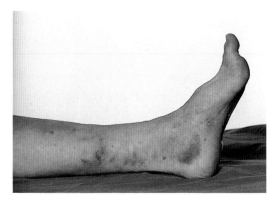

Plate 40. *Ruptured Baker's cyst.* A ruptured Baker's cyst is an important differential diagnosis of deep vein thrombosis. The bruising and discoloration of the skin in the groove behind and above the medial malleolus shown here, is diagnostic of this condition.

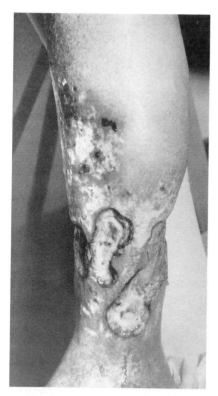

Fig. 14.5 A rapidly enlarging infected venous ulcer with a punched-out edge and a base covered by thick yellow slough. No granulation tissue can be seen and there are no signs of healing.

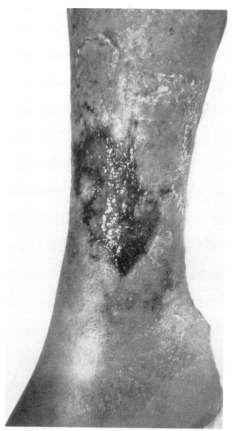

Fig. 14.7 This venous ulcer has a base of healthy 'red' granulation tissue and a gently sloping edge. It is likely to heal rapidly.

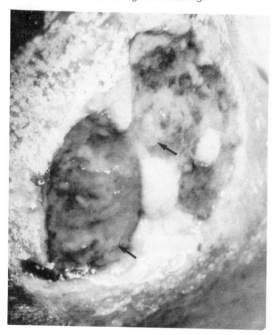

pigmented, thickened and indurated skin and sub-cutaneous fat (Colour plate 7). In the past these changes have been called 'post-phlebitic', even though they can occur in the absence of clear-cut evidence of deep vein damage (see Chapter 11), or 'fat necrosis', even when in the majority of cases there is no histological evidence of fat necrosis (in our view this term should be reserved for the rare situation when there is histological confirmation of dead fat cells, a complication which does undoubtably occur in a few limbs with venous ulceration), or 'panniculitis', even though there is often no inflammatory response either clinically or histologically.

Fig. 14.6 This venous ulcer has a base of pale fibrous tissue (arrowed), indicating that it has been present for some time and that it will be very slow to heal unless the fibrous tissue is excised.

For these reasons we coined the term 'lipodermatosclerosis' to described the pre-ulcer state.[5,7,8] The word implies that the process is sclerotic and involves both the skin and the fat, and we have shown that the deposition of pericapillary fibrin which leads to fibrosis and collagen deposition is invariably found in biopsies from this abnormal tissue (see Chapters 11 and 12). The term lipodermatosclerosis can be shortened to liposclerosis or abbreviated to LDS.

The absence of the characteristic changes of lipodermatosclerosis around an ulcer should immediately raise the suspicion that the ulcer is not caused by venous disease (Fig. 14.8).

Dilated intradermal venules at the ankle

The significance of a patch of dilated intradermal venules, usually in the ankle skin below the ulcer, the 'ankle flare', was stressed by Cockett (Fig. 6.10).[14] It is called the 'corona phlebectatica' in Europe and is the clinical manifestation of a persistently high venous pressure transmitted through incompetent lower leg communicating veins, which causes dilatation and elongation of

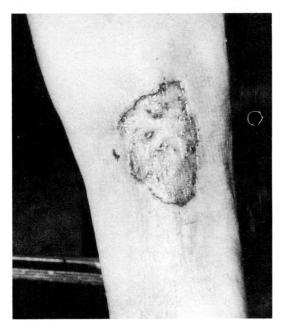

Fig. 14.8 An ulcer of the leg arising in 'normal' surrounding skin. It is very difficult to decide on clinical grounds, in the absence of any pigmentation or lipodermatosclerosis in the adjacent skin, whether this ulcer is venous or not.

the capillaries and venules (Chapters 12 and 13).[10] Lipodermatosclerosis is commonly associated with an ankle flare.

The subcutaneous veins

Large subcutaneous varicosities may be seen close to an ulcer but, thought their presence lends support to a diagnosis of venous ulceration, it is not diagnostic, and the absence of abnormal veins certainly does not exclude the diagnosis. The presence of 'blow-out veins', large varices overlying an incompetent communicating vein (Fig. 6.11),[14] is usually significant, but superficial venous dilatation is often only seen some distance from an ulcer because the lipodermatosclerosis prevents most local veins from dilating, with the exception of those veins that are very close to the skin. Ulcers on the lateral side of the leg are often associated with short saphenous incompetence.[17]

Long saphenous, short saphenous and calf communicating vein incompetence must be sought and excluded in every limb with ulceration. Tourniquet tests and Perthe's walking test (see Chapter 6 page 182) should be performed to ascertain the major sites of venous incompetence in all limbs with superficial varicosities.

When an ulcer is associated with oedema, lipodermatosclerosis and dilated veins (Colour plate 10), the cause is likely to be venous, but venous ulcers can develop in an apparently normal limb (Fig. 14.8). In these circumstances an abnormality of the veins must be confirmed with objective tests (see Chapters 4 and 6) and other causes of ulceration must be excluded.

Regional lymph glands

The lymph glands in the groin and popliteal fossa should always be palpated. If they are enlarged and hard, the possibility of malignant change in the ulcer must be considered but this is a rare event; the most common cause of inguinal lymphadenopathy is infection from the ulcer.

Arterial circulation

All the pulses of the limb should be palpated, especially the dorsalis pedis and posterior tibial pulses, though the latter may be difficult to feel if it lies directly beneath the ulcer. If the pulses are difficult to feel, a Doppler ultrasound flow detector should be used to measure the ankle to arm pressure index. The normal pressure index is between 1 and 1.2 (the pressure in the leg being equal to or slightly higher than that in the arm) but the level which is indicative of arterial insufficiency is open to dispute. Some investigators have proposed that a pressure index below 0.9 is indicative of an arterial influence in the development of ulceration.[16,45] A pressure index of less than 0.7 is certainly significant and, in the absence of any venous abnormality, may indicate that arterial insufficiency is the sole cause of the ulceration.

Doppler ultrasound pressure measurements are undoubtely helpful in assessing the role of the arterial supply of the leg but venous disease may still be the main cause of an ulcer, even when the pressures are significantly reduced.[45] It can be extremely difficult to decide which factor is playing the major role in the genesis of an ulcer, and it can be still more difficult to decide which abnormality to correct first, though a pressure index below 0.7 usually means that the arterial problem must be corrected before the venous abnormality can be properly assessed.

It is important to differentiate between venous and arterial ulcers as standard compression treatment is contra-indicated if there is evidence of arterial insufficiency. Stress has therefore been laid on the Doppler pressures as an important aid to clinical diagnosis and management.[45]

Comment In the absence of severe ischaemia or another obvious cause, ulcers can be treated as 'venous' while awaiting the results of further investigations.

Investigations

An erythrocyte count should be obtained to exclude anaemia or polycythaemia. Sickle cell disease or trait should be considered in all patients likely to be susceptible to this erythrocyte abnormality. The Rose-Waller, latex, autoantibodies and antinuclear factor levels should be measured if there is a suspicion of rheumatoid arthritis, vasculitis or any other auto-immune disease.

Serological tests for syphilis (e.g. TPHA, Treponema pallidum haemagglutination) must be obtained if the ulceration is typical of syphilis (a 'punched-out' edge with a 'wash leather' base),

or if a syphilitic aetiology is suspected from the history, or if the ulcer simply appears 'atypical'.

If it is felt that the ulcer is neither venous nor arterial, a biopsy of it may have to be taken under local anaesthetic, and the patient should be considered for in-patient hospital admission to elucidate the cause and accelerate healing. *When in doubt a biopsy should be performed*; it will often provide a definite diagnosis and will not cause any harm provided there is no arterial insufficiency. Eaglestein[18] has suggested that the presence of perivascular fibrin in the skin around an ulcer may be diagnostic of a venous ulcer (see Chapters 11 and 13).

Tests of venous function (see Chapters 4, 5 and 6)

There is no single test that will diagnose venous ulceration with total confidence but the demonstration of a functional or anatomical abnormality of the calf pump will strengthen the certainty of the diagnosis and help in planning treatment. Our present preference in order of simplicity and cost effectiveness is given below.

1. *Venous directional Doppler ultrasound* This is a quick, easy outpatient method for confirming long saphenous vein incompetence but it is not accurate enough to assess the state of the deep or communicating veins (see Chapters 4 and 6).

2. *Foot volume measurements during exercise* This method is cheap, simple to perform and non-invasive. Other clinicians prefer photoplethysmography or strain-gauge plethysmography. We think foot volume measurements are closer to foot vein pressure studies than the other methods and are quantitative not just qualitative (see Chapters 4 and 6).

3. *Ascending and descending phlebography* These give important information about the pathology of the deep veins, the communicating veins and an indication of deep valve competence (see Chapters 4 and 6) (Fig. 14.9).

4. *Varicography* This is useful when the anatomy of the superficial veins is in doubt, or abnormal superficial-to-deep communications are suspected. It is particularly useful when planning short saphenous vein surgery and before operating on patients with recurrent varicose veins (see Chapters 4 and 6).

5. *Duplex ultrasound/Doppler scanning* It is hoped that the newer, though much more expen-

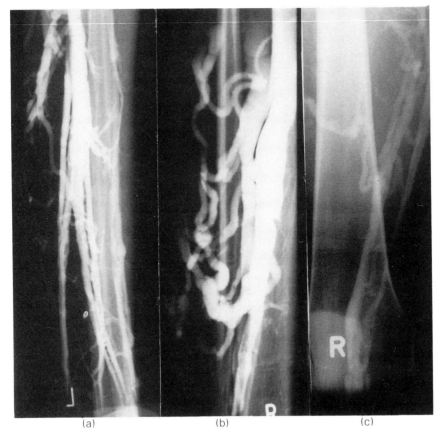

Fig. 14.9 Three ascending phlebograms showing the changes that may accompany venous ulceration.
(a) Normal deep veins and no incompetent communicating veins.
(b) Incompetent lower leg communicating veins.
(c) Severe post-thrombotic deep vein damage with synaechiae and collaterals.

sive, ultrasound venous-imaging equipment will give a better assessment of the deep vein valves than the standard directional Doppler methods but its role is likely to be confined to assessing difficult or recurrent ulcers (see Chapters 4 and 6).

Comment Apart perhaps from the Doppler assessment of long saphenous vein incompetence, all these confirmatory tests are best performed when the ulcer is healed. This means that a diagnosis of venous ulceration and its subsequent treatment must be conducted on the basis of the clinical findings and preliminary tests with final confirmation awaiting more complex investigations after the ulcer has healed.

Differential diagnosis of leg ulcers

Although the preceding section on the diagnosis of venous ulcers has alluded to some of the other causes of leg ulceration, the following paragraphs discuss these causes in detail.

Ulcers caused by arterial insufficiency

An ischaemic ulcer on the tip of a toe which is itself blue and painful offers little difficulty in diagnosis, but the diagnosis is less obvious when the ulcer is in an area of lipodermatosclerosis in a leg with impalpable foot pulses (Fig. 14.10). As already discussed, assessing the relative importance of combined venous and arterial disease can be extremely difficult.

A history of intermittent claudication, rest

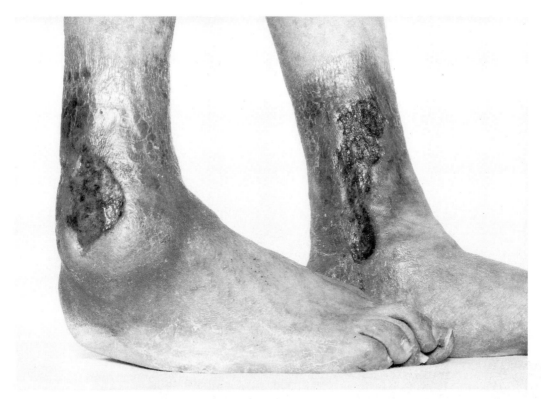

Fig. 14.10 These ulcers in the 'gaiter' region of the leg were caused by arterial ischaemia. The deep and superficial veins were normal but the arterial ankle pressures, measured by Doppler ultrasound, were severely reduced. Arteriography confirmed severe arterial disease.

The appearance of these ulcers and the skin surrounding them made them clinically indistinguishable from venous ulcers but objective tests excluded venous disease and confirmed the presence of severe arterial insufficiency.

pain, or of other symptoms of vascular disease in other systems, indicates that vascular insufficiency may be the cause of the ulcer.

Pain made worse by elevation of the leg is often a feature of ischaemic ulceration, whereas the discomfort of venous disease is almost always relieved by elevation. Ischaemic ulcers are often on the feet and toes (Fig. 14.11a and b) an uncommon site for venous ulcers, but they can develop anywhere on the leg and have no truly specific features except that the granulation in the ulcer base may be pale (Fig. 14.12) and show little evidence of proliferation. The diagnosis is usually suspected when the pulses are found to be absent and the Doppler arterial pressure at the ankle is reduced.

If the ankle/brachial pressure index is reduced, arteriography is often indicated to confirm the diagnosis and decide upon the best method of management. Femoral arteriography may be sufficient if there is a good femoral pulse and distal disease is suspected but it is always wise to obtain information about the aorta and iliac arteries by direct aortography or digital subtraction arteriography (Fig. 14.12), even when the femoral pulse feels normal.

A vascular reconstruction or a lumbar sympathectomy may be required to improve the blood flow to an ischaemic ulcer to enable skin grafts to take or encourage natural healing. Once the arterial circulation of the limb has been improved, it is safe to treat any venous abnormality that is causing symptoms.

Traumatic ulcers

This diagnosis is easy to make when there is a clear history of a direct injury followed immediately by

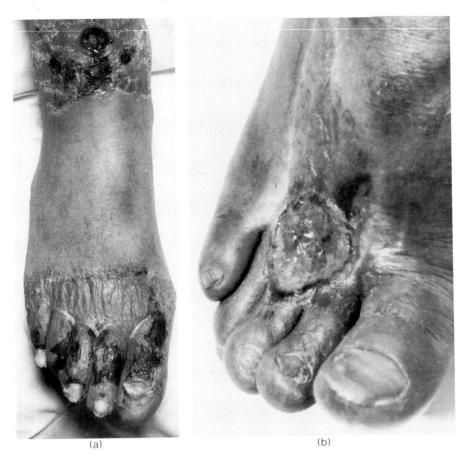

(a)   (b)

Fig. 14.11   Ischaemic ulcers are often on the feet and toes.

(a)   This diabetic patient has gangrene of the toes and ischaemic ulceration around the ankle. There were also ulcers on the outer side of the heel. Ulceration such as this is almost always ischaemic in origin.

(b)   The ulcer at the base of the toes and on the dorsum of the foot of this patient was not in the typical site for an ischaemic ulcer, but arterial insufficiency had to be excluded. The phlebograms were normal. Arteriography showed a superficial femoral occlusion and an additional occlusion of the anterior tibial artery.

obvious damage to the skin (e.g. bruising, laceration). Examination usually reveals a sharply demarcated area of ulceration in otherwise normal skin (Fig. 14.13). The combination of pre-existing venous or arterial disease in association with trauma must, however, always be born in mind, and the presence of lipodermatosclerosis, obvious surface varices or absent foot pulses demands further investigation.

Minor trauma is often the initiating factor in the development of both venous and arterial ulcers. For a confident diagnosis of traumatic ulcer to be made, the patient with a traumatic ulcer must give a clear history of the accident and have no other cause for ulceration.

The common site for a traumatic ulcer is the front of the shin. Ulcers frequently follow a shearing injury which produces a distally based V-shaped flap which undergoes ischaemic necrosis. The skin and subcutaneous tissues of the shin are known to have a poor blood supply and heal slowly.[13] Traumatic ulcers can follow an injury to normal skin but the frail tissues of the elderly, and patients with thin skin following treatment with systemic steroids are especially susceptible to minor injury. In this latter category there are

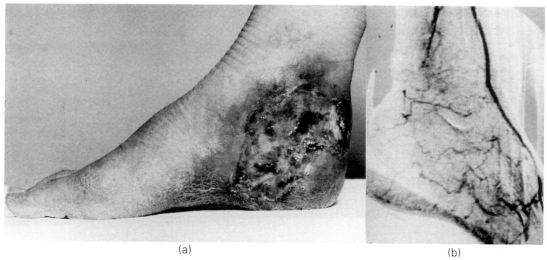

(a) (b)

Fig. 14.12 (a) An ischaemic ulcer of the heel. The patient was referred with a diagnosis of self-mutilation because the ulcer was in an unusual site and had failed to heal with elastic compression and skin grafting.

(b) The digital subtraction arteriogram showed a total occlusion of the posterior tibial artery, confirming the diagnosis of an ischaemic ulcer.

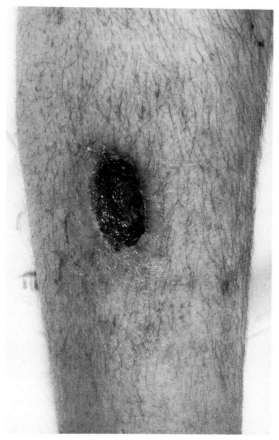

Fig. 14.13 A traumatic ulcer on the front of the shin. The ulcer is surrounded by normal skin and in a site which is frequently injured. This ulcer followed a football injury and healed rapidly.

many patients with rheumatoid arthritis.

The cause of the trauma varies but the supermarket trolley is now high on the list of injurious agents.

Treatment is by compression bandaging or skin grafting. Healing of the ulcer should not be followed by recurrence unless further injuries occur or other abnormalities coexist.

Basal cell carcinoma (rodent ulcers)

Basal cell carcinomata are most often found on the face, in the triangle between the eye, the ear and the mouth; a rodent ulcer that develops on a limb is therefore often misdiagnosed because it is not considered in the differential diagnosis. Every year we see at least two basal cell carcinomata on the legs in which the correct diagnosis has never been considered; an error which has resulted in a considerable delay in initiating treatment.[1]

If the patient has closely observed the lesion during its early stages, he or she will describe the typical behaviour of a basal cell carcinoma – intermittent episodes of ulceration and healing. If the lesion is not treated, it continues to grow and becomes a persistent ulcer; often, however, it does not have the classical 'rolled, pearly' edge seen on the face (Fig. 14.14). Careful inspection may reveal some of the typical appearances with overlying telangiectasis but the centre is often slightly raised and covered with bright red granulation tissue which bleeds easily. This change can sometimes be so prominent that it leads to a misdiagnosis of pyogenic granuloma, even though the long history of the lesion belies this diagnosis.

The skin surrounding the ulcer is normal and the foot pulses are invariably palpable.

If a basal cell carcinoma is suspected a biopsy should be taken of the edge of the ulcer unless the diagnosis is beyond doubt when it should be treated by an excision biopsy with skin grafting if necessary, or by incisional biopsy and radiotherapy, if this treatment is more appropriate. It is important to think of the possibility of basal cell carcinoma when examining any atypical ulcer that has failed to heal. It can occasionally arise in a long-standing venous ulcer[58] or after radiotherapy.

Squamous cell carcinoma

This diagnosis must also be considered as a

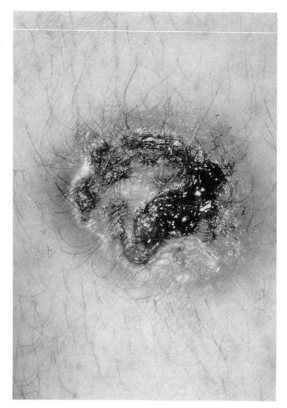

Fig. 14.14 A basal cell carcinoma producing an ulcer on the calf. The surrounding skin is normal, the edge is rolled and appears 'pearly' but there are no telangiectases. This ulcer had scabbed over and broken down several times before the patient presented. The diagnosis was suspected on the basis of the clinical appearance and the ulcer was therefore treated by excision biopsy. Histology confirmed a basal cell carcinoma.

possible cause of any leg ulcer of doubtful aetiology. A squamous cell carcinoma usually presents as an ulcer with a raised everted edge arising in normal skin (Fig. 14.15a) but like basal cell carcinomata this typical appearance is often not seen in the leg and a high level of suspicion must be maintained if the correct diagnosis is to be made.

Squamous cell carcinomata on the leg may be nodular, irregular, often have a sloping edge, grow insidiously, and do not respond to treatment (Fig 14.15b). They are not usually painful even when being dressed but they produce an excessive amount of exudate and slough. The inguinal lymph nodes are often enlarged, sometimes as a result of tumour deposits, but more commonly as a result of secondary infection.

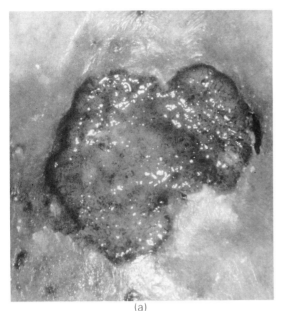

(a)

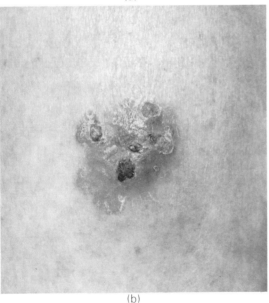

(b)

When a squamous cell carcinoma develops in a chronic venous ulcer it is traditionally called a Marjolin's ulcer,[4,31] though Marjolin[35] originally reported squamous cell carcinomata arising in the scars of old burns. Malignant change in a venous ulcer is a rare complication. A recent review reported only three cases out of 2000 ulcers,[46] and we have only seen 5 cases in 25 years. A Marjolin's ulcer should be suspected if one area of a venous ulcer starts to proliferate and rise above the surface of the rest of the ulcer (Fig. 14.16) (Colour plate 24) or if the nature of the ulcer changes so that it starts to exude and smell.[33] A biopsy should be taken of any long-standing ulcer that displays an unusual appearance or enlarges despite apparently satisfactory treatment.[1]

Squamous cell carcinomata are treated by wide excision and skin grafting, or radiotherapy.

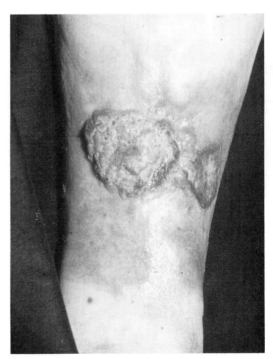

Fig. 14.15 (a) A squamous cell carcinoma arising in the skin of the calf. It has the raised everted edge which is typical of a squamous cell carcinoma. This ulcer arose in normal skin and no predisposing factor could be found.

(b) A squamous cell carcinoma arising in a patch of Bowen's disease. It was mis-diagnosed clinically as a basal cell carcinoma because it had a rolled, not a raised everted edge.

Fig. 14.16 This patient had a long-standing chronic ulcer of the leg which suddenly enlarged, became offensive and developed exuberant 'granulations'. The whole change represented a squamous cell carcinoma developing in a chronic venous ulcer, the so-called Marjolin's ulcer.

The chronic lipodermatosclerosis and dilated veins caused by the long-standing calf pump failure are clearly visible.

Rheumatoid ulcers

These ulcers are discussed separately from the other forms of vasculitis which cause ulceration because they are common and extremely difficult to manage.[2,11,40,51,57]

Ulcers may appear at any site on the legs of patients with rheumatoid arthritis but, interestingly, they still most commonly occur in the gaiter region and therefore often have to be distinguished from venous ulcers (Fig. 14.17). They are not usually surrounded by lipodermatosclerosis and, if this change is present, the ulcer may be of mixed aetiology. Rheumatoid ulcers have no special characteristics but look more like ischaemic ulcers with poor quality granulation tissue in their base, than like venous ulcers.

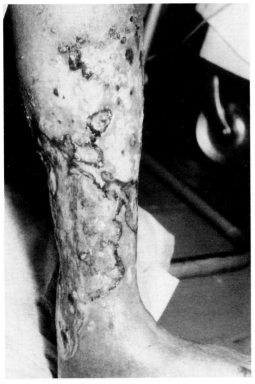

Fig. 14.17 A rheumatoid ulcer. This extensive ulcer developed in a woman who had severe rheumatoid arthritis affecting all her joints, producing almost total immobility. There was no obvious venous abnormality, the phlebograms were normal, and the ankle pressures measured by Doppler ultrasound were normal. Rheumatoid ulcers are presumably caused by arteriolar arteritis and thrombosis.

The diagnosis is made by finding the characteristic changes of rheumatoid arthritis in the hands and other joints and no evidence of venous or large artery disease in the legs. Very rarely, these ulcers occur in the absence of abnormalities of the joints and soft tissues; it is therefore our policy to request serological tests for rheumatoid disease on all new patients presenting with ulceration. The erythrocyte sedimentation rate (ESR) is commonly elevated. For similar reasons we refer those patients who have a sero-negative arthritis to a rheumatologist for confirmation of the diagnosis. Histology of a rheumatoid ulcer has no specific features, it usually shows small vessel endarteritis and round cell infiltration.

The arterial blood supply of the leg must be carefully assessed as severe rheumatoid arthritis may affect the small arteries of the calf and foot and produce distal ischaemia. If the blood supply appears to be satisfactory, an attempt may be made to heal the ulcer by compression but great care must be taken to avoid making the ulcer worse. Many rheumatoid ulcers fail to respond to conservative treatment, and patients have to be admitted for long periods of bedrest, cleansing and repeated skin grafting. Skin grafts often fail to take, and procedures that increase blood flow such as an adjuvant prostacyclin infusion or chemical sympathectomy may help.[51] Unfortunately, bedrest makes joint stiffness worse and often causes a prolonged decrease in mobility despite intensive physiotherapy.

Elastic stockings should be worn once the ulcer is healed, as much for protection as to prevent breakdown. It is not known if anti-inflammatory drugs reduce the risk of re-ulceration.

Neuropathic ulcers

Neuropathic ulcers occur wherever there is pressure on the skin. The areas subjected to the most pressure lie under the first metatarsophalangeal joint and the heel, over the base of the fifth metatarsal where the shoes press and rub against the toes, and over the malleoli (Fig. 14.18). The gaiter region of the leg is rarely affected. These ulcers are painless, punched-out and deep and, though they often have a slough in their base, they are rarely heavily infected. A neurological examination should confirm absence of pain sensation which is often accompained by other sensory

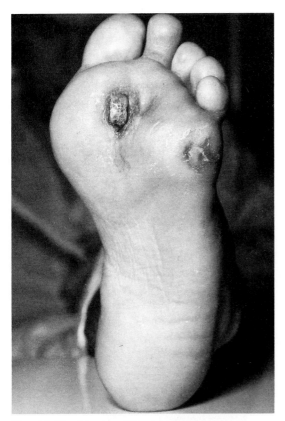

Fig. 14.18 Neuropathic ulcers on the plantar surface of the foot. This patient sustained a traumatic division of the sciatic nerve in a previous accident. Neuropathic ulcers are found in skin which bears weight during standing.

abnormalities such as a loss of vibration or position sense.

Diabetes is one of the most common causes of neuropathy, but even when a diabetic patient presents with an ulcer which is thought to be neuropathic in site and appearance, it is important to exclude infection and arterial insufficiency, both of which commonly coexist. The urine of all patients presenting with leg ulcers should be routinely tested for sugar, and we also routinely request a random blood glucose.

Treatment consists of avoiding further trauma, usually by prescribing complete bedrest, treating infection, controlling the diabetes and improving the blood supply, if it is necessary or possible.

Spina bifida, spinal injury, syringomyelia, tertiary syphilis, transverse myelitis, peripheral neuropathy and stroke are among the numerous other causes of neuropathic damage. In many patients with these diseases it is the pressure of calipers (Fig. 14.19) or wheelchairs that causes the ulceration. The presence of a large, painless ulcer over an area which is subjected to pressure when the patient is in bed (e.g. the back of the heel, the side of knee or over the greater trochanter) should arouse suspicion of a neuropathic ulcer.

If neurological disease has not been previously diagnosed, the patient should undergo a detailed clinical examination to confirm the neurological lesion. Electromyography, spinal radiographs, myelography, and computerized tomography may be required to elucidate the underlying pathology.

The skin and subcutaneous tissues should be protected against further trauma; this can be extremely difficult. Neuropathic ulcers will heal if protected from further pressure but healing may be accelerated by applying split skin grafts or by bringing in new skin by the plastic surgical techniques of rotation flaps or vascularized free flap grafts.

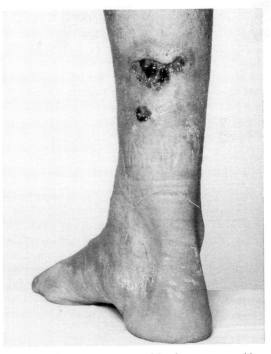

Fig. 14.19 These neuropathic ulcers occurred in a patient who had to wear calipers because the limb had been partially paralysed by poliomyelitis. The calipers had rubbed against the skin and caused the ulceration.

Tuberculous ulcers

Tuberculosis of the skin is now rare in Europe and North America but it is still common in Africa, India and the Far East.

Primary tuberculosis of the skin presents as an indurated plaque which has a transparent appearance which makes it look like 'apple jelly' (Fig. 14.20) but it is rarely seen in the lower leg.[19] True tuberculous ulcers of the skin (scrofula) are uncommon on the legs. These ulcers have an irregular, bluish, friable, undermined edge and a grey–pink base. The ulcers are often multiple, and the patient usually has evidence of systemic, pulmonary, abdominal or skeletal tuberculosis (Fig. 14.20).

Erythema induratum scrofulosorum (Bazin's disease) occurs in the skin of the calf of middle-aged women. It starts as either a single nodule or multiple nodules which gradually turn purple and then break down to form deep undermined ulcers. The regional lymph nodes may enlarge and caseate. It tends to occur on the back of the calf, and this gives the best clue to the diagnosis. Patients with Bazin's disease show hypersensitivity to Mantoux testing. A biopsy of the ulcer edge shows tuberculous granulomata containing Langerhan's giant cells. Tubercle bacilli may be found by Ziehl–Nielsen staining of the biopsy, or may be isolated from the surface of the ulcer if great care is taken with the sample collection. Treatment is by a combination of specific anti-tuberculosis agents.

Erythrocyanosis frigida (curum puellarum) and chilblains (lupus pernio)

Chilblains characteristically occur on the tips of the ears, the fingers and the toes but they can also occur over the Achilles tendon. They normally develop during cold weather and represent the effect of a prolonged period of cutaneous ischaemia, usually transitory, but sometimes permanent (an infarct), caused by excessive vasospasm of the arterioles. Chilblains begin as an area of induration and oedema but then the over-

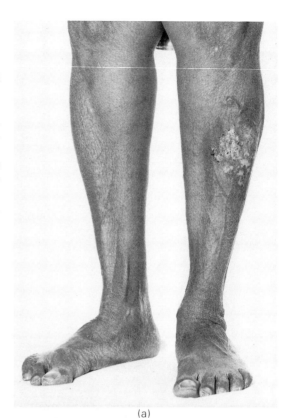

(a)

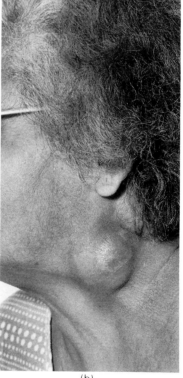

(b)

Fig. 14.20   'Apple jelly' nodules in the skin of the leg (a) in a lady with a proven tuberculous node in the neck (b). The skin lesion resolved when the patient was treated with systemic antituberculosis drugs.

lying skin may ulcerate. If they develop in warm weather, the possibility of sarcoidosis should be considered. This can be confirmed by biopsy and Kveim testing.

Erythrocyanosis frigida is a condition which is found in young women with fat legs and rather thick ankles. It consists of thickened patches of erythematous skin that are mottled and cyanotic at all times (not only in cold weather), and which may very occasionally break down to form areas of superficial, painful ulceration (Fig. 14.21). This ulceration is not preceded by oedema. The diagnosis is based on the clinical appearance of a cool-reddish/blue patch of indurated skin and fat over the lower posterior third of the leg (Fig. 14.21). Although the skin discoloration is similar to that seen over a chilblain, this condition is persistant, not spasmodic and is not closely related to temperature changes. Its cause is unknown. It may be vasospastic, but it is not always relieved by sympathectomy and may therefore have a different aetiology.

The diagnosis may be more difficult to make when the skin has ulcerated but it may be suspected if the surrounding skin shows the characteristic appearances described above. The rest of the limb may have a bluish discoloration (acrocyanosis), a mixture of red and blue changes (erythrocyanosis) or may undergo the white, blue and red changes of Raynauds' phenomenon.

Similar appearances develop in limbs with neurological abnormalities particularly after poliomyelitis. These changes often occur 10 or 20 years after the attack of poliomyelitis and are particularly liable to cause ulceration over the Achilles tendon on the posterior aspect of the leg.

The object of treatment is to keep the limb warm and to encourage healing with conservative measures. Recurrent ulceration and ulcers that will not heal may be improved by vasodilator drugs or sympathectomy. Sympathectomy produces a prolonged almost permanent improve-

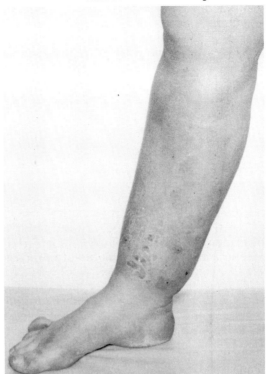

(a)

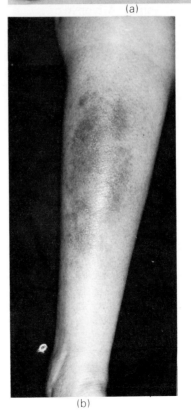

(b)

Fig. 14.21 (a) Small superficial areas of ulceration in a limb with erythrocyanosis frigida. The thickened skin felt cold. The leg is fat, and the foot is slightly oedematous.

(b) Red–purple discolored skin on the back of the calf typical of erythrocyanosis. These areas get chilblains and sometimes ulcerate.

We are grateful to Dr David McGibbon for this illustration.

ment in patients with chilbains and post-poliomyelitis vasospasm but does not always help the patient with idiopathic erythrocyanosis and may make this type of leg oedematous.

Vasculitic ulcers (scleroderma, polyarteritis nodosa)

The common vasculitic ulcer, the 'rheumatoid ulcer' has been discussed on page 384; the other diseases associated with cutaneous vasculitis are far less common than rheumatoid disease but are equally resistant to treatment and it is equally important to diagnose them.

The most common collagen disease causing leg ulceration is scleroderma. Ulceration rarely precedes the other manifestations of this disease but these may have passed unnoticed. Close questioning may reveal that the patient has suffered from Raynaud's phenomenon, arthritis, dysphagia or constipation, and clinical examination may detect spindle-shaped fingers, telangiectases on the face, a puckered mouth and a shiny skin tightly drawn over the facial muscles destroying facial expression.

Ulceration on the lower limb usually appears in a reddened area of skin with surrounding telangiectases (Fig. 14.22a). The ulcers are small, often multiple, painful, penetrate through the full thickness of the skin and show little evidence of healing. They are usually on the toes but may extend onto the foot. Isolated ulcers on the lower limb can also occur (Fig. 14.22b).

The diagnosis is usually confirmed if there are high titres of antinuclear antibodies in the serum, and other autoantibodies may also be present. The erythrocyte sedimentation rate is invariably elevated, and a barium swallow may show defective peristalsis with a rigid oesophagus.

There is no definitive treatment for scleroderma. Some ulcers can be healed by regular cleansing, dressing, and compression bandaging. Other ulcers need prolonged periods of bedrest and may be helped by prostacyclin infusions, sympathectomy and skin grafting. The role of plasmapheresis and immunosupressive agents in treatment is not yet established. Unfortunately, sclerodermatous ulcers have a great tendency to break down, and there is little evidence that elastic support or systemic steroids prevent this from happening.

Small, chronic, recurrent and multiple cutane-ous ulcers also complicate Systemic Lupus Ery-thematosus (SLE) and polyarteritis nodosa. These ulcers may appear anywhere on the leg in otherwise normal skin, though there may be evidence of abnormal skin vessels (telangiectases) and other stigmata of vasculitis. In SLE there may be a butterfly rash across the face and evidence of multisystem disease. Polyarteritis nodosa is often associated with cardiac and renal abnormalities and muscle tenderness.

Cutaneous vasculitis often starts as a nodule or collection of nodules which coalesce before developing intradermal haemorrhages. The skin over the nodules then breaks down to form single or multiple small ulcers (Fig. 14.22b).

Skin biopsies show an arteriolitis with a non-specific round cell infiltration through the whole thickness of the vessel wall. Lupus antibodies may be present in the blood of patients with SLE, and muscle biopsies in patients with polyarteritis may show microaneurysms on the small blood vessels. Treatment is as ineffective for these conditions as it is for scleroderma, though the ulcers sometimes heal with prolonged bedrest.

Dermatologists recognize another type of non-specific cutaneous vasculitis in which there is no systemic disorder (Fig. 14.22c). Skin biopsies show the round cell infiltration of the vessel wall described above with a perivascular deposit of gammaglobulin. The aetiology of this condition remains obscure and there is no specific treatment. Areas of non-specific vasculitis can break down to form small painful ulcers on the legs and feet. The diagnosis is made from immunohisto-chemical stains of skin biopsies.

Ulcers over osteomyelitis

Chronic osteomyelitis of the tibia may discharge through single or multiple sinuses which may be misdiagnosed as ulcers and referred to an ulcer clinic (Fig. 14.23). The patient will often give a history of bone infection and treatment with anti-biotics. The skin surrounding a sinus in the lower leg is usually firmly attached to the underlying bone and, if the tract is probed, bone may be felt beneath the granulation tissue. A plain X-ray will show evidence of bone destruction and new bone formation (Fig. 14.23).

Difficulty occasionally occurs in distinguishing the periosteal reaction that can occur beneath a

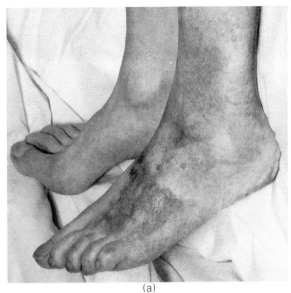

(a)

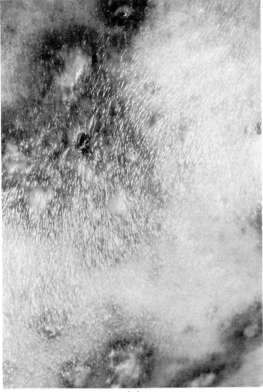

(c)

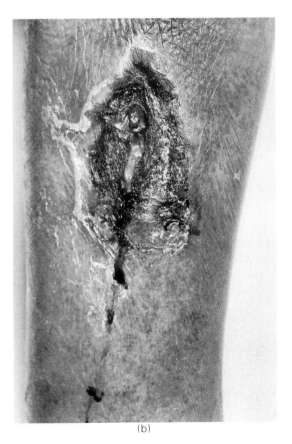

(b)

Fig. 14.22 (a) The clinical features of vasculitis on the dorsal surface of the foot. The skin is red and thickened, and the skin capillaries are dilated.

(b) An ulcerated and gangrenous patch of skin on the anterior surface of the calf. This proved to be caused by a severe vasculitis which extended over the whole of the lower leg and, despite all forms of treatment, the patient rapidly deteriorated and died.

(c) An abnormal area of skin on the calf; biopsy of this area revealed an allergic vasculitis.

We are grateful to Dr Martin Black for this illustration.

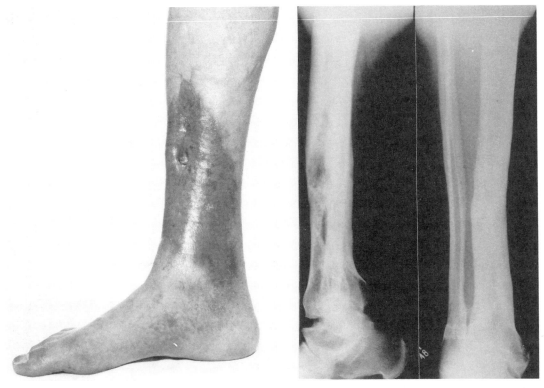

Fig. 14.23 This ulcer looked like a venous ulcer surrounded by severe lipodermatosclerosis, but the skin appeared to be adherent to the front of the tibia. The patient's history revealed that he had had a previous bone infection, and the X-ray of the tibia showed clear evidence of past osteomyelitis. The phlebograms obtained to exclude a post-thrombotic syndrome (which may be a complication of osteomyelitis) were normal.

long-standing chronic venous ulcer from the periostitis over osteomyelitis. An isotope bone scan will shown an increased uptake in bones with osteomyelitis but will be normal with simple periostitis.

Since the advent of antibiotics, ulceration over an old compound fracture of the tibia is more likely to be the result of an associated venous thrombosis or the local skin damage that occurred at the time of the fracture than of long-standing osteomyelitis.

Syphilitic ulcers

Syphilis is now a rare cause of leg ulceration, though it has been an important cause in past centuries. Syphilitic ulcers are usually the result of the skin breaking down over a subcutaneous gumma. The rash that accompanies secondary syphilis is widespread and rarely ulcerates, it should therefore not be mistaken for a venous ulcer. Primary chancres on the leg do not occur.

Gummata begin as red, painless nodules. If the overlying skin becomes necrotic and sloughs, it leaves a circular punched-out ulcer through the whole thickness of the skin, with a 'wash-leather' slough in its base (Fig. 14.24a). Despite the depth of the ulcer, it is always painless and must be distinguished from a neuropathic ulcer. The nodules and ulcers may be multiple and may coalesce to produce a serpiginous lesion. Syphilitic ulcers tend to occur on the upper outer aspect of the lower leg or high on the calf, sites not commonly frequented by venous ulcers.

We still request serological tests for syphilis on all patients with new ulcers but this is probably unnecessary because they are invariably negative. In countries where syphilis is rare, serological tests should probably only be requested when an ulcer is atypical in appearance or site (Fig. 14.24b).

Antibiotic treatment produces rapid healing of syphilitic ulcers leaving the patient with the characteristic 'tissue paper' scars.

Martorell's ulcer

There is considerable doubt about the specificity and even the existence of this ulcer. Martorell[36] claimed that it was an ulcer that occurred in the lower leg of patients with severe hypertension, which resulted from local skin ischaemia produced by the arteriolar narrowing that accompained and perhaps caused the hypertension.

An alternative suggestion is that it is similar to, 'trash foot' which results from inadvertent embolization of arterial debris into the skin of the lower limb at the time of peripheral vascular reconstruction; if so, it would simply be the result of arterial disease in the vessels of the lower limb, in patients likely to be hypertensive.

The ulcer is said to present as a dark red area of skin on the back of the lower leg which becomes black (gangrenous) and then ulcerates (Fig. 14.25). The ulcer has a sloping edge and a red base. We have not seen an ulcer in this site that we have been able to attribute solely to hypertension, and we therefore doubt that the condition exists.

Ulcers associated with blood dyscrasias

Several 'blood-diseases' are associated with ulceration of the legs. In many instances the mechanism that causes the ulceration is obscure but in some cases it is probably venous thrombosis or capillary sludging. The ulcers of sickle cell disease, thalassaemia, thrombotic thrombocythaemia and polycythaemia rubra vera are all probably caused by a combination of venous thrombosis and local capillary thrombosis.

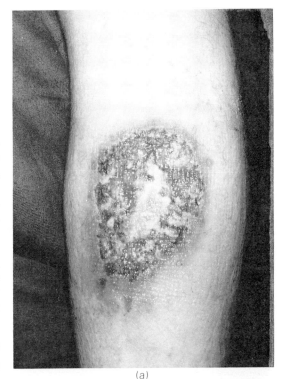

(a)

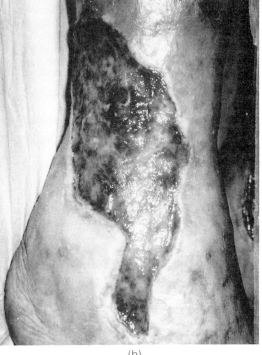
(b)

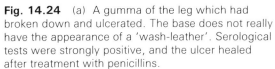

Fig. 14.24 (a) A gumma of the leg which had broken down and ulcerated. The base does not really have the appearance of a 'wash-leather'. Serological tests were strongly positive, and the ulcer healed after treatment with penicillins.

(b) An ulcer which looked like a venous ulcer but serological tests confirmed active syphilis and the ulcer healed after antibiotic treatment.

We are grateful to Dr Martin Black for these illustrations.

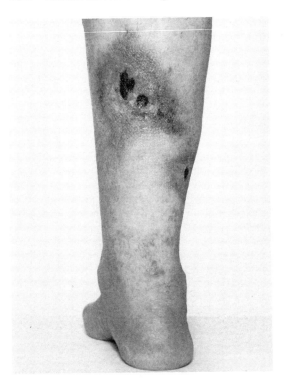

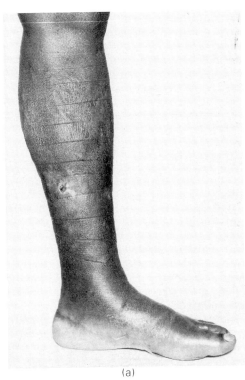

(a)

Fig. 14.25 This ulcer developed on the back of the calf of an obese woman who had hypertension. Phlebograms and physiological tests of calf pump function were normal, and there was no evidence of arterial insufficiency. Some clinicians would classify this as a Martorell's ulcer, others would just consider it to be the result of a local vasculitis or embolism.

Fig. 14.26 Ulcers associated with haematological disease.
(a) An ulcer in a young girl with sickle cell disease. Ascending phlebography did not reveal any post-thrombotic changes or incompetent calf communicating veins.

Leukaemia may also cause local capillary sludging, but the mechanisms by which congenital spherocytosis (acholuric jaundice), elliptocytosis, and pernicious anaemia cause ulceration are unknown.

Leg ulcers associated with abnormalities of the blood have no diagnostic features (Fig. 14.26). They are usually on the lower third of the leg, superficial, painful and multiple. Lipodermatosclerosis is rarely present unless post-thrombotic changes coexist. Koilonychia, a smooth tongue, peripheral neuropathy, a palpable spleen or lymphadenopathy may all be detected on general examination.

We routinely examine the blood and check for sickle cell trait when appropriate in all patients with new or obscure ulcers.

In many instances the main causative factor is a previous deep vein thrombosis; this should be investigated in the usual way while correcting the blood abnormality. Ulcers that are healed conservatively or by skin grafting will break down again if the blood abnormality remains untreated. An exchange transfusion may improve the healing time of ulcers associated with capillary sludging or abnormal plasma constituents. Elastic stockings may be of benefit in preventing reulceration but we do not know why.

Self-induced (artefactual) ulceration

The psychological abnormality that drives patients to self-mutilation is not understood. Depression or a craving for attention in a hysterical personality are two possible mechanisms. We see one or two patients every year with this diagnosis but there are probably others who, by

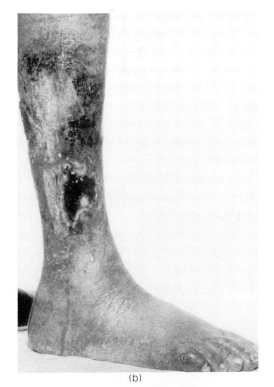

(b)

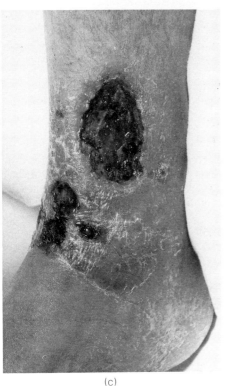

(c)

tampering with their dressings, prevent their genuine ulcers from healing.

Suspicion is often first aroused by the shape and position of the ulcer, and is supported by finding dressings that have been loosened or removed. Bizarre ulcer shapes with normal surrounding skin (Fig. 14.27), often on the anterior surface of the leg at a site which can be easily reached, is highly suggestive. A long history with multiple admissions to other hospitals for treatment of an ulcer that defies all attempts at healing should also arouse suspicion.

Oedema may be produced by applying a tourniquet around the limb, and this may eventually cause ulceration.

Healing beneath a plaster of Paris cast, in hospital, under close inspection is the only way to give credence to the diagnosis which can be extremely difficult if not impossible to confirm.

Psychiatrists seem to agree that confronting the patient with the suspected diagnosis is not advisable but they rarely give positive advice about the correct course of action. When we are certain of the diagnosis, we favour some form of confrontation but only in close consultation with the family doctor who has a detailed knowledge of the patient's home and personal circumstances. Care must be taken not to diagnose self-mutilation in error, as nothing is more certain to upset the doctor–patient relationship and lead to litigation. It is better to delay making a diagnosis and await events than to make a wrong diagnosis of artefactual ulceration.

Pyoderma gangrenosum

Some patients with severe ulcerative colitis develop collections of pustules and areas of skin necrosis on their calves. The lesions begin as pustules but then coalesce and develop into boggy indurated ulcers (Fig. 14.28). At other times the skin becomes necrotic and secondarily infected beneath and around the necrotic skin.

Fig. 14.26 (b) This ulcer, which looks like a typical venous ulcer, was associated with haemosiderosis. The veins were normal.

(c) These ulcers developed in a patient who was known to suffer from polycythaemia. The normal looking skin around the ulcer suggests that a venous abnormality is unlikely. Ulcers associated with polycythaemia sometimes heal after treatment with venesection.

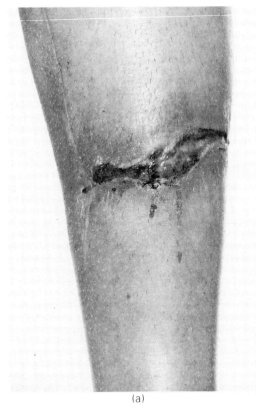

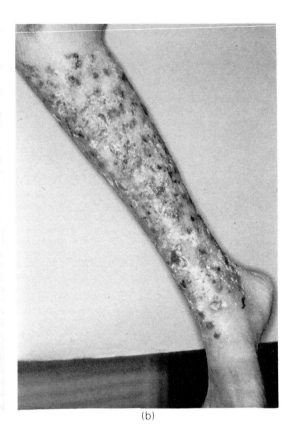

(a)   (b)

Fig. 14.27   Artefactual ulcers.

(a) This ulcer failed to respond to all attempts at healing in a local hospital, but it healed when the dressings were protected with plaster of Paris. The strange horizontal linear appearance is not compatible with any form of pathological ulcer.

(b) This leg has the appearance usually associated with self-inflicted multiple cigarette burns, but the patient was actually producing caustic burns on the leg. The reason for this self-mutilation was obscure.

We are grateful to Dr Martin Black for this illustration.

Pyoderma is almost always associated with ulcerative colitis but it occasionally occurs in patients with Crohn's disease. If the patient gives a history of frequent loose bowel actions, blood and slime in the stool or is known to suffer from or has even had ulcerative colitis, pyoderma must be suspected. Confirmation of colitis by a rectal biopsy supports the diagnosis.

Successful treatment of the colitis is usually associated with an improvement in the pyoderma.

Pressure ulcers on the legs (bed sores or decubitus ulcers)

Pressure ulcers occur at sites where the weight of the body is transmitted through skin that is not adapted to weight bearing. These ulcers are most common in immobile patients in bed, hence the term 'bed sores'. They occur in the same positions on the leg as the neuropathic ulcers of bedridden patients (i.e. over the back of the heel, the head of the fifth metatarsal and the malleoli) but they are painful. While the diagnosis of an ulcer over the heel is rarely in doubt, pressure ulcers in other sites have to be differentiated from venous ulcers.

The diagnosis is usually obvious if the ulcer develops after the patient has had a period of prolonged bedrest but in an elderly demented patient this history may be difficult to obtain, and a history taken from a relative or nurse may be very helpful. The diagnosis depends upon the history because, apart from its site, the appearance of the ulcer is not specific.

Pressures ulcers should not occur. They should

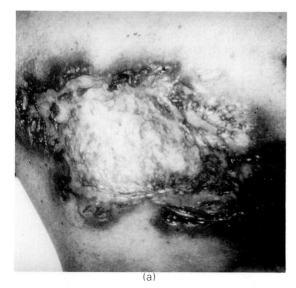

(a)

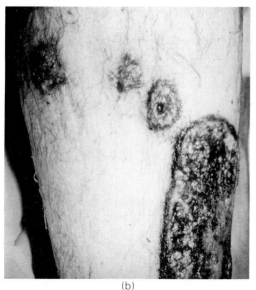

(b)

Fig. 14.28 (a, b) Pyoderma gangrenosum. Both patients had diarrhoea and were passing blood and mucus. A diagnosis of ulcerative colitis was confirmed by sigmoidoscopy and biopsy. The skin lesions improved when the colitis responded to treatment.

We are grateful to Dr Martin Black for these illustrations.

be prevented by frequent position changes and careful nursing. This council of perfection is not always achieved in hospital and can never apply to the frail elderly person living alone.

Most pressure ulcers will heal spontaneously if further damage can be prevented. Deep ulcers may have to be excised and grafted, the choice of skin replacement depending upon the site and size of the ulcer. Ulcers on the legs will usually accept a split-skin graft, whereas ulcers on the buttocks can sometimes only be covered by complex rotation flaps.

Ulcers in lymphoedematous limbs

Skin ulceration in lymphoedematous limbs is rare. When ulceration does occur, it may be associated with defective fibrinolysis.[54] Inadequate clearance of lymph leads to the accumulation of plasma proteins within the interstitial spaces and, if tissue fibrinolysis is defective, lipodermatosclerosis develops. Subsequent trauma or infection may lead to skin breakdown (Fig. 14.29).

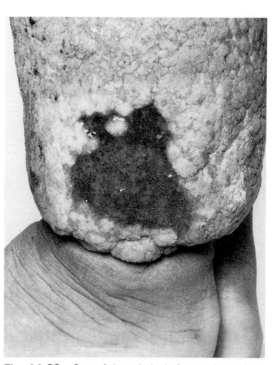

Fig. 14.29 One of the relatively few patients that we have had under our care who have extensive ulceration complicating gross lymphoedema. There was no evidence of venous disease.

An ulcer in an oedematous limb must be differentiated from a post-thrombotic ulcer. The absence of subcutaneous varicosities and dilated intradermal venules, an increased skin thickness, and oedema of the toes should suggest a diagnosis of lymphoedema.

The diagnosis of lymphoedema can be confirmed by isotope or X-ray lymphography[53] but, though the presence of normal lymphatic function excludes lymphoedema, the finding of abnormal lymphatics does not necessarily exclude an alternative cause for the ulceration. Post-thrombotic deep vein damage and lymphoedema can occur in the same leg, and in such patients the venous anatomy and venous function must be studied with phlebography and plethysmography before a final diagnosis can be made.

Ulcers in lymphoedematous limbs can be treated by occlusion and compression in the same way that venous ulcers are treated. Once the ulcers have healed, the lymphoedema can be alleviated by compression, bypass surgery, or by an excisional operation.[26,28,30]

Tropical ulcers

Texts on the differential diagnosis of venous ulceration all contain a reference to tropical ulceration. A number of organisms have been incriminated as a cause of these ulcers but the evidence supporting these suggestions has been mainly anectodal. Actinomycosis, epidermophytosis, blastomycosis, myecytoma (Madura foot), leishmaniasis, monilia, syphilis and yaws can all cause ulceration and are all more common in, but not exclusive to, tropical climates.[17,24]

'Beruli boil' is a particularly virulent form of ulcer, otherwise known as 'Oriental sore' or 'Baghdad boil', which is caused by *Leishmania tropica*, an organism transmitted by the bite of the sand-fly. It begins as an indurated papule which later ulcerates. Scrapings of the ulcer reveal the organism and confirm the diagnosis.

Quist[43] states that 'tropical ulcers are common in barefoot young men (and women)' and are 'the result of trauma in the presence of chronic malnutrition and anaemia'. Recently, work from Papua New Guinea has suggested that a fusiform organism living in salt water lagoons or in the shallow water inside coral reefs may be responsible for tropical ulceration. Colour plate 21 shows a typical circular tropical ulcer in an area of normal skin.

Ulceration following burns or insect bites

Any area of damaged skin can necrose and so become an ulcer.

Burns are usually remembered but a hot water bottle burn occurring during deep sleep may pass unnoticed and this can cause difficulties in diagnosis.

Insect bites are often not recalled by the patient; this makes a diagnosis at the stage of secondary infection and ulceration difficult. As in traumatic ulcers, the surrounding skin is normal and the ulcer is usually small with no specific features. Diagnosis relies on surmize or an appropriate history.

Necrobiosis lipoidica

This condition is found in diabetic patients (Fig. 14.30 and Colour Plate 20) and represents an area of fat necrosis followed by infection and necrosis of the overlying skin. The underlying pathological cause of the fat necrosis is uncertain. Treatment is by antibiotics and dressings, with appropriate control of the diabetes.

Meleney's ulcer[37] (synergistic bacterial gangrene)

This is a rapidly progressive superficial gang-

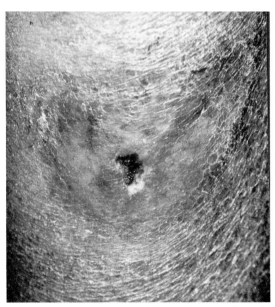

Fig. 14.30 This ulcer could have been attributed to any cause but it occurred in a diabetic patient and was thought to be caused by necrobiosis lipoidica.

rene produced by a synergistic infection of a micro-aerophilic non-haemolytic streptococcus combined with either a staphylococcus, a gram-negative bacillus, a bacteroides, or a clostridial organism. The combination of the two species of bacteria has a synergistic effect causing a rapid extension of the infection through the skin and subcutaneous tissues. The infection causes thrombosis of the small vessels in the skin which in turn causes gangrene.

The initial infection is often trivial but it spreads rapidly along the fascial planes with the overlying erythematous skin quickly becoming insensitive and gangrenous before it necroses

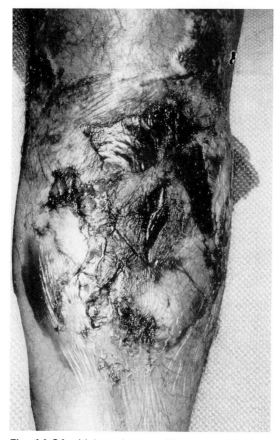

Fig. 14.31 Meleney's ulcer. This patient had been holding a road-breaking drill against his calf and developed an area of erythematous skin which necrosed and then became a large area of superficial spreading gangrene. Bacteriological cultures grew a micro-aerophilic streptococcus and a bacteroides. The patient was treated by wide excision of the skin and subcutaneous tissue followed by skin grafting.

(Fig. 14.31) and separates to leave large areas of ulceration. There are signs of toxaemia, pyrexia, malaise, poor cerebration and prostration. Treatment is urgent and consists of giving large doses of penicillin and excising the gangrenous tissues. Once the infection is under control, the large areas which have been denuded of skin can be covered with skin grafts.

Ulceration caused by arteriovenous fistulae

Arteriovenous fistulae may be either congenital or acquired. The lower limb is the most common site for congenital fistulae. Fistulae may be localized (single) or diffuse (multiple). A cutaneous vascular abnormality (a naevus) may have been present for many years before the ulcer developed.

Ulceration may occur without overt signs of a fistula. Clinical suspicion should be aroused by the youth of the patient, the presence of a capillary or cavernous naevus in the skin, and an increase in the length of the limb. Peripheral oedema, an increase in skin temperature, prominent or pulsatile surface veins, a palpable thrill, an audible bruit and a positive Branham's sign may also be present.

Acquired fistulae are often caused by trauma at the groin or knee but may occasionally follow the spontaneous rupture of an atheromatous artery into its accompanying vein. Accidental iatrogenic fistulae are uncommon but they sometimes complicate arterial catheterization or arterial surgery.

Fistulae deliberately formed to produce venous dilation suitable for venepuncture and renal dialysis or to provide an increased venous flow after a venous reconstruction are the most common forms of iatrogenic fistula. The histological changes of lipodermatosclerosis (see Chapter 13) have been seen in the skin surrounding ulceration of the hand that occasionally develops after the formation of a Bresnia–Cimeno fistula at the wrist.[60] This suggests that pericapillary fibrin, acting as a diffusion block, is a possible mechanism for the ulceration which occurs with arteriovenous fistulae and, interestingly, confirms our observation of the effect of canine arteriovenous fistulae.[9] Other causes of skin ischaemia may be the shunting of blood away from the skin through multiple arteriovenous fistulae[41] or the high venous pressure impairing calf pump function

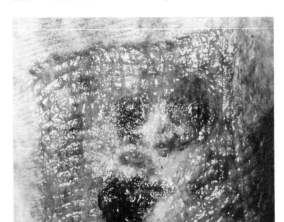

Fig. 14.32 An ulcer on the leg of a lady who had varicose veins and lipodermatosclerosis but the skin on her calves was abnormally warm on palpation. The limb contained multiple arteriovenous fistulae. Part of the ulcer was also abnormal in appearance – it had an area with a raised edge. Biopsy of this area revealed a basal cell carcinoma. This may be an example of malignant change in a chronic venous ulcer or of malignant change in skin subjected to the irradiation which was part of the patient's treatment 20 years previously.

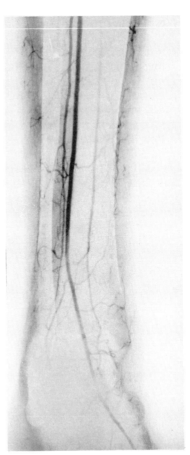

Fig. 14.33 The arteriogram of the leg shown in Fig. 14.32. It shows multiple small arteriovenous fistulae in the skin and subcutaneous tissues.

and producing ulceration by some other, as yet unidentified, mechanism.

The ulcers that develop in a limb containing arteriovenous fistulae have the appearance of venous ulcers (Fig. 14.32). They often occur outside the gaiter region of the leg because their site depends upon the location of the fistula. Although the increased blood flow may make the limb hot and hypertrophic, the ulcers have poor granulation tissue, do not always bleed vigorously and are usually very painful.

The raised limb blood flow can be measured with plethysmography, and arteriography may show the sites of abnormal arteriovenous communications and early filling of the veins (Fig. 14.33).

These ulcers heal when the fistula or fistulae are closed. Localized fistulae may be treated by direct surgical excision of the abnormal vessels or therapeutic embolization. Diffuse fistulae are difficult to treat, but operations designed to remove all the side branches (skeletonization) may be beneficial. Amputation should be reserved for diffuse fistulae which occur throughout the limb and cause congestive cardiac failure or painful incurable ulceration.

Primary skin diseases

We see many patients with contact dermatitis, psoriasis, bullous pemphigoid, impetigo and tinea who have been referred with a diagnosis of venous ulceration (Fig. 14.34a–d). The opinion of a dermatologist should be sought whenever the nature of an ulcer is in doubt, and skin biopsies should be obtained from all atypical ulcers. Livido reticularis (Fig. 14.35) and atrophie blanche (Fig. 14.36) are two forms of cutaneous

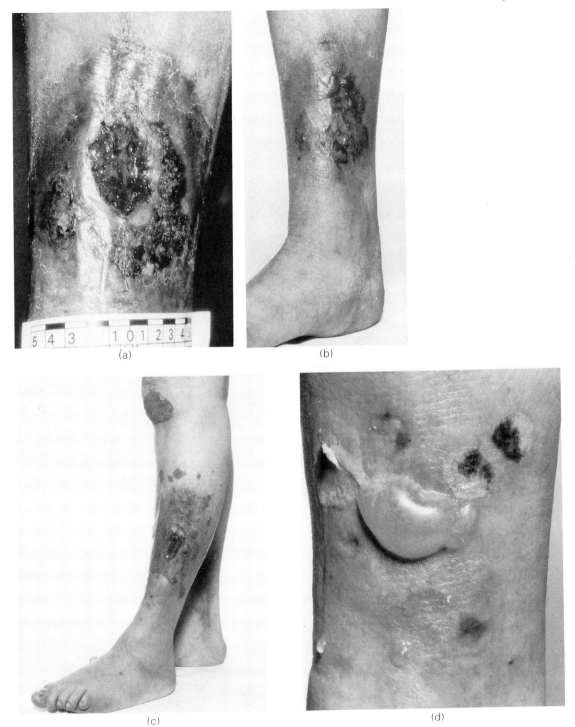

Fig. 14.34 Ulcerated skin disease.
   This ulcer (a) of unknown aetiology was treated by skin grafting. When the ulcer had healed, the leg had the appearance shown in (b). A biopsy revealed the diagnosis to be pemphigoid.
   (c) A leg with severe psoriasis in which one area had become infected and ulcerated.
   (d) A bullous skin eruption which had progressed to ulceration.

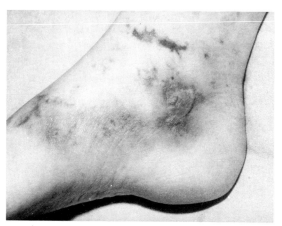

Fig. 14.35 This limb has livido vasculitis. There are patches of red-brown localized vasculitis, one of which has broken down behind the medial malleolus to form a shallow ulcer.

We are grateful to Dr Martin Black for this illustration.

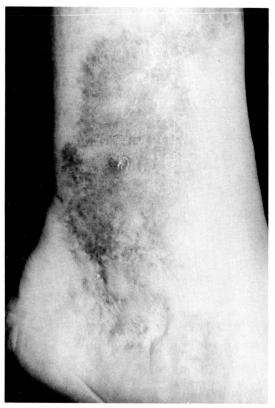

Fig. 14.36 Areas of atrophie blanche throughout a wide area of cutaneous vasculitis. The white areas are scars which have slowly replaced dead skin without going through a phase of ulceration.

We are grateful to Dr Martin Black for this illustration.

vasculitis which may break down to give small painful superficial ulcers[52] in areas of red–brown or white skin. These conditions are common around the ankle, and the ulcers are often misdiagnosed as being venous.

The newly recorded disease of superoxide dismutase defiency and the rare Ehlers-Danlos' syndrome have now been suggested as unusual causes of ulceration. These conditions, together with the cutaneous vasculitides, should be referred to a dermatologist for both diagnosis and treatment.

Summer ulcers

Summer ulcers appear in the summer months on the ankle and dorsum of the feet in young women. They are sometimes associated with areas of livido reticularis and Raynaud's phenomenon. They heal in the cold weather. The aetiology is obscure but we have found that some of these patients have exceptionally high plasma fibrinogen levels and a reduced plasma fibrinolysis. In three of our patients summer ulceration has been prevented by the pharmacological enhancement of fibrinolysis with stanozolol.

Pyogenic granuloma

This usually presents as a raised rapidly growing patch of exuberant granulation tissue but it may be difficult to diagnose if attempts have been made to remove the proud tissue. Diagnosis and treatment consists of excision biopsy.

Gouty tophi and subcutaneous calcification

We have recently seen a persistent ulcer over the Achilles tendon which developed from pressure on an underlying gouty tophus (Fig. 14.37). The uric acid crystals presumably delayed healing by acting as a foreign body.

Subcutaneous calcification[48,56] may act in a similar manner. This may occur in long-standing lipodermatosclerosis or may be the result of metastatic calcification in systemic sclerosis (CREST syndrome) or rheumatoid arthritis.

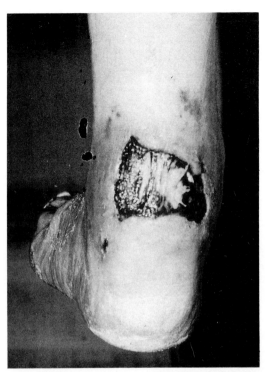

Fig. 14.37 A biopsy of this unusual ulcer over the Achilles tendon showed evidence of urate crystals in the skin. The patient's serum urate level was elevated, and the cause of the ulcer was cutaneous necrosis over a gouty tophus.

The crystals or calcification must be excised before healing can occur.

Infected blisters

Patients who develop gross oedema of the lower limbs as a result of congestive cardiac failure, nephrotic syndrome, hyperalbuminaemia, or pelvic tumours, occasionally develop large intra-dermal blisters. When the outer layer of the blister seperates it leaves a shallow but sometimes an extensive area of ulceration which often becomes infected (Fig. 14.38).

Treatment of the oedema and any secondary infection produces rapid healing, unless there has been full-thickness skin loss in which case skin grafting is required.

Ulcerating mesodermal tumours and lymphomas

Kaposi's sarcoma (Fig. 14.39), histiocytic sar-coma, lymphangiosarcoma (Fig. 14.40), and bone tumours can all rarely present as cutaneous ulceration. Only occasionally do they give rise to problems in diagnosis, provided a biopsy is performed as part of the routine investigation of all atypical ulcers. Lymphomas may also present as ulceration of the leg.

Injection ulcers

The most common 'injection ulcer' on the lower leg follows extravasation of sclerosant during injection sclerotherapy for varicose veins. Sodium tetra decyl sulphate (3%) is probably the most popular sclerosant used in the United Kingdom. The newer sclerosants 'Variglobin' and 'Sclerovein' are said to cause fewer problems if they are injected outside the vein.

Injection ulcers will not occur if care is taken to ensure that the needle is inside the vein at the time of injection. If the needle slips out of the vein, further injection of sclerosant must be abandoned. Once a sclerosant has been injected outside the vein, there is no evidence that its effects can be minimized by dilution with water or saline, or dispersed by hyaluronidase.

Injection ulcers are often indolent and can take many months to heal. It may be best to advise the patient to accept a local excision of the ulcer with a sutured primary closure.

Other hypertonic solutions can also cause ulceration if delivered outside the vein. These include hyperosmolar radiographic contrast media and cytotoxic drugs (Fig. 14.41), though it is unusual for cytotoxic drugs to be injected into leg veins. Healing of these ulcers may also be slow, and excision with or without a skin graft may be necessary.

Nutritional ulcers

Patients with severe deficiency disease such as beri-beri, scurvy, pellagra or kwashiorkor, may develop leg ulcers which will not heal until the nutritional deficiency has been corrected. The mechanism that causes the skin to necrose is obscure but it may be poor cellular regeneration after a minor injury.

Cryoglobulinaemia and macroglobulinaemia

These conditions cause small vessel 'sludging'

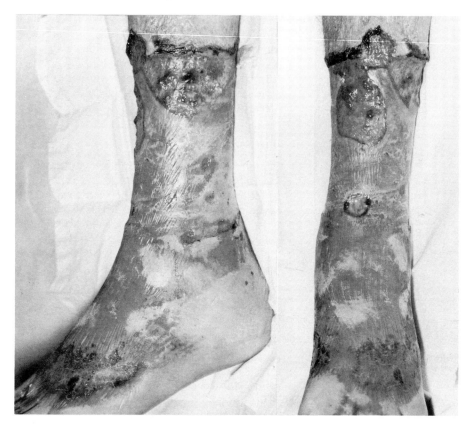

Fig. 14.38 This patient developed massive ankle oedema secondary to congestive cardiac failure. The skin blistered. The blisters became secondarily infected and then broke down to expose areas of superficial ulceration. These ulcers usually heal quickly, unless there has been full-thickness skin loss.

accompanied by vasospasm which occasionally causes ulceration. These ulcers rarely occur on the leg and are usually found on the upper limb. The blood of any patient with Raynauds' syndrome and unusual skin ulceration should be sent for a cryoglobulin assay and protein electrophoresis to exclude these abnormalities.

Yaws, leprosy and anthrax

These are uncommon causes of ulceration of the legs. Yaws usually affects the lower limb and often starts before puberty (Colour plate 22). The Wasserman reaction is positive and the condition has to be differentiated from syphilis.

Lepromatous ulceration is usually neuropathic and associated with thickened nerves and the cutaneous changes of lepromatous or tuberculoid leprosy. Acid-fast bacilli are seen on skin biopsy.

Anthrax or woolsorters' disease presents as a black (malignant) pustule but rarely occurs on the lower limb. The bacillus should be seen in fluid aspirated from the vesicle.

Tularaemia, blastomycosis and sporotrichosis

These are all theoretical rather than real causes of ulceration of the leg. They can be distinguished on bacteriological examination.

Investigation of a venous ulcer

The tests designed to exclude other diagnoses have been mentioned in the previous section on differential diagnosis and are summarized in Table 14.2. Once the diagnosis of venous ulceration has been made, the investigations have two objectives.

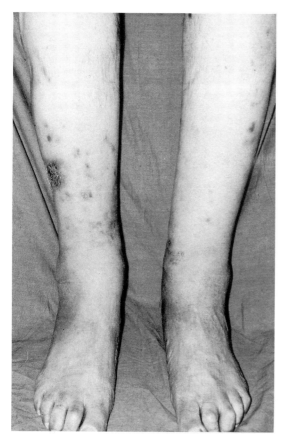

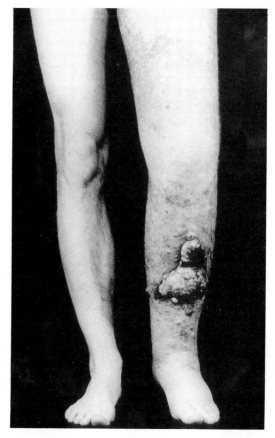

Fig. 14.39 Kaposi's sarcoma is becoming an important differential diagnosis in patients with leg ulceration since the advent of AIDS. Multiple cutaneous red–purple nodules in a known homosexual are an indication for HIV antibody screening. Suspicious lesions should be biopsied to confirm the diagnosis. In this patient one lesion on the lateral side of the right leg and one on the medial side of the left leg have broken down and become ulcers.

We are grateful to Dr Martin Black for this illustration.

Fig. 14.40 This young man had long-standing lymphoedema of the leg. He developed an area of cutaneous erythema which was initially thought to be cellulitis but this rapidly extended and ulcerated. The skin of the rest of the leg then developed multiple small haemorrhagic vascular nodules; biopsies showed these to be Stewart Treves lymphangiosarcoma.

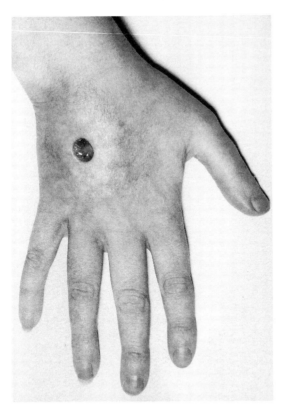

Fig. 14.41 An injection ulcer on the dorsum of the hand following the extravenous extravasation of cytotoxic drugs. Similar lesions can occur when sclerosant escapes from a vein when injecting varicose veins. Injection ulcers may take many weeks to heal and are sometimes best treated by excision and primary suture.

(A) Assessment of the ulcer
    1. size
    2. bacteriology
    3. nutrition
    4. histology
(B) Assessment of the nature and the severity of the venous disease (Table 14.3)

(A) Tests designed to assess the ulcer

Whatever the cause of the ulcer, certain tests must be carried out so that the initial state of the ulcer can be described and the effect of treatment can be assessed.

Table 14.2 Tests that are helpful when investigating the cause of a leg ulcer

Blood investigations
    Haemoglobin*
    White cell count*
    Packed cell volume (PCV)*
    Erythrocyte sedimentation rate (ESR)*
    Rheumatoid factor*
    Rose-Waller
    Latex
    Anti-nuclear factor*
    Blood sugar
    TPHA (Treponema pallidum haemagglutination)*
    Cryoglobulins*
    Plasma protein and strip*
    LE (lupus erythematosus)cells
Urine test (sugar)*
Bacteriological swabs*
Arm and ankle blood pressure index (Doppler
    ultrasound)*
Arteriography
Barium swallow
Isotope lymphography
Nerve conduction studies
Biopsy

*These are routine tests; the others are only performed if clinically indicated.

Table 14.3 The tests that we routinely use to assess the presence and severity of venous disease

Full clinical examination
Tourniquet tests
Doppler ultrasound flow detection of superficial vein
    reflux
Ascending phlebography
Foot volumetry
and in some cases
Varicography
Descending phlebography

1. Size

The only absolute measurement of healing is the time taken for the ulcer to heal completely. This measurement has the advantage of a reasonably clear end-point. All the crust and scab must be removed to allow direct inspection and confirmation of complete epithelialization before healing is accepted. Inadequate inspection will blur the end-point.

The larger the area of the ulcer at the start of treatment, the longer will be the healing time (Fig. 14.42),[50] an initial assessment of the ulcer area is

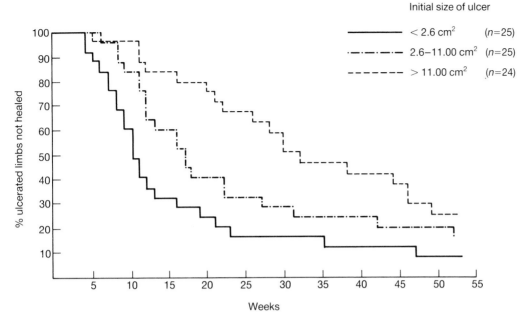

Fig. 14.42 The relationship between ulcer size and ulcer healing. Ulcers have been divided into three groups based on their size at presentation. It can be seen that the largest ulcers take longer to heal but there is considerable variation in the time taken by individual ulcers to heal.

therefore desirable for prognosis and stratification if the patient is participating in a clinical trial. The methods available for this are as follows

(a) Tape measurement of the two largest diameters If the measurements of the two largest diameters (at right angles to each other) are multiplied together, the area of the ulcer is converted to the equivalent of a rectangle. This overestimates the area of most ulcers, as the majority are oval or irregular in shape (Fig. 14.1), but it has a surprisingly good correlation with more accurate methods of measurement described below and is probably adequate for most clinical trials.[50]

(b) Tracing out the perimeter The perimeter of the ulcer area can be traced on to transparent paper or polythene sheeting using an indelible pen. The marked out area on the paper can then be cut out and weighed if the paper is of standard thickness, or converted into square centimeters using a planimeter.

Alternatively, an ultrasonic digitizer can be used with a light pen linked to a computer programme to convert the traced ulcer area to square millimetres.[50]

(c) Photography Serial photographs against a

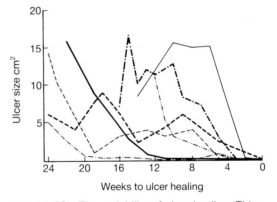

Fig. 14.43 The variability of ulcer healing. This graph plots the healing of seven different ulcers and reveals how variable it can be. This variability means that assessment of treatment by measuring ulcer healing over a short period is a meaningless exercise. The only reliable method of describing healing is the time taken from the commencement of treatment to complete healing.

scale can be used in association with one of the techniques described above to measure the exact surface area of the ulcer.[39] A normal camera does not allow for the convexity of the limb, and therefore this method of measurement will be inaccurate if the ulcer extends on to more than one surface of the leg. A complicated and expensive system of stero-photogrammatory has been introduced to overcome the distortion caused by the convex limb surface and which, in the hands of its users, is claimed to give highly reproducible results.[6]

(d) Mould None of the methods described above makes any attempt to measure the depth of the ulcer. Some investigators have advocated the use of quick-setting moulds to take account of all three dimensions of the ulcer. This technique has not been adopted because it is debatable whether it provides much additional information to the measurement of surface area.

Comment Ulcer measurements allow the doctor or nurse to assess treatment from week to week. It is important that measurements are made to avoid the standard comment 'healing well' which often appears month after month in the patient's records. Some workers have suggested that the healing rate in the first 6 weeks is an indication of successful treatment[6] but this has not been our experience (Fig. 14.43). We find that the initial measurements do no more than allow us to make a crude estimate of the time to total healing.

Other methods used to assess ulcer healing capability, based on the measurement of skin blood flow, have usually been used to assess ischaemic ulcers. These methods include injection of radioactive microspheres, skin fluorescence, and ^{99m}Tc phosphate imaging.[32] They have not yet found a place in the assessment of venous ulcer healing.

(2) Bacteriology

Little is known about the role of bacteria in the genesis and maintainence of venous ulcers. It is assumed that high concentrations of organisms are associated with delayed healing and the rejection of skin grafts but there is little evidence that the elimination of infection or a reduction in the number of bacteria enhances healing.

Several studies[20,21,22,34,38,44,45,46,57] have shown that the organisms listed in Table 14.4 are commonly found on ulcers, and our own findings in 62 new ulcers are shown in Table 14.5. These organisms may simply be surface contaminants. Our own cultures of tissue biopsies taken from the ulcer base have not shown consistent evidence of infection spreading deeply into the granulation tissue. We have specifically looked for anaerobic organisms and found them in 44 per cent of ulcer cultures; this is a much greater incidence than reported in other studies. It may be that anaerobic organisms adversely affect healing because metronidazole (Flagyl) has been reported to speed the healing of some ulcers.[3] These findings await confirmation.

We recommend regular bacteriological examination of ulcers for aerobic and anaerobic organisms and suggest treatment with antibiotics if there is a heavy growth of a single organism or in the rare case where cellulitis or lymphangitis arises from the ulcer.

Hopkins and Jamieson[27] have shown that systemically administered antibiotics can reach the surface of the ulcer but we do not know if they are of benefit when they arrive. Ryan[47] has argued that all organisms are not necessarily bad. For example, he has suggested that coliforms which use up oxygen may encourage the growth of anaerobes, which in turn may protect the aerobes from phagocytosis. Some organisms may remove slough while others may prevent invasion by more virulent microbes.

Comment The bacteriology of venous ulcers deserves closer study. At present, no firm conclusions can be drawn from the published work about the significance of bacteria on ulcer-healing or the value of their eradication.

3. Nutrition

An association between certain anaemias and ulceration has already been discussed but all varieties of chronic ulceration may cause anaemia. Blood loss and chronic infection can combine to give a mixed picture of bone marrow depression and iron deficiency anaemia. Schraibman and Stratton[49] found significantly lower haemoglobin and ferritin levels in 30 patients with leg ulcers compared to a similar number of age and sex matched controls. The patients with ulcers also had lower levels of protein and albumin but these reductions did not reach statistical significance.

Table 14.4 Bacteriology of venous ulcers

Organisms	Study 1 (62 ulcers)* No. ulcers infected	Study 2 (47 ulcers)† No. ulcers infected
Staphylococcus aureus	15	27
Staphylococcus epidermidis	12	—
Streptococcus		
Group A	—	2
Group B	1	2
Group C	—	3
Group D	4	—
Viridans	3	—
Escherichia coli	4	1
Proteus mirabilis	1	2
Enterobacter	3	1
Pseudomonas aeruginosa	5	1
Pseudomonas maltiphola	1	1
Clostridium perfringens	—	1
Corynebacterium	4	—
Acinetobacter calcoaceticus	3	—
Klebsiella pneumoniae	3	—
Citrobacter freundi	1	—
Yeast	2	—
Normal skin flora	—	4
No growth	—	2

*Study 1 – Friedman S J, Su W P D. Management of leg ulcers with hydrocolloid occlusive dressing. *Arch Dermatol* 1984; **120**: 1329.
†Study 2 – Eriksson G. Bacterial growth in venous leg ulcers – its clinical significance in the healing process. In: *Royal Society of Medicine, International Congress and Symposium Series*, 1985; No **88**: 45.

Table 14.5 Bacterial flora of 63 consecutive new leg ulcers

Organism	No. ulcers with organism	Percentage
Staph. aureus	32	51
Strep. faecalis	20	31
Staph. epidermidis	12	19
P. mirabilis	12	19
Ps. aeruginosa	12	19
β-haemolytic strep.	10	16
Diphtheroid	10	16
E. coli	4	6
P. vulgaris	4	6
Non-haemolytic strep.	3	5
Ent. cloacae	3	5
Klebsiella	3	5
α-haemolytic strep.	2	3
Ac. anitratus	2	3
M. morganii	2	3
Strep. milleri	1	2
Ps. putrefaciens	1	2
H. parainfluenzae	1	2

The nutritional status of all patients with ulcers should be assessed from anthropomorphic measurements and blood studies.

4. Trace elements

Much attention has been paid to the effect of zinc deficiency and its replacement in leg ulceration.[23,25,59] Serum zinc levels have been found to be low in some patients but it has been shown that serum zinc does not correlate well with total body zinc which is better assessed by measuring intracellular leucocyte zinc.[29] Confirmation that patients with venous ulcers have a true tissue zinc depletion is essential before attempting to show that systemically or locally administered zinc improves healing.

Biopsy

The principal object of ulcer-biopsy is to exclude non-venous causes of ulceration. We are not aware of any studies which have used repeated biopsies to access ulcer healing or healing potential.

Clinicians are naturally averse to performing a biopsy when an ulcer is showing signs of healing, in case it delays or reverses the healing process. If, however, oxygenation and healing are related to the presence of pericapillary fibrin, an initial assessment of the amount of extravascular protein which is present might indicate the likelihood of healing and the need for prolonged rest, elevation, or fibrinolytic enhancement. A further biopsy when an ulcer fails to show signs of healing might explain why this is happening. Ultimately, the clinical behaviour of ulcers must be related to a knowledge of the pathological changes occurring in the skin, some of which can only be assessed by biopsy.

(B) Tests to assess the nature and severity of the calf pump failure

These tests are discussed in detail in Chapter 4. The tests that we commonly use are listed in Table 14.3.

References

1. Ackroyd JS, Young AE. Leg ulcers that do not heal. *Br Med J* 1983; **286**: 207.
2. Anning ST. *Leg Ulcers. Their Causes and Treatment.* London. J & A Churchill. 1954.
3. Baker PG, Haig G. Metronidazole in the treatment of chronic pressure sores and ulcers. A comparison with standard treatments in general practice. *Practitioner* 1981; **225**: 569.
4. Black W. Neoplastic disease occurring in varicose ulcers or eczema: A report of 6 cases. *Br J Cancer* 1952; **6**: 120.
5. Browse NL, Jarett PEM, Morland M, Burnand KG. Treatment of liposclerosis of the leg by fibrinolytic enhancement: a preliminary report. *Br Med J* 1977; **2**. 434.
6. Bulstrode CJK, Goode AW, Scott PJ. Stereophotogrammetry for measuring rates of cutaneous healing: a comparison with conventional techniques. *Clin Sci* 1986; **71**: 437.
7. Burnand KG, Browse NL. The postphlebitic limb and venous ulceration. In Russell RCG (Ed) *Recent Advances in Surgery* Edinburgh. Churchill Livingstone 1982.
8. Burnand KG, Clemenson G, Morland M, Jarrett PEM, Browse NL. Venous lipodermatosclerosis: treatment by fibrinolytic enhancement and elastic compression. *Br Med J* 1980; **280**: 7.
9. Burnand KG, Clemenson G, Whimster I, Gaunt J, Browse NL. The effect of sustained hypertension in the skin capillaries of the canine hind limb. *Br J Surg* 1982; **69**: 41.
10. Burnand KG, Whimster IW, Clemenson G, Lea Thomas M, Browse NL. The relationship between the number of capillaries in the skin of the venous ulcer bearing area of the lower leg and the fall in foot vein pressure during exercise. *Br J Surg* 1981; **68**: 297.
11. Callum MJ, Ruckley CV, Dale JJ, Harper DR. Chronic leg ulcer. The incidence of associated non-venous disorders. In Negus D, Jantet G (Eds) *Phlebology '85* London. Libbey 1986.
12. Callum MJ, Ruckley CV, Harper DR, Dale JJ. Chronic ulceration of the leg: extent of the problem and provision of care. *Br Med J* 1985; **290**: 1855.
13. Cockett FB, Elgan Jones DE. The ankle blow out syndrome. A new approach to the varicose ulcer problem. *Lancet* 1953; **1**: 17.
14. Cockett FB. Diagnosis and surgery of high pressure venous leaks in the leg. A new overall concept of surgery of varicose veins and venous ulcers. *Br Med J* 1956; **2**: 399.
15. Coleridge-Smith PD, Scurr JH. A direct method for measuring venous ulcers. *Br J Surg* 1986; **73**: 320.
16. Cornwall JV, Lewis JD. Leg ulcer revisited. *Br J Surg* 1983; **70**: 681.
17. Dodd H, Cockett FB. *The Pathology and Surgery of the Veins of the Lower Limb.* Edinburgh. Livingstone 1965.
18. Eaglestein WH. Personal communication. 1985.
19. Ellis H. Leg, ulceration of. In Hart FD (Ed) *French's Index of Differential Diagnosis* 12th edition. Bristol. Wright 1985.
20. Freidman SA, Gladstone JL. The bacterial flora of peripheral vascular ulcers. *Arch Dermatol* 1969; **100**: 29.
21. Friedman SJ, Su WP. Management of leg ulcers with hydrocolloid occlusive dressings. *Arch Dermatol* 1984; **120**: 1329.
22. Geronemus RG, Mertz PM, Eaglestein WG. Wound healing: the effects of topical antimicrobial agents. *Arch Dermatol* 1979; **115**: 1311.
23. Greaves MW, Boyde TR. Plasma zinc concentrations in patients with psoriasis, other dermatoses, and venous leg ulceration. *Lancet* 1967; **2**: 1019.
24. Haegar K. Leg ulcers. In Haegar K (Ed) *Venous and Lymphatic Disorders of the Leg.* Lund. Scandinavian University Books 1966.
25. Halsted JA, Smith JC. Plasma zinc in health and disease. *Lancet* 1970; **1**: 322.
26. Homans J. Treatment of elephantiasis of the legs. *N Engl J Med* 1936; **215**: 1099.

27. Hopkins NFG, Jamieson CW. Antibiotic concentration in exudate in venous ulcers; the prediction of ulcer healing rate. *Br J Surg* 1983; **70**: 532.

28. Hurst PA, Kinmonth JB, Rutt DL. A gut and mesentery pedicle for bridging lymphatic obstruction. *J Cardiovasc Surg* 1978; **19**: 589.

29. Keeling PWN, Jones RB, Hilton PJ, Thompson RPH. Reduced leucocyte zinc in liver disease. *Gut* 1980; **21**: 561.

30. Kinmonth JB, Hurst PA, Edwards JM, Rutt DL. Relief of lymph obstruction by use of a bridge of mesentery and ileum. *Br J Surg* 1978; **65**: 829.

31. Knox LC. Epithelioma and chronic venous ulcer. *JAMA* 1925; **85**: 1046.

32. Lawrence PF, Syverud JB, Disbro MA, Alazraki N. Evaluation of Technetium-99m phosphate imaging for predicting skin ulcer healing. *Am J Surg* 1983; **146**: 746.

33. Liddell K. Malignant changes in chronic varicose ulceration. *The Practitioner* 1975; **215**: 335.

34. Lookingbill DP, Miller SH, Knowles RC. Bacteriology of chronic leg ulcers. *Arch Dermatol* 1978; **114**: 1765.

35. Marjolin JN. *Ulcere diet de med (practique)* 2nd edition. Paris. 1846.

36. Martorell F. Hypertensive ulcer of the leg. *Angiology* 1950; **1**: 133.

37. Meleney FL. *Clinical Aspects and Treatment of Surgical Infections*. London. Saunders 1949.

38. Mitchell AAB, Pettigrew JB, MacGillvray D. Varicose ulcers as reservoirs of hospital strains of *Staph. aureus* and *Pseudomonas pyocyanea*. *Br J Clin Pract* 1970; **24**: 223.

39. Myers MB, Cherry G. Zinc and the healing of chronic leg ulcers. *Am J Surg* 1984; **120**: 77.

40. Negus D, Friedgood A. The effective management of venous ulceration. *Br J Surg* 1983; **70**: 623.

41. Piulacks P, Vidal-Barraquer F. Pathogenic study of varicose veins. *Angiology* 1953; **4**: 59.

42. Prentice AG, Lowe GDO, Forbes CD. Diagnosis and treatment of venous thromboembolism by consultants in Scotland. *Br Med J* 1982; **285**: 630.

43. Quist G. *Surgical Diagnosis*. London. Lewis 1977.

44. Ramsey LE. Impact of venography on the diagnosis and management of deep vein thrombosis. *Br Med J* 1983; **286**: 698.

45. Ruckley CV, Callum MJ, Harper DR, Dale JJ. The Lothian and Forth valley leg ulcer survey. Part 4 Arterial disease. In Negus D, Jantet G (Eds) *Phlebology '85*. London. Libbey 1986.

46. Ryan TJ, Wilkinson DS. Diseases of the veins and arteries – Leg ulcers. In Rook A, Wilkinson DS, Ebling FJG (Eds) *Textbook of Dermatology*. 4th edition Oxford. Blackwell Scientific Publications 1985.

47. Ryan TJ. *The Management of Leg Ulcers*. Oxford. Oxford Medical Publications 1983.

48. Sarkany I, Kreel L. Subcutaneous ossification of the legs in chronic venous stasis. *Br Med J* 1966; **2**: 27.

49. Schraibman IG, Stratton FJ. Nutritional status of patients with leg ulcers. *J R Soc Med* 1985; **78**: 39.

50. Stacey M, Pattison M, Layer G, Burnand KG. Measurement of the healing of venous ulcers. *Br J Surg* 1987; (in press).

51. Stacey-Clear A, Cornwall JV, Lewis JD. Intravenous prostacyclin (PE1$_2$) and skin grafting for rheumatoid leg ulcers. In Negus D, Jantet G (Eds) *Phlebology '85*. London. Libbey 1986.

52. Stevanovic DV. Atrophie blanche: a sign of dermal blood flow occlusion. *Arch Dermatol* 1974; **109**: 858.

53. Stewart GJ, Gaunt JI, Croft DN, Browse NL. Isotope lymphography: a new method of investigating the role of the lymphatics in chronic limb oedema. *Br J Surg* 1985; **72**: 906.

54. Stewart GJ, Pattison M, Burnand KG. Abnormal fibrinolysis: the cause of lipodermatosclerosis or 'chronic cellulitis' in patients with primary lymphoedema. *Lymphology* 1984; **17**: 23.

55. Thurtle OA, Cawley MID. The frequency of leg ulceration in rheumatoid arthritis; a survey. *J Rheumatol* 1983; **10**: 507.

56. Van der Molen HR. Calcifications sous-cutanees phlebopathiques. *Phlebologie* 1976; **28**: 551.

57. Van Duyn J. Proteus/staphylococcal synergism in punched out ulcers. *Plast Reconst Surg* 1967; **40**: 86.

58. Walkden V, Black MM. Basal cell carcinomatous changes of the lower leg: an association with chronic venous stasis. *Br J Dermatol* 1981; **105** Suppl 9: 9.

59. Withers AFD, Baker H, Musa M, Dormandy TL. Plasma-zinc in psoriasis. *Lancet* 1968; **2**: 278.

60. Wood ML, Reilly GD, Smith GT. Ulceration of the hand secondary to a radial arteriovenous fistula: a model for varicose ulceration. *Br Med J* 1983; **2**: 1167.

15

Venous ulceration: natural history and treatment

Natural history

Epidemiological studies[35,46] have shown that some patients live in symbiosis with their leg ulcers for many years without much discomfort but without achieving any period of healing, whereas other patients have ulcers that are so painful and extensive that they beg for an amputation. In the United Kingdom approximately 100 limbs are amputated for venous disease every year,[103] 1 in every 700 000 of the population.

Many studies have described excellent early results of ulcer treatment by a number of different techniques but there are few long-term follow-up studies. We have been unable to find any studies reporting the results of ulcer treatment over periods of 10 or 20 years with adequate follow-up. The position is similar to that for breast carcinoma 20 years ago when there were many 5-year follow-up studies but none of 10 or 20 years.

The need for long-term studies is highlighted by our own experience in a trial of ulcer treatment that we are conducting. Only venous ulcers which have been confirmed by special investigations have been entered into the study. Over 80 per cent of ulcerated legs have been healed within 1 year of presenting to the clinic by a combination of paste bandages and elastic compression. The remainder have been successfully healed with split skin grafts. Thus if patients with venous ulceration agree to treatment, it is possible to achieve healing by conservative or surgical means in almost every case. The problem is how to maintain healing. Ten of the ulcers referred to above have broken down within 18 months of healing.

Why do some ulcers break down when others remain healed?

The logical answer is that venous ulcers will recur if the underlying pathophysiological abnormality is not corrected. This explanation is probably not the whole answer as the physiological tests of calf pump function in patients whose ulcers remain healed are often similar to those of patients whose ulcers broke down. We need to know much more about the factors that cause ulceration, as well as improving our methods of correcting calf pump function, before we can hope to treat all venous ulcers successfully.

The natural history studies of venous ulceration reveal the following information.

1. They represent a potentially insoluble problem from the moment they first develop until the patient dies.[25,99,100]

2. The number of patients presenting for treatment is the tip of an iceberg.[35]

3. In only a small group of patients, those with ulceration caused by superficial vein incompetence, is long-term cure possible.[27]

4. We need long-term follow-up studies to assess which of the treatments for post-thrombotic ulcers is the most successful in preventing recurrence.

5. Untreated venous ulcers will remain unhealed for many years.[35]

6. Without permanent prophylactic measures many venous ulcers will recur.[27,31]

7. Almost all venous ulcers can be healed with good medical treatment but universal prevention of recurrence cannot yet be achieved.[25]

8. Our immediate aim must be to develop treatments that will prevent ulcer recurrence. Our long-term aim must be to prevent the occurrence of the venous and tissue changes that precede ulceration by preventing deep vein thrombosis

and developing techniques that fully correct calf pump dysfunction.

Effect on the patient

Ulcers are often painful and smelly. They require frequent dressings and visits to or by medical personnel. They therefore interfere with work and holidays and restrict the lifestyle of the patient. As a result patients with this problem may develop personality disorders, even severe depression and paranoia.

The patient's daily life may come to revolve around the ulcer and it may provide the only reason for contact with the inhabitants of the world outside the home for a depressed, aged and immobile patient. Chronic ulcers cause shorten-ing of the Achilles tendon with the development of an equinus deformity (Fig. 15.1). This in turn may cause pain and further reduce mobility. Chronic anaemia is another reason for loss of general well being.[138]

Bathing is a problem when the leg is wrapped with dressings making it difficult to maintain personal hygiene. This may add to a sense of social isolation. The significance of ulceration of the leg is clouded by ignorance and hearsay. Some patients still believe that healing of an ulcer leads to certain death; this belief is presumably a relic from the theory that ulcers let out evil humours, a theory that was in vogue from the time of Hippocrates to the end of the Dark Ages.[4]

An inability to stay at work because of frequent visits to the doctor or the hospital may inflict a

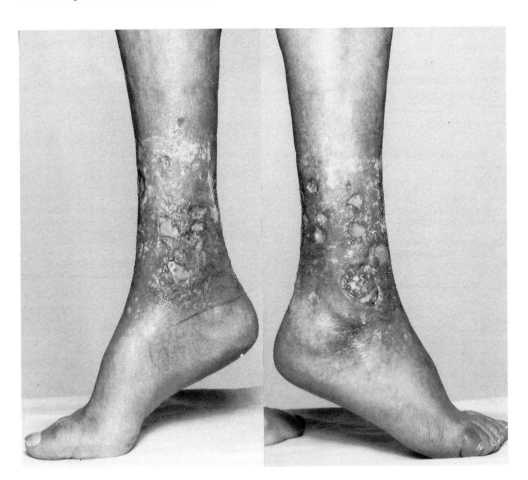

Fig. 15.1   Medial and lateral views of an ulcerated leg showing an equinus deformity causing 4 cm of apparent shortening as a result of periarticular inflammation, fibrosis, and shortening of the Achilles tendon.

considerable economic burden on the patient. The cost of drugs, dressings and elastic stockings is an additional financial burden. All these factors make venous ulceration a miserable experience which is the reason why many patients are so grateful when their doctor shows some enthusiasm and interest in their care. When ulcer care is delegated to junior doctors whose knowlege and experience does not compare with that of their seniors, many patients are given conflicting and wrong advice; not surprisingly, the patients decide to take over the management of their ulcers themselves.

Effect on medical services

It has been estimated that every unhealed ulcer costs the community £1200/ulcer/year in dressings and medical time.[80] In-patient admissions costing over £100/day are also expensive, making ulcer treatment a major drain on scarce medical resources. Any measures which successfully prevent recurrence are bound to be cost effective.

Many hospitals have now developed ulcer clinics to concentrate expertise at a single site, and it is hoped that improvements in treatment will follow. At present most ulcer treatment is undertaken by overworked general practitioners, and community nurses.[35] These workers must become involved in research and understand the new methods of diagnosis and treatment if progress is to be made.

Treatment

The treatment of venous ulceration has two objectives:

  (a) to heal the ulcer
  (b) to prevent recurrence of the ulcer

Treatments designed to heal the ulcer are as follows.

1. Compression (normally by bandages or stockings) combined with dressings
2. Bedrest with leg elevation
3. Surgical excision of slough
4. Topical application
    (a) antiseptics
    (b) antibiotics
    (c) cleaning agents to dissolve slough
    (d) agents to promote healing

5. Applications for the surrounding skin
6. Systemic medication
    (a) to promote healing
    (b) to sterilize the surface of the ulcer
7. Physical methods
    (a) to promote healing
    (b) to clean the ulcer
8. Application of skin substitutes to promote healing
    (a) human amnion
    (b) lyophylized pigskin
9. Skin grafting
    (a) split skin grafts
    (b) pinch grafts
    (c) full-thickness grafts
    (d) pedicle grafts
    (e) vascularized free flap grafts
10. Ulcer excision followed by skin grafting
11. Correction of calf pump malfunction
    (a) injection/compression sclerotherapy
    (b) surgical ligation of the superficial and lower leg communicating veins
    (c) surgical reconstruction of the deep veins or valves
    (d) elastic compression stockings
12. Miscellaneous treatments

1. Compression with bandages over dressings

The value of compressing the limb with bandages has been recognized for many years. In addition to its therapeutic value, it helps to avoid hospital admissions and is therefore inexpensive. This treatment also allows the patient to continue his normal life, apart from the time devoted to changing the dressings and re-applying or adjusting the compression bandages or stocking.

Celsus[37] described the use of plasters and linen roller bandages to treat leg ulcers in AD 25; many other dressings and many different methods of bandaging have been described since that time. In 1783 Underwood[154] described the first use of modified elastic (Welsh flannel) but this was not generally accepted. In 1866 Spender[146] wrote 'the proper application of the bandage is of such great importance in the treatment of varicose ulcers of the legs that it should, when possible, be executed by the surgeon in attendance'. He felt that 'compression answers every objective to be gained by the recumbent posture'. Widespread use of 'elastic compression' followed the description of an adhesive elastic bandage by Dickson Wright[56] in 1930, and the development of the strong elastic webbing bandage described by Bisgaard[16] in 1948.

Stockings offer an alternative means of compression. Richard Wiseman[165] described a compression stocking for treating leg ulceration in 1676 (Fig. 15.2). It was made of soft leather and could be laced up to differing degrees of tightness to alter the degree of compression. As it was also shaped to the contour of the leg, it probably represents the first attempt to produce a graduated compression stocking. It was not, however, until the advent of elastic fibres that could be woven into stockings that true elastic stockings became widely used as an alternative to bandages.

Since bandaging began, dressings have been placed over the ulcer to absorb the ulcer exudate and prevent soiling of the compressing bandage. The earliest dressings were leaves soaked in wine[68] but leaves were replaced by linen, wool and gauze as these materials became freely available. More recently, colloidal silver, aluminium foil[75,76] and living membranes[13,79] have all been used with varying degrees of success.

Modern methods of compression

Sigg[142] credited Van der Molen[157] with the idea of progressively reducing (graduating) the degree of compression along the leg so that the maximum compression is applied at the ankle and minimum compression is applied to the knee or thigh. Graduated compression stockings aim to prevent venous capillary transudation for different degrees of venous pressure fall during exercise.[149,150] Pressures of 40–50 mmHg are required at the ankle to balance the Starling equation[148] in limbs with a severe post-thrombotic syndrome and no reduction in superficial vein pressure during exercise (see Chapter 12). Graduated compression also increases the velocity of blood flow in the deep veins.[141] All methods of compression stimulate the release of fibrinolytic activity[39] and reduce discomfort by preventing oedema and venous distension. These beneficial effects of graduated compression are lost if the compression weakens or is poorly applied, or if a tourniquet effect develops anywhere along the leg.

The history of compression has been fully reviewed by Marmasse.[105]

The methods of compression currently available are:

- compression bandages
- elastic stockings
- inflatable pneumatic leggings

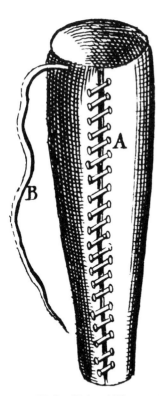

Fig. 15.2 Richard Wiseman's laced leather stocking. It was shaped to be narrower at the ankle and wider over the calf. The lace allowed the stocking to be tightened to apply the correct amount of pressure; this was the forerunner of the modern elastic stocking. (From Heister L. 1768. A General System of Surgery. London. Whiston 1768).

Compression bandages

Bandages are probably the most popular form of compression because they are relatively inexpensive and can therefore be discarded when they become soiled by ulcer exudate. The problems associated with their use include:

- failure to stay in place
- variations in the skill (and consequently the compression) with which they are applied
- loss of compression after washing

It has been shown that bandaging techniques vary considerably from doctor to doctor and from nurse to nurse.[51] The use of a stocking tester may help the development of greater uniformity in bandaging techniques,[126] but a recent attempt to produce a standard amount of compression by printing rectangles on the surface of a bandage which become square when the bandage is pulled to its correct tension (STD, Thusane) did not appear to reduce variability when we tested the bandaging efficiency of inexperienced volunteers.[126] Despite this, the concept of a 'built in' regulator of compression seems attractive.

The compression bandages most commonly used are:

- The red-line Bisgaard bandage (Marlowe)
- Elastocrepe (Smith and Nephew)
- Lestraflex (Seton)
- J-press (Johnson and Johnson)
- Coban (Layman)
- Tubigrip (Seton)
- Thusane (STD)
- Tensopress (Smith and Nephew)

The Blue- or Red-line bandages, which are made of elastic webbing, give very good compression but tend to slip and are unsightly because they are very thick.

Elastocrepe is widely used but has been shown to lose its elasticity when washed[51] or reapplied.[126] It only provides an adequate amount of compression when it is combined with a paste bandage or covered by Tubigrip.

Lestraflex is an inelastic self-adhesive bandage that can cause sensitivity rashes when applied directly to the skin but its adhesive property does prevent it from slipping. It is now seldom used because of skin reactions, unless it is applied over the top of another bandage.

J-press provides a very low degree of compression and is of doubtful value for ulcer treatment.

Coban also provides low levels of compression and is difficult to apply correctly.

Tubigrip provides poor compression on its own but is useful if used with Elastocrepe and paste bandages.

Thusane is a new elastic bandage which provides good levels of compression but has not yet been tested in ulcer-healing trials.

Tensopress is a new elastic bandage which also provides a good level of compression but has also not been used in any ulcer-healing studies.

Application of a compression bandage[51]

The art of bandaging has almost disappeared as surgical wound dressings have become lighter or non-existent. The one place where bandaging skill is essential is in the ulcer clinic. In 1859 Hunt[88] wrote that the problems with bandaging arose because 'the application of a bandage is looked upon as an easy and simple operation which may be satisfactorily entrusted to a nurse or the patient'. He went on to state that 'a correctly applied bandage on an ulcer patient must be applied from the toes to the knee, with all parts of the leg being equally supported'. Hunt was the first person to suggest including pads beneath the bandage to fill out any depressions in the leg (Fig. 15.3), and he also said that if a bandage caused pain, it should be taken off and re-applied.

Dale has shown that bandaging is an acquired skill.[51] She recommends that the first turn should

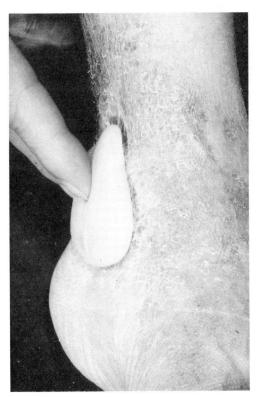

Fig. 15.3 This ulcer was situated in the natural hollow just behind and below the medial malleolus. In order to compress this area of skin after the ulcer had healed the hollow was filled with a silastic pad applied beneath the stocking.

be around the ankle before working down to the foot. This starts the bandage well and prevents slipping at the ankle (Fig. 15.4).

The three basic rules of bandaging are – apply the outside of the roll to the leg, bandage from the medial to the lateral side and bandage from below upwards. The bandage should roll away from the hand and must be evenly spaced with, if possible, a slightly greater tension (compression) applied at the ankle. A figure of eight overlaping technique (Fig. 15.4) prevents the bandage slipping down. A layer of stockinette (Tubigrip) applied over the bandage prevents the edges of the bandage rucking up. Simple crepe bandages or stockinette used on their own do not apply satisfactory compression.

The elastic bandages currently available that can be recommended are the Bisgaard bandage, a combination of Elastocrepe and Tubigrip, Tensopress and Thusane.

Elastic stockings

It is usually not practical to use elastic stockings when there is an open ulcer because it is difficult to pull a stocking up over a dressing without disturbing the dressing. Also, the exudate soils the stocking which consequently has to be washed frequently and elasticity is lost. Some stains are not easily removed and the elastic fibres of the

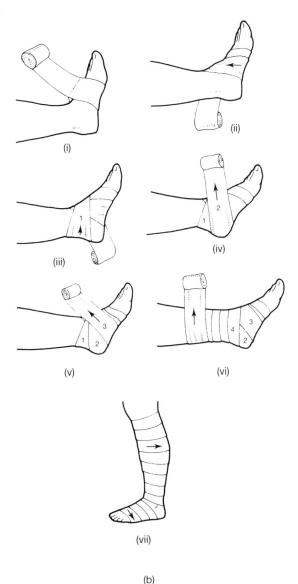

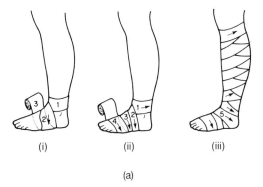

Fig. 15.4 (a) Dale's technique for applying a bandage to the leg.

  (i) The first turn is placed around the ankle to fix the bandage.

  (ii) The bandage is then taken down over the ankle to compress the foot.

  (iii) The bandage is then taken up over the initial turn to cover the lower leg to knee level using an overlapping figure-of-eight technique.

(b) The standard bandaging technique.

  (i) The first turn is placed around the dorsum of the foot.

  (ii) The bandage is then brought up over the ankle.

  (iii–v) The ankle is then enclosed as shown.

  (vi) The remainder of the leg is bandaged by simple overlapping turns.

  (vii) The final appearance.

stocking may be weakened by the exudate. We only replace bandages with a stocking when the ulcer reaches an advanced stage of healing or becomes covered by a firmly fixed dry scab. The advantages of stockings are that the degree of compression they apply is known and constant and that they do not slip down or become loose as easily as bandages. The types of elastic hosiery available and the methods of testing stockings is discussed in detail in the section on the prevention of ulcer recurrence (see page 433) and in Chapter 12.

Pneumatic compression

Intermittent positive pressure applied by inflatable leggings has been advocated for ulcer healing. These boots were originally designed to prevent the development of post-operative deep vein thrombosis[84] but it has been suggested that they might enhance ulcer healing.[12,128,166] Their use usually entails the admission of the patient to hospital because the equipment is expensive, and this together with the risk of cross-infection has prevented their routine use for the treatment of ulcers. There are no controlled trials of this technique in ulcer healing.

Ulcer dressings

Dressings applied directly to ulcers should ideally exhibit certain properties. They should be non-adherent so that removal is painless and does not damage new fragile epithelium which is beginning to grow in across the surface of the ulcer. The dressing should be highly absorbent while maintaining the moisture of the wound and not degrading or altering its characteristics in response to changes in temperature or humidity, or when soaked with exudate. The dressing should be safe, non-toxic and non-antigenic. Dressings must be easily available, sterile, conformable and cost effective.[80,92] Morgan[108] has pointed out that a dressing fulfilling all these characteristics does not exist.

There are four main types of dressing that can be applied to an ulcer.

(i)   Absorbent dressings
(ii) Impregnated dressings
(iii) Occlusive dressings
(iv) Impregnated bandages

(i) Absorbent dressings

The materials that have been used to absorb ulcer exudate include: linen, cotton wool, gauze (open-weave cotton), non-adherent dressings (carbonet) (Johnson and Johnson), melolin (Smith and Nephew), and gamgee pads.

Gauze is the only dressing that is universally acceptable as it is non-allergic and does not produce sensitivity reaction. Unfortunately, it commonly adheres to the surface of the ulcer and is painful to remove.

Melolin (Smith and Nephew) is a non-adherent dressing but has poor absorbing properties and can cause allergy, rashes and skin maceration.

N–A (non-adherent) dressings (Johnson and Johnson) are also relatively poor at absorbing exudate and can cause skin maceration.

Perfron and *Releasell* (Johnson and Johnson) are two new low adherent dressings which are alternatives to melolin and gauze.

Telfa (Kendall) is a similar to Perfron and Releasell.

Tricotex (Smith and Nephew) is similar to N–A dressings.

Actisorb (Johnson and Johnson) is charcoal cloth enclosed in a porous envelope.

Mesalt (Mölnlycke) is a crystalized salt dressing.

(ii) Impregnated dressings

The majority of impregnated dressings are made of gauze coated with petroleum jelly (vaseline) often with the addition of an antibacterial agent.

Paraffin gauze, plain (Jelonet, Tulle gras) (Smith and Nephew)
Paraffin gauze + chlorhexidine (Bactigras) (Smith and Nephew)
Paraffin gauze + Framycetin (Sofra-Tulle) (Roussell)
Paraffin gauze + Fusidic acid (Fucidin, Intertulle) (Leo)

There is little evidence to justify the addition of an antibacterial agent to dressings. All the antibiotic and antiseptic tulles can cause local sensitivity reactions and encourage colonization by resistant bacteria. In our opinion they should never be used.

A single layer of paraffin gauze covered by

ordinary gauze has good non-adherent and absorbent qualities and is painless on removal. It can be used at any stage in the management of an ulcer but is most suitable when the ulcer is clean and healing. The paraffin gauze must be applied to the ulcer, not to the surrounding skin, to avoid skin maceration. There is no evidence that the petroleum jelly delays or enhances healing. This is one of the most popular forms of dressing.

(iii) Absorbent and occlusive dressings

There are many occlusive wound dressings which have been devised as ulcer dressings. They are all absorbent but in some the fluid in the dressing is prevented from evaporating so the dressing stays moist and does not adhere. Examples of occlusive wound dressings are given below.

Hydrogels
Scherisorb – a starch copolymer/gel (Schering)

Vigilon – an insoluble cross-linked polyethylene oxide copolymer (Baird)

Geliperm – a polyacrylamide composite hydrogel, which comes in wet, dry and granulated gel forms (Geistlich)

Sorbsan – a biodegradable, hydrophilic gel of an alginate (NI Medical)

Kaltostat – a calcium alginate fibre (Cair)

Synthaderm – a polyurethane foam, hydrophilic on one side and hydrophobic on the other side (Armour)

Covaderm – a modified polyurethane which is an improvement on Synthaderm (Armour)

Hydrocolloids
Granuflex – a polymeric dressing with an adhesive face and a water-proof backing which makes it impermeable (Squibb, Surgicare)

Dermiflex – a methylcellulose base with a foam backing (Johnson and Johnson)

Comfeel – an impermeable polymeric dressing (Coloplast)

Polyurethane sheets
Opsite (Smith and Nephew), Bioclusive (Johnson and Johnson), Steridrape (3M), Transigen (Smith and Nephew), and Tegaderm (3M), are all semipermeable and non-absorbent.

Foam-dressings
Silastic foam – a silicon base with a catalyst (Calmic)

Lyofoam – a polyurethane foam which can be made with added carbon (Ultra Laboratories)

The majority of these dressings have been developed over the past 10 years. They have not been tested in large scale controlled clinical trials of ulcer-healing, and their acceptance must therefore await further studies. The use of these dressings is supported by the results of animal wound healing studies but such studies may not be relevant to human venous ulceration.

(iv) Impregnated bandages

These are gauze bandages impregnated with zinc, calamine, ichthyol, oxyquinoline or tar. Although they are sold on the basis of their incorporated medicament, they probably work because they set into a semi-hard cast which acts as a very effective form of external compression. The paste simply allows the bandage to mould to the shape of the limb. Whether the medicament has any intrinsic effect on ulcer healing is debatable.

Impregnated bandages are marketed as:

Calaband (calamine), (Seton)
Viscopaste PB7 (zinc oxide), (Smith and Nephew)
Quinaband (oxyquinoline), (Dalmas)
Uroband (zinc paste, ichthammol and urethane), (Dalmas)
Zincaband (zinc oxide), (Seton)
Ichthoband (icthyol), (Seton)

Paste bandages are amongst the most popular form of ulcer dressing in the United Kingdom and have replaced the Unna paste boot.[155] There are no controlled clinical trials of the use of paste bandages but in our experience a combination of Calaband covered with elastrocrepe and Tubigrip heals between 70 and 80 per cent of venous ulcers within 1 year of beginning treatment (Fig. 15.5). Many other workers have reported similar results, for example only 19 out of 173 patients required hospital admission for failed treatment in Monroe-Ashman and Wells' series.[112] Nevertheless, it is desirable to undertake controlled studies to compare paste bandages with some of the newer forms of dressing described above.

Paste bandages can cause damage to the leg if they are incorrectly applied, and they can also cause sensitivity reactions (Fig. 15.6). If a sensiti-

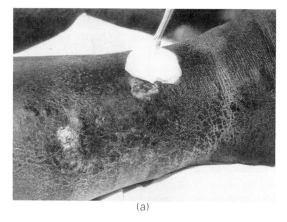

(a)

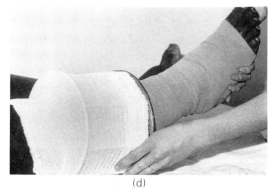

(d)

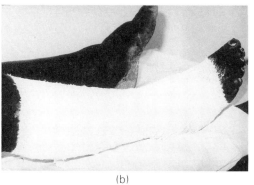

(b)

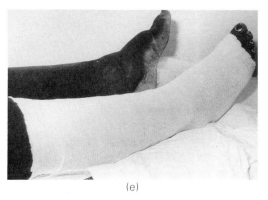

(e)

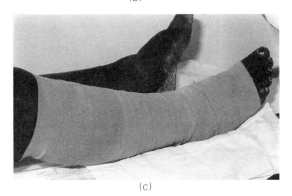

(c)

Fig. 15.5 (a) Before applying a paste bandage (Calaband, Seton), the exudate must be wiped off the ulcer. If the base contains soft slough it should be removed.

(b) The paste bandage is then applied directly onto the ulcer and covered by Elastocrepe, (c) and Tubigrip bandages, (d and e). Thusane or Tensopress bandages are alternatives.

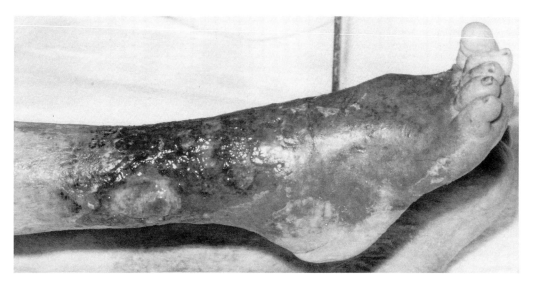

Fig. 15.6   The skin of this leg has developed an allergy to a paste bandage. The skin is erythematous and ezcematous. The paste bandage must not be used again. Propaderm should be applied and the paste bandage replaced with gauze dressings and a simple bandage.

vity reaction occurs, the bandage must be removed immediately and replaced by a simple dressing with compression bandages.

Comment   Despite the multiplicity of bandages, stockings and dressing materials that are available, there have been few trials comparing their clinical value. This is partly because controlled trials on ulcer healing are difficult and expensive and partly because it has been suggested by some workers that comparisons between groups of ulcers are invalid on the grounds of individual ulcer heterogeniety.[2] It is essential that these problems are overcome and that good studies on the value of different ulcer treatments are conducted.

2. Bedrest with leg elevation

Hippocrates[85] stated that 'in the case of an ulcer it is not expedient to stand, more especially if the ulcer be situated in the leg', and Ambrose Paré[123] also felt that those who have 'an ulcer in the leg ought neither to stand or sit but lie on a bed'. Both Petit in 1790[127] and Hunter in 1835[89] suggested that bedrest at home or in a hospital was beneficial to healing. Sharpe[140] and Brodie[24] suggested that the leg should be kept horizontal with the body. Anning[4] recognized that elevation of the leg

above the level of the heart was even more effective but Foote[67] while agreeing with this approach pointed out its high cost, if it meant admitting all patients with ulcers into hospital beds.

Dodd and Cockett[59] regarded bedrest as an essential preliminary to successful grafting of a venous ulcer, and Fegan[64] and Bourne[22] both advocated periods of leg elevation as part of their outpatient treatment regimen. We are not aware of a comparison of bedrest *alone* against bedrest plus local ulcer dressings but we accept that a period of bedrest with leg elevation is a highly successful way of healing ulcers. The main objection to this regimen is the lack of hospital beds and the cost. Cottonot *et al.*[47] showed that the cost of healing an ulcer by hospital admission was 20 times greater than the cost of outpatient treatment. In 1849 Crichett[49] had pointed out that there were many practical objections to prolonged in-patient treatment, not only social and economic disadvantages but the risk of joint stiffness and the development of a further deep vein thrombosis.

The policy of most clincians supervising ulcer care is to continue outpatient treatment for as long as possible, but there is a group of patients whose ulcers will never heal while they are walking about and who have to be admitted to hospital.[74] When this group with intractable ulceration is added to the group in whom surgical treatment (e.g. skin grafting) is indicated to speed up the healing process, we find that a significant number of patients still need to be admitted to hospital for the treatment of venous ulceration. Bedrest with maximal leg elevation is an integral part of our initial management of these patients.

3. Surgical excision of slough

Hippocrates[85] suggested that ulcers healed better after they were 'scarified'. Since then many other workers have suggested that the excision of all dead tissue speeds ulcer healing.[59,67,136] Excision can be done with a scalpel or a sharp pair of scissors, but this may be very painful. If excision is done with care when the slough is ready to separate, it can be done without anaesthesia, but if the slough is firmly adherent, a local or general anaesthetic is required. Local anaesthetics applied topically to the ulcer base or infiltrated by a fine needle through the base of the ulcer are usually effective but may fail to produce analgesia because of fibrosis in the ulcer base. For ulcer excision under general anaesthesia the patient should normally be admitted to hospital. This procedure should be reserved for ulcers that either fail to heal or enlarge during outpatient management.

4. Topical applications

Many agents have been applied topically in an attempt to improve the healing of ulcers. These substances tend to fall into three major categories – antiseptics, antibiotics and desloughing (cleansing) agents. A fourth minor category consists of miscellaneous agents thought to stimulate ulcer healing.

(a) Antiseptics

These include:

- hypochlorite solutions (Eusol, Milton and Chlorasol) (Schering)
- cetrimide (Savlon, Savloclens, Savlodil)
- chlorhexidine (Hibitane)
- hydrogen peroxide 3% (Hioxyl, Quinoderm) (Stuart Pharmaceuticals)
- benoxyl peroxide (Benoxyl) (Stiefel)
- povidone iodine (Betadine, Napp Laboratories; Disadine Stuart Pharmaceuticals)

- cadexomer iodine (Iodosorb) (Stuart Pharmaceuticals)
- aqueous gel containing brilliant green and lactic acid (Variclene)
- mercurochrome 1–2 %
- potassium permanganate 1:10 000
- gentian violet
- gentian violet in alcohol
- proflavine
- acetic acid
- ethylalcohol
- phenoxyethanol
- silver nitrate

Hypochlorite, hydrogen peroxide, and even chlorhexidine have been shown in a series of animal studies[23] to damage granulation tissue and slow wound healing. Antiseptics have never been shown to promote ulcer healing and they can cause allergic skin reactions.[119]

The reports on the efficacy of povidone iodine are purely anecdotal.[26] Iodosorb appeared to reduce healing time in two controlled trials in patients with venous ulcers,[118,144] but this conclusion has been challenged by other investigators[45,111] because the standard treatment used in the original trials may have delayed healing in the control group in which ulcers appeared to take an excessively long time to heal.

(b) Topical antibiotics

A number of antibiotics have been applied to the surface of ulcers but there is little justification for their use because there are few controlled trials that show them to be beneficial. Bacterial resistance and skin sensitivity reactions are real risks, and topical antibiotics should be abandoned as a treatment for venous ulceration.

Some topical antibiotics that have received anecdotal support include:

- silver sulphadiazine (Flamazine) (Smith and Nephew)
- neomycin–bacitracin (Cicatrin) (Wellcome)
- mupirocin 2% (Bactroban) (Beecham)
- neomycin and gramicidin (Graneodin) (Squibb)

(c) Cleansing agents used to dissolve slough

These substances are mainly chemicals or naturally derived enzymes that are proteolytic or fibrinolytic.

- Aserbine – a mixture of malic, benzoic and salicylic acids (Bencard)
- Malatex – similar to Aserbine (Norton)
- Varidase – a mixture of streptokinase and streptodornase (Lederle)
- Travase – a fibrinolytic agent with a liquifying agent (Sutilains)
- Debrisan – a hydrophilic dextranomer (Pharmacia)

The active ingredient of Aserbine and Malatex is a malic acid ester. Varidase is a streptokinase–streptodornase mixture,[32] and Travase is a fibrinolytic agent mixed with a substance that liquifies pus.[43] Debrisan, a three-dimensional network of dextran polymers, showed some encouraging early results in cleansing ulcers[110,137] but failed to heal them more swiftly than standard treatments.[72,73] The cost of Debrisan makes its general acceptance into clinical practice unlikely unless it can be shown to significantly reduce the healing time.

All these preparations can be used to deslough dirty ulcers if patients will not tolerate surgical cleansing because of pain. They must be applied two or three times each day and can be extremely effective; sloughs will liquify in 2 or 3 days. There is no firm evidence that they promote ulcer healing.

(d) Agents thought to encourage ulcer healing

Many agents have been thought to promote ulcer healing by a local or general action but all the published studies contain serious flaws. Agents that have been claimed to promote healing include:

> Hyaluronic acid, N-acetyl hydroxyprolene, collagen gel, lysozyme, napthaquinine, anthrocyanosides, Paw-Paw, zinc, steel foil, aluminium foil and amino acid solution

Little can be said about most of these preparations when the evidence justifying their use is mostly anecdotal and unconfirmed.[53,63,69,91,104,106,121,122]

5. Dermatological preparations for the surrounding skin

The skin around the ulcer may be treated for eczema and contact sensitivity with Lassar's paste, potassium permanganate, gentian violet or local steroids (Propaderm, Betnovate, Hydrocor-

tisone or Clobetasol).[136] We use Propaderm ointment to treat excoriated eczematous skin around an ulcer. It is highly effective in resolving eczema but great care must be taken to avoid applying the cream to the ulcer surface, because steroids may delay ulcer healing.[62] Excessive and continuous use of corticosteroids on eczematous skin may cause thinning and atrophy and should be avoided.[158]

6. Systemic medications

(a) Medicaments thought to promote healing

The process of healing is extremely complex and needs an adequate supply of protein, vitamins, trace metals and oxygen. Medicaments that have been tried include:

- zinc
- stanozolol
- oxpentifylline
- prostaglandins
- oxyrutosides
- diuretics
- vasodilators

Zinc   Serum zinc has been found to be low in some patients with chronic venous ulceration,[70,71,78,113] and systematically administered zinc has been reported to improve ulcer healing in patients with low serum zinc levels.[129] Serum zinc does not, however, correlate well with cellular zinc deficiency, and therefore the relevance of serum zinc levels is extremely doubtful.[96] Zinc can be given as effervescent zinc tablets and does no harm but probably does little good.

Stanozolol (Stromba)   We have reported the use of this fibrinolytic enhancing agent in the treatment of pre-ulcerative lipodermatosclerosis[28] but have *not* examined its effect on venous ulceration.

Oxpentifylline (Trental)   Oxpentifylline is known to enhance fibrinolysis but it also increases capillary perfusion by reducing blood viscocity and increasing red cell deformability. It has been examined in one open study of venous ulcer healing which revealed apparently good results,[160] though the percentage of ulcers healed is similar to the number healed in other studies using paste bandages. In a double blind trial,[161] 44 per cent of the ulcers in the control group improved compared with 86 per cent of the ulcers of the patients receiving Trental, but the end points of this trial are weak and the healing rate in the control group is extremely poor. This drug requires further study.

Prostaglandins The prostaglandins are powerful vasodilators. Prostaglandin infusions are claimed to improve the healing of severe rheumatoid ulcers[147] and prostaglandin El is said to be of value in both venous and arterial ulcers;[11] 4 out of 5 patients with venous ulcers responding to prostaglandin infusion compared with 1 out of 5 who responded to a saline infusion. These new powerful agents need detailed investigation. Much more information is required concerning the route of administration (intravenous or intra-arterial), the dose, the duration of treatment, and the type of ulcer that will respond.

Oxyrutosides (Paroven) Paroven reduces capillary permeability and white blood cell migration and has been shown, in controlled trials, to reduce the symptoms of chronic venous insufficiency[133] but there is no evidence that it promotes ulcer healing.

Diuretics Diuretics may be of occasional value in patients with an ulcer in a very swollen leg, usually caused by congestive cardiac failure. They do not directly promote ulcer healing but reduction of the oedema probably improves the capillary circulation and the efficacy of the calf muscle pump.[114]

Vasodilators There is no evidence that vasodilators help the healing of venous ulcers.

Systemic antibiotics

Virtually every antibiotic that has ever been produced has been used to treat venous ulcers but there is very little evidence that they help healing unless the ulcer is contaminated by a single pathogenic organism (see page 406, Chapter 14) or there is associated cellulitis, which in our experience is extremely rare. The organisms most commonly found colonizing venous ulcers include staphylococci, streptococci, pseudomonas, klebsiella, E. coli and E. proteus (see Tables 14.4 and 14.5).

The role of anaerobic organisms in delaying ulcer healing has been neglected. Our own data suggests that these organisms are much more common than the results of standard bacteriological tests suggest, and good controlled trials of antibiotics known to be effective against anaerobic bacteria should be encouraged. Our clinical impression is that metronidazole reduces both the odour and the purulent exudate of dirty ulcers.

7. Physical methods of treatment

Physical methods of treatment include:

- massage
- short-wave diathermy
- ultraviolet light
- vibratory electromagnetic waves

Massage This was first recommended by White[163] but was later championed by Bisgaard[16] as an adjunct to compression bandaging. We are not aware of any control trials of its use. Gentle massage around an ulcer disperses oedema and may increase blood flow but some authors have reported poor results from massage.[7,50]

Ultraviolet light Anning[4] states that ultraviolet light may stimulate healing and kill bacteria. Like may other remedies that can be shown to have an effect in an experimental model, it has not been specifically tested on venous ulceration. Dodd *et al.*[57] have suggested that ultraviolet light may also cause vasodilatation and increase skin oxygen tension which may be beneficial and could theoretically improve the healing of venous ulcers.

Ultrasound This increases the local blood flow and may break down interstitial fibrin and fibrous tissue. There are controlled trials which suggest that ultrasound accelerates ulcer healing[34,60] but the rate of healing of the 'control arm' ulcers was poor in these trials and further studies are required. Ultrasound may prove to be a promising adjunct to standard treatment.

Electromagnetic waves There is one publication[36] of the value of this treatment in leg ulcers. It is difficult to draw any conclusions from one enthusiastic report.

8. Skin substitutes

(a) Human amnion

Human amnion was first used to dress venous ulcers by Hansen[79] who claimed that it promoted healing if left in undisturbed contact with the ulcer for 6–10 weeks. It has not been widely used, perhaps because of difficulties in procurement as it has to be applied relatively fresh.[153] Amnion has the advantage of being a biological tissue whose lack of surface tissue antigens protect it from rejection,[5] and it is thought to contain substances that stimulate angiogenesis.[61]

Three studies[13,61,145] in the last 5 years have reported the value of amnion in healing ulceration of the lower limb but all these studies have been uncontrolled and are therefore of doubtful validity. Further controlled studies are required before the value of amnion can be accepted.

(b) Porcine dermis (lyophylized freeze dried porcine epidermis) (Corethium; Ethicon)

The initial open studies[94,134] with porcine skin suggested that it doubled the healing rate of venous ulcers when compared with conventional treatment of Calaband or Quinaband with elastic support.

The subsequent double blind trial showed a 33 per cent reduction in the healing time of the porcine-treated ulcers which only just reached statistical significance.[135] The sample size in both these studies was small, and a type II error is possible. The cost of this material can hardly justify its use if the time saved in healing is so small.[131] Further studies are required to confirm the efficacy of porcine dermis before its routine use can be recommended.

9. Skin grafts (autografts)

Skin grafting is the treatment of choice for ulcers that will not heal with conservative treatment, but few clinicians would feel that skin grafting should be the primary method of treatment for *all* venous ulcers.

When a decision has been taken to graft an ulcer, the choice has to be made between pinch grafts and split skin grafts. Each method has its advocates.[3,9,33,38,59,101,102,107,115,130,131] If split thickness grafts are selected as the means of treatment, they should be cut into postage stamp size or shredded before being laid on the ulcer bed.

Pinch grafts are usually taken and applied under local anaesthetic in an out-patient clinic.[38,131] Although split skin grafting can be managed in this way, it is more usual to give the patient a general anaesthetic.[101,115] General anaesthesia has the advantage of allowing the ulcer to be simultaneously excised, thus the skin graft can be applied to healthy tissue and there is a better chance of achieving satisfactory 'graft take'.

(a) Split skin grafts (Thiersch grafts)[3,59,101,102,115,131]

Small split skin grafts can be taken after local anaesthetic infiltration in the out-patient clinic. For large grafts the patient is usually given a general anaesthetic before being prepared with chlorhexidine and draped to expose the ulcer. The front of the thigh of the same leg, which is the normal donor site, is also prepared. The base of the ulcer is lightly curretted or excised, unless it is very clean. Bleeding is controlled by firm pressure. Persistent bleeding may require careful diathermy coagulation or catgut ligation. The skin graft is then taken with a mini-Humby knife containing an ordinary razor blade, a full-sized Humby knife or an electric dermatome. For all except the smallest ulcers we prefer to use the dermatome because it cuts a more even graft than we can achieve by hand. We always take more skin than is required to cover the ulcer. Grafts should be approximately 0.1 mm thick as thin grafts take better than thick ones. When the graft has been cut it is spread out, epidermis down, on paraffin gauze. It is then cut to the shape of the ulcer or into small squares ('postage stamps') and applied to the ulcer providing the base is clean, healthy and not bleeding excessively.

If the graft is applied as a single sheet, a few slits are made in it to allow serum to escape and it is held in place with a few silk or nylon sutures. The ends of these sutures can be tied over a pad of flavine wool or silastic foam to press the graft on to the ulcer base and reduce the possibility of exudate or blood collecting beneath it which can prevent adherence.

If the ulcer base is bleeding excessively or is not as clean as anticipated, we wrap the graft in a moistened saline swab, place it in a sterile air-tight container and keep it in a refrigerator at 4°C until the ulcer base is considered to be satisfactory. The ulcer is inspected daily, and when it is clean enough the graft is applied in the ward without anaesthesia.

Alternatively, grafts may be glued down with tissue glue,[86] or simply held in place by a firm dressing or left completely uncovered. When grafts are left uncovered it is preferable to build a padded plaster of Paris boot, with a window over the graft, to prevent the patient inadvertently rubbing off or damaging the fragile skin during the night. The window can be covered with bandages at night to protect the graft while still allowing air to circulate around it. The advantage of this method is that the graft can be inspected each day and collections of fluid which accumulate beneath it can be aspirated; the disadvantage is that this complication is more likely to develop because of the absence of firm pressure on the graft. We have not performed a proper comparison of these two methods of application but prefer to apply to grafts at operation and keep them covered with dressings and bandages.

The donor site is covered by Opsite (Smith and Nephew), Steridrape (3M), or paraffin gauze, cotton wool and a crepe bandage.

Grafts are not inspected for 5–7 days unless the patient is in pain or develops a pyrexia. When the dressings are taken off, the grafted area is cleaned, any pieces of skin that have failed to adhere are removed and new pieces of split skin from the excess stored in the refrigerator are applied, unless further cleansing of the ulcer base is necessary. Skin will remain viable in the refrigerator for up to 2 weeks, and we have occasionally found that skin that has been kept for 3 weeks has been accepted. Patience and perseverence are demanded to obtain complete skin cover. Refractory ulcers may require three or four applications, over a 3–4 week period.

Until complete healing has been achieved the patient must remain on strict bedrest with the foot of the bed elevated. The ulcer must be *completely* healed before the patient is allowed to stand up or walk (Fig. 15.7).

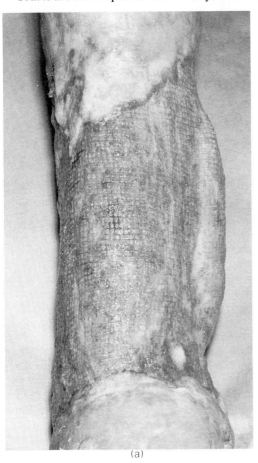
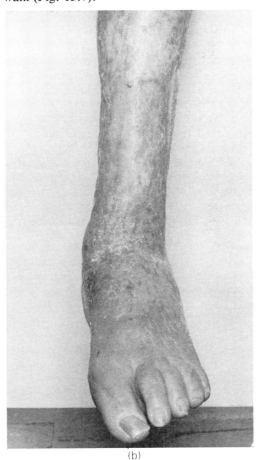

(a) (b)

Fig. 15.7 (a) A large circumferential venous ulcer that is obviously too large to treat conservatively.
(b) The base of the ulcer was excised and covered with split skin grafts, this resulted in complete healing.

Results　There are few reports which detail the success of split skin grafting in healing venous ulcers. Holm and Holmsted[86] reported 75 per cent success (32 out of 40) with tissue glue. We have had much better results (effectively 100 per cent) with persistence and repeated applications of skin. We have only failed when an element of arterial ischaemia has been present.

(b) Pinch grafts[9,33,38,107,131]

The skin of the thigh is prepared with chlorhexidine 0.5% in 70% spirit and draped. The ulcer is then cleaned and prepared in the same manner. The ulcer base may have to be anaesthetized with topical analgesic jelly before being gently freshened with a currette to remove all the slough and necrotic tissue. For a full excision of the ulcer base a general anaesthetic is often needed.

A strip of skin along the anterior surface of the thigh is infiltrated with an intradermal local anaesthetic. A medium-sized hypodermic needle is then inserted into the anaesthetized skin to 'pick it up' before a circular slither of skin beneath the needle is cut off with a sharp scalpel.

The centre of each circle of skin is between 0.5 mm and 1.0 mm thick and the diameter of each piece is approximately 1 cm. It is important not to cut through the full thickness of the dermis at the centre of the 'circle', but at this point the graft should be almost full thickness. Multiple pinch grafts are applied to cover the whole of the ulcer, leaving less than 1 mm between each circle of skin if possible (Fig. 15.8).

When the grafts are in place the whole ulcer is covered with paraffin gauze, cotton dressing gauze, cotton wool and a firmly applied Elastocrepe bandage. The donor site is similarly covered. Patients are allowed to be mobile at home but are encouraged to rest with the leg up as much as possible before returning in 7–10 days for the grafted ulcer to be inspected. Any grafts which have not taken may be replaced with additional pinch grafts.

Once the ulcer is covered with grafts that have 'taken', it should be covered with dry dressings and bandages which should be renewed at weekly intervals until complete healing has occurred.

Results　Using this technique, Monk and Sarkany[107] and Poskitt *et al.*[131] were able to obtain early healing of between 60 per cent and 90 per cent of their venous ulcers. However, Monk and

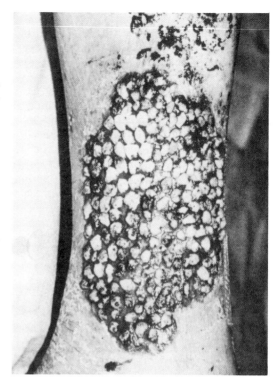

Fig. 15.8　An ulcer covered with pinch grafts taken from the thigh as 1 cm discs. (We are indebted to Dr T Ryan for this illustration).

Sarkany[107] found that nearly 80 per cent of ulcers treated in this way recurred within 1 year, compared with a 60 per cent recurrence rate in those healed by conservative methods; both groups of patients were given elastic stockings after successful healing. The high recurrence rate is probably related to the fact that only a small proportion of their patients underwent surgical correction of their *underlying venous abnormality*.

Comment　We reserve skin grafting for ulcers that are resistant to orthodox out-patient compression bandaging techniques. We admit such patients to hospital, keep them on strict bedrest (except for toilet requirements once or twice a day) and apply antiseptic dressings of dry gauze soaked in hydrogen peroxide, hibitane or normal saline four times a day until the ulcer is clean. These regular dressing changes are combined with mechanical cleaning by scraping and cutting off slough and necrotic debris.

This technique cleans most ulcers in 5–14 days and, if the granulation tissue in the base looks healthy and clean, we proceed to apply skin grafts directly to the ulcer base but if the granulation tissue is sparse or exuberant, we currette the ulcer with the patient anaesthetized. If the ulcer base fails to produce healthy granulation tissue after repeated dressings and currettage, we excise the whole ulcer including the unhealthy surrounding skin and all the subcutaneous tissue.

We prefer to apply 'postage stamp' grafts at the time of ulcer currettage or excision and bandage the grafted leg rather than use the delayed application technique. We continue to apply further grafts until the ulcer is healed.

We have successfully healed all the venous ulcers of patients who we have admitted to our wards over the last 5 years by diligently following this regimen, but because we have sometimes been unable to correct the underlying venous abnormality, a proportion of these, 'healed ulcers' have recurred.

(c) Full-thickness skin grafts

We have not used full-thickness skin grafts on venous ulcers. It is of interest to note that Bergan[15] recommended removal of irreparably damaged skin and its replacement with firm and elastic skin; the illustration in this publication appears to show a full-thickness graft.

This technique has not, to our knowledge, been recommended by any other investigator.

(d) Pedicle grafts

When a patient has had repeated ulcers which have irreparably damaged the skin and subcutaneous tissues which are scarred, and avascular, we combine with our plastic surgical colleagues to excise the abnormal tissues and replace them within full-thickness normal skin from another site.

Figure 15.9 shows a patient who underwent a *cross-leg flap* for persistent venous ulceration lasting for more than 15 years that had not been helped by communicating vein ligation, deep venous reconstruction or continuous use of graduated elastic stockings. After the cross-leg flap was performed the ulcer remained healed and the transfered skin remained in good condition after 2 years. Then lipodermatosclerosis developed in the 'good' skin which has broken down and ulcerated!

The cross-leg flap is ideal when the venous disease is unilateral. If both legs are abnormal, a tubed pedicle graft can be used. These operations are not always successful. No large series with long-term results has been published. Pedicle grafts should be used sparingly because they require a long stay in hospital, considerable patient co-operation and patience, and will probably give long-term success in only approximately 50 per cent of the cases.

(e) Vascularized free flap grafts

Most patients who have chronic venous ulceration that fails to respond to the medical and surgical

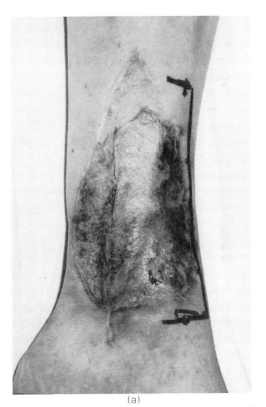

(a)

Fig. 15.9 This post-thrombotic venous ulcer failed to respond to out-patient treatment. Surgery to the communicating veins and deep veins had failed, and the ulcer kept recurring even though the patient wore elastic support stockings constantly.

(a) The ulcers were healed by split skin grafting after a period of bedrest and cleaning. The abnormal lipodermatosclerotic skin was then marked out and excised.

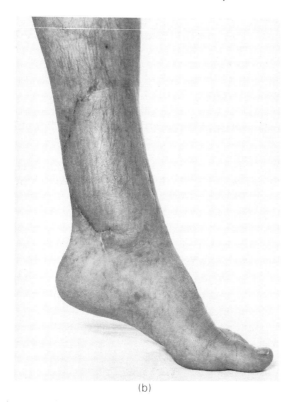

(b)

Fig. 15.9 (b) A cross leg flap from the opposite calf was used to cover the skin defect. After separation of the flap the defect on the healthy limb was covered with split skin grafts.

treatments outlined above, have got post-thrombotic deep vein damage. This makes the use of vascularized free flap grafts[95] questionable because it is difficult to find a healthy deep vein for the venous anastomosis and there is an increased risk of thrombosis of the pedicle vein.

Nevertheless, we have successfully treated two patients with severe intractable post-thrombotic ulceration in this way. Both patients were given anticoagulants postoperatively. One patient developed a large haematoma beneath the flap which required repeated aspiration but the flap survived. This type of operation is a major under-taking and should only be used as a last resort when there is no other skin available for the well-established cross-leg or pedicle grafts.

(f) Tissue expansion

The use of inflatable plastic tissue expanders can be a useful method of increasing the amount of tissue available before transferring it to replace an area of damaged abnormal skin.

10. Ulcer excision followed by skin grafting

Skin grafts only 'take' when they have an adequate supply of blood and oxygen. The changes that precede ulceration affect the sub-cutaneous tissues as well as the skin (see Chapters 11 and 13). After many years of calf pump mal-function, the skin and subcutaneous tissues can be completely replaced by fibrous tissue with a minimal, almost non-existent, blood supply. Ulcers in this type of tissue have a grey-white base peppered with a few pale pink capillary loops (Fig. 14.6). They will never produce sufficient granulations to nuture and hold a skin graft. This is the type of ulcer that fails to heal with medical treatment and rejects split skin grafts applied to its surface.

Once the lack of blood supply is recognized, it is wise to accept that all the diseased tissue beneath and around the ulcer must be excised in order to find tissue with an adequate blood supply. Some-times the excision has to include the deep fascia.[130] After such an excision has been performed, split skin grafts can be applied in the manner already described.

Total excision of an ulcer and its base has a major advantage; any incompetent communicat-ing veins beneath the ulcer are automatically ligated and divided. The excision can also be combined with a full communicating vein ligation operation (see Chapter 7, page 225); this treats the immediate cause of the ulceration and improves the chance of long-term success.

Ligating communicating veins, days, weeks or months after healing an ulcer is associated with a significant incidence of both ulcer and wound breakdown. Excising the ulcer, ligating the com-municating veins and grafting the defect (Fig. 15.10) avoids this problem, though the patient may have to stay in hospital a little longer than would be necessary after a simple skin graft.

We do not know of any trials comparing direct application of split skin to the ulcer base against excision and grafting.

11. Correction of calf pump malfunction

The techniques used to diagnose and correct calf pump malfunction are described in Chapter 7 and Chapter 9.

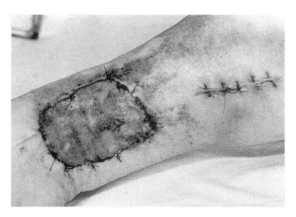

Fig. 15.10 This ulcer has been excised and covered with a split skin graft. The medial calf communicating veins have been ligated at the same time. An additional incision above the ulcer (combined with the ulcer excision) has allowed all the communicating veins to be explored. A small skin bridge has been left between the two incisions.

Some investigators have advocated the use of these methods to accelerate healing of the ulcer while other workers have only used them to prevent recurrence once the ulcer has healed. This latter policy is discussed in the section on ulcer prophylaxis (page 431). As other methods of ulcer healing are invariably combined with some definitive treatment of the venous abnormality, an assessment of the independent value of the correction of calf pump malfunction is extremely difficult.

The methods used to correct the venous abnormality include:

(a) sclerotherapy
(b) surgical ligation of the superficial and lower leg communicating veins
(c) surgical reconstruction of the deep veins or valves
(d) elastic compression stockings

(a) Sclerotherapy

Fegan's group[83] claimed that injection compression sclerotherapy (see Chapter 7 page 239 for the technique) combined with ulcer dressing successfully maintained ulcer healing for more than 4 years in 82 per cent of a consecutive group of 82 women presenting with venous ulcers. There was no control group treated by compression and dressings without injections, and we are not told how many ulcers healed, broke down and were then healed by a second course of treatment. Henry *et al.*[83] imply, however, that dressings in their hands were totally ineffective unless combined with sclerotherapy. It is difficult to interpret these results in view of the implied poor results of standard treatment and the lack of controls. There are other anecdotal reports[41,109] on the value of injection compression in the healing of ulcers but we are unaware of any controlled studies which prove that the use of sclerotherapy increases the rate of healing that can be achieved by simple compression and dressings.

(b) Surgical ligation of the superficial and lower leg communicating veins

Linton and Hardy,[99] in a review of the surgical treatment of the post-thrombotic syndrome, advocated healing all ulcers before ligating the communicating veins and treating any other superficial vein incompetence (see Chapter 7, page 225 for techniques). In 1953 Linton reiterated this opinion[100] but in the same year Cockett and Elgan Jones[40] reported, in the *Lancet*, two cases in whom they had simultaneously ligated the lower leg communicating veins and grafted an associated venous ulcer with good results. In a postscript to this publication they recorded 20 additional successes.

In 1955 Cockett[41] was advocating ulcer excision combined with communicating vein ligation followed 4 or 5 days later, by the application of split skin grafts to the granulating area left by the ulcer excision. No results of this change in policy were presented. In the same year Dodd *et al.*[58] reported their results of ankle communicating vein ligation for the venous ulcer syndrome. Unfortunately, it is impossible to ascertain from this paper whether the ulcers were healed or open at the time of the surgery.

Lofgren's[101] review of 129 patients with 'stasis' ulcers treated by skin grafting and surgery to the superficial veins does not clearly state whether the skin grafts and the surgery were performed simultaneously or if the vein surgery was carried out after the ulcer had healed. In a further review in 1974 Lofgren[102] commented that 'vein surgery and skin grafting can be done as a combined procedure or vein surgery alone may be sufficient if the ulcer is small or nearly healed'. A follow-up of between 3 years and 12 years showed that 70 per cent of the ulcers treated in this way had remained healed, but the majority of patients were wearing elastic stockings as an additional treatment.

Cockett's idea of operating on the veins before healing the ulcer[41] was taken up by Pickerill *et al.* in 1970.[130] They suggested that 1 week after 'appropriate surgery to the superficial veins and perforating veins the patient should be taken back to the operating theatre for a radical excision of the ulcer including the damaged surrounding skin with immediate application of split skin grafts'. No numbers or results are quoted in this paper.

In 1974 De Palma[54] again described a synchronous operation to ligate the communicating veins and apply split skin grafts to the ulcer. Yet again, neither the long-term nor the short-term results of this treatment on ulcer healing are recorded.

In a more recent survey on the ligation of incompetent ankle communicating veins in the treatment of venous ulceration,[115] the majority of ulcers (87–80 per cent) were healed with conservative treatment before the operation. In those that were not healed (20 per cent), split skin grafts were applied at time of surgery to the veins. The success rates of the sequential and simultaneous procedures are not presented separately.

In another report[152] on the results of ankle communicating vein ligation in preventing recurrence of venous ulcers, it was stated that some patients with extensive ulceration were treated through subfascial explorations which were left unsutured and subsequently closed by the application of split skin grafts. Again it is impossible to separate this group of patients from those who were treated by staged procedures, and therefore the success of this approach cannot be assessed.

Comment   This review of some of the publications on the effect of combining the treatment of venous ulceration and calf pump malfunction shows that surgical correction of superficial venous incompetence can be satisfactorily performed in the presence of an ulcer, but there is little evidence that this accelerates the healing of the ulcer, unless the ulcer is treated by simultaneous or subsequent split skin grafting. There is, however, no evidence that split skin grafts are less likely to adhere when they are applied at the same time as venous surgery, and we have already mentioned our own satisfactory results with this method of healing ulcers that are resistant to conservative forms of treatment.

Why then do we *not* follow this policy for all patients with venous ulceration that have proved resistant to dressings and compression? The main reason why we prefer to heal the ulcer first is that it is often difficult to define the disorder of the calf pump in the presence of an active ulcer and it is therefore difficult to decide on the best method of treatment until the ulcer is healed. Furthermore, if the ulcer is healed, we are able to operate in a sterile field thus avoiding the high risk of wound infection which occurs with simultaneous operations (Fig. 15.10).[94,107]

It is essential that proper comparisons are made between the many combinations of sclerotherapy, surgery to the superficial veins, surgery to the communicating veins, surgery to both the superficial and communicating veins, and pre-operative, peroperative and postoperative skin grafting. Such studies would allow the best combination of these procedures to be selected and, if only the saphenous system or communicating veins were treated, it would be possible to discover which has the major role in the genesis of ulceration.

(c) Surgical reconstruction of the deep veins or valves

The operations used to reconstruct the deep veins or repair the valves include:

- femoral valve reconstruction[98]
- valve transposition operations[97]
- popliteal to femoral vein, saphenous vein bypass operations[90,159]
- sapheno-femoral bypass operations[120]
- femoro-caval bypass operations[52]
- brachial valve transplantation[151]
- the gracilis sling operation[132]
  (see Chapters 8 and 9 for details)

These operations have all been used to reconstruct or bypass damaged deep veins and have all been claimed to heal ulcers or prevent recurrence of ulcers.[14] They have almost always been combined with other operations on the superficial veins of the lower leg or with prolonged periods of bedrest. All these procedures require further evaluation[1] but if they are to be used, it is probably preferable that any ulceration should be healed first. They may have a place in the prevention of ulcer recurrence but they do not yet have a role in accelerating ulcer-healing.

Few investigators still consider that ligation of the femoral vein to prevent deep venous reflux promotes ulcer healing.[10,55,99]

(d) Elastic compression stockings

The role and value of elastic stockings is discussed in the section on the prevention of ulcer recurrence.

12. Miscellaneous treatments

Many ancillary treatments have been tried, for example

    (a) hyperbaric oxygen
    (b) lumbar sympathectomy
    (c) weight reduction, diuretics and vitamins
    (d) acidification

(a) Hyperbaric oxygen The low tissue oxygen found in association with venous ulceration has already been described (Chapter 13, pages 354–359). Bass[8] reported a series of patients with venous ulcers who were treated with hyperbaric oxygen given for 2 hours every day, 5 days of the week. The only additional treatment was a gauze dressing. Seventeen of the ulcers treated this way healed in a mean of 6 weeks but, unfortunately, the initial ulcer size is not given, and there was no control group. A similar study[55] without controls also reported good results. A properly controlled study is required to assess the value of this treatment; until this has been carried out it cannot be recommended.

(b) Lumbar sympathectomy Opinions concerning the value of lumbar sympathectomy in the treatment of venous ulceration are conflicting. Fontaine[66] gave an anecdotal report of the value of lumbar sympathectomy as an adjuvant treatment in the management of chronic ulcers of the leg, but both Linton and Hardy[99] and Dodd and Cockett[59] strongly condemned its use for venous ulceration.

In contrast, a recent paper has suggested that lumbar sympathectomy is effective in healing venous ulcers which have proved resistant to treatment by conventional means.[125] Eighty of these ulcers remained healed between 2 years and 11 years after treatment. A controlled trial is required before sympathectomy can be advocated

for the treatment of venous ulceration.

(c) Weight reduction, diuretics and vitamins Haeger[77] has championed the value of diuretics and weight reduction in the healing of ulcers, but there is little hard evidence to justify the value of either form of treatment. The administration of extra vitamins to patients who are not suffering from vitamin deficiency is of no value and may even do harm.

(d) Acidification One study suggests that acidification of the ulcer surface promotes healing.[164] This was a controlled but small study that used a healing equation rather than reporting the total number of ulcers healed. We are not aware that this work has been repeated.

Prevention of ulcer recurrence

A review of all the treatments presented above shows that most studies report that between 60 per cent and 90 per cent of all 'new ulcers' can be healed within 3–12 months of presentation with conservative treatment. The factors which may influence this time period include:

- size of the ulcer at presentation
- number of years that the ulcer has been present
- time that the ulcer has remained unhealed
- nature of the underlying venous disease

The ulcers that do not heal with medical treatment can be healed by skin grafting. The challenge is to maintain healing.

Methods of preventing ulcer recurrence

The techniques used to prevent ulcer recurrence are given below.

1. Sapheno-femoral or sapheno-popliteal ligation with stripping and local avulsions
2. Ligation of the lower leg communicating veins
3. A combination of 1 and 2
4. Deep vein bypass or reconstruction
5. Injection compression sclerotherapy
6. Elastic stockings
7. Fibrinolytic enhancement
8. Permanent use of compression bandages

Superficial vein surgery

The value of occluding incompetent superficial-to-deep communications depends upon the role that each site of incompetence plays in calf pump malfunction. Most patients have long or short saphenous vein incompetence but the value of correcting this abnormality alone is not known. Our own clinical experience suggests that saphenous ligation on its own, in the presence of lower leg communicating vein incompetence, does not prevent ulcer recurrence, but other investigators would not agree with us.[139]

None of the proponents of ligation of the lower leg communicating veins[40,41,99,100,115,116] has carried out this operation without simultaneously correcting incompetence of the saphenous veins, if this is present. We have found that ligation of incompetent communicating veins alone fails to restore the foot vein pressure fall during exercise to normal,[30] and Bjordal[17,18,19,20,21] has shown that saphenous incompetence has a greater influence on calf pump function than communicating vein incompetence.

The inadequacy of the studies that have been published on this subject has been discussed already but a prospective trial of ligation of the communicating veins *alone* without saphenous surgery would be unlikely to obtain the approval of an ethical committee, despite its apparent importance.

The operation chosen by most surgeons is the combination of communicating vein ligation with sapheno-femoral and sapheno-popliteal ligation.[6,40,41,48,54,58,59,99,100,115,116,152]

In our experience[27] this is a good operation to perform in limbs with phlebographically 'normal' deep veins but it is relatively ineffective in limbs with clear-cut phlebographic evidence of deep vein damage. All the patients with post-thrombotic ulcers in one of our series treated by operation alone developed at least one ulcer recurrence within 5 years of operation. The patients in this study were not provided with elastic stockings. Negus's prospective, but uncontrolled, study[115,116] of identical surgery combined with permanent elastic stocking support[7] revealed a much lower incidence of recurrence during a following period of approximately 3 years.

We are now comparing the results superficial vein surgery followed by elastic stockings, after healing, with the results achieved in a randomly selected group of control patients treated with stockings and stanozolol (fibrinolytic enhancement) after ulcer healing.

The evidence suggests that a combination of surgery followed by permanent support with elastic stockings is more certain to prevent ulcer recurrence than surgery alone, particularly in limbs which have severe post-thrombotic deep vein damage.

The cause of ulcer recurrence after surgery Finding the cause of an ulcer that has recurred after surgery is a difficult clinical problem because it is always possible that the initial surgery was inadequate or incorrect (e.g. an incompetent communicating vein or the long saphenous vein may have been missed or not properly divided) or that the surgery was adequate and a new cause of ulceration has developed.

Nielubowitcz and Szostek[117] investigated a small group of 11 patients whose ulcers recurred with phlebography to try to discover if communicating veins had been missed at the original operation. They found evidence of communicating vein incompetence in four limbs, but it was impossible to distinguish between new communicating veins that had developed and communicating veins that had been missed at the original operation.

Recurrent incompetent communicating veins should be treated surgically and we have many patients on whom we have performed this operation three or four times over 10–15 years. We also have some patients where re-exploration has failed to reveal any incompetent communicating veins and we have been unable to define the cause of their recurrent ulcer.

Deep vein bypass or reconstruction

A description of these techniques[14] is given in Chapter 9 and their place in accelerating the healing of ulcers has also been briefly mentioned. As most of these techniques have been developed within the last 5–10 years their role in the prevention of ulcer recurrence has not yet been established.

Before deep vein reconstruction can be used for preventing ulcer recurrence it is necessary to prove that it permanently cures the deep vein abnormality it is designed to correct.

Injection compression sclerotherapy

Nothing has been added to the uncontrolled study of Henry *et al.*[83] which suggested that sclerotherapy sustained the long-term healing of ulcers.

Elastic support stockings

Many authors[6,15,48,99,100] have recommended the continued use of permanent elastic support in limbs with severe post-thrombotic damage, but this recommendation has been based more on theoretical considerations than on proven efficacy.

The older type of compression stocking has now been superceded by the graduated compression stocking, but this change is also the result of theoretical arguments rather than practical experience.[143,157] Stemmer[149,150] has calculated that the ideal external compression should exactly match, and therefore overcome, the increase in venous pressure that causes the loss of capillary transudate into the tissues.[148] The higher venous pressure at the ankle therefore demands a greater external compression pressure to prevent transudation than the lower venular pressure at the knee. Sigg's argument[142,143] for graduated compression was more straightforward; he simply believed that the greatest pressure should be applied over the 'ulcer bearing skin'.

A number of measurements of calf pump function have shown that graduated compression is more effective in promoting venous return than standard uniform compression stockings.[44,87,93,124]

Indirect evidence of the value of graduation is provided by two studies. Firstly, graduated compression stockings alone or in combination with fibrinolytic enhancement have been shown to reduce areas of lipodermatosclerosis.[28] Secondly, surgery to the communicating veins combined with graduated compression has produced better results than those reported with surgery alone,[27,115,116] but there are still no studies of the ability of elastic stockings alone to prevent ulcer recurrence.

External compression has two other effects, it increases the rate of blood flow in the deep veins[141] and it may encourage the release of fibrinolytic activator from the venous endothelium.[39]

Standardization of stockings A number of methods are used to test the elastic tension at different sites in a stocking. The tension can then be converted to a compression pressure by Laplace's equation (pressure = tension × radius). Techniques which use testing rigs are indirect methods; direct methods measure the pressure beneath the stocking when it is on the patient's leg.

Indirect measurements of tension

(i) *The Ingstron tester* measures the tension in a section of a stocking held between two moveable T-pins. It is simply a standard form of tensiometer.

(ii) The Hatra tester involves placing the stocking on a 'leg former' and then stretching it by pulling out a movable bar to a predetermined site. A measuring head is then applied to the stretched stocking to obtain the fabric tension at the desired position.

(iii) *The Hohenstein tester* is a computerized device which measures the tension between numerous points marked on a stocking stretched over an expandable leg former.

Direct measurements of tension

The original Sigg balloon tester[143] has been superceded by the testing system devised by Borgnis and Bollinger.[156] The Borgnis system overcomes the defect of the original balloon tester which gave false results because the inflated balloon between the leg and the stocking increased the curve (reduces the radius) of the leg thus artificially increasing the measured tension.

The Borgnis medical stocking tester (The MST) consists of a long thin plastic envelope containing four pairs of carbon electrodes on its two inside opposing surfaces which make contact when the envelope is empty (Fig. 15.11). When the probe is placed on the limb beneath the stocking the carbon contacts meet and complete four independent circuits which light four indicator lights on the pump. Air is then slowly pumped into the plastic envelope by an electric pump. When the pressure in the envelope exceeds the pressure applied by the stocking, the contacts separate, the circuit is broken and the indicator light is extinguished. The pressure in the envelope at the moment that each of the contacts break is recorded on a digital dial which provides a series of pressure measurements from four points beneath the stocking. The amount of air required to separate the contacts within the envelope is so small that the curvature of the overlying stocking is not changed and the true tension which the stocking is imparting to the limb can be recorded.

Which tester? Which stocking? It is important to state the type of test used when publishing data on stocking tensions because the indirect

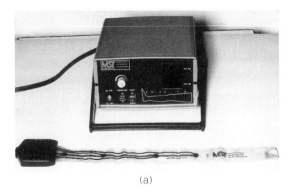

(a)

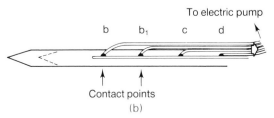

(b)

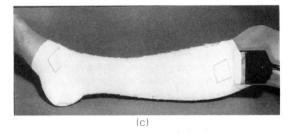

(c)

Fig. 15.11 The Borgnis Tester.

(a) The envelope (probe) containing the four circular carbon contacts is in the foreground; the pump with the pressure dial is behind. When the pump is turned on, air is blown into the envelope. The pressure at which the contacts separate is equal to the compression pressure of the stocking at the point of measurement. This is recorded on the digital display.

(b) This diagram shows the circuits inside the envelope.

(c) The Borgnis Tester beneath a Thusane bandage.

methods give different values to those of the direct methods.[162] The British Standards Committee have chosen the Hatra system as their reference test.[29]

The advantage of the Borgnis tester is that it measures the actual pressure developed by the stocking on an individual limb which often differs from the manufacturer's specification;[32] this is hardly surprising as artificial formers are very different from real legs. The MST probe is, however, very temperamental. It can be markedly affected by minor adjustments to the overlying stocking and, unfortunately, has a short life; the carbon wears off the contacts after approximately 100 tests. The MST probe is, however, a valuable tool for testing the accuracy of stocking fitting and for carrying out studies on the durability of stockings.[32]

We have found that stockings tested by this method rarely achieve the pressures claimed by the manufacturers using their laboratory methods of testing and that stockings which are subjected to normal wear and tear and regular washing loose their elasticity after 6–12 months. We now give each patient four pairs of stockings every year so that each pair is used for no more than 6 months.

There is no substitute for a good quality, inevitably expensive, elastic stocking. Each clinician must decide which stockings provide the best compression, using the Borgnis tester, and which are the most cosmetically acceptable. In the United Kingdom we prescribe either Sigvaris 503 or 504 (Ganzoni), or Venosan 2000 (Credenhill) because we have tried and tested these two makes of stocking against others and found them to be superior in quality and acceptability.

We prescribe only below the knee stockings for patients with the calf pump failure syndrome (Fig. 15.12) because we are unaware of any studies that show that full length stockings are more effective, though some patients with oedema of the whole leg caused by iliac vein obstruction prefer full length stockings. Stockings must be put on before getting out of bed every morning and worn every day, all day, until the patient goes to bed. This must be impressed upon each patient. Pulling on a stocking is quite difficult, especially for the patient who is elderly or who has arthritis of the hands. If possible, we arrange for these patients to be helped with application, removal, washing and re-application of their stockings by their spouse, other relatives, a neighbour or even regular visits from the community nurse. Although continuous use of stockings may be dangerous in ischaemic limbs, the inability to put on stockings may well allow the development of another ulcer. Under these circumstances it may be better for the patient to wear the stockings constantly, day and night.

Stocking care Elastic stockings must be

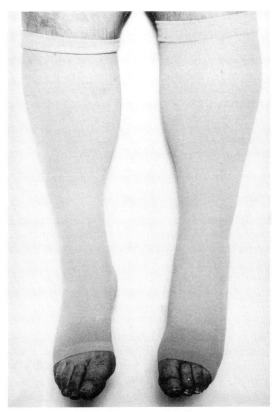

Fig. 15.12 A patient fitted with a pair of below-knee medium compression (503) Sigvaris stockings. These provide good quality graduated compression and, with normal care and usage, last approximately 6 months.

looked after properly otherwise they do not retain their elasticity. They must be washed in soap not in detergent, and each patient needs to have at least two pairs if each pair is to be washed after it has been worn. Patients are provided with a silk sock to help the stocking slide over the foot, and they should wear rubber gloves when pulling the stocking up the leg to avoid damaging the stocking with the finger nails.

When a stocking is easy to apply, it needs to be replaced. If a stocking tester is not available, feeling the tension by picking up the stocking off the leg and inspecting its external appearance is often enough to indicate the need for replacement. It is better to err towards unnecessary replacement than to have a patient with a recurrent ulcer.

Comment Although there is circumstantial evidence to support the belief that elastic stock-

ings prevent ulcer recurrence, there is an absence of hard supporting facts. There is also no evidence that wearing a graduated compression stocking after a deep vein thrombosis prevents the development of lipodermatosclerosis and ulceration. Much more information is required on the role of elastic stockings in ulcer prevention.

If rubber sensitivity develops, stockings made of 'man-made' elastic should be prescribed for the patient.

Some patients who have severe post-thrombotic syndrome get an unbearable amount of pain and discomfort when wearing a high-compression stocking. These patients are very difficult to treat.

Fibrinolytic enhancement

The value of the anabolic steroid stanozolol, which enhances blood and tissue fibrinolytic activity, in the treatment of lipodermatosclerosis is discussed in Chapter 12 (page 342). A review of a group of patients with lipodermatosclerosis treated with a course of fibrinolytic enhancement has shown that they developed statistically fewer ulcers in the 5 years following treatment than in the 5 years preceding the treatment.[31] All these patients, however, wore elastic stockings for the second 5 years, and it is possible that the stockings rather than the fibrinolytic enhancement may have prevented the ulcers recurring. Nevertheless, these observations indicate that we need to find out whether the resolution of lipodermatosclerosis does reduce the risk of subsequent ulceration or re-ulceration.

Permanent use of compression bandages

We have some patients who are incapable of wearing elastic stockings and who we treat with 'permanent' paste bandages (usually a Calaband, covered by Elastocrepe and Tubigrip bandages) which are changed at weekly or monthly intervals by the community nurse. This regimen has been extremely effective in keeping the skin healthy and the oedema under control.

Commentary on ulcer healing and prevention

In 1953 Cockett and Elgan Jones[40] argued that ligation of the communicating veins, when post-thrombotic skin changes were just appearing, would reduce the incidence of ulceration. This approach seems to be logical but there have not been any prospective studies which have scientifically tested whether elastic stockings or early venous surgery prevents ulceration in limbs with post-thrombotic deep vein damage. We recommend that all patients who have had an extensive deep vein thrombosis, involving more than just one or two calf veins, should wear below-knee, graduated, compression stockings for the rest of their lives.

If lipodermatosclerosis develops, we prescribe a course of stanozolol for 6–9 months while continuing to wear stockings until the maximum resolution has been achieved (Colour plates 30–32).

If the patient presents with an ulcer, we try to heal it conservatively, with Calaband, Elastocrepe and Tubigrip or with dry dressings and compression, before investigating the limbs to ascertain whether the superficial, communicating, or deep veins are at fault.

If the deep veins are normal, we operate to eradicate long and short saphenous vein incompetence and routinely ligate all medial lower leg communicating veins through a subfascial approach.

If there is evidence of severe post-thrombotic deep vein damage, we assess the role of the superficial veins by using tourniquet tests in association with foot volumetry and tailor our surgery according to the findings of these tests in combination with the anatomical information provided by phlebograms. If the post-thrombotic damage is mainly in the calf veins and there is superficial vein or communicating vein incompetence with improvement in the expelled foot volume with tourniquets, we attempt to ligate the sources of superficial reflux and prescribe permanent stockings. If there is severe post-thrombotic damage in the thigh or pelvis with no improvement in the expelled foot volume with tourniquets and poor collateral vessels, we would consider a 'Palma' bypass[120] or a femoro-caval reconstruction,[52] if this is possible, together with ligation of the incompetent communicating veins.

If there is extensive post-thrombotic damage at all levels, we try to avoid surgery and rely on elastic stockings and fibrinolytic enhancement for severe lipodermatosclerosis.

We consider that this is a logical approach to ulcer prophylaxis but other clinicians would simply ligate all the incompetent communicating veins of all patients with ulcers and provide elastic stockings. These clinicians must, however, expect a 10–15 per cent incidence of recurrence. Careful identification of those situations likely to cause a recurrence should lead to better treatment of these patients and possibly a lower incidence of recurrence.

Treatment of the complications of venous ulceration and its associated conditions

Eczema

Venous ulcers are commonly associated with eczema in the skin near the ulcer or at distant sites around the body (e.g. the opposite leg, the upper limb, and even the face and the trunk). The aetiology of the eczema is obscure. It may be the result of local skin sensitivity to lesser degrees of the damage which causes lipodermatosclerosis and ulceration.

The eczema may be treated with local or systemic steroids, and it usually disappears when the ulcer heals or the venous abnormality is repaired.

Contact dermatitis

Although this dermatitis is similar to venous eczema it is worth thinking of contact dermatitis as a separate entity because it is often caused by the treatment of the ulcer[81] rather than by the underlying skin abnormality. Eighty per cent of patients who have had an ulcer for more than 5 years are sensitive to at least one agent that has been applied to the skin during this period.[136] The presence of contact dermatitis appears to delay the healing of the ulcer.

Causes of contact dermatitis include:[136]

Bandages containing dyes or rubber, adhesive plasters, antibiotics, antiseptics, coal-tars, local anaesthetics, antihistamines, soaps, spirits, ointment preservatives and stabilizers (e.g. lanolin), wood alcohols, diachylon, parabens, mercuric chloride, chlorocresol, and methylate.

Patients who have contact dermatitis that does not subside when the allergen is withdrawn should be referred for a dermatological opinion and possible patch testing.

Treatment of contact dermatitis is by withdrawal of the sensitizer and application of local steroid creams. Systemic steroids may occasionally be required.

Cellulitis, lymphangitis and septicaemia

Ulcers can serve as the portal of entry of bacteria that cause cellulitis, but this is surprisingly rare. Acute lipodermatosclerosis is often misdiagnosed as cellulitis.

Treatment with systemic antibiotics is indicated if a patient develops a hot, red, tender area of skin or swollen subcutaneous tissue, sometimes associated with lymphangitis, lymphadenitis and pyrexia. The exudate from the ulcer and the blood should be cultured but antibiotics should be started before the results of the cultures and bacteriological sensitivities are available. We favour a combination of amoxycillin and flucloxacillin. Amoxycillin alone, Septrin, or cephalosporins are alternatives.

Haemorrhage

A brisk spontaneous haemorrhage may arise from a venous ulcer (see Chapter 6, page 173). The ulcer is often small and relatively uncontaminated. Treatment is by applying pressure on the bleeding point and elevation of the limb until the bleeding stops. The patient should lie down with the leg elevated on a bed or chair, and a pad should be applied to the ulcer with a firm bandage. If the patient has no help, he or she should raise the leg and press on the bleeding point. Occasionally, the haemorrhage is profuse and the patient has to be admitted to hospital for a blood transfusion. The definitive treatment is to heal the ulcer. If the bleeding recurs during treatment, the ulcer is best treated by excision and skin grafting.

'Champagne bottle' legs, ankylosis and equinus deformity of the ankle

The contraction of the fibrous tissue that follows the healing of severe lipodermatosclerosis or ulceration often constricts the tissues around the ankle to give the leg the shape of an inverted 'champagne' bottle. This affects the function of the calf muscle pump by interfering with ankle movements and causes oedema of the foot.

Dodd and Cockett[59] described a 'gusset' operation for this condition, in which a vertical incision is made through the thickened tissue to allow it to retract and the resulting gap is closed by a split skin graft. This operation gives the limb a better shape but there is no evidence that it leads to better calf pump function.

The combination of persistent pain, recurrent ulceration and fibrosis often causes plantar flexion at the ankle (equinus) and eventually a fibrous ankylosis in plantar flexion (Fig. 15.1). Movement of the ankle joint is painful and the patient therefore walks on the ball of the foot, with the ankle and knee flexed and without contracting the calf muscles at all. If the Achilles tendon is involved in the base of the ulcer, the fibrosis may extend into the tendon and the development of the equinus deformity is accelerated.

If the deformity is mild, it may be simply treated by raising the heel of the shoe. If the deformity is severe, the function of the ankle joint may only be regained by lengthening the Achilles tendon; it is preferable to heal the ulcer before undertaking such an operation. Skin breakdown at the site of the incision is common. If the tendon can be successfully lengthened and joint mobility regained, the calf muscle pump will improve.

Anaemia

This topic has been discussed in Chapter 14 (page 406). Anaemia may be the result of iron deficiency or marrow depression. It responds to oral administration of iron and healing of the ulcer.[138] Blood transfusions are rarely required.

Malignant change

This problem is discussed in detail in Chapter 14 (page 383). Marjolin's ulcer is extremely rare but over-growth of any part of a long-standing ulcer with the development of a foul smelling odour should arouse suspicion. If a biopsy shows a squamous cell or even a basal cell carcinoma, the ulcer should be widely excised and the defect in the skin covered with a skin graft. Radiotherapy to skin damaged by chronic venous insufficiency may cause skin necrosis.

Amputation

More than 50 limbs are amputated, each year, for

chronic painful venous ulcers in the United Kingdom.[103] If all medical and surgical measures fail in a leg severely damaged by deep vein thrombosis which is the cause of constant pain, amputation may have to be considered. Artificial legs are never as satisfactory as natural limbs, and most natural limbs even with a large chronic ulcer are preferable to a prosthesis. We try to avoid amputation, but have had to resort to this treatment on two occasions in the past 20 years.

Conclusion The care of venous ulcers is often delegated to junior surgeons who are commonly ill-equipped to cope with their care. Ulcers require careful assessment, and their management must be carefully monitored. When an ulcer is healed, the venous abnormality must be defined and corrected. There is truth in both of the following statements.

'The clinical evaluation of the patient's leg is more satisfactory than any artificial means. The patient's history is written on the skin of his leg. It is there to be read by those who wish to read it' (Bergan).[15]

'Correct anatomical and pathophysiological diagnosis of leg ulcers leads to better treatment. The patient may have the problem for life' (Browse).[25]

Our aim must be to achieve palliation, to look for a cure and hope that better methods of preventing and treating deep venous thrombosis will eventually lead to the eradication of venous ulceration.

References

1. Ackroyd JS, Browse NL. The investigation and surgery of the post-thrombotic syndrome. *J Cardiovasc Surg* 1986; **27**: 5.
2. Allen S. Varicose ulcers: preliminary report on a new material to assist regranulation. *Curr Med Res Opin* 1973; **1**(10): 603.
3. Anderson MN, Donald KE. Results of surgical therapy of severe stasis ulceration of the legs. *Ann Surg* 1963; **157**: 281.
4. Anning ST. *Leg Ulcers. Their Causes and Treatment*. London. Churchill 1954.
5. Arkle CA, Adinolfi M, Welsh KI, Leibowitz S, McColl I. Immunogenicity of human amniotic epithelial cells after transplantation into volunteers. *Lancet* 1981; **2**: 1003.
6. Arnoldi CC, Haeger K. Ulcus cruris venosum – crux medicorum? *Läkartidningen* 1967; **64**: 2149.
7. Bartholomew A. Short account of the treatment by physiotherapy of gravitational ulcers. *Br J Phys Med* 1952; **15**: 289.
8. Bass BH. The treatment of varicose leg ulcers by hyperbaric oxygen. *Postgrad Med J* 1970; **46**: 407.
9. Battle R. *Plastic Surgery*. London. Butterworths 1964.
10. Bauer G. The etiology of leg ulcers and their treatment by resection of the popliteal veins. *J Int Chir* 1948; **8**: 937.
11. Beitner H, Hammar H, Olsson AG, Thyresson N. Prostaglandin El treatment of leg ulcers caused by venous or arterial incompetence. *Acta Derm Venereol (Stockh)* 1980; **60**: 425.
12. Belcaro GV, Coen F. Pneumatic intermittent compression treatment of venous ulcerations caused by venous hypertension. In Negus D, Jantet G (Eds) *Phlebology '85*. London. Libbey 1986.
13. Bennett JP, Mathews R, Page-Faulk W. Treatment of chronic ulceration of the legs with human amnion. *Lancet* 1980; **1**: 1153.
14. Bergan JJ, Yao JST, Flinn WR, McCarthy WJ. Surgical treatment of venous obstruction and insufficiency. *J Vasc Surg* 1986; **3**: 174.
15. Bergan JJ. Ulcers of the leg. *Ind Med Surg* 1967; **36**: 253.
16. Bisgaard H. *Ulcers and Eczema of the Leg Sequels of Phlebitis*. Copenhagen. Munksgaard 1948.
17. Bjordal RI. Simultaneous pressure and flow recordings in varicose veins of the lower extremity. *Acta Chir Scand* 1970; **136**: 309.
18. Bjordal RI. Pressure patterns in the saphenous system in patients with venous leg ulcers. *Acta Chir Scand* 1971; **137**: 495.
19. Bjordal RI. Blood circulation in varicose veins of the lower extremities. *Angiology* 1972; **23**: 163.
20. Bjordal RI. Circulation patterns in incompetent perforating veins in the calf and in the saphenous system in primary varicose veins. *Acta Chir Scand* 1972; **138**: 251.
21. Bjordal RI. Circulation patterns in the saphenous system and the perforating veins of the calf in patients with previous deep venous thrombosis. *Vasa* 1974; Suppl **3**: 1.
22. Bourne IHJ. Vertical leg drainage of oedema in treatment of leg ulcers. *Br Med J* 1974; **2**: 581.
23. Brennan SS, Leaper DJ. Antiseptics and wound healing. *Br J Surg* 1985; **72**: 780.
24. Brodie BC. *Lectures Illustrative of Various Subjects in Pathology and Surgery*. London. Longmans 1846.
25. Browse NL. Venous ulceration. *Br Med J* 1983; **286**: 1920.

26. Burke H B, Kuglar W, Oriti J, Seidenspinner C, Lockwood B, Buskey A. The use of gelfoam powder and betadine-saturated gauze in treatment of chronic ulcerations. *J Foot Surg* 1981; **20**: 76.

27. Burnand K G, O'Donnell T F, Lea Thomas M, Browse N L. Relation between post-phlebitic changes in the deep veins and results of surgical treatment of venous ulcers. *Lancet* 1976; **1**: 936.

28. Burnand K G, Clemenson G, Morland M, Jarrett PEM, Browse N L. Venous lipodermatosclerosis: treatment by fibrinolytic enhancement and elastic compression. *Br Med J* 1980; **280**: 7.

29. Burnand K G, Layer G. Graduated elastic stockings. *Br Med J* 1986; **293**: 224.

30. Burnand K G, O'Donnell T F, Lea Thomas M, Browse N L. The relative importance of incompetent communicating veins in the production of varicose veins and venous ulcers. *Surgery* 1977; **82**: 9.

31. Burnand K G, Pattison M, Browse N L. The results of a course of Stromba treatment on lipodermatosclerosis: a five year follow-up. In Davidson J F, Bachmann F, Bouvier C A, Kruithof EKO (Eds) *Progress in Fibrinolysis*. Vol 6. Edinburgh. Churchill Livingstone 1983; 526.

32. Burnand K G, Pattison M, Layer G T. How effective and long lasting are elastic stockings? In Negus D, Jantet G (Eds) *Phlebology '85*. London. Libbey 1986.

33. Burns D A, Sarkany I. Management of stasis ulcers by pinch graft. *Br J Dermatol* 1976; **95** Suppl 14: 82.

34. Callam M J, Dale J J, Ruckley C V, Harper D R. Trial of ultrasound in the treatment of chronic leg ulceration. In Negus D, Jantet G (Eds) *Phlebology '85*. London. Libbey 1986.

35. Callam M J, Ruckley C V, Harper D R, Dale J J. Chronic ulceration of the leg: extent of the problem and provision of care. *Br Med J* 1985; **290**: 1855.

36. Carion J, Debelle M, Goldschmidt J P. New therapeutic measures for the treatment of ulcers. *Phlebologie* 1978; **31**: 4: 339.

37. Celsus A C. *Of Medicine in Eight Books*. Trans Grieve J. London. Wilson 1756.

38. Chilvers A S, Freeman G K. Outpatient skin grafting of venous ulcers. *Lancet* 1969; **2**: 1087.

39. Clarke R L, Orandi A, Cliffton E E. Tourniquet induction of fibrinolysis. *Angiology* 1960; **11**: 367.

40. Cockett F B, Elgan Jones D. The ankle blow-out syndrome; a new approach to the varicose ulcer problem. *Lancet* 1953; **1**: 17.

41. Cockett F B. The pathology and treatment of venous ulcers of the leg. *Br J Surg* 1955; **43**: 260.

42. Conrad P. Treatment of varicose veins and venous ulcers. *Med J Aust* 1977; **1**: 144.

43. Coopwood T B. Evaluation of a topical enzymatic debridement agent. Sutilains Ointment: a preliminary report. *South Med J* 1976; **69**: 834.

44. Cornwall J V, Doré C, Lewis J D. To graduate or not? The effect of compression garments on venous refilling time. In Negus D, Jantet G (Eds) *Phlebology '85*. London. Libbey 1986.

45. Cornwall J V, Gilliland E L. Controlled trial of Iodosorb in chronic venous ulcer (Letter). *Br Med J* 1985; **291**: 902.

46. Cornwall J V, Lewis J D. Leg ulcers re-visited. *Br J Surg* 1983; **70**: 681.

47. Cottonot F, Carton F X, Tessler L, Lamoure B, Denoeux J P, Ceccaldi F, Kerner S. Incidences economiques du mode de traitement des ulceres de jambe. *Phlebologie* 1979; **32**: 333.

48. Cranley J J, Krause R J, Strasser E S. Chronic venous insufficiency of the lower extremity. *Surgery* 1961; **49**: 48.

49. Crichett G. *Lectures on the Cause and Treatment of Ulcers of the Lower Extremity*. London. Churchill 1849.

50. Curwen I H M, Scott B O. The ambulant treatment of the complications resulting from varicose veins and allied conditions. *Arch Phys Med Rehabil* 1953; **1**: 17.

51. Dale J, Callam M, Ruckley C V. How efficient is a compressive bandage? *Nursing Times* 1983; **Nov 16**: 49.

52. Dale W A. Peripheral venous reconstruction. In Dale W A (Ed) *Surgical Problems*. New York. McGraw Hill 1985; 493.

53. Daniel F, Foix C, Zaegel R. Le collagene approche physiologique de la cicatrisation cutanee. Son application dans la traitement partique des ulceres de jambe. *Sem Hop Paris* 1978; **54**: 833.

54. De Palma R G. Surgical therapy for venous stasis. *Surgery* 1974; **76**: 910.

55. de Takats G, Graupner G W. Division of the popliteal vein in deep venous insufficiency of the lower extremities. *Surgery* 1951; **29**: 342.

56. Dickson Wright A. Treatment of varicose ulcers. *Br Med J* 1930; **2**: 996.

57. Dodd H J, Tatnall F M, Gaylarde P M, Sarkany I. The effect of ultraviolet irradiation on skin oxygen tension and its potential role in the management of venous leg ulcers. In Negus D, Jantet G (Eds) *Phlebology '85*. London. Libbey 1986.

58. Dodd H, Calo A R, Mistry M, Rushford A. Ligation of the ankle communicating veins in the treatment of the venous ulcer syndrome of the leg. *Lancet* 1957; **2**: 1249.

59. Dodd H, Cockett FB. *The Pathology and Surgery of the Veins of the Lower Limb.* London. Churchill Livingstone 1976.

60. Dyson M, Franks C, Suckling J. Stimulation of healing of varicose ulcers by ultrasound. *Ultrasonics* 1976; **14**: 232.

61. Egan TJ, O'Driscoll J, Thakar DR. Human amnion in the management of chronic ulceration of the lower limb: a clinico-pathological study. *Angiology* 1983; **34**: 197.

62. Evans CD, Harman RRM, Warin RP. Varicose ulcers and the use of topical corticosteroids. *Br Med J* 1967; **2**: 482.

63. Famulari C, Monaco M, Versaci A, Perri S, Terranova ML, Cuzzocrea D. L'azione della N-acetil-idrossiprolina nella guarigione della lesioni ulcerative cutanee. *Ann Ital Chir* 1979; **51**: 527.

64. Fegan WG. *Varicose Veins and Compression Sclerotherapy.* London. Heinemann 1971.

65. Fischer BH. Treatment of ulcers of the legs with hyperbaric oxygen. *J Dermatol Surg* 1975; **1**: 55.

66. Fontaine R. Remarks concerning venous thrombosis and its sequelae. *Surgery* 1957; **41**: 6.

67. Foote RR. *Varicose Veins.* London. Butterworths 1954.

68. Galen C. *Ad Scripti Libri.* Venice. Vincentium Valgrisium 1562.

69. Gallaso U, Fiumano F, Cloro L, Strati V. L'uso dell'acido ialuronico nella terapia delle ulcere varicose degli arti inferiori. *Minerva Chir* 1978; **33**: 1581.

70. Greaves MW, Ive FA, Skillen AW. Effects of long continued ingestion of zinc sulphate in patients with venous leg ulceration. *Lancet* 1970; **2**: 889.

71. Greaves MW, Ive FA. Double blind trial of zinc sulphate in the treatment of chronic venous leg ulceration. *Br J Dermatol* 1972; **87**: 632.

72. Groenewald JH. An evaluation of Dextranomer as a cleansing agent in the treatment of postphlebitic stasis ulcer. *S Afr Med J* 1980; **57**: 809.

73. Groenewald JH. The treatment of varicose stasis ulcer. A controlled trial. *Praxis* 1981; **70**: 1273.

74. Gupta PD, Saunders WA. Chronic leg ulcers in the elderly treated with absolute bedrest. *Practitioner* 1982; **226**: 1611.

75. Haeger K. Preoperative treatment of leg ulcers with silver spray and aluminium foil. *Acta Chir Scand* 1963; **125**: 32.

76. Haeger K. Topical treatment of varicose ulcers. *Br J Med* 1930; **2**: 996.

77. Haeger K. *Venous and Lymphatic Disorders of the Leg.* Copenhagen. Scandinavian University Books 1966.

78. Hallböök T, Lanner E. Serum-zinc and healing of venous leg ulcers. *Lancet* 1972; **2**: 780.

79. Hansen ET. Amniotic grafts in chronic skin ulceration. *Lancet* 1950; **1**: 850.

80. Harkiss KJ. Cost analysis of dressing materials used in venous leg ulcers. *Pharm J* 1985; **31**: 268.

81. Harms W. Lokale therapie insbensondere der Ulzera. *Hautarzt* 1979; **30**: 210.

82. Hellgren L. Cleansing properties of stabilized trypsin and streptokinase-streptodornase in necrotic leg ulcers. *Eur J Clin Pharmacol* 1983; **24**: 623.

83. Henry MEF, Fegan WG, Pegum JM. Five year survey of the treatment of varicose ulcers. *Br Med J* 1971; **2**: 493.

84. Hills NH, Pflug JJ, Jeyasingh K, Boardman L, Calnan JS. Prevention of deep vein thrombosis by intermittent compression of calf. *Br Med J* 1972; **1**: 131.

85. Hippocrates 460 BC. *"De Ulceribus" – The genuine works of Hippocrates.* Adams F (Trans and Ed). London. Sydenham Society 1849.

86. Holm J, Holmstedt B. Skin transplantation of venous ulcers using a fibrinogen glue. In Negus D, Jantet G (Eds) *Phlebology '85.* London. Libbey 1986.

87. Horner J, Fernandes e Fernandes J, Nicolaides AN. Value of graduated compression stockings in deep venous insufficiency. *Br Med J* 1980; **280**: 820.

88. Hunt T. *A Guide to the Treatment of Diseases of the Skin: with Suggestions for their Prevention* 4th edition. London. Richards 1859.

89. Hunter J. *The works of John Hunter FRS.* Palmer JF (Ed) London. Longman 1835.

90. Husni EA. Venous reconstruction in postphlebitic disease. *Circulation* 1971; **43** Suppl: 147.

91. Hutinel B, Raider P. Le gel de collagene: un nouveau traitment dans la cicatrisation des ulceres de jambe. *Phlebologie* 1977; **30**: 317.

92. Johnson A. The economics of modern wound management. *Br J Pharm Pract* 1985; **7**: 294.

93. Jones NAG, Webb PJ, Rees RI, Kakkar VV. A physiological study of elastic compression stockings in venous disorders of the leg. *Br J Surg* 1980; **67**: 569.

94. Kaisary AV. A temporary biological dressing in the treatment of varicose ulcers and skin defects. *Postgrad Med J* 1977; **53**: 672.

95. Kartik I, Gulyas G. A lab boerhianyainak potolasa arteria dorsalis pedis szigetlebennyl. *Magy Traumatol Orthop* 1979; **22**: 146.

96. Keeling PWN, Jones RB, Hilton PJ, Thompson RPH. Reduced leucocyte zinc in liver disease. *Gut* 1980; **21**: 561.

97. Kistner RL, Sparkuhl MD. Surgery in acute and chronic venous disease. *Surgery* 1979; **85**: 31.

98. Kistner RL. Surgical repair of the incompetent femoral vein valve. *Arch Surg* 1975; **110**: 1336.

99. Linton RR, Hardy IB. Post-thrombotic syndrome of the lower extremity. Treatment by interruption of the superficial femoral vein and ligation and stripping of the long and short saphenous veins. *Surgery* 1948; **24**: 452.

100. Linton RR. The post-thrombotic ulceration of the lower extremity: its etiology and surgical treatment. *Ann Surg* 1953; **138**: 415.

101. Lofgren KA, Lauvstad WA, Bonnemaison MFE. Surgical treatment of large stasis ulcer: review of 129 cases. *Mayo Clin Proc* 1965; **40**: 560.

102. Lofgren KA. Stasis ulcer: Diagnosis and treatment. *Minn Med* 1974; **57**: 135.

103. Luff R. Personal Communication. 1986.

104. Margraf HW, Covey TH. A trial of silver-zinc-allantoinate in the treatment of leg ulcers. *Arch Surg* 1977; **112**: 699.

105. Marmasse J. La methode compressive a travers les ages. *Phlebologie* 1979; **32**: 119.

106. Mian E, Currie SB, Lietti A, Bombardelli E. Antocianosidi e parete dei microvasi nuovi aspetti sul modo d'azione dell effetto protettivo nelle sindromi da abnorme fragilita a capillare. *Minerva Med* 1977; **68**: 3565.

107. Monk BE, Sarkany I. Outcome of venous stasis ulcers. *Clin Exp Dermatol* 1982; **7**: 397.

108. Morgan DA. *The Care and Management of Leg Ulcers*. UKCPA Boot's Award. 1984.

109. Morris WT, Lamb AM. The Auckland hospital varicose veins and venous ulcer clinic: a report on six years work. *NZ Med J* 1981; **93**: 350.

110. Morrison JD. Debrisan. An effective new wound cleanser. *Scott Med J* 1979; **23**: 277.

111. Moss C, Taylor A, Shuster S. Controlled trial of Iodosorb in chronic venous ulcers. *Br Med J* 1985; **291**: 902.

112. Munro-Ashman EJ, Wells RS. The treatment time for varicose ulcers. *Br J Clin Pract* 1968; **22**: 129.

113. Myers MB, Cherry G. Zinc and leg ulcers. *Am J Surg* 1970; **120**: 77.

114. Myers MB, Richter M, Cherry G. Relationship between edema and the healing rate of stasis ulcers of the leg. *Am J Surg* 1972; **124**: 666.

115. Negus D, Friedgood A. The effective management of venous ulceration. *Br J Surg* 1983; **70**: 623.

116. Negus D. Prevention and treatment of venous ulceration. *Ann R Coll Surg Engl* 1985; **67**: 144.

117. Nielubowitcz J, Szostek M. Recurrences after the Linton flap operation. *J Cardiovasc Surg* 1979; **20**: 49.

118. Ormiston MC, Seymour MTJ, Venn GE, Cohen RI, Fox JA. Controlled trial of Iodosorb in chronic venous ulcers. *Br Med J* 1985; **291**: 308.

119. Osmundsen PE. Contact dermatitis to chlorhexidine. *Contact Dermatitis* 1982; **8 (2)**: 81.

120. Palma EC, Esperon R. Sapheno-femoral bypass. Vein transplants and grafts in the surgical treatment of the post-phlebitic syndrome. *J Cardiovasc Surg* 1960; **1**: 94.

121. Palmieri B, Boraldi F. Trattamento topico di alcune lesioni distrofiche a flogistiche della cute e dei tissuti molli. *Arch Sci Med (Torino)* 1977; **134**: 481.

122. Papageorgiou VP. Wound healing properties of naphthaquinone pigments from Alkanna tinctoria. *Experientia* 1978; **34**: 1499.

123. Paré A. (trans and ed Johnson T). *The works of the Famous Chirurgian Ambrose Paré*. London. Cotes et Du Gard 1649.

124. Partsch H. Do we need firm compression stockings exerting high pressure? *Vasa* 1984; **13**: 52.

125. Patman RD. Sympathectomy in the treatment of chronic venous leg ulcers. *Arch Surg* 1982; **117**: 1561.

126. Pattison M, Stacey MC, Layer GT, Burnand KG. Which elastic bandage gives the best compression? *Phlebology* 1987; in press.

127. Petit JL. *Traites des Maladies Chirurgicales* Vol II. Paris. Mequignon 1790.

128. Pflug JJ. Intermittent compression of the swollen leg in general practice. *The Practitioner* 1975; **215**: 69.

129. Phillips A, Davidson M, Greaves MW. Venous leg ulceration: Evaluation of zinc treatment, serum zinc and rate of healing. *Clin Exp Dermatol* 1978; **2**: 395.

130. Pickrell K, Thompson L, Nichol T, Kasdan M. The surgical treatment of varicose ulcers. *Am Surg* 1970; **36**: 55.

131. Poskitt KR, James AJ, Lloyd-Davies ERV, Walton J, McCollum CN. Pinch grafting of porcine dermis in venous ulcers. A randomised trial. *Br Med J* 1987. In press.

132. Psathakis N. Has the "substitute valve" at the popliteal vein solved the problem of venous insufficency of the lower extremity? *J Cardiovasc Surg* 1968; **9**: 64.

133. Pulvertaft T. Paroven in the treatment of chronic venous insufficiency. *The Practitioner* 1979; **223**: 838.

134. Rundle JSH, Cameron SH, Ruckley CV. New porcine dermis dressing for varicose and traumatic leg ulcers. *Br Med J* 1976; **2**: 216.

135. Rundle JSH, Elton RA, Cameron SH, Watson N, Gunn AA, Ruckley CV. Porcine dermis in

varicose ulcersa clinical trial. *Vasa* 1981; **10**: 246.

136. Ryan T. *The Management of Leg Ulcers*. Oxford. Oxford Medical Publishers 1983.

137. Sawyer PN, Dowbak G, Sophie Z, Feller J, Cohen L. A preliminary report of the efficacy of Debrisan (Dextranomer) in the debridement of cutaneous ulcers. *Surgery* 1979; **85**: 201.

138. Schraibman I, Stratton FJ. Nutritional status of patients with leg ulcers. *J R Soc Med* 1985; **78**: 39.

139. Sethia KK, Darke SG. Long saphenous incompetence as a cause of venous ulceration. *Br J Surg* 1984; **71**: 754.

140. Sharp S. *A Treatise on the Operations of Surgery* 7th edition. London. Tonson 1758.

141. Sigel B, Edelstein AL, Savitch L, Hasty JH, Felix WR. Types of compression for reducing venous stasis. *Arch Surg* 1975; **110**: 171.

142. Sigg K. Compression with pressure bandages and elastic stockings for prophylaxis and therapy of venous disorders of the leg. *Fortschr Med* 1963; **15**: 601.

143. Sigg K. *Varizen, Ulcus Cruris and Thrombose* 3rd edition. Berlin. Springer 1968.

144. Skog E, Arnesjö B, Troëng T, Gjöres JE, Bergljung L, Gundersen J, Hallböök T, Hessman Y, Hillström L, Mansson T, Eilard U, Eklöf B, Plate G, Norgren L. A randomized trial comparing cadexomer iodine and standard treatment in the out-patient management of chronic venous ulcers. *Br J Dermatol* 1983; **109**: 77.

145. Somerville PG. The possible use of amniotic membrane in chronic leg ulcers. *Phlebologie* 1982; **35**: 223.

146. Spender JK. *A Manual of the Pathology and Treatment of Ulcers and Cutaneous Diseases of the Lower Limbs*. London. Churchill 1866.

147. Stacey-Clear A, Cornwall JV, Lewis JD. Intravenous prostacyclins (PGI₂) and skin grafting for rheumatoid leg ulcers. In Negus D, Jantet G (Eds) *Phlebology '85*. London. Libbey 1986.

148. Starling EH. On the absorbtion of fluid from the connective tissue spaces. *J Physiol (Lond)* 1896; **19**: 312.

149. Stemmer R, Marescaux J, Furderer C. Compression treatment of the lower extremities particularly with compression stockings. *The Dermatologist* 1980; **31**: 355.

150. Stemmer R. Ambulatory elasto-compressive treatment of the lower extremities particularly with elastic stockings. *Der Kassenarzt* 1969; **9**: 1.

151. Taheri SA, Lazar L, Elias SM, Marchand P. Vein valve transplant. *Surgery* 1982; **91**: 28.

152. Thomas AMC, Tomlinson PJ, Boggon RP. Incompetent perforating vein ligation in the treatment of venous ulceration. *Ann R Coll Surg Engl* 1986; **68**: 214.

153. Trelford JD, Trelford-Sauder M. The amnion in surgery, past and present. *Am J Obstet Gynecol* 1977; **134**: 835.

154. Underwood M. *A Treatise upon Ulcers of the Legs*. London. Mathews 1783.

155. Unna PG. *Die Histopathologie der Hautkrankheiten*. Berlin. Verlag Hirschwald 1894.

156. Van den Berg E, Borgnis FE, Bollinger AA, Wupperman Th, Alexander K. A new method for measuring the effective compression of medical stockings. *Vasa* 1982; **11**: 117.

157. Van der Molen HR. The choice of compressive methods in phlebology. *Phlebologie* 1982; **35**: 73.

158. Vin F. Corticotherapie locale ablusive en phlébologie. A propos d'une observation. *Phlebologie* 1982; **35**: 819.

159. Warren R, Thayer TR. Transplantation of the saphenous vein for post-phlebitic stasis. *Surgery* 1954; **35**: 867.

160. Weitgasser H, Schmidt-Modrow G. Trental forte in der ulcus cruris-therapie. Ergebnis einer feldstudie. *Z Hautkr* 1982; **57**: 1574.

161. Weitgasser H. The use of pentoxifylline (Trental 400) in the treatment of leg ulcers: results of a double-blind trail. *Pharmatherapeutica* 1983; **3**: 143.

162. Westlake BC, Hasty JH. An analysis of factors to be addressed in the measurement of elastic compression. In Negus D, Jantet G (Eds) *Phlebology '85*. London. Libbey 1986.

163. White RP. Ulcers of the legs, miscalled varicose: a clinical review. *Br J Dermatol* 1918; **30**: 138.

164. Wilson IAI, Henry M, Quill RD, Byrne PJ. The pH of varicose ulcer surfaces and its relationship to healing. *Vasa* 1979; **8**: 339.

165. Wiseman R. *Eight Chirurgical Treatises*. London. Tooke & Meredith 1676.

166. Zelikowski A, Argranat A, Sternberg A, Haddad M, Urca I. The conservative treatment of stasis ulcer. *Angiology* 1978; **29**: 832.

16

Deep vein thrombosis: pathology

A thrombus is a semi-solid mass, formed from the components of the blood, which has developed in the bloodstream within the heart or blood vessels. A clot is blood which has coagulated *in vitro* (i.e. in a test tube). A deep vein thrombosis is a thrombus which has formed in the veins beneath the deep fascia of the leg. Thrombus within the pelvic or abdominal veins that carry blood from the legs is also commonly classified as 'deep vein thrombosis' and some authorities would include thrombus in the communicating veins of the lower limb within the definition (Fig. 16.1).

Prevalence and incidence of deep vein thrombosis

The true prevalence of deep vein thrombosis in the population is unknown, as many cases without symptoms pass undetected.[319]

Clinical evidence

In 1956 Gjöres[107] attempted to assess the prevalence of deep vein thrombosis in Sweden. As this study relied on clinical diagnosis, it undoubtedly underestimated the occurrence of deep vein thrombosis, but it suggested that 2–3 per cent of the population had had a deep vein thrombosis at some time.

In a large survey of 158,200 medical, surgical and gynaecological patients who were admitted to hospital, Barker *et al.*[19] found an overall incidence of deep vein thrombosis of 0.95 per cent, and a 0.57 per cent incidence of pulmonary embolism, which was fatal in 0.22 per cent.

Among 334,355 patients admitted to the Charity Hospital in New Orleans, USA, in 1951, 590 patients had the clinical signs of deep vein thrombosis, an incidence of 0.02 per cent.[234]

Forty-five per cent of these patients had pulmonary emboli.

In 1941 Welch and Faxton[319] suggested that clinical tests were very insensitive after finding that only 5.5 per cent of 128 cases of fatal pulmonary embolism had clinical evidence of a preceding thrombosis. This was confirmed by the work of Gibbs[106] and Sevitt and Gallagher[266,267] who found no physical signs in two-thirds of the patients who were shown to have a deep vein thrombosis at autopsy. Further confirmation was provided when the fibrinogen uptake test was developed.[96,139,215] Consequently none of the clinical studies of the incidence of deep vein thrombosis or pulmonary embolism has any scientific validity, and it is now accepted that surveys of this condition must be based upon objective methods of diagnosis.

Phlebographic evidence

In 1976 Nylander and Olivecrona[230] performed phlebograms on all patients presenting to the only hospital in Malmö with any symptoms in the legs suggestive of deep vein thrombosis. Evidence of thrombosis was seen in 231 of these phlebograms. The population served by this hospital was 263,000; the incidence of deep vein thrombosis was therefore of 0.9/1000/year (0.09 per cent). As the indications for phlebography were clinical signs, this study suffers from the same defects as the other clinical studies mentioned above, but it does give an indication of the incidence of 'clinical' deep vein thrombosis in the 'normal' population.

Extrapolating from all the postoperative surveys that have been made,[32,68] it is reasonable to assume that at least twice as many patients are having silent thromboses and that the true inci-

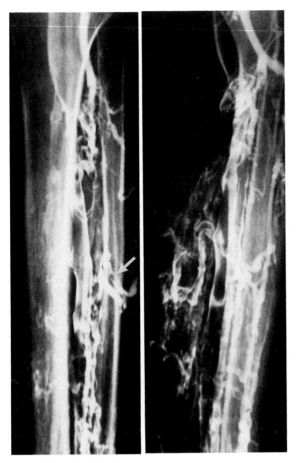

Fig. 16.1 An ascending phlebogram showing extensive thrombus throughout the deep veins of the calf. Thrombus is seen in the tibial and peroneal veins, and on the lateral projection there is extensive thrombus within the soleal sinusoids. The arrow points to a small thrombus within a calf communicating vein which is seen as a small circular filling defect.

dence of deep vein thrombosis is nearer 0.27 per cent. This figure takes no account of all the patients who are admitted to hospital with a serious illness or for an operation; one-third of these patients will develop a thrombosis.

In 1977 Nylander and his colleagues[229] found that 24 per cent of the phlebograms which showed evidence of recent or old thrombosis came from patients who had had an operation and 8 per cent came from patients who had had a major injury. These percentages agree surprisingly well with the survey by Gjöres[107] of patients with 'clinical' thrombosis. Surgery and trauma has therefore been shown to be responsible for approximately one-third of all deep vein thromboses in Scandinavia over the last 30 years.

The prevalence of thrombosis in the general population will be increased by a number which is approximately equivalent to one-third of all the operations and major injuries occurring in the population. This is a figure which is not available and which will vary considerably from decade to decade and between countries.

Autopsy evidence

Autopsy only provides the incidence of deep vein thrombosis in patients who have died as a result of pulmonary embolism or other causes. Autopsy does not determine the incidence of thrombosis in those patients with the same diseases who have not died. In 1961 Sevitt and Gallagher[267] reported that 60 per cent of all autopsies in patients who had died after injuries or burns showed thrombosis in the deep veins; pulmonary embolism was found in 20 per cent of these examinations and in 16 per cent the emboli were considered to be large enough to have caused death.

Morrell and Dunhill[206] found an incidence of pulmonary embolism at autopsy of 63 per cent in surgical patients and 45 per cent in medical patients. Havig[129] found a similar incidence (55 per cent) of macroscopic evidence of pulmonary embolism in a randomly selected group of autopsies, and evidence of microscopic emboli was found in another 14 per cent of autopsies; the overall incidence was therefore 69 per cent. Pulmonary embolism was thought to be the cause of death in 33 per cent of patients and to be a major factor in 19 per cent. These figures must be accepted with caution because it is extremely difficult for a pathologist to estimate the significance of a pathological finding in the event of death from pulmonary embolism, which is primarily a pathophysiological abnormality. In Havig's study two-thirds of the deep vein thrombi were within the ilio-femoral segment, and only one-third were confined to the calf or foot. Embolism appeared to be the immediate cause of death in 7 of the 31 patients who died postoperatively.

The incidence of fatal pulmonary embolism after surgery, based on a few large series of patients who had autopsies because they died after a surgical operation,[16,156,172,253] has been found to be between 0.4 per cent and 1.6 per cent.

Two studies in 1981 suggested that the incidence of pulmonary embolism was beginning to decline.[82,252] It is not clear whether this decline is the result of effective prophylactic regimens which have been used with increasing vigour over the past 20 years or the result of a real change in the natural history of the disease.

All the autopsy studies show that pulmonary embolism complicates at least one in every 30 cases of deep vein thrombosis (see Chapter 21).

Deep vein thrombosis and surgery

Incidence of postoperative deep vein thrombosis

Our knowledge of the incidence of postoperative deep vein thrombosis is much better than our knowledge of the incidence of deep vein thrombosis in the general population who may be forming and lysing small thrombi all the time. The incidence of postoperative thrombosis does, however, depend upon the method used for its detection (see Chapter 4).

The radioactive fibrinogen uptake test has been extensively employed as a screening test but bipedal ascending phlebography remains the gold standard for diagnosis. The fibrinogen uptake test,[59,169] plethysmography,[76,327] Doppler ultrasound[257] and thermography[256] each have areas of inaccuracy. Even phlebography relies on interpretation, and studies have shown that radiological reports may differ by as much as 10 per cent.

The ideal method for assessing the incidence of postoperative thrombosis is pre-operative and postoperative phlebography but only a few such studies, involving small numbers of patients, have been carried out.[30] Several studies have used postoperative phlebography alone,[32] and in many studies phlebography has been employed to confirm the accuracy of a positive fibrinogen uptake test.[32,168]

The ^{125}I fibrinogen uptake test is the most commonly used method for assessing the effect of prophylactic regimens. Although it probably detects small calf thrombi more efficiently than phlebography,[54,169] it cannot be used in the presence of superficial thrombophlebitis, wounds, fractures, ulcers, cellulitis or arthritis in the leg – all of which produce false-positive scans (see Chapter 4, page 102). Unfortunately, we do not know the clinical significance of very small calf

thrombi,[36,87] though there is a correlation between the risk of pulmonary embolism and a positive fibrinogen uptake test.[48,250,253,316] Nevertheless, the fibrinogen uptake test remains the best simple, almost non-invasive test that is available and, despite its disadvantages, it has been instrumental in expanding our understanding of the factors that affect the incidence of post-operative thrombosis.

Incidence of pre-operative deep vein thrombosis

The majority of thrombi develop in the deep veins of the calf in the first 5 days after an operation but some thrombi begin to develop before the operation.

Four studies have used phlebography to screen patients awaiting an operation. Thrombi were found in 5 out of 60 patients awaiting prostatectomy,[23] in 3 out of 40 patients awaiting hip replacement,[30] in 10 out of 50 patients awaiting operations on the gastrointestinal tract[131] and in 7 out of 47 patients awaiting operation on hip fractures.[285] Thus between 5 and 15 per cent of patients begin their operation with a thrombus already present in their calf veins.

Deep vein thrombosis after general surgery

Bergqvist[32] has summarized the published data and has computed an average incidence of thrombosis of 29 per cent from 28 studies on 1081 general surgical patients in whom the fibrinogen uptake test has been used for screening. This figure of 29 per cent for general surgical patients *not* given any form of prophylaxis has been confirmed.[68,251] Malignant disease appears to increase the risk of developing a postoperative thrombosis[31] but the effect of splenectomy, which was thought to be associated with a higher incidence of thrombosis, remains unproven as the results are conflicting.[56,78]

Deep vein thrombosis after urological surgery

There is a significantly greater incidence of thrombosis after open prostatectomy (38 per cent) than after general surgical operations[32,69] but a much lower incidence (11 per cent) after transurethral resection of the prostate.[51,132,196,219,275] The administration of epsilon-aminocaproic acid, an antifibrinolytic agent which is commonly given after prostatectomy to reduce bleeding, does not appear to increase the risk of deep vein thrombosis or pulmonary embolism.[308]

Deep vein thrombosis after gynaecological surgery

The incidence of thrombosis after gynaecological surgery varies between 29 per cent[18] and 14 per cent.[314] Thrombosis appears to be less common after gynaecological operations than after general surgical operations (19 per cent)[32] even after making an allowance for the younger age of many of the gynaecological patients. The adverse effect of malignancy on thrombosis was confirmed when thrombosis was found in 35 per cent of a group of patients who had a hysterectomy for carcinoma, compared with 12 per cent when the hysterectomy was performed for benign disease.[314]

Deep vein thrombosis after vascular surgery

In a group of patients who had phlebograms after *femoro-popliteal bypass surgery* 43 per cent had evidence of a deep vein thrombosis;[124] other investigators have found a lower incidence of approximately 8 per cent.[155,211]

The incidence of thrombosis, estimated by the fibrinogen uptake test, following *aorto-iliac surgery* has varied between 21 per cent and 32 per cent.[8,26,126] When Doppler flow detection was combined with the fibrinogen uptake test, the incidence was 13 per cent.[243] This figure is closer to the 4 per cent incidence reported by Satiani *et al.*,[259] who used a combination of the fibrinogen uptake test with impedance plethysmography, and reported that the fibrinogen uptake test gave many false-positive results.

Operations on *varicose veins* are reported to carry a low incidence of deep vein thrombosis[83,194] but objective studies have not been performed, perhaps because of the fear of inducing venous thrombosis in a recently traumatized venous system. The incidence after compression sclerotherapy is also reputed to be low.[140]

Deep vein thrombosis after fractures and orthopaedic surgery

Most of the studies involving the incidence of thrombosis in orthopaedic surgery have used

phlebography rather than the fibrinogen uptake test because leg wounds cause false-positive fibrinogen uptake tests and this test is inaccurate above the middle of the thigh. Since Bauer in 1944[21] showed a relationship between the site of thrombosis and the site of the fracture, it has been recognized that patients with fractures of the lower limb have an increased risk of thrombosis. Sevitt and Gallagher[266] showed that 29 (83 per cent) of 35 patients on whom an autopsy was performed after a fractured hip had evidence of deep vein thrombosis (Fig. 16.2).

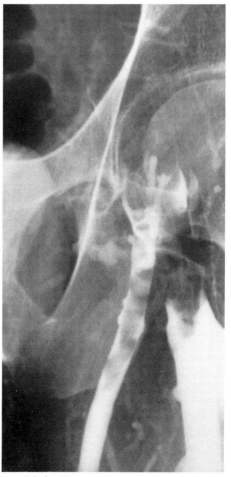

Fig. 16.2 Thrombus is seen as a filling defect within the common femoral and long saphenous vein in relation to a fracture of the neck of the femur (not visible on this film). The thrombus was localized to the area of the injury, the calf and popliteal veins did not contain any filling defects.

Most recently, with the advent of total hip replacement and the vast increase in these operations, it has been recognized that cold orthopaedic surgery also carries a high risk of thrombosis (see Chapter 19). It has been suggested[222,281] that the increased incidence of femoral vein thrombosis on the side of a hip replacement operation is caused by local trauma to the femoral vein when the hip is dislocated during the operation. The incidence of thrombosis beginning in the calf is, however, similar in both legs and Bergqvist's compilation[32] based on nine studies of the risk of venous thrombosis after hip fracture, shows that though 40 per cent of the thrombi occurred on the side of the fractured limb, 23 per cent developed in the opposite limb.

Deep vein thrombosis after neurosurgery

The incidence of thrombosis after neurosurgical operations is said to be approximately 30 per cent.[32]

Deep vein thrombosis after renal transplantation

Although this operation is thought to carry a high risk of thrombosis, there have been no good prospective, large-scale studies to confirm or refute this hypothesis.[32]

Deep vein thrombosis during pregnancy

Almost all the studies on thrombosis in pregnancy have been based on clinical signs because X-rays and radioactive isotopes are contra-indicated; the true incidence of thrombosis during pregnancy is therefore unknown.[10]

A pregnant woman is reported to have a five times greater risk of developing a deep vein thrombosis than a non-pregnant age-matched control,[264] and proximal left-sided thrombi are reputed to be more common in pregnancy.[29].

Aetiology of deep vein thrombosis

The above section on the incidence of thrombosis shows the important role of surgery, trauma and intercurrent illness in the development of thrombosis. These factors, together with a number which will be discussed at the end of this section, are contributory rather than truly causative factors in the development of thrombosis.

The mechanisms that cause blood to coagulate *in vivo* are still poorly understood. The mechanism responsible for thrombosis in arteries appears to be different to that responsible for thrombosis in veins, and there may even be differences in the composition of thrombi in various parts of the vascular system.[239] Thrombus in arteries with little or no blood flow consists of a fibrin mesh and red cells; the thrombus in a free-flowing system consists of a laminate of platelets and fibrin (the white head) with fibrin and red cells in its propagating tail.

Although Wiseman described pulmonary embolism in 1676[333] and Hunter[154] described 'phlebo-thrombosis' in his *Treatise on the blood, inflammation and gun-shot wounds*, it was Rudolph Virchow[309] who recognized the association between the two conditions and went on to propose the famous triad of causes for thrombosis.

1. Changes in the lining of the vessel wall (wall damage)
2. Changes in the flow of blood (stasis)
3. Changes in the constituents of the blood (hypercoagulability)

Much time and energy has been expended to try to discover which of these mechanisms, alone or in combination, is the most important in the generation of a thrombus.

It was known as early as 1922 that the blood fibrinogen increased in response to trauma[99] but it was not until the discovery of the coagulation cascade,[34,186] that the modern era of thrombosis research began. Early experimental work showed that platelets accumulated on the walls of damaged vessels,[35,321] particularly during periods of low blood flow.[88]

Von Recklinghausen[313] suggested that the deposition of thrombus was related to eddy currents, a fact that was confirmed when deposits of platelets were found at sites of turbulent flow in arteriovenous shunts.[249] In 1929 Evans[93] associated the postoperative increase in circulating platelets, with an increased risk of thrombosis.

In 1922 Aschoff[12] described the pathological changes that occurred in a developing thrombus and suggested that this process could only occur if there was an associated slowing of blood flow. He chose to ignore a considerable number of earlier studies[22,108,134,179,265] which showed that blood trapped in a vessel between two ligatures did not clot immediately but remained fluid for several hours.

In 1934 Homans[143] recognized the high incidence of thrombosis in the deep veins of the lower limb and proposed the role of 'stasis' in its development. He produced thrombosis by injecting a mixture of saline and 'muscle juice' into a segment of a dog's femoral vein that had been occluded by ligatures, and he noticed that a thrombus did not form if a collateral vein draining the occluded segment was left untied.

In 1942 Wright[337] reported an increase in the number of circulating platelets and their adhesiveness in the postoperative period, and several other workers described increases in blood coagulability that were associated with a clinical deep vein thrombosis.[81,201,235,271,272,318]

In 1950 Ochsner, DeBakey and Decamp,[234] in their large survey of venous thrombosis, suggested that the shortened prothrombin times and high antithrombin levels found in some of their patients might lead to thrombosis when combined with 'circulatory stasis'.

In 1956 Wright et al.,[336] using a radioisotope clearance technique, showed that the velocity of venous flow was reduced in limbs that were horizontal at rest, and increased with elevation or movement. This provided a rationale for the practice of early ambulation after operation[37,58,177,240] and the wearing of elastic stockings,[329,330] both these practices have been reported to reduce the incidence of thrombosis.

At the end of the 1950s two important autopsy studies on the location of thrombi in the deep veins of the lower limb were carried out.[106,267] These investigations observed that the majority of thrombi developed in the venous sinusoids of the soleus muscle.

By the end of the 1950s most investigators believed that stasis was the major factor responsible for the development of venous thrombosis, but, apart from some simple studies on coagulation factors, the relationship between coagulation and thrombosis remained largely unexplored. The role of vein wall damage was largely discredited by the failure to find any endothelial abnormalities beneath the origins of thrombi, even though the limitations of the histological techniques available at the time were clearly recognized.[197,233,255]

During the last 30 years more information about coagulation and wall abnormalities has appeared and, though the role of stasis is still widely accepted as a major contributory factor in the development of venous thrombosis, most of the current arguments concern the significance of vessel wall abnormalities and hypercoagulability of the blood.

Endothelial damage

Prostacyclin, bradykinin, angiotensin, adenonucleotides, plasminogen activator, tissue urokinase, factor VIII related protein, and glycosamino glycans are synthesized by the endothelial cell.[192] Some or all of these substances may help to prevent the deposition of thrombi, control local permeability or have some local effect on blood coagulation and fibrinolysis.

Although it is readily accepted that ulceration or rupture of an atheromatous plaque in an artery leads to exposure of collagen which stimulates platelet and fibrinogen deposition,[13,100,208,209,210,239] there is little evidence that endothelial damage and subendothelial collagen exposure occurs in veins.[152,238,309] Many of the attempts to discover venous endothelial changes beneath thrombus, have, however, used standard transmission microscopy, a technique now accepted as severely limited.[197,233,255]

The high incidence of thrombosis found in the veins of the lower limb in patients who have sustained tibial fractures,[138,231] supports the hypothesis that endothelial injury can cause deep vein thrombosis. The distortion of the femoral vein that occurs during total hip replacement is also associated with a high incidence of femoral vein thrombosis close to the site of injury.[281]

Many of the experimental systems for producing deep vein thrombosis in animals have relied on causing severe endothelial damage, often by introducing noxious materials into the vein.[153,203] Some systems produce a red propagating thrombus;[79,123] other systems induce a platelet thrombus[11,28,148,149,343] and their relevance to human deep vein thrombosis is therefore questionable. Ligation of the femoral vein of rabbits rarely induces thrombosis, unless it is combined with local or distant trauma, when the incidence of thrombosis is proportional to the extent of the trauma.[40] The animal models of Day et al.[79] and Hamer and Malone[123] appear to relate more closely to clinical deep vein thrombosis, and they may enable more detailed studies of the role of endothelial changes in thrombogenesis to be performed.

In a series of studies using scanning electron microscopy Stewart *et al.* have re-examined the role of the endothelium in thrombosis.[286,291] Stasis was produced in the jugular and femoral veins of the dog by gentle finger occlusion of the vein,[287] and in some experiments coincidental distant trauma was applied to another part of the animal.[290] Stewart showed that neither distant trauma nor stasis alone were capable of producing consistent changes in the endothelium but a combination of the two factors caused large numbers of white blood cells to adhere to the endothelial surface of the occluded vein.[288] These white cells then migrated through the intercellular junctions to accumulate between the endothelium and basement membrane. This migration was followed by patchy endothelial desquamation, exposing large areas of subendothelial collagen.

White cell migration in response to acute inflammation has been recognized for many years[59,67,97,335] but it had never before been ascribed a role in the production of venous thrombosis. The endothelial cells appeared be intact on scanning electron microscopy suggesting that the damage was produced by the white cells, rather than the endothelial cell damage resulting in white cell invasion.

Stewart *et al.*[288] also studied the consequences of white cell invasion at 6 and 24 hours, and at 3, 7, 15 and 28 days after the initial insult. At 6 hours white cell invasion was still apparent and amorphous material had accumulated on the areas of vein wall denuded of epithelium. One vein was said to contain a 'typical' venous thrombus consisting of red cells enmeshed with fibrin. By 24 hours the subendothelial white cells were no longer visible but the endothelium was extensively damaged with amorphous material scattered over its surface. After 28 days the appearances were returning to normal but the amorphous material and giant cells could still be seen.

Stewart[291] has emphasized the importance of 'early' examination of experimentally thrombosed veins, as many of the minor changes which she observed could easily have been missed because they disappeared within 24 hours. These changes were only clearly seen with scanning electron microscopy and would not have been detected by standard histological preparations.

The endothelial damage is patchily distributed, and leucocytes have a short life span and rapidly disappear.[62]

The jugular vein that had not been occluded showed a few adherent white cells without evidence of migration or endothelial shedding; this indicated that extensive distant tissue damage was capable of producing only minor local vessel wall changes if stasis was absent. Stewart suggested[291] that the leucotactic stimulus might be a component of the complement system activated by the release of antigen–antibody complexes[44] or endotoxins,[104,148,286] though any factor capable of increasing endothelial permeability might be responsible. She[291] felt that the stasis effect was not the result of ischaemic damage, but that stasis increased the leucotactic gradient thus enhancing white cell migration. Stasis may also alter the activity of coagulation factors and, if these factors accumulate on the vessel wall as a result of the injury, stasis may promote thrombosis.

Collagen is one of the best known stimuli of platelet activation and adhesion.[13,42,43,100,145,146,147,148,247,248,278,279,342] The small gaps in the endothelium described by Stewart *et al.*,[288] which may also be caused by the venous distension, may be sufficient to initiate thrombosis.

Anoxia is also known to produce endothelial damage,[189] and it has been suggested that relative anoxia within the valve cusps may render endothelial cells anoxic and cause them either to malfunction or to be shed.[122]

Regardless of whether thrombosis is the result of venous distension, mild anoxia or leucocyte migration, it may develop without overt macroscopic or histological signs of endothelial damage (Table 16.1).

Stewart has provided further support for her theory by showing that white cells are capable of binding fibrin and producing a red 'fibrin' venous type of thrombus rather than the platelet (arterial) thrombus that usually occurs on exposed collagen.

Doubt has been cast on Stewart's theory by Thomas *et al.*,[298] who recently re-examined the effect of a severe local venous crushing injury on the development of thrombosis in the jugular veins of rabbits. They found that though platelets rapidly adhered to the damaged surface, there was no fibrin formation at the injured site and the subsequent addition of stasis failed to generate stasis thrombi. They therefore failed to confirm

Table 16.1   Agents which are noxious to endothelium

Anoxia
Distension
Antibodies against endothelium
Sensitized lymphocytes
Circulating immune complexes
Complement and leucocytes
Oxygen free radicals
Platelet aggregations
Serotonin (5-hydroxytryptamine)
Adenosine diphosphate
Histamine
Prostaglandins
Increased wall shear
Thrombin

Stewart's findings and concluded that even severe vessel wall injury was a poor stimulus to fibrin formation at the site of injury.

Comment   Stewart's experiments have given considerable support to the concept of endothelial injury but there remain misgivings about the role of this mechanism in the genesis of human deep vein thrombosis, and a more subtle change of endothelial cell function remains a credible alternative. Improved methods of producing experimental thrombi may help to define the role of endothelial injury.[166]

Endothelial cell malfunction

Tissue plasminogen activators

The vein wall synthesizes and stores tissue plasminogen activator (Fig. 16.3).[14,183,300] Tissue plasminogen activator is released in response to a number of different stresses which include stasis, adrenaline, desmopressin, exercise and food.[15,44,94,226] Defective production or release of activator from the vein wall has been found to be associated with recurrent deep vein thrombosis.[70,157,163,165,181,283,292,294]

The tissue plasminogen activator activity of the vein wall is known to be depressed after prostatectomy[182] but is increased by other types of trauma.[338] Reduced levels of vein wall activator are found in patients with severe lipodermatosclerosis or post-thrombotic deep vein damage; it is not clear, however, if this is the cause or the

result of the initial thrombotic episode.[49,334]

Reduced levels of fibrinolytic activity have been detected in the soleal veins which are often the first veins to develop thrombus[216] but this finding has not been confirmed.[80,180] The fibrinolytic activity of the vein wall declines with age,[164] as the risk of postoperative deep vein thrombosis increases.

Nilsson *et al.*[225] studied plasminogen activator release in a group of patients with recurrent deep vein thromboses; they found reduced levels of activator production in some patients and normal levels of activator release with elevated levels of inhibitor in others. They have suggested that high levels of tissue plasminogen activator inhibitor might be responsible for recurrent thromboses in some patients. Doubt has been cast on the validity of this study[176] because activator and inhibitor levels were measured after the thrombosis had occurred and might be an effect of repeated thromboses rather than the cause.

All these observations on the association between alterations in fibrinolysis and venous

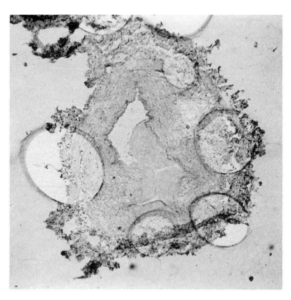

Fig. 16.3   The 'Todd' technique for detecting tissue plasminogen activator activity released from a vein wall.[300] Thin sections of fresh frozen vein are incubated on a film of fibrin placed on a microscope slide. Tissue plasminogen activator released from the vein wall during incubation initiates fibrinolysis seen as clear zones in the sheet of stained fibrin. The amount of lysis in individual sections can be compared by a scoring system.

thrombosis support the hypothesis that endothelial malfunction may alter the release of plasminogen activator or inhibitor, and may therefore be an important cause of venous thrombosis.

Prostacyclin

The pathway for prostacyclin production and degradation is shown in Table 16.2.

Prostacyclin (PGI_2) is a very unstable prostaglandin with a half life in serum of approximately 2 min. PGI_2 was first isolated, from arterial walls, in 1976 by Moncada and his colleagues.[204] It is a potent inhibitor of platelet aggregation and a smooth muscle relaxant.[205] It is thought to prevent platelet aggregation by increasing the intracellular concentration of cyclic adenosine diphosphate[297] which in turn blocks the synthesis of thromboxane by the platelets. It is conceivable that defective prostacyclin production by the endothelial cells of the vein wall could lead to deep vein thrombosis.

There is a report[174] of a single patient who experienced recurrent deep vein thromboses and spontaneous abortions and who later developed ovarian infarction and aortic thrombosis. No prostacyclin activity was detectable in tissue biopsies of this patient's arterial wall, and a sample of the patient's plasma abolished prostacyclin production by a rat aorta. Further studies may determine whether prostacyclin plays an important role in the aetiology of venous thrombosis.

The lupus anticoagulant

The lupus antiocoagulant is an immunoglobulin that may act by binding the phospholipid portion of the prothrombin activator complex thus prolonging the partial thromboplastin time.[39] It is also thought to interfere with release of arachadonic acid and the phospholipids from the cell membrane thus inhibiting the production of prostacyclin.[60,61] It seems that a reduced activity of prostacyclin is the result of a circulating inhibitor complex rather than a failure of the synthesis of PGI_2 by the endothelial cells.

Adenosine diphosphatase deficiency

Adenosine diphosphatase is the enzyme which converts adenosine-diphosphate to adenosine-monophosphate and adenosine, which both inhibit platelet aggregation. Theoretically, changes in enzyme activity could lead to an increased risk of thrombosis,[135,136] but this seems likely to be more important in the arteries than in the veins.[71,178]

Glycosoaminoglycans (GAGS)

These compounds are thought to be synthesized and stored in the walls of blood vessels.[112,159,213] Approximately 80 per cent of the glycosoaminoglycans stored in the vessel walls are in the form of heparan sulphate[55,173,207] which is a weaker anticoagulant than heparin itself. Smaller quantities of hyaluronic acid, chondroitin sulphate and heparin are also present in the vessel wall and are of doubtful significance. Heparan sulphate may act by accelerating the inactivation of thrombin by antithrombin III, but it also carries a strongly negative surface charge (as found on heparin), and this may help to maintain the ability of the endothelium to act as a continuous membrane and to resist thrombus forming on its surface.[260] There is insufficient information to justify attributing a role of intracellular glycosoaminoglycans in the development of venous thrombosis.

Table 16.2 Prostacylin and thromboxane metabolism*

Vessel wall	Platelet
Membrane phospholipids	Membrane phospholipids
$1 \rightarrow \quad \downarrow \quad \leftarrow A$	$1 \rightarrow \quad \downarrow \quad \leftarrow A$
Arachidonic acid	Arachidonic acid
$2 \rightarrow \quad \downarrow \quad \leftarrow B$	$2 \rightarrow \quad \downarrow \quad \leftarrow B$
Endoperoxides	Endoperoxides
$3 \rightarrow \quad \downarrow \quad \leftarrow C$	$4 \rightarrow \quad \downarrow \quad \leftarrow D$
Prostacylin	Thromboxane A_2
$\downarrow$	$\downarrow$
6-keto $PGF_{1\alpha}$	Thromboxane B_2

Enzyme activators	*Inhibitors*
A = Phospholipase A_2	1 Chloroquine and hydrocortisone
B = Cyclo-oxygenase	2 Acetylsalicylic acid and indomethacin
C = Prostacyclin synthetase	3 Tranylcypromine and 15-hydroperoxyarachidonic acid
D = Thromboxane synthetase	4 Nictindole and imidazole

* Modified from Bergqvist[32]

Antithrombin III

There is some evidence that this important inhibitor of coagulation may be present in endothelial cells.[17,63] Antithrombin III inhibits prothrombin activation to thrombin and also inhibits the activation of factor X. The significance of reduced tissue levels of antithrombin III in the genesis of venous thrombosis is not known.

Factor VIII

This factor, which has Von Willebrand-like activity, is known to be important in haemostasis and has been found in endothelial cells[38,141,160] where it can be localized by histochemical techniques. Factor VIII related antigen can be detected in the blood, and levels of this antigen have been found to rise after trauma.[56,227] This elevation may be important in the development of postoperative thrombosis but this has not yet been confirmed, and no relationship has been established between a rise in the level of antigen and the subsequent development of thrombosis.

Comment Endothelial malfunction may be important in the genesis of thrombosis but further evidence must be produced before this mechanism is generally accepted. Until recently the function of the endothelium has not been studied extensively, and the production of prostacyclin, tissue plasminogen activator, glycosoaminoglycans, coagulation factors and their inhibitors by the endothelial cell may be very important in the development of thrombosis. Alterations in the production of these substances (and others not yet discovered) may disturb the delicate balance between thrombosis and thrombolysis and may initiate a deep vein thrombosis.

Stasis

There are a number of clinical conditions in which obstructed or defective venous drainage is known to be associated with an increased risk of thrombosis; supporting the hypothesis that stasis is a causal agent for thrombosis. These conditions include partial caval obstruction during pregnancy,[171] iliac vein obstruction by a transplanted kidney,[162] the left common iliac vein compression syndrome,[66,195] and paralysed calf muscles.[72,105,315]

Any assessment of the role of postoperative venous stasis in the genesis of deep vein thrombosis is affected by the technique used to measure venous blood flow. All the techniques shown in Table 16.3 have been used to measure the velocity of venous return from the lower limbs after surgery. Most of these techniques, however, measure superficial vein blood flow from the skin and subcutaneous tissues which may not be the same as deep vein blood flow. In an attempt to separate blood flow changes in the deep and superficial veins Nicolaides *et al.*[217,218] combined serial phlebography with isotope clearance studies. They found a rapid rate of flow in the major limb veins and a reduced flow from the soleal sinusoids. This study has, however, been criticized on the grounds that flow measured by the serial phlebography is affected by the density of the contrast medium.[32]

After drawing attention to the development of thrombi in the apices of the valve pockets (Fig. 16.4), McLachlin and his colleagues,[200] using cine-phlebography, showed that contrast medium remained in the valve sinuses for 30–60 min if the calf muscles were not exercised. This finding was confirmed by Cotton and Clark[73] who suggested that eddy currents within the valve pocket might encourage the deposition of platelets and thrombus (Fig. 16.5). The presence of vortices within the valve pockets is known to increase the risk of thrombus deposition.[170,277,284] Although McLachlin[200] and Sevitt[269] found that thrombi may develop in any valve sinus of the lower limb (Fig. 16.6), the fibrinogen uptake test has shown that the majority of thrombi begin in the calf veins or soleal sinusoids below the knee; this observation has been confirmed by phlebography (Figs. 16.1 and 16.7).[52,221]

The calf pump does not function during general anaesthesia with muscle relaxation,[4] calf blood flow, and consequently venous velocity, therefore falls. The reduction of calf blood flow may persist

Table 16.3 Techniques that have been used for measuring venous blood flow

Sodium[24] clearance[335]
I[125] Hippuran clearance[128]
Xenon clearance[32]
Thermodilution[32]
Plethysmographic venous emptying[32]
Serial phlebography[217]
Arterial inflow[51]

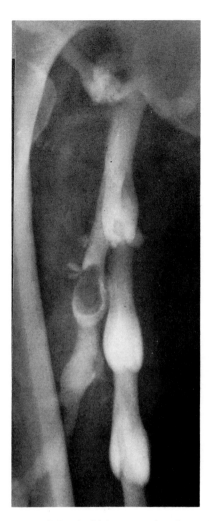

Fig. 16.4 A phlebogram showing a thrombus within a valve cusp. The valve sinus was thought, by McLachlin *et al.*[200] to be the site of origin of all deep vein thrombi.

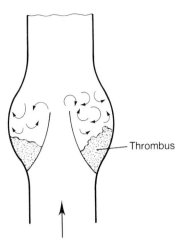

Fig. 16.5 A diagram showing blood flow past a venous valve with the arrows showing the 'vorticeal' flow setting up 'eddy currents' which allow platelet and thrombus deposition within the valve cusp.

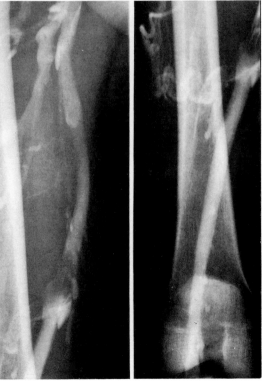

Fig. 16.6 A thrombus seen as a filling defect originating within a valve cusp in the femoral vein and extending through a small branch vein which joins the deep femoral vein.

for 7 days after an operation (Fig. 16.8),[53,85] and any increase in blood viscosity will reduce the flow rate still further.[86,320]

The studies of Wessler,[322,326] and those of Stewart,[286,291] have shown that stasis is not the prime cause of experimental venous thrombosis but that stasis is undoubtedly a strong potentiating factor which, when combined with one of the other two major mechanisms, will cause thrombosis.

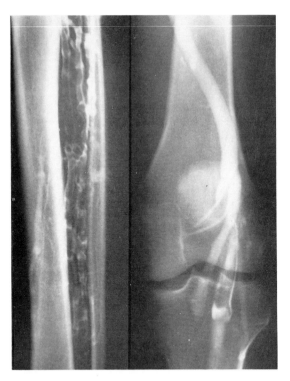

Fig. 16.7 Extensive thrombosis in the calf veins extending up to the popliteal vein. There is no thrombus within the femoral vein.

Abnormalities of coagulation

Although intravascular thrombosis does not readily occur in an occluded segment of vein, Wessler[326] showed that thrombosis did accompany stasis if it was preceded by activation of the clotting mechanism; he achieved this experimentally by infusing heterologous serum before producing venous stasis. Thrombus was not produced by either the serum infusion or the stasis alone, but only by their combination and then only if the serum infusion preceded the stasis. The thrombi that formed within the veins in response to these combined stimulae bore a closer resemblance to red propagated thrombus than to the laminated platelet/fibrin thrombus that appears to initiate deep vein thrombosis in man. If, however, these 'stasis thrombi' were left in a free-flowing circulation, fibrin, platelets and leucocytes adhered to their surface.[299]

The results of these experiments suggest that hypercoagulability, at either a local or distant site, is an essential factor in the initiation of deep vein thrombosis. Activated Factor X[322] or low levels of antithrombin III[263] may be responsible for the development of this hypercoagulable state.[322]

Other agents which have been shown to potentiate 'stasis thrombi' include ellegalic acid which

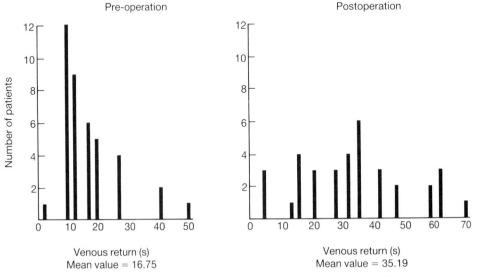

Pre-operation

Postoperation

Venous return (s)
Mean value = 16.75

Venous return (s)
Mean value = 35.19

Fig. 16.8 The effect of operation on venous blood flow measured by the [24]sodium clearance technique.[85] Pre-operatively, venous blood flow from the ankle to the groin took 16 s; postoperatively, venous blood flow took 35 s. 'Venous stasis' is one of the factors that encourages postoperative deep vein thrombosis. Modified from Doran.[85]

activates the Hageman factor, long chain saturated fatty acids[41] and Gram-negative endotoxins.

Viruses[328] and malignant cells[84,103] may also stimulate hypercoagulability and may induce disseminated intravascular coagulation.

Changes of coagulation can be considered under three headings:

- changes in the coagulation factors and their inhibitors,
- changes in the number and behaviour of the platelets,
- changes in plasminogen activators and their inhibitors.

Changes in the coagulation factors and their inhibitors

The concentration of fibrinogen in the blood rises after surgery,[99] fibrinogen synthesis and turnover increases and its half-life decreases.[77,137] The rise in plasma fibrinogen concentration increases blood viscosity which in turn slows venous blood flow.[193] Abnormalities of the blood such as polycythaemia rubra vera, leukaemia, multiple myeloma and other macroglobulinaemias, all of which raise blood viscosity, are associated with an increased risk of deep vein thrombosis.

Factors II, V, VII and XIII become elevated after surgery, and there is a coincidental rise in the platelet count.[91,109,340] Wessler and Yin[322] have drawn attention to the greater risk of thrombosis associated with increased activation of factor X, which may be the result of a deficiency of factor Xa inhibitor. Antithrombin III is a naturally occurring α_2-globulin, present in the blood, which prevents the activation of factor Xa and inhibits the conversion of prothrombin to thrombin.[263,339]

In 1965 Egeberg[90] described a Norwegian family that had suffered from recurrent venous thromboses in whom low levels of antithrombin III were found. The antithrombin III levels in those members of the family (and some of their near relatives) who had had a thrombosis were found to be half the normal value. Antithrombin III deficiency appears to be transmitted as an autosomal dominant. Since the original report many other families who have this deficiency have been described,[118,119,188,258,311,312] and the abnormality has been estimated to occur in one in every 2000 families.[245,246]

Antithrombin III levels have also been reported to be lower in patients with an acute venous thrombosis,[311] after operation[236,282] and in women who are taking the contraceptive pill;[310] all these conditions are known to predispose to venous thrombosis. Any insult such as an operation or phlebography,[322] in the presence of antithrombin III deficiency, appears to increase the risk of thrombosis.

Surprisingly, 'low-normal' pre-operative antithrombin III levels do not correlate with the development of postoperative thrombosis,[2,158] and the level of factor Xa inhibitor[339] does not correlate with the development of postoperative thrombosis.[117]

The blood levels of the fibrinolytic inhibitors, α_2-antiplasmin, α_2-macroglobulin and α_2-antitrypsin, are also unable to predict the development of postoperative thrombosis.[295] The pre-operative blood level of fibrinopeptide A, which is released in the late stages of the coagulation, also appears to be unrelated to the development of thrombosis[301] but the level of this substance has been found to rise postoperatively, indicating that thrombin activation is taking place.

Levels of factor XII (Hageman factor) and factor XIIa, which are thought to be interrelated, are also reduced postoperatively.[133] It is of some interest that Hageman, though defective in factor XII, died from a massive pulmonary embolism following a pelvic fracture.[241]

A battery of coagulation tests have been examined in an effort to detect 'hypercoagulability' but no convincing relationship with postoperative thrombosis has been found. The indicators of coagulability that have been studied are:

- shortening of the activated partial thromboplastin time[151]
- low antithrombin III levels[90]
- reduction in fibrinolytic activity[49]
- thromboelastography[130]
- fibrinopeptide A levels[228]
- platelet factor IV[64]
- β-thromboglobulin[185]
- fibrin degradation[101]

Although the concept of 'hypercoagulation' is attractive, there is little evidence that the tests of coagulation, in contrast to tests of fibrinolysis, can detect patients at increased risk of developing a deep vein thrombosis.

Recently, protein-C deficiency, protein-S deficiency and hereditary heparin co-factor II deficiency have all been reported to increase the risk of recurrent deep vein thrombosis in certain families.[33,47,113,144,191,237,302]

Perhaps, as more sophisticated tests of coagulation become available, the role of inherited defects of the coagulation factors in the development of spontaneous or recurrent venous thrombosis will become clearer. Antithrombin III deficiency is the only coagulation abnormality that is generally accepted as a cause of venous thrombosis.

Changes in the platelets

Platelets do not appear to play such a dominant role in the development of venous thrombosis as they do in arterial thrombosis,[209,210,269,343] and anti-platelet drugs have not been shown to reduce the risk of venous thrombosis in the postoperative period.[50,150]

After any injury there is an initial fall in the platelet count but it then rises above normal levels.[27,317] This increase in platelets is accompanied by an increase in platelet activity.[92,317,337] Despite these changes, no relationship has been found between the alteration in platelet behaviour and the risk of developing a postoperative thrombosis.[25,214] The platelet specific β-thromboglobulin, which can be measured in blood samples, does not rise significantly with the onset of thrombosis.[276]

It is possible that prostacyclin deficiency and the lupus anticoagulant may increase the level of platelet thromboxane, thus inducing thrombosis. Thromboxane, like prostacyclin, is derived from the phospolipids but instead of being produced in the endothelial cells, it is produced by the platelet membrane.[121,331] Thromboxane is the most powerful platelet aggregating agent known but there are no reports that increased thromboxane synthesis is a cause of venous thrombosis.

Although thrombocytosis is frequently stated to be associated with an increased risk of deep vein thrombosis,[127] the association has not been proven.[57] The role of the platelet in the genesis of deep vein thrombosis remains obscure.

Changes in plasminogen activators and their inhibitors

The changes in plasminogen activator and its inhibitors within the endothelial cell have already been described (see page 450). It is difficult to know whether the blood fibrinolytic activity represents a separate and independent function of plasminogen activators or whether it mirrors the endothelial production on which it is dependent.

Blood fibrinolytic activity rapidly increases after trauma[6,27,187,232] and then falls over the next 24–48 hours.[190,232,340] The extent of this fall was shown by Browse *et al.*[49] to relate to the presence of malignancy and to the presence, rather than the development, of a thrombosis. Becker[24] and Reilly *et al.*[242] were unable to correlate the preoperative fibrinolytic status of the blood with the risk of postoperative thrombosis but in retrospective and prospective studies other workers have found that patients developing postoperative thrombi have significantly lower levels of blood fibrinolytic activity.[1,98,110,190]

An increase in tissue plasminogen activator inhibitor has also been related to an increased risk of thrombosis,[224,225] but the published studies have not determined whether this is a cause or an effect.[176]

Comment Interest in the genesis of venous thrombosis is now moving away from the relatively simple concepts of stasis, damage to the vessel wall, and changes in coagulation. More attention is being focused on the balance between activator and inhibitor substances secreted by the vessel wall and circulating levels of procoagulants and anticoagulants. Many of these compounds exist in a delicate balance in which inhibition and activation are evenly matched. Alteration of this balance may encourage thrombosis. The development of methods capable of measuring minute quantities of activators and inhibitors will allow the role of these compounds in the development of thrombosis to be determined. The factors discussed above are the prime elements in the initiation of thrombosis. These effects are potentiated by many well recognized risk factors which are discussed in the next section.

Factors that increase the risk of deep vein thrombosis

The factors that increase the risk of deep vein thrombosis are listed in Table 16.4.

Table 16.4 Risk factors for deep vein thrombosis

Age
Sex
Season
Race
Occupation
Type of operation
Type of anaesthetic
Length of operation
Pregnancy and puerperium
General injury
Local injury
Immobilization
Bedrest
Malignancy
Previous venous thrombosis
Varicose veins
Obesity
Cardiac failure
Myocardial infarction
Arterial ischaemia
Contraceptive pill
Intravenous saline (haemodilution)
Haemostatic drugs
Other drugs
Vasculitis (Buerger's disease, Behçet's syndrome)
Congenital venous abnormalities, Klippel–Trenaunay syndrome

Age and sex

Many studies have shown that the risk of deep vein thrombosis increases with age[19,107,234,273] but between the sexes there is no obvious difference in this risk. The majority of large series show that the incidence of deep vein thrombosis is equal in men and women.[127]

Climate

It is difficult to separate the geographical and climatic factors which may influence deep vein thrombosis from racial factors but some studies suggest that thrombosis is less common in warmer countries[114,175] and during the summer months. Other investigators have suggested that there is a seasonal variation in the incidence of deep vein thrombosis with peaks in the spring and autumn,[3,234] and more pulmonary emboli have been reported during these periods.[95,129] These observations have not, however, been confirmed by studies using more objective forms of diagnosis.[7]

Race

There are definite differences in the incidence of deep vein thrombosis between racial groups (e.g. between the Caucasians of the United States and the Japanese,[111] and between the Negroes and Caucasians of South Africa).[161] The reason for these differences is not known.

Occupation

Little is known about the influence of occupation on deep vein thrombosis but prolonged episodes of sitting during aeroplane flights, watching television, or being confined in an air raid shelter have been reported to predispose to thrombosis.[142,212,220,274] (We have all seen patients who have suffered a pulmonary embolism as they walked away from an aeroplane.)

Operations

The type and the length of surgical operations affect the incidence of postoperative deep vein thrombosis.[32]

Pregnancy

The high incidence of deep vein thrombosis during pregnancy and the puerperium has been recognized for many years.[10,303,337]

Vein trauma

The role of local vein damage and of distant trauma in deep vein thrombosis has been confirmed by a number of studies which have already been discussed (see page 448).

Prolonged immobility

The adverse effect of prolonged immobility and bedrest has been well documented.[53,58,106]

Malignant disease

In a series of autopsies in which a deep vein thrombosis was found,[280] 10 per cent had a coincidental carcinoma of the pancreas. In 1941 Barker *et al.*[19] also found an increased risk of venous thrombosis in patients with malignant disease. These clinical studies have been confirmed by studies using the fibrinogen uptake test.[167,244]

Previous thrombosis

A history of a previous episode of venous thrombosis and embolism is associated with an increased risk of a further deep vein thrombosis. (Fig. 16.9).[167,261] This is particularly apparent if it is combined with another risk factor (e.g. operation or pregnancy).

Varicose veins

The association of varicose veins and deep vein thrombosis is probably the result of superficial thrombophlebitis (a recognized risk in patients with varicose veins) spreading through communicating veins into the deep veins (see Chapter 22). This association is not universally accepted because the published evidence is conflicting.

Obesity

Obesity has been shown to confer an additional risk of thrombosis on patients taking the contraceptive pill,[305] and increases the risk of postoperative deep vein thrombosis.[129,167] In three studies of predictive indices, obesity has consistently appeared as a major indicator increasing the chance of thrombosis (Fig. 16.10).

Medical illness

Ochsner *et al.*[234] reported a high incidence of deep vein thrombosis in medical patients, and Short[273] subsequently drew attention to the increased incidence of deep vein thrombosis in patients with heart failure. Patients suffering from an acute myocardial infarction also have a high incidence of deep vein thrombosis and pulmonary embolism;[125,316] this may explain the reduction in mortality effected by treatment with anticoagulants.[202]

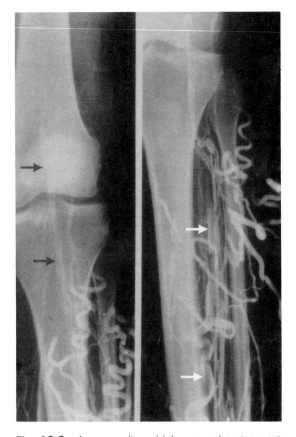

Fig. 16.9   An ascending phlebogram showing post-thrombotic deep vein damage in the popliteal and calf veins (black arrow) and fresh thrombus in the stem veins (white arrow) and in a subcutaneous varicose vein (white arrow). Post-thrombotic deep vein damage increases the risk of further thrombosis.

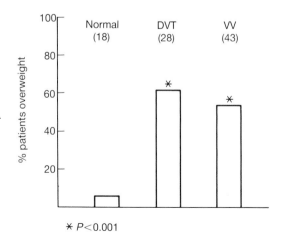

Fig. 16.10   This figure shows the percentage overweight of 18 normal control subjects, 28 patients with deep vein thrombosis (DVT), and 43 patients with varicose veins (VV), compared against the ideal maximum weights of an age and sex matched normal population taken from the Ciba–Geigy tables. The patients with deep vein thrombosis or varicose veins can be seen to be more than 50% overweight.

Oral contraceptives

In the 1960s it was recognized that the contraceptive pill increases the risk of thrombo-embolic disease.[304,305,306] Large scale prospective epidemiological studies have continued to confirm this association.[307] Oestrogens are known to increase the permeability of rabbit aortic wall, and this suggests that they may initiate a thrombosis by causing endothelial damage.[5] Low levels of antithrombin III have also been found in patients taking oestrogen-based oral contraceptives.[254]

Haemodilution

It has been suggested that the administration of intravenous saline may increase the risk of deep vein thrombosis.[130]

Vasculitis

In Buerger's disease, (thrombo-angiitis obliterans) and in Behçet's syndrome there is a vasculitis of unknown etiology. Both conditions are associated with superficial and deep vein thrombosis, and patients with these conditions who are undergoing surgical operations probably have a higher risk of thrombotic complications.

Congenital venous abnormalities

Patients with the Klippel–Trenaunay syndrome (and probably venous angioma) have an increased incidence of spontaneous venous thromboembolism and a higher incidence of postoperative deep vein thrombosis.[20]

Comment

All the conditions discussed in this section are accepted risk factors for deep vein thrombosis and are not primary causes. They are important because recognition of these factors in the presence of other major risk factors (e.g. surgery) may affect the type of prophylactic measures that are considered. Whenever possible, the summation of risk factors should be avoided. For example, patients should stop taking the contraceptive pill before surgery,[9,116] obese patients should try to lose weight before surgery, and a prolonged period of bedrest before an operation should be avoided if possible.

A number of predictive indices of deep vein thrombosis have been developed; these are based on the risk factors and laboratory tests of coagulability and thrombolysis. The purpose of these indices is to identify patients at high risk so that they can be given suitable prophylaxis and to avoid giving unnecessary prophylaxis to patients who are unlikely to develop a thrombosis.

Predictive indices

Lister in 1862[179] and Ochsner *et al.* in 1951,[234] recognized that a number of factors (e.g. age, operations, fractures and cardiac disease) increased the risk of deep vein thrombosis.

In the 1960s Hume[151] attempted to predict thrombosis from a series of coagulation tests but in 1973 Gallus[102] found that the partial thromboplastin time was the only coagulation test of predictive value.

Nilsen *et al.*[223] showed that a high plasma fibrinogen and a low antithrombin III level were indicative of an increased risk of deep vein thrombosis, and they produced a formula from these tests to aid prediction. Breeneman[45,46] devised a predictive assessment from a discriminate analysis of retrospective data.

Clayton *et al.*[65] developed an extremely complicated scoring system from an analysis of the results of a number of tests of coagulation and fibrinolysis which had been carried out on a large cohort of patients undergoing operations. The presence or absence of postoperative thrombosis was diagnosed in these patients by the fibrinogen uptake test. Clayton found that the five variables which had the best predictive value were: the euglobulin clot–lysis time, age, the presence of varicose veins, fibrin-related antigen (fibrin degradation products) and the percentage overweight. This index was then examined prospectively. Nine out of 10 patients who developed a deep vein thrombosis were correctly identified[74] but the index incorrectly identified 7 patients to be at 'high' risk who did not develop a thrombosis. The index was then used to determine prophylaxis;[75] patients who were predicted to develop a thrombosis were given subcutaneous heparin. The incidence of thrombosis in the 'high' risk group who were treated with 5000 units of heparin twice a day was 3.8 per cent; this was similar to the incidence of 4 per cent which was found in the 'low' risk group who were not given heparin. This was the first study to test the efficacy of a predictive index in a prospective study. It shows that this approach can be highly effective but it has not been generally adopted because of the time and cost involved in performing the laboratory tests.

Another study by Lowe *et al.*[184] on 63 patients, who had upper gastrointestinal surgery, found that five clinical variables had predictive value while the laboratory tests were unhelpful. The useful predictors were age, percentage over-weight for age, sex, the presence of varicose veins and cigarette smoking. Lowe *et al.* also tested their index prospectively on 41 patients, and then used it to give selective prophylaxis to a further 40 patients. Deep vein thrombi developed in 2 of the 24 'high' risk, treated patients (8 per cent) and in 2 out of 16 'low' risk, untreated patients (14 per cent). This study shows that anthropomorphic measurements can be used to predict deep vein thrombosis.

In the most recent study by Sue-Ling *et al.*[293] seven factors were identified which were then used to construct a predictive index. In descending order of predictive power these factors were: age, the euglobulin clot–lysis time, previous abdominal surgery, varicose veins, antithrombin III concentration, cigarette smoking and platelet count. Pre-operatively, the predictive index correctly indentified 91 per cent of patients who developed a deep vein thrombosis and wrongly allocated 19 per cent of patients who did not. A shortened version of this index, based on age and euglobulin lysis time, was 91 per cent sensitive and 63 per cent specific. In a prospective study of 43 patients, this shortened predictive index correctly identified 93 per cent of the patients who developed a thrombosis and wrongly allocated 17 per cent of those who did not.

Comment   It is interesting that each of the studies searching for predictive indices has found different risk factors to be of value. The main object of these studies has been to find a way of abandoning universal deep vein thrombosis prophylaxis and replacing it by selective prophylaxis for those patients who are really at risk.

The concept is financially attractive and will reduce the incidence of side-effects; few surgeons have, however, introduced any of these indices to their clinical practice, and most rely on clinical experience (the clinical factors of the various indices). Another interesting feature of these studies has been the regular appearance of a test of fibrinolysis among the useful tests of predictive value. This suggests that an abnormality of the control of coagulation is of major importance in the aetiology of deep vein thrombosis.

Pathological features of a deep vein thrombus

The pathological features of a deep vein thrombus have been described in detail by Aschoff, Hadfield, and Sevitt (Fig. 16.11).[12,120,268]

Aschoff described the initial platelet cluster on the vessel wall as a grey amorphous thickening.[12] The next stage is the development of Aschoff's 'coral reef' or corralline thrombus produced by the deposition of more platelets on the surface of the initial platelet clump, presumably in response to adenosine diphosphate or thromboxane release. The thrombus then grows towards the centre of the vessel lumen; alternate layers of fibrin and red cells are trapped between layers consisting mainly of platelets, giving the laminated appearance known as the 'lines of Zahn' (Fig. 16.11).[341] As the thrombus grows out into the bloodstream it is bent in the direction of flow making the lines of Zahn appear curved or oblique. If this type of thrombus is viewed from its surface, it appears to have a number of ridges which are the platelet layers; the troughs in between correspond to the 'red thrombus' which is made up from fibrin and red cells and is slower to develop and earlier to retract.

As the coralline thrombus extends across the lumen, the flow beyond it becomes turbulent and gradually decreases. Red thrombus, a mixture of fibrin and red cells, then forms on the surface of the coralline thrombus and extends in the direction of flow (Fig. 16.11). This 'propagated' thrombus develops when blood flow in the vessel has been critically reduced. Propagated thrombus can form in flowing blood but when the vein is completely occluded there is usually rapid extension of this jelly-like red thrombus up to the mouth of the next major tributary. If this tributary becomes occluded, the propagated thrombus continues to extend proximally and may reach several feet in length.

When the vein becomes totally occluded by the thrombus, the thrombus begins to adhere to the endothelium. The process of organization, invasion with granulation tissue, and replacement of the fibrin by fibrous tissue, occurs wherever

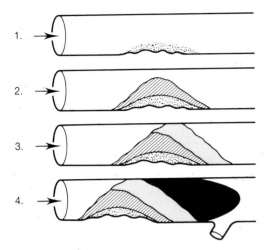

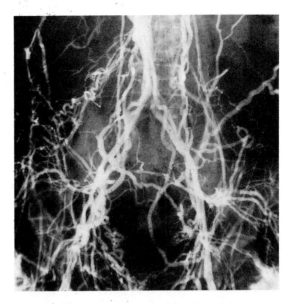

Fig. 16.11 Stages in the development of a venous thrombosis.

1. The initial platelet cluster adheres to the vein wall as a grey amorphous thickening.

2. Laminated coralline thrombus develops on the surface of the platelet cluster, with alternate layers of fibrin and red cells trapped between layers of fibrin and platelets (the lines of Zahn).[341]

3. As the thrombus grows across the flowing blood, it bends in the direction of the blood flow making the lines of Zahn oblique.

4. When the vein is totally occluded non-adherent, jelly-like, soft, propagated thrombus spreads up the vessel as far as the next major tributary. This thrombus is dark red and consists only of fibrin and red cells.

Fig. 16.13 A phlebogram of a patient obtained 6 months after a massive ileocaval thrombosis. Considerable recanalization has occurred but many collateral channels have also developed. It is not possible to assess whether these vessels are vena venora, anatomical collaterals, a reopened vein or a recanalized thrombus (see Fig. 16.11).

the thrombus has become adherent. Where the thrombus remains loose within the lumen, the polymerization and maturation of the fibrin within the thrombus causes it to retract (Fig. 16.12). Thrombus retraction and organization eventually leads to recanalization and re-endothelialization (Fig. 16.13).[115,262,296] This process destroys all the valves in the affected segment of vein[89] (Fig. 16.14) and is accompanied by an enlargement of the collateral venous channels. There is a considerable danger of embolization until a non-adherent non-occlusive thrombus begins to contract. Contraction

Fig. 16.12 Contraction and retraction of a thrombus. The phlebogram on the left shows a large, 7–10 day old popliteal vein thrombus which is beginning to retract and adhere to the vein wall. The phlebogram on the right was performed on the same limb 1 month later. The thrombus has contracted considerably but remains as a central strand in the centre of the vein lumen.

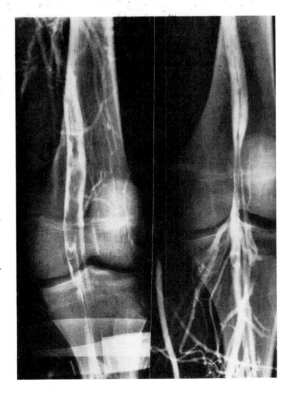

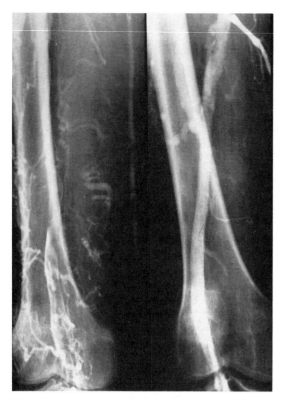

Fig. 16.14 This phlebogram (left) showed an extensive superficial femoral vein thrombus. A second phlebogram obtained 6 months later (right) shows good reopening but a totally valveless channel.

normally occurs 5–10 days after thrombus formation, and is caused by the contraction of polymerizing strands of fibrin. If a thrombus has not fragmented by this stage, it usually becomes adherent to one side of the vein, and organization occurs as if the thrombus was fully adherent.

There is no value in distinguishing phlebothrombosis from thrombophlebitis[268] because though septic thrombophlebitis was common during the last century,[154] it is rarely seen today, and the inflammatory changes that are found in a thrombosed deep vein are almost certainly the result of the thrombosis and not the cause of the thrombosis. A venous thrombus is usually sterile and is only mildly irritant.

Site of origin of deep vein thrombosis

In extensive autopsy studies on the occurrence of deep vein thrombosis, Gibbs[106] drew attention to the large number of thrombi that appear to involve or originate in the calf veins. Sevitt and Gallagher[267] confirmed Gibb's findings but observed that in burnt and injured patients thrombus could also develop in isolation in the iliac, femoral (superficial and deep), and popliteal veins (Fig. 16.15). The advent of phlebography and the use of the fibrinogen uptake test has confirmed both these post-mortem observations.[52,96,215,221,281] Most deep vein thrombi develop in the calf veins but they can develop at other sites, particularly if there is local tissue damage. The soleal sinusoids and the valves of the calf veins are the common sites of origin of deep vein thrombi. Sevitt has suggested that the eddy currents that occur as blood passes a valve[270] encourage the deposition of thrombus within the valve cusp with the 'formed elements' especially the red cells, being sifted out into the valve pocket by the turbulence (Fig. 16.5). Compression by exercising muscles may wash these small deposits away but if thromboxane (which stabilizes the aggregation of any platelet clumps) is released, the nidus for the growth of thrombus will persist. The subsequent chain reaction, with the generation of thrombin and fibrin, produces a growing thrombus.

Sevitt[268] described the platelet clump with its fibrin fringe as the foundation stone and building blocks of the growing thrombus (Fig. 16.16). Propagation then depends on the balance between the coagulation and fibrinolytic mechanisms; the coagulation mechanisms favour extension and the fibrinolytic mechanisms favour thrombolysis. Growth is by the deposition of layers of aggregated platelets and fibrin containing red and white cells; this becomes the visible propagating head and tail of the thrombus. The original platelet nidus is usually transformed into a fibrin thrombus containing many red cells and a few platelets.

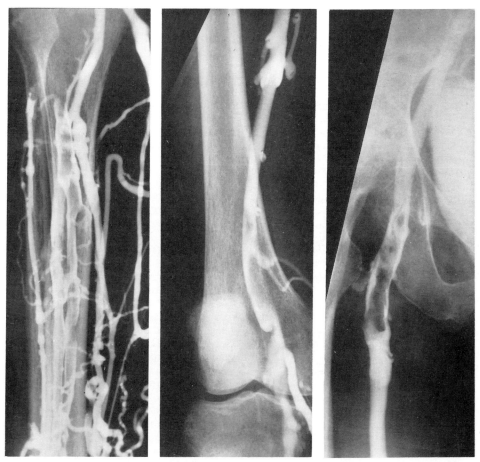

Fig. 16.15 An ascending phlebogram showing separate and distinct areas of thrombosis – in the calf, in the popliteal vein and in the femoral vein. There is no connection between the thrombi at these different sites.

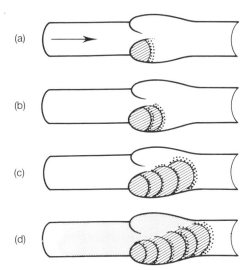

(a)

(b)

(c)

(d)

Fig. 16.16 This diagram illustrates Sevitt's platelet clumps with fibrin fringes (building blocks). The first diagram shows thrombus being laid down in the valve sinus. The subsequent diagrams show the thrombus extending across the vessel wall to occlude flow and allow propagation of thrombus. Modified from Sevitt.[268]

References

1. Aberg M, Isacson S, Nilsson IM. The fibrinolytic system and postoperative thrombosis following operation of rectal carcinoma. A preliminary report. *Acta Chir Scand* 1974; **140**: 352.
2. Aberg M, Nilsson IM, Hedner U. Antithrombin III after operation. *Lancet* 1973; **2**: 1337.
3. Allen A, Linton R, Donaldson G. Venous thrombosis and pulmonary embolism. *JAMA* 1945; **128**: 397.

4. Almen T, Nylander G. Serial phlebography of the normal lower leg during muscular contraction and relaxation. *Acta Radiol* 1962; **57**: 264.

5. Almen T, Hartel M, Nylander G, Olivecrona H. Effect of estrogen on the vascular endothelium and its possible relation to thrombosis. *Surg Gynec Obstet* 1975; **140**: 938.

6. Anderson L, Nilsson IM, Olow B. Fibrinolytic activity in man during surgery. *Thromb Diath Haemorrh* 1962; **7**: 391.

7. Andreasen C, Krieger-Lassen H. Fatal pulmonary embolism in a surgical department during a period of 15 years. *Acta Chir Scand* (Suppl) 1965; **343**: 42.

8. Angelides NS, Nicolaides AN, Fernandes J, Gordon-Smith I, Bowers R, Lewis JD. Deep venous thrombosis in patients having aortoiliac reconstruction. *Br J Surg* 1977; **64**: 517.

9. Anon. Elective surgery and the pill. *Br Med J* 1976; **2**: 546.

10. Anon. Thromboembolism in pregnancy. *Br Med J* 1979; **1**: 1661.

11. Apitz K. Die Bedeutung der Gerinnung und Thrombose für die Blutstillung. *Virchows Arch Path Anat* 1942; **308**: 540.

12. Aschoff L. Thrombose und Sandbankbildung. *Beitr Pathol Anat* 1912; **52**: 207.

13. Ashford TP, Freiman DG. The role of the endothelium in the initial phases of thrombosis. *Am J Pathol* 1967; **50**: 257.

14. Astedt B, Pandolfi M. On release and synthesis of fibrinolytic activators in human organ culture. *Eur J Clin Biol Res* 1972; **17**: 261.

15. Astrup T. Tissue activators of plasminogen. *Fed Proc* 1966; **25**: 42.

16. Atik N, Broghamer W. The impact of prophylactic measures in fatal pulmonary embolism. *Arch Surg* 1979; **114**: 366.

17. Awbrey BJ, Hoak JC, Owren WG. Binding of human thrombin to cultured human endothelial cells. *J Biol Chem* 1979; **254**: 4092.

18. Ballard RM, Bradley-Watson PJ, Johnstone FD, Kenney A, McCarthy TG, Campbell S, Weston J. Low doses of subcutaneous heparin in the prevention of deep vein thrombosis after gynaecological surgery. *J Obstet Gynaecol Br Commonw* 1973; **80**: 469.

19. Barker NU, Nygaard K, Walters W, Priestly JT. A statistical study of post operative venous thrombosis and pulmonary embolism. III. Time of occurrence during the postoperative period. *Proc Mayo Clin* 1941; **16**: 17.

20. Baskerville PA, Ackroyd JS, Lea Thomas M, Browse NL. The Klippel-Trenaunay syndrome: Clinical, radiological and haemodynamic features and management. *Br J Surg* 1985; **72**: 232.

21. Bauer G. Thrombosis following leg injuries. *Acta Chir Scand* 1944; **90**: 229.

22. Baumgarten P. *Die sogennaute Organization des Thrombus*. Leipzig. O Wigand. 1877.

23. Becker J, Borgström S, Saltzman CF. Incidence of thrombosis associated with epsilon-aminocaproic acid administration and with combined epsilon-aminocaproic acid and subcutaneous heparin therapy. II A clinical study with the aid of intravenous phlebography. *Acta Chir Scand* 1970; **136**: 167.

24. Becker J. Fibrinolytic activity of the blood and its relation to postoperative venous thrombosis of the lower limbs. A clinical study. *Acta Chir Scand* 1972; **138**: 787.

25. Becker J. The relation of platelet adhesiveness to postoperative venous thrombosis in the legs. *Acta Chir Scand* 1972; **138**: 781.

26. Belch JJF, Lowe GDO, Pollock JG, Forbes CD, Prentice CRM. Subcutaneous heparin in the prevention of venous thrombosis after elective aortic bifurcation graft surgery. *Thromb Haemost* 1979; **42**: 303.

27. Bergentz S-E, Nilsson IM. Effect of trauma on coagulation and fibrinolysis in dogs. *Acta Chir Scand* 1961; **122**: 21.

28. Berman HJ, Fulton GP. Platelets in the peripheral circulation. In Johnson SA (Ed) *The Henry Ford Hospital Symposium on Blood Platelets*. Boston. Little Brown 1961.

29. Berqvist A, Berqvist D, Hedner U. Clinical manifestations of thrombosis during pregnancy. *Läkartidningen* 1982; **79**: 901.

30. Berqvist D, Elvelin R, Eriksson U, Hjelmstedt A. Thrombosis following hip arthroplasty; a study using phlebography and the[125]I fibrinogen test. *Acta Orthop Scand* 1976; **47**: 549.

31. Berqvist D, Hallböök T. Prophylaxis of postoperative venous thrombosis in a controlled trial comparing dextran 70 and low-dose heparin. A study with the[125]I fibrinogen test. *World J Surg* 1980, **4**: 239.

32. Berqvist D. *Postoperative Thromboembolism*. Berlin. Springer 1983.

33. Bertina RM, Broekmans AW, Van Der Linden IK, Mertens K. Protein C deficiency in a Dutch family with thrombotic disease. *Thromb Haemost* 1982; **48**: 1.

34. Biggs R. *Human Blood Coagulation, Haemostasis and Thrombosis*. Oxford. Blackwell Scientific Publications 1972.

35. Bizzozero J. Über einen neuen formbestandtheil des bluts und dessen rolle bei der Thrombose und der Blutgerinnung. *Virchows Arch Path Anat* 1882; **90**: 261.

36. Blaisdell FW. Low dose heparin prophylaxis of venous thrombosis. *Am Heart J* 1979; **97**: 685.

37. Blodgett JB, Beattie EJ. Early post-operative rising: A statistical study of hospital complications. *Surg Gynec Obstet* 1946; **82**: 485.

38. Bloom AL, Giddings JC, Wilks CJ. Factor VIII on the vascular intima: possible importance in haemostasis and thrombosis. *Nature* 1973; **241**: 217.

39. Boey LM, Colaco CB, Gharavi AE, Elkon KB, Loizou S, Hughes GRV. Thrombosis in systemic lupus erythematosus: striking association with the presence of circulating "lupus anti-coagulant" *Br Med J* 1983; **287**: 1021.

40. Borgström S, Gelin E. The formation of vein thrombin following tissue injury. An experimental study in rabbits. *Acta Chir Scand* (Suppl) 1959; **247**.

41. Botti RE, Ratnoff OD. The clot promoting effect of long chain saturated fatty acids. *J Clin Invest* 1963; **42**: 1569.

42. Bounameaux Y. The adherance of blood platelets to subendothelial fibers. *Thromb Diath Haemorrh* 1961; **6**: 504.

43. Bounameaux Y. The coupling of platelets with subendothelial fibers. *C R Soc Biol* 1959; **153**: 865.

44. Boyden S. The chemotactic effect of mixtures of antibody and antigen on polymorphonuclear leucocytes. *J Exp Med* 1962; **115**: 453.

45. Breneman J. A formula for predicting and a device for preventing postoperative thromboembolic disease. *Angiology* 1963; **14**: 437.

46. Breneman J. Postoperative thromboembolic disease. Computer analysis leading to statistical prediction. *JAMA* 1965; **193**: 576.

47. Broekmans AW, Veltkamp JJ, Bertina RM. Congential protein C deficiency and venous thromboembolism. A study of three Dutch families. *N Engl J Med* 1983; **309**: 340.

48. Browse NL, Clemenson G, Croft D. Fibrinogen detectable thrombosis in the legs and pulmonary embolism. *Br Med J* 1974; **1**: 603.

49. Browse NL, Gray L, Morland M, Jarrett PEM. Blood and vein wall fibrinolytic activity in health and vascular disease. *Br Med J* 1977; **1**: 478.

50. Browse NL, Hall JH. Effect of dipyridamole on the incidence of clinically detectable deep vein thrombosis. *Lancet* 1969; **2**: 718.

51. Browse NL, Jackson BT, Mayo ME, Negus D. The value of mechanical methods of preventing postoperative calf vein thrombosis. *Br J Surg* 1974; **61**: 219.

52. Browse NL, Lea Thomas M. Source of non-lethal pulmonary emboli. *Lancet* 1974; **1**: 258.

53. Browse NL. Effect of bedrest on resting calf blood flow of healthy adult males. *Br Med J* 1962; **1**: 1721.

54. Browse NL. The ^{125}I fibrinogen uptake test. *Arch Surg* 1972; **104**: 160.

55. Buonassisi V. Sulfated mucopolysaccharide synthesis and secretion in endothelial cell cultures. *Exp Cell Res* 1973; **76**: 363.

56. Butler MJ, Britton BJ, Smith M, Hawkey C, Irving MH. Coagulation and fibrinolytic response during operative surgery. *Br J Surg* 1975; **62**: 666.

57. Butler MJ, Mathews F, Irving MH. The incidence of post-operative deep vein thrombosis after splenectomy. *Clin Oncol* 1977; **3**: 51.

58. Canavarro K. Early post-operative ambulation. *Ann Surg* 1946; **124**: 180.

59. Cappell DF. In *Muir's Textbook of Pathology*. London. Edward Arnold 1958.

60. Carreras LO, Defreyn G, Makin SJ, Vermylen J, Deman R, Spitz B, Van Assche A. Arterial thrombosis, intrauterine death and "lupus" anti-coagulant: Detection of immunoglobulin interfering with prostacylin formation. *Lancet* 1981; **1**: 244.

61. Carreras LO, Vermylen JG. "Lupus" anti-coagulant and thrombosis: possible role of inhibition of prostacyclin formation. *Thromb Haemost* 1982; **48**: 38.

62. Cartwright GE, Athens JW, Boggs DR, Wintrobe MM. The kinetics of granulopoiesis in normal man. *Blood* 1965; **24**: 780.

63. Chan V, Chan TK. Antithrombin III in fresh and cultured human endothelial cells: a natural anticoagulant from the vascular endothelium. *Thromb Res* 1979; **15**: 209.

64. Chesterman CN, McGready JR, Doyle DJ, Morgan FJ. Plasma levels of platelet factor 4 measured by radio-immunoassay. *Br J Haematol* 1978; **40**: 489.

65. Clayton JK, Anderson JA, McNichol GP. Pre-operative prediction of post-operative deep vein thrombosis. *Br Med J* 1976; **2**: 910.

66. Cockett FB, Lea Thomas M. The iliac compression syndrome. *Br J Surg* 1965; **52**: 816.

67. Cohnheim J. In: McKee AB (Ed) *Lectures in General Pathology*. London. New Sydenham Society 1889.

68. Colditz GA, Tuden RA, Oster G. Rates of venous thrombosis after general surgery: combined results of randomized clinical trials. *Lancet* 1986; **2**: 143.

69. Collins R, Klein L, Skillman J, Salzman E. Thromboembolic problems in urologic surgery. *Urol Clin North Am* 1976; **3**: 393.

70. Conard J, Veuillet-Duval A, Horellou MH, Samama M. Etude de la coagulation et de la fibrinolyse dans 131 cas de thromboses veineuses récidivants. *Nouv Rev Fr Hematol* 1982; **24**: 205.

71. Cooper DR, Lewis GP, Lieberman GE, Webb H, Westwick J. ADP metabolism in vascular tissue, a possible thrombo-regulating mechanism. *Thromb Res* 1979; **14**: 901.

72. Cope C, Reyes T, Skversky N. Phlebographic analysis of the incidence of thrombosis in hemiplegia. *Radiology* 1973; **109**: 581.

73. Cotton LT, Clarke C. Anatomical localization of venous thrombosis. *Ann R Coll Surg Engl* 1965; **36**: 214.

74. Crandon AJ, Peel KR, Anderson JA, Thompson V, McNichol GP. Post-operative deep vein thrombosis: indentifying high risk patients. *Br Med J* 1980; **281**: 343.

75. Crandon AJ, Peel KR, Anderson JA, Thompson V, McNicol GP. Prophylaxis of postoperative deep vein thrombosis: selective use of low-dose heparin in high-risk patients. *Br Med J* 1980; **281**: 345.

76. Cranley JJ, Canos AJ, Sull WJ, Grass AM. Phleborheographic technique for diagnosis of deep vein thrombosis of the lower extremities. *Surg Gynec Obstet* 1975; **141**: 331.

77. Davies JWL, Liljedahl SO, Reizenstein P. Fibrinogen metabolism following injury and its surgical treatment. *Injury* 1970; **1**: 178.

78. Dawson AA, Bennett B, Jones PF, Munro A. Thrombotic risks of staging laparotomy with splenectomy in Hodgkin's disease. *Br J Surg* 1981; **68**: 842.

79. Day TK, Cowper SV, Kakkar VV, Clarke KGA. Early venous thrombosis: a scanning electron microscopic study. *Thromb Haemost* 1977; **37**: 477.

80. de Cossart L. Plasminogen activator in soleal veins. *Phlebology* 1986; **1**: 119.

81. de Takats G. Heparin tolerance. A test of the clotting mechanism. *Surg Gynec Obstet* 1943; **77**: 31.

82. Dismuke SE. Declining mortality from pulmonary embolism in surgical patients. *Thromb Haemost* 1981; **46**: 17.

83. Dodd H, Cockett F. *The Pathology and Surgery of the Veins of the Lower Limb.* Edinburgh. Churchill Livingstone 1976.

84. Donati MB, Poggi A, Mussoni L, de Gaetano G, Garattini S. Hemostasis and experimental cancer dissemination. In Day SB, Myers WPL, Stansly P, Garratini S, Lewis MG (Eds) *Cancer Invasion and Metastasis: Biologic Mechanisms and Therapy.* New York. Raven Press 1977.

85. Doran FSA, Drury M, Sivyer A. A simple way to combat the venous stasis which occurs in the lower limb during surgical operations. *Br J Surg* 1964; **51**: 486.

86. Dormandy J, Edelman J. High blood viscosity: an aetiological factor in venous thrombosis. *Br J Surg* 1973; **60**: 187.

87. Douss TW. The clinical significance of venous thrombosis of the calf. *Br J Surg* 1976; **63**: 377.

88. Eberth CJ, Schimmelbusch C. *Die Thrombose nach Versuchen und Leichenbefunden.* Stuttgart. F Enke 1888.

89. Edwards AE, Edwards JE. The effect of thrombophlebitis on the venous valve. *Surg Gynec Obstet* 1937; **65**: 310.

90. Egeberg O. Inherited antithrombin deficiency causing thrombophilia. *Thromb Diath Haemorrh* 1965; **13**: 516.

91. Egeberg O. Changes in the coagulation system following major surgical operations. *Acta Med Scand* 1962; **171**: 679.

92. Emmons PR, Mitchell JRA. Postoperative changes in platelet-clumping activity. *Lancet* 1965; **1**: 71.

93. Evans WH. Discussion on post-operative thrombosis. *Proc R Soc Med* 1929; **22**: 729.

94. Fearnley GR. *Fibrinolysis.* London. Edward Arnold 1965.

95. Feinleib M. Venous thrombosis in relation to cigarette smoking, physical activity and seasonal factors. *Millbank Med Fund Q* 1972; **50**: 123.

96. Flanc C, Kakkar VV, Clarke MB. The detection of venous thrombosis of the legs using ^{125}I labelled fibrinogen. *Br J Surg* 1968; **55**: 742.

97. Florey HW. *General Pathology.* London. Lloyd-Luke 1962.

98. Flute PT, Kakkar VV, Renney JTG, Nicolaides AN. The blood and venous thromboembolism. In Kakkar VV, Jouhar AJ (Eds) *Thromboembolism.* Edinburgh. Churchill Livingstone 1972.

99. Foster DP, Whipple CH. Blood fibrin studies. Fibrin influenced by cell injury, inflammation, intoxication, liver injury and the Eck fistula. Notes connecting the origin of fibrin in the body. *Am J Physiol* 1922; **58**: 407.

100. French JE, Macfarlane RG, Sanders AG. The structure of haemostatic plugs and experimental thrombi in small arteries. *Br J Exp Pathol* 1964; **45**: 467.

101. Gaffney PJ, Joe F, Mahmoud M. Giant fibrin fragments derived from cross-linked fibrin: structure and clinical application. *Thromb Res* 1980; **20**: 647.

102. Gallus AS, Hirsh J, Gent M. Relevance of preoperative and postoperative blood tests to postoperative leg vein thrombosis. *Lancet* 1973; **2**: 806.

103. Gasic GJ, Boettiger D, Catalfamo JL, Gasic TB, Stewart GJ. Platelet interactions in malignancy and cell transformation: functional and

biochemical studies. In de Gaetano G, Garattini S (Eds) *Platelets: A Multidisciplinary Approach.* New York. Raven Press 1978.

104. Gaynor E. The role of granulocytes in endotoxin-induced vascular injury. *Blood* 1973; **41**: 797.

105. Gibbard F B, Gould S R, Marks P. Incidence of deep vein thrombosis and leg oedema in patients with strokes. *J Neurol Neurosurg Psychiatry* 1976; **39**: 1222.

106. Gibbs N M. Venous thrombosis in the lower limbs with particular reference of bedrest. *Br J Surg* 1957; **45**: 209.

107. Gjöres J-E. The incidence of venous thrombosis and its sequelae in certain districts of Sweden. *Acta Chir Scand* (Suppl) 1956; **206**: 1.

108. Glennard F. Contribution a l'étude des causes de la coagulation spontanee du sang a son issue de l'organisme application a la transfusion. *Paris Thesis* 1875.

109. Godal H C. Quantitative and qualitative changes in fibrinogen following major surgical operations. *Acta Med Scand* 1962; **171**: 687.

110. Gordon-Smith I C, Hickman J A, LeQuesne L P. Postoperative fibrinolytic activity and deep vein thrombosis. *Br J Surg* 1974; **61**: 213.

111. Gore I, Hirst A, Tanaka K. Myocardial infarction and thromboembolism. A comparative study in Boston and in Kyushu, Japan. *Arch Intern Med* 1964; **113**: 323.

112. Gore I, Larkey B J. Functional activity of aortic mucopolysaccharides. *J Lab Clin Med* 1960; **56**: 839.

113. Griffin J H, Evatt B, Zimmerman T S, Kleiss A J, Widemann C. Deficiency of protein C in congenital thrombotic disease. *J Clin Invest* 1981; **68**: 1370.

114. Groote Schuur Hospital Thromboembolus Study Group. Failure of low-dose heparin to prevent significant thromboembolic complications in high-risk surgical patients. Interim report of a prospective trial. *Br Med J* 1979; **1**: 1447.

115. Gryner L. Activity of anchonitic surface compounds in producing vascular obliteration. *Proc Soc Exp Biol Med* 1946; **62**: 49.

116. Guillebaud J. Surgery and the pill. *Br Med J* 1985; **291**: 498.

117. Gunn I. Anti-Xa factor as a predictor of postoperative deep vein thrombosis in general surgery. *Br J Surg* 1979; **66**: 636.

118. Gyde O H B, Littler W A, Stableforth D E. Familial antithrombin III deficiency. *Br Med J* 1978; **1**: 508.

119. Gyde O H B, Middleton M D, Vaughan G R, Fletcher D J. Antithrombin III deficiency hypertriglyceridaemia and venous thromboses. *Br Med J* 1978; **1**: 621.

120. Hadfield C. Thrombosis. *Ann R Coll Surg Engl* 1950; **6**: 219.

121. Hamberg M, Svensson J, Samuelsson B. Thromboxanes: a new group of biologically active compounds derived from prostaglandin endoperoxides. *Proc Natl Acad Sci USA* 1975; **72**: 2994.

122. Hamer J D, Malone P C, Silver I A. The pO_2 in venous valve pockets: its possible bearing on thrombogenesis. *Br J Surg* 1981; **68**: 166.

123. Hamer J D, Malone P C. Experimental deep venous thrombogenesis by a noninvasive method. *Ann R Coll Surg Engl* 1984; **66**: 416.

124. Hamer J D. Investigation of oedema of the lower limb following successful femeropopliteal bypass surgery: the role of phlebography in demonstrating venous thrombosis. *Br J Surg* 1972; **59**: 979.

125. Handley A. Low-dose heparin after myocardial infarction. *Lancet* 1972; **2**: 623.

126. Hartsuck J, Greenfield L. Postoperative thromboembolism. A clinical study with ^{125}I fibrinogen and pulmonary scanning. *Arch Surg* 1973; **107**: 733.

127. Harvey-Kemble J V. The incidence of deep vein thrombosis. *Br J Hosp Med* 1971; **6**: 721.

128. Harvey-Kemble J V. The effect of surgical operation on leg venous flow measured with radioactive hippuran. *Postgrad Med J* 1971; **47**: 773.

129. Havig Ö. Deep vein thrombosis and pulmonary embolism. An autopsy study with multiple regression analysis of possible risk factors. *Acta Chir Scand* (Suppl) 1977; **478**.

130. Heather B, Jennings S, Greenhalgh R. The saline dilution test – a preoperative predictor of DVT. *Br J Surg* 1980; **67**: 63.

131. Heatley R V, Hughes L E, Morgan A, Okwonga W. Preoperative or postoperative deep-vein thrombosis? *Lancet* 1976; **1**: 437.

132. Hedlund P O. Postoperative venous thrombosis in benign prostatic disease. A study of 316 patients with the ^{125}I fibrinogen uptake test. *Scand J Urol Nephrol* (Suppl) 1975; **27**.

133. Hedner U, Martinsson G, Bergqvist D. Influence of operative trauma on factor XII and inhibitor of plasminogen activator. *Haemostasis* 1983; **13**: 219.

134. Hewson W. *Experimental Enquiries: 1 An Enquiry into the Properties of Blood with Some Remarks on its Morbid Appearances and an Appendix Relating to the discovery of the Lymphatic System in Birds, Fish and the Animals Called Amphibians.* London. T Cadell 1771.

135. Heyns A P, Badenhorst C J, Retief F P. ADPase

activity of normal and atherosclerotic human aorta intima. *Thromb Haemost* 1977; **37**: 429.

136. Heyns AP, Van Den Berg DJ, Potgieler FP, Retief FP. The inhibition of platelet aggregation by an aorta intima extract. *Thromb Diath Haemorrh* 1974; **32**: 417.

137. Hickman JA. A study of the metabolism of fibrinogen after surgical operations. *Clin Sci* 1971; **41**: 141.

138. Hjelmstedt A. *Deep Venous Thrombosis in Tibial Fracture. A Clinical Phlebographic and Physiological Study.* Uppsala. *Thesis Almquist and Wiksell* 1968.

139. Hobbs JT, Davis JWL. Detection of venous thrombosis with ^{131}I labelled fibrinogen in the rabbit. *Lancet* 1960; **2**: 134.

140. Hobbs JT. Compression sclerotherapy of varicose veins. In Bergan JJ, Yao JST (Eds) *Venous Problems.* Chicago. Year Book Medical Publishers 1978.

141. Holmberg L, Mannucci BM, Turesson I, Ruggeri ZM, Nilsson IM. Factor VIII antigen in the vessel wall in von Willebrand's disease and haemophilia. A *Scand J Haematol* 1974; **13**: 33.

142. Homans J. Thrombosis of deep leg veins due to prolonged sitting. *N Engl J Med* 1954; **250**: 148.

143. Homans J. Thrombosis of the deep veins of the leg, causing pulmonary embolism. *N Engl J Med* 1934; **211**: 993.

144. Horellou MH, Conard J, Bertina RM, Samama M. Congenital protein C deficiency and thrombotic disease in nine french families. *Br Med J* 1984; **289**: 1285.

145. Hovig T. The effect of calcium and magnesium on rabbit blood platelet aggregation *in vitro*. *Thromb Diath Haemorrh* 1963; **12**: 179.

146. Hovig T. The ultrastructure of rabbit blood platelet aggregates. *Thromb Diath Haemorrh* 1962; **8**: 455.

147. Hugues J, Lapière M. Nouvelles researches sur l'accolment des plaquettes aux fibères de collagère. *Thromb Diath Haemorrh* 1964; **11**: 327.

148. Hugues J. Accolement des plaquettes aux structures conlonctives perivascularies. *Thromb Diath Haemorrh* 1962; **8**: 241.

149. Hugues J. Contribution a l'étude des facteurs vasculaires et sanguins dans l'hemostase spontanee. *Arch Int Physiol* 1953; **61**: 565.

150. Hull R, Hirsh J. Prevention of venous thrombosis and pulmonary embolism with particular reference to the surgical patient. In Joist JH, Sherman LA, (Eds) *Venous and Arterial Thrombosis. Pathogenesis, Diagnosis, Prevention and Therapy.* New York. Grune & Stratton 1979.

151. Hume M, Chan YK. Examination of the blood in the presence of venous thrombosis. *JAMA* 1967; **200**: 747.

152. Hume M, Sevitt S, Thomas DP. *Venous Thombosis and Pulmonary Embolism.* Cambridge, Massachusetts. Harvard University Press 1970.

153. Hunt PS, Reeves TS, Hollings RM. A 'standard' experimental thrombus: Observations on its production, pathology, response to heparin and thrombectomy. *Surgery* 1966; **59**: 812.

154. Hunter J. In: Palmer JF (Ed) *A treatise on Blood, Inflammation and Gunshot wounds.* London. Longman 1834.

155. Husni EH. The oedema of arterial reconstruction. *Circulation* (Suppl 1) 1967; **35**: 169.

156. International Multi-centre Trial. Prevention of fatal post-operative pulmonary embolism by low doses of heparin. *Lancet* 1975; **2**: 45.

157. Isacson S, Nilsson IM. Defective fibrinolysis in blood vein walls in recurrent "idiopathic" venous thrombosis. *Acta Chir Scand* 1972; **138**: 313.

158. Ishak M, Morley K. Deep venous thrombosis after total hip arthroplasty: a prospective controlled study to determine the prophylactic effect of graded pressure stockings. *Br J Surg* 1981; **68**: 429.

159. Izuka K, Murata K. Inhibitory effects of human aortic and venous acid glycosaminoglycans on thrombus formation. *Atherosclerosis* 1972; **16**: 217.

160. Jaffe EA, Hoyer LW, Nachman RL. Synthesis of antihemophilic factor antigen by cultured human endothelial cells. *J Clin Invest* 1973; **52**: 2757.

161. Joffe SN. Racial incidence of postoperative deep vein thrombosis in South Africa. *Br J Surg* 1974; **61**: 982.

162. Joffe SN. Deep vein thrombosis after renal transplantation. *Vasc Surg* 1976; **10**: 134.

163. Johansson L, Hedner U, Nilsson IM. A family with thromboembolic disease associated with deficient fibrinolytic activity in vessel wall. *Acta Med Scand* 1978; **203**: 477.

164. Johnson RH, Mansfield A. A new method for the detection of plasminogen activator content of vein walls. *Acta Haematol* 1978; **60**: 243.

165. Jorgensen M, Mortensen JZ, Madsen AG, Thorsen S, Jacobsen B. A family with reduced plasminogen activator activity in blood associated with recurrent venous thrombosis. *Scand J Haematol* 1982; **29**: 217.

166. Kakkar VV, Day TK. The vessel wall and venous thrombosis. In Neville Wolfe (Ed) *Biology and Pathology of the Vessel Wall.* New York. Praeger 1983.

167. Kakkar VV, Howe CT, Nicolaides AN, Renney

JTG, Clarke MB. Deep vein thrombosis of the leg: Is there a "high-risk" group? *Am J Surg* 1970; **120**: 527.

168. Kakkar VV, Sasahara AA. Diagnosis of venous thrombosis and pulmonary embolism. In Bloom AL, Thomas DP (Eds) *Haemostasis and Thrombosis*. Edinburgh. Churchill Livingstone 1981.

169. Kakkar VV. The diagnosis of deep vein thrombosis using fibrinogen test. *Arch Surg* 1972; **104**: 152.

170. Karino T, Motomiya M. Vortices in the pockets of a venous valve. *Microvasc Res* 1981; **21**: 247.

171. Kerr MG, Scott DB, Samuel E. Studies of the inferior vena cava in late pregnancy. *Br Med J* 1964; **1**: 532.

172. Klein A, Hughes LE, Campbell H, Williams A, Zlosnick J, Leach KG. Dextran 70 in prophylaxis of thrombo-embolic disease after surgery: A clinically orientated randomized double blind trial. *Br Med J* 1975; **2**: 109.

173. Kraemer PM. Heparin releases heparan sulfate from the cell surface. *Biochem Biophys Res Commun* 1977; **78**: 1334.

174. Lanham JG, Levin M, Brown Z, Gharavi AE, Thomas PA, Hanson GC. Prostacyclin deficiency in a young woman with recurrent thrombosis. *Br Med J* 1986; **292**: 435.

175. Lawrence JC, Xabregas A, Gray L, Ham JM. Seasonal variation in the incidence of deep vein thrombosis. *Br J Surg* 1977; **64**: 777.

176. Layer G, Burnand KG. Two different mechanisms in patients with venous thrombosis and defective fibrinolysis. *Br Med J* 1985; **291**: 56.

177. Leithauser OJ. Early ambulation and related procedures in surgical management. Springfield Illinois. Charles C Thomas 1946.

178. Lieberman GE, Lewis GP, Peters TJ. A membrane-bound enzyme in rabbit aorta capable of inhibiting adenosine-diphosphate-induced platelet aggregation. *Lancet* 1977; **2**: 330.

179. Lister J. On the coagulation of blood. Croonian Lecture. *Proc R Soc Lon* 1862; **12**: 580.

180. Ljungnér H, Berqvist D, Isacson S, Nilsson IM. Comparison between the plasminogen activator activity in walls of superficial, muscle and deep veins. *Thromb Res* 1981; **22**: 295.

181. Ljungnér H, Berqvist D, Isacson S. Plasminogen activator activity of superficial veins in acute deep venous thrombosis. *Vasa* 1982; **11**: 174.

182. Ljungnér H, Isacson S. The fibrinolytic activity in vein walls in patients undergoing prostatectomy. *Sven Läkaresällsk Förh* 1979; **88**: 23.

183. Loskutoff DJ, Edgington T. Synthesis of a fibrinolytic activator and inhibitor by endothelial cells. *Proc Nat Acad Sci USA* 1977; **74**: 3903.

184. Lowe GDO, Osborne DH, McArdle BM, Smith A, Carter DC, Forbes CD, McLaren D, Prentice CRM. Prediction and selective prophylaxis of venous thrombosis in elective gastrointestinal surgery. *Lancet* 1982; **1**: 409.

185. Ludlam CA, Cash JD. β-thromboglobulin: a new tool for the diagnosis of hypercoagulability? In: Neri Serner GG, Prentice CRM (Eds) *Haemostasis and Thrombosis*. London. Academic Press 1978; 159.

186. MacFarlane RG. An enzyme cascade in the blood clotting mechanism and its function as a biochemical amplifier. *Nature* 1964; **202**: 498.

187. Macintyre IMC, Webber RG, Crispin JR, Jones DRB, Wood JK, Allan NC, Prescott RJ, Ruckley CV. Plasma fibrinolysis and postoperative deep vein thrombosis. *Br J Surg* 1976; **63**: 694.

188. Mackie M, Bennett B, Ogston D, Douglas AS. Familial thrombosis inherited deficiency of antithrombin III. *Br Med J* 1978; **1**: 136.

189. Malone PC, Morris CJ. Margination and sequestration of platelets and leucocytes on hypoxic endothelium. *J Path* 1978; **125**: 119.

190. Mansfield A. Alteration in fibrinolysis associated with surgery and venous thrombosis. *Br J Surg* 1972; **59**: 754.

191. Marlar RA, Endres-Brooks J. Recurrent thromboembolic disease due to heterozygous protein C deficiency. *Thromb Haemost* 1983; **50**: 331.

192. Mason R, Sharp D, Chuang H, Mohammed F. The endothelium. Roles in thrombosis and haemostasis. *Arch Pathol Lab Med* 1977; **101**: 61.

193. Matsuda T, Murakami M. Relationship between fibrinogen and blood viscosity. *Thromb Res* 1976; Suppl (**II**): 25.

194. May R. *Surgery of Veins of the Leg and Pelvis*. Stuttgart. Thieme 1979.

195. May R. Thurner J. Ein Gefässsporn in der Vena iliaca com. sin. als wahrscheinliche Ursache der überwiegend linksseitigen Beckenvenenthrombosen. *Z Kreislaufforsch* 1956; **45**: 912.

196. Mayo ME, Halil T, Browse NL. The incidence of deep vein thrombosis after prostatectomy. *Br J Urol* 1971; **43**: 738.

197. McGovern VJ. Reactions to injury of vascular endothelium with special reference to the problems of thrombosis. *J Path Bacteriol* 1955; **69**: 283.

198. McGrath JM, Stewart GJ. The effects of endotoxin on vascular endothelium. *J Exp Med* 1969; **129**: 833.

199. McLachlan MSF, Thompson JG, Taylor DW, Kelly M, Sackett DL. Observer variation in the interpretation of lower leg venograms. *Am J Radiol* 1979; **132**: 227.

200. McLachlin AD, McLachlin JA, Jory TA,

Rawling EG. Venous stasis in the lower extremities. *Ann Surg* 1960; **152**: 678.

201. Meyers L, Poindexter CH. A study of the prothrombin time in normal subjects and in patients with arteriosclerosis. *Am Heart J* 1946; **31**: 27.

202. Mitchell JRA. Can we really prevent postoperative pulmonary emboli? *Br Med J* 1979; **1**: 1523.

203. Mitchell JRA. Experimental thrombosis. In Chalmers DG, Gresham GA (Eds) *Biological Aspects of Occlusive Vascular Disease*. London. Cambridge University Press 1964.

204. Moncada S, Gryglewski R, Bunting S, Vane JR. An enzyme isolated from arteries transforms prostaglandin endoperoxides to an unstable substance that inhibits platelet aggregation. *Nature* 1976; **263**: 663.

205. Moncada S, Vane JR. Unstable metabolites of arachidonic acid and their role in haemostasis and thrombosis. *Br Med Bull* 1978; **34**: 129.

206. Morrell MT, Dunhill MS. The post mortem incidence of pulmonary embolism in a hospital population. *Br J Surg* 1968; **55**: 347.

207. Murata K, Nakazawa K, Hamai A. Distribution of acidic glycosaminoglycans in the intima, media and adventitia of bovine aorta and their anticoagulant properties. *Atherosclerosis* 1975; **21**: 93.

208. Mustard JF, Hegardt B, Rowsell HC, MacMillan RL. Effect of adenosine nucleotides on platelet aggregation and clotting time. *J Lab Clin Med* 1964; **64**: 548.

209. Mustard JF, Murphy EA, Rowsell HC, Downie HG. Factors influencing thrombus formation in vivo. *Am J Med* 1962; **33**: 621.

210. Mustard JF. Function of blood platelets and their role in thrombosis. *Trans Am Clin Climatol Assoc* 1976; **87**: 104.

211. Myhre HO, Stören EJ, Ongre A. The incidence of deep venous thrombosis in patients with leg oedema after arterial reconstruction. *Scand J Thor Cardiovasc Surg* 1974; **8**: 73.

212. Naide M. Spontaneous venous thrombosis in the legs of tall men. *JAMA* 1952; **148**: 1202.

213. Nakazawa K, Murata K. Acidic glycosamino glycans in three layers of human aorta: their different constitution and anticoagulant function. *Paroi Arterielle* 1975; **2**: 203.

214. Negus D, Pinto DJ, Brown N. Platelet adhesiveness in postoperative deep vein thrombosis. *Lancet* 1969; **1**: 220.

215. Negus D, Pinto DH, LeQuesne LP, Brown N, Chapman M. [125]I labelled fibrinogen in the diagnosis of deep vein thrombosis and its correlation with phlebography. *Br J Surg* 1968; **55**: 835.

216. Nicolaides AN, Clark CT, Thomas RD, Lewis JD. Soleal veins and local fibrinolytic activity. *Br J Surg* 1972; **59**: 914.

217. Nicolaides AN, Kakkar VV, Field ES, Renney JTG. The origin of deep vein thrombosis: a venographic study. *Br J Radiol* 1971; **44**: 653.

218. Nicolaides AN, Fernandez JF, Pollack AV. Intermittent sequential compression of the legs in prevention of venous stasis and postoperative DVT. *Surgery* 1980; **87**: 69.

219. Nicolaides AN, Field ES, Kakkar VV, Yates-Bell AJ, Taylor S, Clarke MB. Prostatectomy and deep-vein thrombosis. *Br J Surg* 1972; **59**: 487.

220. Nicolaides AN, Irving D. Clinical factors and the risk of deep venous thrombosis. In Nicolaides AN (Ed) *Thromboembolism, Aetiology, Advances in Prevention and Management* Lancaster. NTP 1975.

221. Nicolaides AN, Kakkar VV, Field ES, Fish P. Soleal veins, stasis and prevention of deep vein thrombosis. In Kakkar VV, Jouhar AJ (Eds) *Thromboembolism*. Edinburgh. Churchill Livingstone 1972.

222. Nillius AS, Nylander G. Deep vein thrombosis after total hip replacement: a clinical and phlebographic study. *Br J Surg* 1979; **66**: 324.

223. Nilsen D, Jeremic M, Weisert O. An attempt at predicting postoperative deep vein thrombosis by preoperative coagulation studies in patients undergoing total hip replacement. *Thromb Haemost* 1980; **43**: 194.

224. Nilsson IM, Krook H, Sternby N-H, Söderberg E, Söderström N. Severe thrombotic disease in a young man with bone marrow skeletal changes and with a high content of an inhibitor in the fibrinolytic system. *Acta Med Scand* 1961; **169**: 323.

225. Nilsson IM, Ljungner H, Tengborn L. Two different mechanisms in patients with venous thrombosis and defective fibrinolysis: low concentration of plasminogen activator or increased concentration of plasminogen activator inhibitor. *Br Med J* 1985; **290**: 1453.

226. Nilsson IM, Pandolfi M. Fibrinolytic response of the vascular wall. *Thromb Diath Haemorrh* (Suppl) 1970; **40**: 231.

227. Nilsson IM. Biochemical and clinical aspects of factor VIII. In Saldeen T (Ed) *The Microembolism Syndrome*. Stockholm. Almqvist & Wiksell 1979.

228. Nossel HL. Radioimmunoassay of fibrinopeptides in relation to intravascular coagulation and thrombosis. *N Engl J Med* 1976; **295**: 428.

229. Nylander G, Olivecrona H, Hedner U. Earlier and concurrent morbidity of patients with acute lower leg thrombosis. *Acta Chir Scand* 1977; **143**: 425.

230. Nylander G, Olivecrona H. The phlebographic

pattern of acute leg thrombosis within a defined urban population. *Acta Chir Scand* 1976; **142**: 505.

231. Nylander G, Semb H. Veins of the lower part of the leg after tibial fractures. *Surg Gynec Obstet* 1972; **134**: 974.

232. O'Brien TE, Woodford M, Irving MH. The effect of intermittent compression of the calf on the fibrinolytic responses in the blood during a surgical operation. *Surg Gynec Obstet* 1979; **149**: 380.

233. O'Neill JF. The effects on venous endothelium of alterations in blood flow through the vessels in vein walls, and the possible relation to thrombosis. *Ann Surg* 1947; **126**: 270.

234. Ochsner A, DeBakey ME, DeCamp PT. Venous thrombosis. Analysis of 580 Cases. *Surgery* 1951; **29**: 24.

235. Ogura JH, Fetter NR, Blankenhorn MA, Glueck HI. Changes in blood coagulation following coronary thrombosis measured by the heparin retarded clotting test (Waugh and Ruddick test). *J Clin Invest* 1946; **25**: 586.

236. Olsson P. Variations in antithrombin activity in plasma after major surgery. *Acta Chir Scand* 1963; **126**: 24.

237. Pabinger-Fasching I, Bertina RM, Lechner K, Niessner H, Korininger CH. Protein C deficiency in two Austrian families. *Thromb Haemost* 1983; **50**: 180.

238. Paterson JC. The pathology of venous thrombi. In Sherry S, Brinkhous KM, Genton E, Stengle JM (Eds) *Thrombosis*. Washington D C. National Academy of sciences USA 1969.

239. Poole JCF, French JE. Thrombosis. *J Atheroscler Res* 1961; **1**: 251.

240. Powers JH. Post-operative thromboembolism: Some remarks on the influence of early ambulation. *Am J Med* 1947; **3**: 224.

241. Ratnoff OD, Busse RJ, Sheon RP. The demise of John Hageman. *N Engl J Med* 1968; **279**: 760.

242. Reilly DT, Burden AC, Fossard DP. Fibrinolysis and the prediction of postoperative deep vein thrombosis. *Br J Surg* 1980; **67**: 66.

243. Riley KN, McCabe CJ, Abbott WM, Brewster DC, Moncure AC, Reidy NC, Darling RC. Deep venous thrombophlebitis following aortoiliac reconstructive surgery. *Arch Surg* 1982; **17**: 1210.

244. Roberts VC, Cotton LT. Prevention of postoperative deep vein thrombosis in patients with malignant disease. *Br Med J* 1974; **1**: 358.

245. Rosenberg RD. Actions and interactions of antithrombin and heparin. *N Engl J Med* 1975; **292**: 146.

246. Rosenberg RD. Heparin, antithrombin and abnormal clotting. *Ann Rev Med* 1978; **29**: 367.

247. Roskam J, Hughes J, Bounameaux Y, Salmon J. The part played by platelets in the formation of an efficient hemostatic plug. *Thromb Diath Haemorrh* 1959; **3**: 510.

248. Roskam J. Role of platelets in the formation of a hemostatic plug. In Johnson SA (Ed) *The Henry Ford Hospital Symposium on Blood Platelets*. Boston, Massachusetts. Little Brown 1961.

249. Rowntree LG, Shionya T. Studies on experimental extracorporeal thrombosis. 1 – A method for direct observation of extracorporeal thrombosis formation. *J Exp Med* 1927; **45**: 7.

250. Ruckley CV. ^{125}I fibrinogen test in the diagnosis of deep vein thrombosis. *Br Med J* 1975; **2**: 498.

251. Ruckley CV. A multi-unit controlled trial of heparin and dextran in the prevention of venous thromboembolic disease. In Kakkar VV, Thomas DP (Eds) *Heparin, Chemistry and Clinical Usage*. London. Academic Press 1976.

252. Ruckley CV. Pulmonary embolism; trends in Edinburgh surgical units over twenty years. *Thromb Haemost* 1981; **46**: 18.

253. Sagar S, Massey J, Sanderson JM. Low dose heparin prophylaxis against fatal pulmonary embolism. *Br Med J* 1975; **4**: 257.

254. Sagar S, Stamatakis JD, Thomas DP, Kakkar V V. Oral contraceptives antithrombin III activity and post-operative deep vein thrombosis. *Lancet* 1976; **1**: 509.

255. Samuels PB, Webster DR. The role of venous endothelium in the inception of thrombosis. *Ann Surg* 1952; **136**: 422.

256. Sandler DA, Martin JF. Liquid crystal thermography as a screening test for deep-vein thrombosis. *Lancet* 1985; **1**: 665.

257. Sandler D, Martin JF, Duncan JS, Ward P, Ramsay LE, Lamont AC, Ross B, Sherriff S, Walton L. Diagnosis of deep-vein thrombosis: Comparison of clinical evaluation, ultrasound, plethysmography and venoscan with X-ray venogram. *Lancet* 1984; **2**: 716.

258. Sas G, Blasko G, Bankegyi D, Jako J, Palos A. Abnormal antithrombin III (antithrombin III "Budapest") as a cause of a familial thrombophilia. *Thomb Diath Haemorrh* 1974; **32**: 105.

259. Satiani B, Kuhns M, Evans WE. Deep venous thrombosis following operations upon the abdominal aorta. *Surg Gynec Obstet* 1980; **151**: 241.

260. Sawyer PN, Srinivasan S. The role of surface

phenomena in intravascular thrombosis. *Bibl Anat* 1973; **12**: 106.

261. Schaub N, Duckert F, Fridrich R, Gruber UF. Häufigkeit postoperative tiefer Venenthrombosen bei Patienten der allgemeinen Chirurgie und Urologie. *Langenbecks Arch Chir* 1975; **340**: 23.

262. Scott GBD. Venous intimal thickenings and thrombosis. *J Path Bact* 1956; **72**: 543.

263. Seeger WH, Marciniak E. Inhibition of autoprothrombin C activity with plasma. *Nature* 1962; **193**: 1188.

264. Seigel DG. Pregnancy, the puerperium and the steroid contraceptive. In Foster D (Ed) The Epidemiology of Venous Thrombosis. *Millbank Memorial Fund Q* 1972; **50**: 15.

265. Senftleben W. Über den verschluss der blutgefässe nach unterbindung. *Arch Path Anat Physiol* 1879; **77**: 421.

266. Sevitt S, Gallagher NG. Prevention of venous thrombosis and pulmonary embolism in injured patients. *Lancet* 1959; **2**: 981.

267. Sevitt S, Gallagher NG. Venous thrombosis and pulmonary embolism. A clinico-pathological study in injured and burned patients. *Br J Surg* 1961; **48**: 475.

268. Sevitt S. Pathology and pathogenesis of deep vein thrombi. In Bergan JJ, Yao JST (Eds) *Venous Problems*. Chicago. Year Book Medical Publishers 1978.

269. Sevitt S. The structure and growth of valve-pocket thrombi in femoral veins. *J Clin Pathol* 1974; **27**: 517.

270. Sevitt S. Venous thrombosis and pulmonary embolism. Their prevention by oral anticoagulants. *Am J Med* 1962; **33**: 703.

271. Shapiro S. Hyperprothrombinemia, a premonitory sign of thromboembolization (Description of a method). *Exper Med Surg* 1944; **2**: 103.

272. Shapiro S, Sherwin B, Gordimer H. Postoperative thrombo-embolization. *Ann Surg* 1942; **116**: 175.

273. Short DS. A survey of pulmonary embolism in a general hospital. *Br Med J* 1952; **1**: 790.

274. Simpson K. Shelter deaths from pulmonary embolism. *Lancet* 1940; **2**: 744.

275. Sinclair J, Forbes CD, Prentice CRM, Scott R. The incidence of deep vein thrombosis in prostatectomised patients following the administration of the fibrinolytic inhibitor, aminocaproic acid (EACA). *Urol Res* 1976; **4**: 129.

276. Smith RC, Duncancson J, Ruckley CV, Webber RG, Allan NC, Dawes J, Bolton AF, Hunter WM, Pepper DS, Cash JD. β-thromboglobulin and deep vein thrombosis. *Thromb Haemost* 1978; **39**: 338.

277. Smith R, Blick E, Coalston J, Stein P. Thrombus production by turbulence. *J Appl Physiol* 1972; **32**: 261.

278. Spaet TH, Ts'Ao CH. Vascular endothelium and thrombogenesis. In Sherry S, Brinkhous KM, Genton E, Stengle JM (Eds) *Thrombosis*. Washington DC. National Academy of Sciences USA 1969.

279. Spaet TH, Erichson RB. The vascular wall in the pathogenesis of thrombosis. *Thromb Diath Haemorrh* (Suppl) 1966; **21**: 67.

280. Sproul EE. Carcinoma and venous thrombosis: the frequency of association of carcinoma in the body or tail of the pancreas with multiple venous thrombosis. *Am J Cancer* 1938; **34**: 566.

281. Stamatakis JD, Kakkar VV, Sagar S, Lawrence D, Nairn D, Bentley PG. Femoral vein thrombosis and total hip replacement. *Br Med J* 1977; **2**: 223.

282. Stathatkis N, Papayannis AG, Gardikas CD. Postoperative antithrombin III concentration. *Lancet* 1973; **1**: 430.

283. Stead NW, Bauer KA, Kinney TR, Lewis JG, Campbell EE, Shifman MA, Rosenberg RD, Pizzo SV. Venous thrombosis in a family with defective release of vascular plasminogen activator and elevated plasma factor VIII, von Willebrand's factor. *Am J Med* 1983; **74**: 33.

284. Stein P, Sabbah H. Measured turbulence and its effect on thrombus formation. *Circ Res* 1974; **35**: 608.

285. Stevens J, Fardin R, Freeark R. Lower extremity thrombophlebitis in patients with femoral neck fractures. A venographic investigation and a review of the early and late significance of the findings. *J Trauma* 1968; **8**: 527.

286. Stewart GJ, Anderson MJ. An ultrastructural study of endotoxin induced changes in mesenteric arteries. *Br J Exp Pathol* 1971; **52**: 75.

287. Stewart GJ, Ritchie WGM, Lynch PR. A scanning and transmission electron microscopic study of canine jugular veins. Scanning electron microscopy (Part III). In *Proceedings of the Workshop on Scanning Electron Micro copy in Pathology*. Illinois. IIT Research Institute Chicago, 1973.

288. Stewart GJ, Ritchie WGM, Lynch PR. Venous endothelial damage produced by massive sticking and emigration of leucocytes. *Am J Pathol* 1974; **74**: 507.

289. Stewart GJ, Stern HS, Lynch PR, Malmud LS, Schaub RG. Response of the canine jugular veins and carotid arteries to hysterectomy: increased permeability and leucocyte adhesions and invasion. *Thromb Res* 1980; **20**: 473.

290. Stewart GJ, Stern HR, Schaub RG. Endothelial alterations, deposition of blood elements and increased accumulation of ^{131}I-albumin in canine jugular veins following abdominal surgery. *Thromb Res* 1978; **12**: 555.

291. Stewart GJ. The role of the vessel wall in deep venous thrombosis. In Nicolaides AN (Ed) *Thromboembolism. Aetiology, Advances in Prevention and Management*. Lancaster MTP 1975.

292. Stormorken H, Lund M, Holmsen I. Vessel wall activator (tPA) as evaluated by poststasis euglobulin lysis time (PELT) in recurrent deep vein thrombosis. In Jespersen J, Kluft C, Korsgaard O (Eds) *Clinical Aspects of Fibrinolysis and Thrombolysis*. Esbjerg. South Jutland University Press 1983.

293. Sue-Ling HM, Johnston D, McMahon MJ, Phillips PR, Davis JA. Pre-operative identification of patients at high risk of deep venous thrombosis after elective major abdominal surgery. *Lancet* 1986; **1**: 1173.

294. Sundqvist S-B, Hedner U, Kullenberg HKE, Bergentz S-E. Deep venous thrombosis of the arm: a study of coagulation and fibrinolysis. *Br Med J* 1981; **283**: 265.

295. Taberner DA, Poller L, Burslem RW. Antiplasmin concentration after surgery: failure of alpha$_2$-antiplasmin to rise in patients with venous thrombosis. *Br Med J* 1979; **1**: 1122.

296. Tanaka K, Hirst AE, Smith LL. Rate of endothelialization in venous thrombi: an experimental study. *Arch Surg* 1982; **117**: 1045.

297. Tateson JE, Moncada S, Vane JR. Effect of prostacyclin (PGX) on cyclic AMP concentration in human platelets. *Prostaglandins* 1977; **13**: 389.

298. Thomas DP, Merton RE, Wood RD, Hockley DJ. The relationship between vessel wall injury and venous thrombosis: an experimental study. *Br J Haematol* 1985; **59**: 449.

299. Thomas DP, Wessler S. Stasis thrombi induced by bacterial endotoxin. *Circ Res* 1964; **14**: 486.

300. Todd AS. The histological localization of fibrinolysis activator. *J Path Bact* 1959; **78**: 281.

301. Törngren S, Norén I, Savidge G. The effect of low-dose heparin on fibrinopeptide A, platelets, fibrinogen degradation products and other haemostatic parameters measured in connection with intestinal surgery. *Thromb Res* 1979; **14**: 871.

302. Tran TH, Marbet GA, Duckert F. Association of hereditary heparin co-factor 2 deficiency with thrombosis. *Lancet* 1985; **2**: 413.

303. Trousseau A. *Phlegmatia alba dolens. In clinique médicale de l'Hotel-Dieu de Paris* 2nd edition. Vol 3. Paris. Baillière 1865; 654.

304. Vessey MP, Doll R, Fairburn AS. Post-operative thromboembolism and the use of oral contraceptives. *Br Med J* 1970; **3**: 123.

305. Vessey MP, Doll R. Investigation of relation between use of oral contraceptives and thromboembolic disease: a further report. *Br Med J* 1968; **2**: 199.

306. Vessey MP, Mann JI. Female sex hormones and thrombosis. *Epidemiological aspects. Br Med Bull* 1978; **34**: 157.

307. Vessey M, Mant D, Smith A, Yeates D. Oral contraceptives and venous thromboembolism: findings in a large prospective study. *Br Med J* 1986; **292**: 526.

308. Vinnicombe J, Shuttleworth KED. Aminocaproic acid in the control of haemorrhage after prostatectomy. Safety of aminocaproic acid – a controlled trial. *Lancet* 1966; **1**: 232.

309. Virchow R. Die Verstopfung den Lungen arteries und ihre Folgen. *Beitr Exp Path Physiol* 1846; **21**.

310. Von Kaulla E, Von Kaulla KM. Oral contraceptives and low antithrombin III activity. *Lancet* 1970; **1**: 36.

311. Von Kaulla E, Von Kaulla KN. Antithrombin III and diseases. *Am J Clin Pathol* 1967; **48**: 69.

312. Von Kaulla E, von Kaulla KN. Deficiency of antithrombin III activity associated with hereditary thrombosis tendency. *J Med* 1972; **3**: 349.

313. Von Recklinghausen F. Handbuch der allgemeinen Pathologie des Kreislaufs und der Ernäbrung. *Deutsche Churgie* 1883; **2**: 52.

314. Walsh JJ, Bonnar J, Wright FM. A study of pulmonary embolism after deep leg vein thrombosis after major gynaecological surgery using labelled fibrinogen, phlebography and lung-scanning. *J Obstet Gynaecol Br Commonw* 1974; **81**: 311.

315. Warlow C, Ogston D, Douglas AS. Deep venous thrombosis of the legs after strokes. Part I. Incidence and predisposing factors. *Br Med J* 1976; **1**: 1178.

316. Warlow C, Ogston D. the ^{125}I-fibrinogen technique in the diagnosis of venous thrombosis. *Clin Haematol* 1973; **2**: 199.

317. Warren R, Lauridsen J, Belko J. Alteration in numbers of circulating platelets following surgical operation and administration of adrenocorticotrophic hormone. *Circulation* 1953; **7**: 481.

318. Waugh TR, Ruddick DW. Studies on increased coagulability of the blood. *Canad M A J* 1944; **51**: 11.

319. Welch CE, Fexon HH. Thrombophlebitis and pulmonary embolism. *JAMA* 1941; **117**: 1502.

320. Wells RE. Rheological aspects of stasis in throm-

bus formation. In Sherry S (Ed) *Thrombosis*. Washington. National Academy of Sciences USA 1969.

321. Welsh WH. The structure of white thrombi. *Trans Path Soc Phil* 1887; **13**: 281.

322. Wessler S, Yin ET. Experimental hypercoagulable state induced by factor X: comparison of the non-activated and activated forms. *J Lab Clin Med* 1968; **72**: 256.

323. Wessler S, Yin ET. On the mechanism of thrombosis. *Prog Hematol* 1969; **6**: 201.

324. Wessler S. Studies in intravascular coagulation. I. Coagulation changes in isolated venous segments. *J Clin Invest* 1952; **31**: 1011.

325. Wessler S. Studies in intravascular coagulation. III. The pathogenesis of serum induced venous thrombosis. *J Clin Invest* 1955; **34**: 647.

326. Wessler S. Thrombosis in the presence of vascular stasis. *Am J Med* 1962; **33**: 648.

327. Wheeler HB, Anderson FA, Cardullo PA, Patwarden NA, Jian-Ming L, Cutler BS. Suspected deep vein thrombosis: management by impedance plethysmography. *Arch Surg* 1982; **117**: 1206.

328. Wigton DH, Kociba GJ, Hoover EA. Infectious canine hepatitis: animal model for viral-induced disseminated intravascular coagulation. *Blood* 1976; **47**: 287.

329. Wilkins RW, Mixter G, Stanton JR, Litter J. Elastic stockings in the prevention of pulmonary embolism: a preliminary report. *N Engl J Med* 1952; **246**: 360.

330. Wilkins RW, Stanton JR. Elastic stockings in the prevention of pulmonary embolism. II. A progress report. *N Engl J Med* 1953; **248**: 1087.

331. Wills AL, Kuhn DC. A new potential mediator of arterial thrombosis whose biosynthesis is inhibited by aspirin. *Prostaglandins* 1973; **4**: 127.

332. Winter JH, Fenech A, Bennett B, Douglas AS. Thrombosis after venography and familial antithrombin III deficiency. *Br Med J* 1981; **283**: 1436.

333. Wiseman R. *Several Surgical Treatises*. London. Norton & Macock 1676.

334. Wolfe JHN, Morland M, Browse NL. The fibrinolytic activity of varicose veins. *Br J Surg* 1979; **66**: 185.

335. Wright G Payling. *An Introduction to Pathology*. London. Longmans Green 1958.

336. Wright H Payling, Osborn SB, Edmonds DG. Effects of post-operative bedrest and early ambulation on the rate of venous blood flow. *Lancet* 1956; **1**: 222.

337. Wright H Payling. Changes in the adhesiveness of blood platelets following parturition and surgical operations. *J Path Bact* 1942; **54**: 461.

338. Wu AVO, Mansfield A. The relationship between the blood and vein wall fibrinolytic activity in response to surgical trauma. *Acta Haematol* 1980; **63**: 191.

339. Yin ET, Wessler S, Stoll PJ. Identity of plasma activated factor X inhibitor with antithrombin III and heparin co-factor. *J Biol Chem* 1971; **246**: 712.

340. Ygge J. Studies on blood coagulation and fibrinolysis in conditions associated with an increased incidence of thrombosis. Methodological and clinical investigations. *Scand J Haematol* (Suppl) 1970; **11**.

341. Zahn W. Untersuchungen über Thrombose. *Zentralbl Med Wissenschaften* 1872; **10**: 129.

342. Zucker MB, Borelli J. Platelet clumping produced by connective tissue suspensions and by collagen. *Proc Soc Exp Biol Med* 1962; **109**: 779.

343. Zucker MB. Platelet agglutination and vasoconstriction as factors in spontaneous hemostasis in normal, thrombocytopenic, heparinized and hypoprothrombinemic rats. *Am J Physiol* 1947; **148**: 275.

17

Deep vein thrombosis: diagnosis

The clinical diagnosis of deep vein thrombosis can be extremely difficult because many patients have no symptoms or signs in the affected limb.

Symptoms

The symptoms that are commonly produced by deep vein thrombosis are pain, swelling, and a faint blue – red discoloration of the skin (Colour plate 37). Profound cyanotic discoloration (phlegmasia cerulea dolens), or pallor (phlegmasia alba dolens) and frank venous gangrene (Colour plate 38) are much less common.

The more proximal and occlusive the thrombus, the more marked are the symptoms and physical signs. Postoperative calf thrombi often do not cause any symptoms,[50] and the clinical significance of small symptomless calf thrombi has been questioned,[15,42,108] there is, however, no doubt that calf thombi can sometimes progress to extensive life-threatening proportions if they are left untreated.

Deep vein thrombosis may also present as a pyrexia of unkown origin or with the symptoms of pulmonary embolism without any evidence of leg symptoms.

A paradoxical embolus (seen only a few times during a surgeon's career) occurs when a venous thromboembolus passes from the right to the left side of the heart through a congenital defect and then impacts in the arterial side of the circulation. The cardiac abnormality is usually a ventricular septal defect or a patent ductus arteriosus. A paradoxical embolus should be suspected if no cause can be found for an arterial embolus in a patient with a cardiac murmur, pulmonary hypertension and a swollen limb.

Many patients who present with the clinical signs of a post-thrombotic limb, confirmed by phlebography, have no previous history of a clinical deep vein thrombosis or pulmonary embolism, the whole process having been completely silent. This finding fits with the fact that half of the patients with a positive fibrinogen uptake test have no symptoms.[50]

Signs

The physical signs of a deep vein thrombosis may be as ephemeral as the symptoms, and they are often non-existent.

Tenderness

The most common but most inaccurate physical sign is tenderness on compressing the calf muscles, or tenderness over the course of the main veins of the thigh. Tenderness should be elicited carefully with firm but gentle manual pressure along the course of the veins and over both bellies of the gastrocnemius muscle with the knee flexed to 150°. Only half the patients with calf muscle tenderness have a thrombosis.[50] Tenderness at other sites (e.g. the lateral part of the thigh) rarely indicates a thrombosis. The aetiology of the tenderness remains obscure, as it does not appear to be related to either the extent or adherence of the thrombus.[23]

Oedema

Deep vein thrombosis often causes mild pitting oedema of the ankle. This is a significant clinical sign and is a true indicator of thrombosis in 70 per cent of cases, especially if it is unilateral.[106] Oedema of the foot and calf indicates that the thrombus has probably extended into the popliteal vein and above (Fig. 17.1). Swelling of

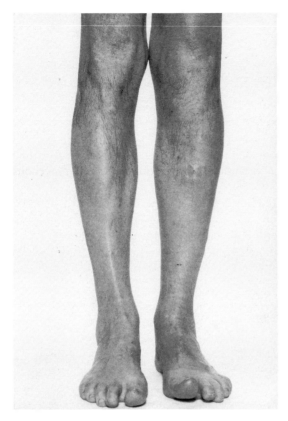

Fig. 17.1 Oedema is the most sensitive of the physical signs of deep vein thrombosis; it correctly indicates the diagnosis in approximately 70 per cent of cases.

This patient complained of minor swelling of the left ankle but the photograph reveals that there was swelling of the whole leg. The left calf was firm but not tender. Phlebography revealed a complete popliteal – femoral – iliac thrombosis.

the whole leg is associated with ilio-femoral or vena caval thrombosis (Colour plate 37).

Muscle induration

The calf muscles may feel 'woody' hard if there is extensive intramuscular thrombosis but it may be possible to palpate small tender patches before this happens; these small areas are presumably related to localized areas of intramuscular thrombosis. As the muscles become stiff, there may be a detectable difference in the mobility (floppiness) of one calf which can be observed by gently shaking the calves with the hand or by flexing the knees to 150° and gently knocking them together.

Warm and distended superficial veins

If there is significant venous outflow obstruction, the skin of the leg may feel warm and the superficial veins may be distended and fail to collapse when the limb is elevated. Distended veins in the affected groin of a limb with an ilio-femoral thrombosis indicate a major degree of venous obstruction.

Homans' dorsiflexion test

Homans' dorsiflexion sign is another method of testing tenderness of the calf but has been disowned by Homans as unreliable.[25] In 1944 Homans made the following statement.[69]

'*Homans' sign*. I prefer to call it the dorsiflexion sign. Actually the dorsiflexion of the feet is intended to bring out, on the side of the venous thrombosis, some degree of irritability of the posterior muscles, the soleus and gastrocnemius. *Discomfort need have no part in this reaction*. Dorsiflexion may be less complete in response to an equal degree of upward pressure on the affected side as compared with the normal, or the patient may involuntarily flex the knee, as the forefoot is forced upwards, to release the tension on the posterior muscles. If one looks at the dorsiflexion sign as evidence of even the faintest irritability of the posterior muscles, (the early stage of the thrombosis occurring within and about them), the sign will be found more frequently than either tenderness or swelling.'

Archer[7] chided Sandler and Martin[138] with this direct quote from Homans when they had defined the sign as 'pain in the calf on passive dorsiflexion of the foot'. Sandler's riposte[139] was to quote four medical textbooks in which pain was included in the definition of Homans' sign, and to carry out a small survey amongst junior doctors in Sheffield all of whom understood Homans' sign to be pain in the calf on dorsiflexion of the foot (but he did not state if he had himself been teaching these students!). A review of three surgical textbooks[3,68,128] shows that Homans' sign is commonly defined as pain on dorsiflexion of the foot, though Hobsley[68] like Browse[21] goes on to point out that Homans tried to disown the sign.

We suspect that pain has crept into the definition of 'Homans' sign' because 'increased resistance' is ill defined and often difficult to judge. We neither use nor recommend the test, irrespective of its definition, because it is inaccurate, and we would happily relegate it to obscurity.

The Loewenberg test

This was an attempt to quantify Homans' sign; it elicited 'tenderness' by inflating a pneumatic tourniquet placed around the calf muscles to different pressures to determine the pressure that caused pain. It has proved as unreliable as the dorsiflexion test.[102]

Skin discoloration

A white leg (phlegmasia alba dolens) is a common and significant appearance. It is more often observed by the clinician than complained of by the patient, as it is always associated with pain or swelling. The pallor is probably caused by extensive oedema which obscures the capillary circulation of the skin,[70] though some investigators have suggested that arterial spasm is also present.[118] A white leg is usually caused by an ilio-femoral thrombosis.

A blue leg (phlegmasia cerulea dolens)[53] is often observed by the patient but is usually associated with a degree of pain and swelling which overshadows the cyanosis. The 'blue' appearance is caused by venous congestion secondary to a thrombosis in both the external and common iliac veins (and often the internal iliac veins) which obstructs the venous drainage of the limb. The skin may be covered with small petechiae, and areas of skin may become gangrenous if the outflow obstruction is not relieved.

Venous gangrene

If the venous outflow of a limb is severely reduced as in phlegmasia cerulea dolens, the arterial inflow may become obstructed. The tips of the toes become deep blue and then black, or the skin blisters (Colour plate 38). These changes usually affect all the toes, unlike arterial gangrene where only one or two toes may be affected, and may spread onto the dorsal and ventral surfaces of the forefoot. The general swelling and blueness of the limb, even when elevated, distinguishes it from the pale, cold, shrivelled limb of acute arterial ischemia.

Loss of peripheral arterial pulses

It is often difficult to palpate the foot pulses in a limb with phlegmasia cerulea dolens or venous gangrene. This observation led Oschner and DeBakey to suggest that an extensive venous thrombosis causes arterial spasm.[118] The arterial inflow to the limb is usually reduced by the massive obstruction to venous outflow, but Lea Thomas and Carty[91] suggested that in some limbs obstruction to arterial inflow might be the prime abnormality, precipitating a secondary venous thrombosis.

Our clinical experience supports the hypothesis that ilio-femoral venous thrombosis initiates arterial spasm that often resolves with rest, limb elevation and anticoagulation. We have performed arteriograms on a few of these patients and found evidence of arterial emboli, possibly arising from the artery adjacent to the primary site of the venous thrombosis and caused by the involvement of the arterial wall in the inflammatory process. As with so many clinical problems, it is probable that all three mechanisms (venous obstruction, arterial spasm and arterial emboli) play a part in different circumstances.

Very occasionally, a paradoxical embolus may be the cause of a blue swollen limb in which the pulses are absent.

Superficial thrombophlebitis

Any patient who presents with a superficial thrombophlebitis may have a deep vein thrombosis (see Chapter 22).[10]

Pyrexia

Patients with a deep vein thrombosis often have a low persistent fever. A patient who is found to have this type of fever in the postoperative period should be carefully screened to exclude a silent deep vein thrombosis. A similar fever is often found in patients who have repeated small pulmonary emboli.

Signs of pulmonary embolism

The clinical features of pulmonary embolism are discussed in detail in Chapter 21. Many patients with a silent deep vein thrombosis present with chest pain, haemoptysis or shortness of breath.

The discriminant value of the symptoms and signs

In a prospective study of deep vein thrombosis diagnosed with the fibrinogen uptake test and confirmed by phlebography, Flanc *et al.*[50] found that 11 per cent of the patients with a proven thrombosis had a marked increase in ankle size, 25 per cent had calf tenderness, 34 per cent had a distinguishable difference in limb temperature, 52 per cent had mild unilateral ankle oedema, and 68 per cent showed some induration of the calf muscles. In a similar study Howe[72] reported that the presenting symptoms of thrombosis were pain and tenderness in 66 per cent of patients, swelling in 10 per cent, and pulmonary embolism in 10 per cent. The remaining 15 per cent of patients presented with massive axial vein occlusion (white or blue legs).

McLachlin *et al.*[106] reported that unilateral leg swelling gave a correct indication of the diagnosis of deep vein thrombosis in 80 per cent of patients, local tenderness and a positive Homans' sign correctly diagnosed thrombosis in only 50 per cent and 8 per cent respectively. Gibbs[52] also found that ankle oedema was a reliable clinical sign of deep vein thrombosis.

The significance of increased skin temperature as a diagnostic indication of deep vein thrombosis was examined by Provan in 1968.[127] Provan concluded that an increased skin temperature was not sufficiently accurate to be used as a basis for diagnosis.

The ankle – brachial arterial pressure index may be used to assess arterial inflow if the pulses are impalpable but it does not assist in making a correct clinical diagnosis of deep vein thrombosis.

Differential diagnosis

As the history and physical signs of deep vein thrombosis are so imprecise, a firm diagnosis depends upon the use of special tests. The 'gold standard' investigation is bipedal ascending phlebography (see Chapter 4, page 103). It is essential to confirm a clinical diagnosis of deep vein thrombosis with an objective investigation because treatment is not without risk,[9,51,88,101,103] and the studies on the accuracy of clinical diagnosis show that it is incorrect 30 – 50 per cent of the time.[50,88,129,144] The particular advantage of phlebography is that it gives information about both the type and the extent of the thrombus. The value of the alternative tests that can be used to

Table 17.1 Conditions which mimic deep vein thrombosis

Torn gastrocnemius muscle
Ruptured Baker's cyst
Calf haematomata
Lymphoedema with cellulitis
Acute arterial ischaemia
Extrinsic obstruction of veins and lymphatics in pelvis
Pathological fracture of femur
Superficial thrombophlebitis
Acute arthritis of the knee
Haemarthrosis of the knee
Torn meniscus
Achilles tendonitis
Oedema from congestive cardiac failure or the nephrotic syndrome
Rapidly growing sarcoma
Myositis ossificans
Munchausen's syndrome

diagnose thrombosis is discussed in the final section of this chapter.

The many conditions which mimic a deep vein thrombosis and require special investigation to be detected are listed in Table 17.1.

Ruptured Baker's cyst

This is now recognized as one of the most important and most difficult conditions to distinguish from acute deep thrombosis.[84] Both conditions present with an acute onset of pain and swelling in the calf, and only a few patients give a prior history of arthritic pains in the knee joint.[144]

Once the cyst has ruptured, there may be few physical signs of arthritis in the knee joint, and there is usually no residual effusion or palpable cyst.[104] There is often some bruising but this commonly appears in the lower part of the leg, anterior to the Achilles tendon, days later and is of no help in making the diagnosis in the acute stage (see Colour plate 40).

Deep vein thrombosis and a ruptured Baker's cyst can occur simultaneously[9,144] or the latter may precipitate the former; these situations make the diagnosis extremely difficult.

If a ruptured Baker's cyst is suspected, arthrography, ultrasound, and phlebography may be required.[9]

Torn gastrocnemius or plantaris muscle

These conditions cause a pain of sudden onset, sometimes followed by swelling of the leg. The pain usually develops faster than the pain of a thrombosis, and the patient is often taking some form of strenuous exercise when the symptoms begin. Unlike a rupture of the Achilles tendon, partial tears of the fibres of gastrocnemius muscle have no physical signs other than some muscle tenderness and pain when the muscle is contracted against resistance.

Lymphoedema with cellulitis

A limb with mild lymphoedema may suddenly develop a severe cellulitis causing pain, redness and swelling. In the early stages this may be quite difficult to differentiate from an acute deep vein thrombosis. The diagnosis usually becomes apparent when the red area of skin extends and the patient develops a high pyrexia with rigors; neither of these signs are really typical of a thrombosis. Nevertheless, every year we see several patients with lymphoedema whose attacks of cellulitis have been mis-diagnosed as deep vein thrombosis, and who have been treated, some for many years, with anticoagulants. A normal phlebogram and an abnormal lymphogram (isotopic or X-ray) [86,146] will differentiate between lymphoedema with cellulitis and deep vein thrombosis.

Acute arterial ischaemia

This usually presents with severe pain but without swelling. Occasionally, however, arterial occlusion and venous thrombosis occur simultaneously[9]; the venous congestion and oedema are the dominant signs. The pallor of the limb and developing muscle weakness and paraesthesiae should quickly indicate the correct diagnosis.

Haemorrhage into the limb

Patients on anticoagulants or patients with coagulation defects may suffer a sudden acute bleed into a joint or the soft tissues following minor trauma. Haemorrhage will be suspected if the coagulation defect is known but may not be diagnosed if the clinician is unaware of the condition. The loss of joint mobility or a localized swelling in a joint or muscle, together with

abnormal coagulation tests should confirm the diagnosis without the need to perform phlebography. Computerized tomography (CT) scanning is occasionally required to confirm the diagnosis.

Pelvic or intra-abdominal tumours obstructing the veins

Patients with pelvic or intra-abdominal tumours are at increased risk of developing deep vein thrombosis, but sometimes the tumour will obstruct the veins without causing a thrombosis (see Fig. 9.9, page 279). This difference, which can only be revealed by phlebography, may be clinically significant when planning the management of the tumour, especially if that treatment may cause tumour regression (Fig. 17.2 a and b).

It is important to perform an abdominal, rectal and/or a vaginal examination on all patients who present with a spontaneous deep vein thrombosis to exclude an abdominal or pelvic malignancy.[33,41,131,145]

Pathological fractures

A history of injury is invariably present in patients with ordinary fractures. In patients with pathological fractures, however, a history of injury may be absent, and these patients often present with an unexplained and sudden onset of severe limb pain and swelling. Pathological fractures should be suspected if the patient is known to have had prior treatment for a malignant disease or has clinical evidence of malignant disease elsewhere. A careful clinical examination will usually reveal localized tenderness, immobility and deformity but these signs may be minimal and easily missed. Radiographs of the bones will confirm the diagnosis and obviate the need for phlebography. A radioactive isotope bone scan may provide evidence of other bony metastases.

Superficial thrombophlebitis

Superficial thrombophlebitis presents as a hot tender linear swelling of the skin and subcutaneous tissues. It is common in patients with varicose veins (see Chapter 22 and Fig. 17.3).

Superficial thrombophlebitis and deep vein thrombosis often coexist,[10] and superficial thrombophlebitis is often mistaken for a deep

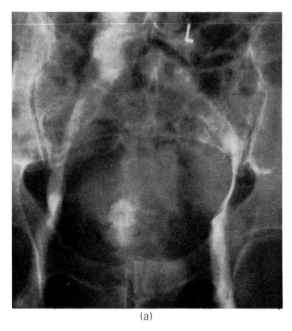

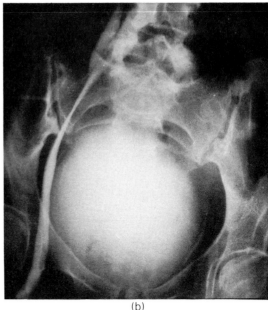

(a)   (b)

Fig. 17.2   Compression of a deep vein causes the same symptoms as a deep vein thrombosis.
  (a) This patient's pain and leg swelling were caused by a large pelvic mass compressing the left external vein.
  (b) This patient's swollen right leg was caused by a large bladder compressing the right iliac vein.

vein thrombosis. As the association between the two types of thrombosis is so common, phlebography should be considered in all patients who do not have visible varicose veins.[10] Some patients who have recurrent superficial thrombophlebitis have a hitherto unsuspected malignancy, particularly if their superficial thrombophlebitis is associated with a deep vein thrombosis (see Chapter 22).[145]

Acute arthritis

Acute arthritis of the knee joint may cause pain, redness and swelling of the calf in the affected limb.[89] The pain is usually in the joint and is exacerbated by joint movement but occasionally it does spread throughout the leg. The diagnosis is easy to make if other joints are affected but even rheumatoid arthritis can be mono-articular. Clinical examination is usually diagnostic but plain radiographs and serological tests may be required. The fibrinogen uptake test should be interpreted with care in patients with acute arthritis because it is an important cause of false-positive readings (see Fig. 4.32, page 102). A positive fibrinogen uptake test in a patient with arthritis should always be checked by phlebography.[126]

Internal derangements of the knee

Many abnormalities of the knee joint (e.g. meniscal tears, meniscal cysts, loose bodies, effusions, chondromalacia patellae, recurrent dislocation of the patella, osteochondritis) can cause swelling and pain, both in and around the knee. These conditions should be distinguishable from deep vein thrombosis by the history and by physical signs related to knee movements.

Achilles tendonitis

This causes pain which is localized to the Achilles tendon. It is usually the result of excessive and unaccustomed exercise but may be associated with Reiter's syndrome. There is usually pain on forcible dorsiflexion of the foot and tenderness over the tendon rather than over the calf.

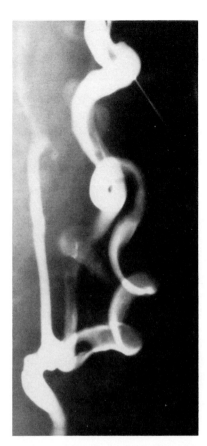

Fig. 17.3 Fresh thrombus in a varicose vein. Superficial thrombophlebitis is a common complication of varicose veins but when it occurs in a normal vein it is often associated with a deep vein thrombosis and is frequently caused by occult malignant disease (see Chapter 22).

Generalized oedema

Patients with congestive cardiac failure, protein depletion, renal failure and fluid overload tend to develop swelling of the legs, which may cause diagnostic difficulties, particularly during the postoperative period. The swelling is invariably bilateral, but deep vein thrombosis is also often bilateral. The absence of calf tenderness or fever does not help because they are often not present when there is a thrombosis. As there is a high incidence of thrombosis in patients with conditions that cause generalized oedema, it is often necessary to confirm or exclude the presence of thrombosis with phlebography.

Soft-tissue sarcoma

A sarcoma of the muscles, fibrous tissue or bone of the leg usually causes a localized swelling in the thigh or lower leg but may cause chronic pain, venous obstruction and generalized swelling of the limb. In the early stages the diagnosis may be very difficult. If the phlebogram of a leg in which there is persistent pain and swelling is normal, CT scanning, arteriography and surgical exploration with biopsy should be considered (see Chapter 26 and Fig. 26.12).

Myositis ossificans

This condition rarely causes diagnostic difficulties, as it invariably follows a well-remembered injury to the thigh. The swelling and pain may occasionally be mistaken for a thrombosis, especially if the patient has forgotten about the original injury. Plain radiographs always show soft-tissue calcification.

Munchausen's syndrome

Some patients deliberately induce swelling of the leg by applying a tourniquet; the swelling is then mistaken for lymphoedema or recurrent deep vein thrombosis.

Practical significance of the symptoms and signs

Deep vein thrombosis occurs in two groups of patients. In most instances the patient has a predisposing condition (e.g. medical illness or a surgical operation) and is in hospital. A few patients, however, present with the symptoms and signs of thrombosis or embolism as the first and only event, and do not have an obvious predisposing cause; most of these patients are seen in the doctor's office as out-patients or require urgent admission to hospital for investigation of their symptoms.

Patients in hospital known to be at risk

If the diagnosis of deep vein thrombosis is not to be missed in patients who are in hospital, it must be considered as a possibility at all times. Screening procedures should be used in patients in the high risk groups (see Chapter 19) if prophylaxis is not universally employed, but as no type of prophylaxis is infallible, a high degree of clinical vigilance must be maintained. It should be part of the routine for all staff (junior and senior) to inspect the temperature charts and to examine the legs of patients for swelling and tenderness every day. Any symptoms or signs which suggest deep vein thrombosis or pulmonary embolism should stimulate a detailed clinical examination followed by the appropriate tests to exclude the diagnosis. Every surgeon must remember that approximately one-third of his patients may develop a deep vein thrombosis. The incidence in medical patients is somewhat less (15–20 per cent) but this is still a significant percentage of the total 'in-patient' population.

Patients who present with symptoms and signs which suggest thrombosis or embolism, de novo

Patients who suddenly develop symptoms in the legs or chest which suggest deep vein thrombosis or pulmonary embolism require a detailed clinical examination and basic investigations in order to answer the following questions.

- Is a deep vein thrombosis the most likely diagnosis?
- If not, what is the cause of the symptoms and signs?
- Is there any evidence of a pre-existing condition which could have caused the deep vein thrombosis?
- Has the patient had a pulmonary embolus?
- If not, what is the cause of the chest symptoms?

These questions are not difficult to answer when the symptoms and signs are typical. For example, a patient who has an aching pain in the calf that has developed over several hours and is associated with leg swelling and a predisposing factor (e.g. a past history of thrombosis, ingestion of the contraceptive pill, a family history of thrombosis, a known malignancy, an haematological disease, a recent illness or an injury) almost certainly has a deep vein thrombosis, especially if a pleuritic chest pain, haemoptysis or shortness of breath is also present.

In many patients, however, the story is less clear-cut, the symptoms and signs are vague, there is no obvious predisposing cause and in some cases the history is so 'atypical' that the diagnosis is merely considered as a differential diagnosis or there may be good evidence for another cause for the symptoms. In this group of patients a meticulous systematic clinical examination may detect another cause of the symptoms.

When the history and examination have been completed it should be possible to place the patient in one of the following four categories and to obtain some indication of an underlying cause.

1. The patient almost certainly has deep vein thrombosis complicated by pulmonary embolism.
2. The patient almost certainly has a deep vein thrombosis.
3. The possibility of a deep vein thrombosis is sufficiently strong to justify its investigation before excluding other causes of the symptoms.
4. It is unlikely that the patient has a deep vein thrombosis, and other causes of the symptoms should be investigated first.

1. The patient almost certainly has had a deep vein thrombosis complicated by pulmonary embolism Treatment with heparin should begin at once, and the patient must be admitted to hospital immediately for confirmation of the diagnosis, to assess the risk of further embolism, and to plan further treatment.

2. The patient almost certainly has a deep vein thrombosis The diagnosis must be confirmed so that appropriate treatment to prevent extension of the thrombus and reduce the risk of embolism can be started.

3. The patient may have had a deep vein thrombosis If there is doubt but a genuine possibility that the patient has had a deep vein thrombosis, the diagnosis should be confirmed as soon as possible using the most accurate and informative test. If patients are treated solely on clinical evidence, two out of three will be given the wrong treatment as a clinical diagnosis has been shown to be incorrect in 63 per cent of patients,[129] and at best carries only a 50 per cent chance of being correct.[50,144] Treatment should not be started without objective evidence of thrombosis.[23,50] The place of the various diagnostic tests in the management of deep vein thrombosis is discussed in the next section.

4. The patient is unlikely to have had a deep vein thrombosis The investigations indicated for this group of patients are those which will help to confirm the cause of the symptoms (e.g. X-rays of the chest and lower limb to confirm a pathological fracture caused by a metastasis from a carcinoma of bronchus).

It is probably not necessary to carry out specific tests to exclude a deep vein thrombosis in these patients, except when all the other tests are negative and the symptoms and signs persist.

Is there a cause for the deep vein thrombosis?

Once the diagnosis of deep vein thrombosis has been confirmed by an objective test, every attempt should be made to detect or exclude an underlying cause. In the absence of obvious symptoms and signs, the major concern is to exclude occult maligant disease.[33,41,131,145] A careful history and physical examination may reveal a neoplasm of the rectum or prostate, or lymphadenopathy which suggests Hodgkin's disease. Examination of the male genitalia may reveal a testicular tumour. If there is a history of weight loss, or a raised erythrocyte sedimentation rate (ESR), or the patient is elderly, then a chest radiograph, an ultrasound scan of the liver, kidneys and pelvis, and probably a barium meal and enema must be arranged, but specific points in the history may indicate other investigations which should be carried out (e.g. upper gastro-intestinal endoscopy, intravenous excretory urography, abdominal CT scanning, colonoscopy and endoscopic retrograde cholangio-pancreatography).

If the results of all these tests are within normal limits, the patient must be followed carefully with regular re-examinations and further specific tests as required. It is sometimes several years before the occult cause of a deep vein thrombosis becomes apparent.

Recurrent deep vein thrombosis

There is a special group of patients who develop recurrent episodes of thrombosis, often despite adequate anticoagulation therapy. In these patients it is important to exclude malignant disease (as outlined above) and any abnormality of coagulation. A coagulation screen should be accompained by specific tests of antithrombin-III,[1,45,54,58,119,134,141,152,153,160] protein-C,[13,54,71,120,142] lupus anticoagulant,[16,28] and heparin cofactor-II levels,[151] with measurements of plasminogen activator and its inhibitors.[18,30,77,79,114,115,159]

Investigations

The techniques used to investigate the venous system have already been described in detail in Chapter 4. This section discusses the accuracy, advantages and disadvantages of each of the methods used to diagnose deep vein thrombosis.

Ascending phlebography (Chapter 4, page 103)

Indications

Phlebograms should be obtained from all patients in whom there is a strong clinical suspicion of deep vein thrombosis or pulmonary embolism, or clear evidence of pulmonary embolism. Bipedal ascending phlebography provides adequate information in 95 per cent of patients.[22] Phlebograms can be obtained even when there are contraindications (e.g. sensitivity to iodine, the early stages of pregnancy and circulatory shock caused by a pulmonary embolism) provided special precautions are taken.[98]

Advantages

1. The diagnosis of deep vein thrombosis can be confirmed with certainty in 95 per cent of limbs.[22,95]
2. The nature of the thrombus, its site, extent, degree of adherence and age can be determined (see Figs. 4.42, 4.43).[19,95]
3. The risks of embolization can be estimated (see Fig. 4.43).[19,95]
4. The clinical diagnosis may be refuted if the phlebogram is normal.[35,50,59,74,75,117,124]

Disadvantages

1. There may be disagreement over the interpretation of some phlebographic appearances,[40,105] but this decreases with the experience of the observer (see Fig. 4.42).[40,92]
2. Not all the veins of the limb can be filled with contrast medium.
   (a) The foot veins are often not examined (Fig. 17.4a).
   (b) Some calf veins will not be opacified (see Fig. 4.34).[22,97,98]
   (c) The deep femoral vein is only displayed in 30 per cent patients (see Fig. 4.35a and Fig. 17.4b).[37]

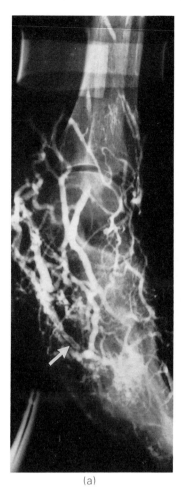
(a)

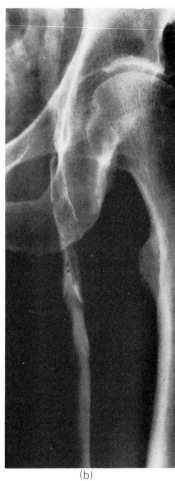
(b)

Fig. 17.4 The three segments of the veins of the lower limb not usually visualized by ascending phlebography are the foot veins, the deep femoral vein and the internal iliac vein and its tributaries but they may all contain thrombus.

(a) A phlebogram showing thrombus in a foot vein (arrowed).

(b) This large thrombus, which is extending up the common femoral vein, has its origin in the deep femoral vein. The superficial femoral vein is normal. The deep femoral vein is only visible in 30 per cent of ascending phlebograms.

(d) The tributaries of the internal iliac vein are never shown with standard ascending phlebography (see Fig. 4.35b and Fig. 17.4c and d).[20,90]

(e) The common iliac veins and inferior vena cava may be poorly opacified if the radiological technique is poor.[17,95,97,98]

3. If the tourniquets are not correctly applied, the superficial veins may fill with contrast medium, making interpretation difficult.[97]

4. Phlebography only shows the state of the veins at the time of the examination. Progression or regresssion of thrombus can only be assessed by repeated examination.[22]

5. The procedure used to be unpleasant and painful but the new hypo-osmolar contrast media have almost abolished these complaints (see Chapter 4).

6. Bilateral ascending phlebography takes 30 minutes and requires standard X-ray equipment and an experienced radiologist. It costs approximately the same as an intravenous excretory urogram (IVU).

7. The complications of the procedure have been discussed in Chapter 4.[94] The new isosmolar contrast media have dramatically reduced the incidence of these complications.[4,5] In particular, the risks of inducing thrombosis and producing tissue necrosis from extravasation have been virtually eliminated. The risk of the injection and manipulation causing a pulmonary embolism is theoretical rather than real.

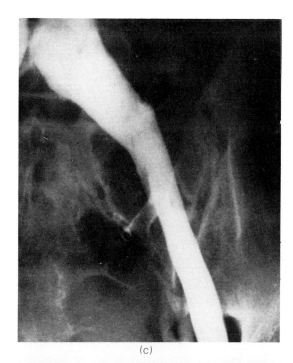

(c)

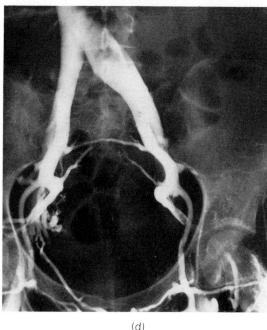

(d)

Fig. 17.4 (c) Fresh thrombus in the internal iliac vein.

(d) The tributaries of the internal iliac vein are only fully visualized by intraosseous phlebography (see Chapter 4). In this example there is fresh thrombus in the left inferior gluteal vein.

Accuracy

It is very difficult to find a precise estimate of the accuracy with which plebography detects deep vein thrombosis. Phlebography appears to detect slightly fewer calf vein thrombi than the fibrinogen uptake test;[24,50,83,112,137,154] this could be because the fibrinogen uptake test is over-sensitive or because phlebography is failing to reveal small thrombi. Phlebography can miss thrombi in the deep femoral vein[37] and internal iliac veins (Fig. 17.4).[90] Thrombi are also easily missed in the foot veins (Fig. 17.4)[96] because these veins are not usually examined during standard ascending phlebography.

There have been few reports in the literature of patients dying as a result of a proven pulmonary embolism after apparently normal phlebograms[73] but there have been no large planned comparisons between phlebography during life and autopsy examination.[109]

The overall accuracy and the positive and negative test accuracy is over 90 per cent,[22] and phlebography remains the gold standard against which other tests must be compared. It is of far greater clinical significance that phlebography provides information about the site, the extent and the age of the thrombus, which the other methods cannot provide.

The role of other phlebographic techniques

Cinephlebography[8,81] This method adds little to the standard screening and cut film techniques.[98] It is useful in the assessment of calf pump function but not in the diagnosis of deep vein thrombosis.

'No-tourniquet' technique This technique, described by Nylander,[6,17,60,116] is associated with a high incidence of false-positive interpretations caused by underfilling of the deep veins and 'knot-hole' effects in the superficial veins. We are not aware of any published comparison between this technique and our standard tourniquet technique.[93]

Perfemoral venography[97,98] This is carried out under local anaesthesia and is frequently used to provide better quality images of the iliac veins and vena cava. If there is a good flow of blood into the syringe before injection is made, there is no danger of disrupting a femoral vein thrombus and causing an embolus. The main indication for the use of this technique is the display of the upper limit of an ilio-femoral thrombosis that is not clearly visible on the ascending phlebogram.

Intraosseous phlebography[97,98] This should only be used in a patient who is considered to be at high risk of embolism and in whom the ascending phlebograms and attempted percutaneous femoral phlebograms have failed to outline the iliac veins and inferior vena cava.[95] It has the disadvantages that it is painful and must therefore be carried out under a general anaesthetic, and it may very occasionally, be complicated by fat embolism. It does, however, always display the whole iliac system and the vena cava.

Fibrinogen uptake test (Chapter 4, page 100)[24,83,100,132,137]

This test was originally devised by Hobbs and Davies[67] but was developed for use as a screening test for deep vein thrombosis by Flanc *et al.*[50] and Negus *et al.*[112]

Ideally, this test should be started before a thrombus develops (e.g. before an operation), as it is much less accurate when detecting established thrombus.[24,122] It is used chiefly to assess different regimens of thrombosis prophylaxis, and it has been abandoned as a universal screening test on the grounds of expense. It is only used for the diagnosis of established deep vein thrombosis when it is known that the thrombus is less than 5 days old and there is no clinical urgency to obtain the result.

Indications

1. Screening of patients at high risk who are undergoing surgical procedures
2. Assessment of new methods of prophylaxis or treatment
3. Diagnosis of deep vein thrombosis when combined with other non-invasive techniques

Contra-indications

1. Pregnancy
2. When operations are to be performed on the legs (e.g. ligation of varicose veins, femoro-popliteal bypass or orthopaedic surgery below the hip joint)
3. The presence of inflammation or recent local injury in the leg (e.g. fractures, bruises,

muscle tears, ulcers, inflammation or acute arthritis) (see Fig. 4.32 page 102)
4. Gross oedema of the legs (e.g. lymphoedema or congestive cardiac failure)

Advantages

1. The approximate extent of the thrombosis can be assessed daily
2. Scanning is painless and the procedure is almost non-invasive
3. There is no risk of causing a thrombosis

Disadvantages

1. It is expensive and time consuming
2. There is a risk of transmitting infectious hepatitis and HIV virus if the fibrinogen is not obtained from tested donors
3. It cannot detect thrombus above the middle of the thigh
4. Failure to detect other causes of fibrinogen deposition before ordering the test (see above) will increase the incidence of false-positive tests
5. It is only very accurate when used proleptically

Accuracy

Both the positive and the negative test accuracies for thrombus below the mid thigh are between 95 per cent and 100 per cent when the test is used proleptically and compared with phlebography, provided all limbs with clinically detectable causes of false-positives are excluded from testing.[24,50,82,83,100,112,137] The positive and negative test accuracies, under similar conditions, for established thrombus less then 7 days old are both 75 per cent.[24,122] The incidence of pulmonary embolism after a negative scan is very low (0 out of 687).[82]

Comment Within its limitations, the ^{125}I-fibrinogen uptake test is a very useful screening test for thrombosis. Expense has stopped it from becoming part of routine clinical practice. It is important that the test procedure and interpretation are standardized.[132] We believe that it still has a role to play in screening a few high risk patients, even when they are given some form of prophylaxis.

Other isotope uptake tests

⁹⁹ᵐtechnetium plasmin uptake test [2,39,44,76]

This test was developed to improve on the accuracy of 75 per cent which was found when the ^{125}I-fibrinogen uptake test was used to examine patients with established thrombosis.[22,24,122] It has been reported to be 97 per cent sensitive, and 55 per cent specific, with a predictive value of 79 per cent in positive cases and 92 per cent in negative cases.[2] However, the isotope has a short half-life and the injectate has to be specially prepared for each test. There is a high false-negative rate in patients with bilateral thrombosis.

⁹⁹ᵐtechnetium streptokinase uptake test [43,85]

The plasmin uptake test and the streptokinase uptake test were both developed so that results could be obtained more quickly than with the fibrinogen uptake test. The early results were encouraging but there have been problems involving sensitivity reactions to streptokinase and the short half-life of the isotope.

⁹⁹ᵐtechnetium-labelled red cells [14]

It has been reported that this test has a sensitivity of 100 per cent and a specificity of 89 per cent.[14] It gives an anatomical picture of the whole venous tree which is imaged by a gamma-camera. The quality of the image is very inferior to those produced by phlebography. This technique has not been adopted because of the time needed to label the red cells and the requirements for highly sophisticated imaging apparatus.

Radio-labelled plasminogen uptake test [63]

This test is identical in principal and accuracy to the plasmin and streptokinase uptake tests described above.

Indium-labelled platelets

This technique was introduced to provide a quicker result than that given by the ^{125}I-fibrinogen uptake test.[49,87] Grimley *et al.*[55] reported that it was 60 per cent accurate for calf thrombi and 66 per cent accurate for thigh thrombi. There were 14 per cent false-positives in the calf and 19 per cent false-positives in the thigh. The test requires time and skill, and technical assistance is needed to prepare the platelets. These disadvantages have restricted its application but a new monoclonal antibody against platelets may improve the efficiency of the labelling.[123]

Technetium-labelled macroaggregates of albumin

This technique is used to provide images which are similar to a phlebogram but their quality is far inferior to the images obtained from a standard X-ray contrast phlebogram.[65,135,136,155] The sensitivity for thigh thrombus has been claimed to be 80 per cent with a specificity of 98 per cent. Unfortunately, this test cannot detect calf vein thrombi.[113] It can be a useful axial vein screening test when performed as part of a perfusion lung scan.

⁹⁹ᵐtechnetium-labelled fibrinogen [80,140]

This test provides a combination of static and dynamic scans of the leg veins following the injection of technetium-labelled fibrinogen into a foot vein. It has been called the 'venoscan' by Sandler *et al.*[140] who claim that it has an 80 per cent accuracy with a sensitivity of 83 per cent and a specificity of 76 per cent. The nature of the equipment needed for this test has inhibited its study by other investigators.

Comment Despite the efforts of the protagonists for each of these newer isotope scans, none has yet displaced the fibrinogen uptake test or phlebography. Their accuracies are only marginally better than that of the fibrinogen uptake test, and they are all more complicated and expensive. False-positive scans always occur in patients who have bruising, haematomata or inflammation in the legs; this makes the clinical decision about whether it is appropriate to use one of these tests the single most important factor in determining their accuracy.

Ultrasound (Chapter 4, page 80)

There are two methods of detecting venous thromboses with ultrasound—*indirectly* by the assessment of the venous flow and *directly* with greyscale ultrasound imaging (echo or sonography).

Blood flow detection

Many investigators [47,48,107,140,143,147,149] have studied the value of the ultrasound flow detector as a means of detecting deep vein thrombosis. They have all found that the blood flow response to calf squeezing or the Valsalva manoeuvre is reduced in patients with extensive thrombus in the popliteal, femoral or iliac veins, and Evans[47,48] claims that there is a reduction in femoral vein blood flow response to squeezing when there is calf vein thrombus. Most of the published studies show that the test is only useful in diagnosing thrombus in the large axial veins (i.e. the popliteal vein and above.)

Indications

1. Screening of the axial veins of patients at high risk, including pregnant women with swollen legs
2. Confirmation of a clinical diagnosis of axial vein occlusion

Contra-indications

None

Advantages

1. Ultrasound flow detectors are inexpensive
2. It is simple, non-invasive and highly acceptable to patients
3. It can be repeated daily, or even more frequently
4. It can be used during pregnancy

Disadvantages

1. It cannot detect isolated calf vein thrombi
2. It often fails to detect thrombi which are only partially occluding the vein
3. It gives a false sense of security. A positive test is an indication for phlebography not the end of the diagnostic investigations
4. It may give false-positive results if the test is performed incorrectly

Accuracy

The slightly exaggerated claims, which were made for the accuracy of this test by the pioneers,[47,48,143,149] have not been substantiated by other investigators.[62,107] For example, in one study when ultrasound was compared prospectively with phlebography[107] only 3 out of 10 calf thrombi were correctly detected and 5 of 34 more extensive axial vein thrombi were missed. Of the 5 axial vein thrombi that were missed, 1 was partially occlusive and 4 had an extensive collateral circulation. Of the 21 false-positive results, 11 had marked oedema of the leg and 4 had haematomata which may have been compressing the veins.

Hanel *et al.*[62] found a specificity and sensitivity of 90 per cent for axial vein thrombi; in calf thrombi the sensitivity was only 40 per cent but the specificity remained high at 97 per cent. Of the 19 false-negative results they obtained, 15 were related to thrombi in the calf veins. The 4 thrombi in the femoral veins that were missed were very small.

Recently, Sandler *et al.*[140] have reported an overall accuracy of this test of 82 per cent when compared with simultaneous phlebography in patients with a mixture of thrombi, many of which were in the calf veins.

Comment Our clinical experience is that a reduced femoral vein blood flow in response to calf squeezing is an accurate indication of the presence of occlusive axial vein thrombosis, especially if there are confirmatory physical signs but a negative test does not exclude significant non-adherent axial vein thrombus.

Ultrasound flow detection is a very useful method for assessing the cause of leg swelling in a pregnant woman when phlebography may be contra-indicated, but it may be replaced by ultrasound imaging which may be more accurate.

Ultrasound imaging

Although B-mode ultrasound imaging of the veins was originally described in 1976,[38] it has only recently been developed as a clinical tool.

Indications

1. Confirmation of the clinical diagnosis of deep vein thrombosis

Contra-indications

None

Advantages

1. It is non-invasive
2. When combined with a Doppler flow detection facility, it is more accurate than the simple flow probe
3. It may give some indication of the precise extent, age and degree of adherence of the thrombus
4. It is safe to use during pregnancy

Disadvantages

1. It is extremely operator-dependent
2. An examination takes quite a long time and considerable skill and anatomical knowledge
3. The apparatus is expensive

Accuracy

In 1976 the technique was shown to detect thrombi in 30 out of 32 limbs with phlebographically proven major vein thrombi,[38] and to confirm the presence of normal veins in 17 out of 18 limbs with normal phlebograms. Since 1976, technical improvements have been made in the probes and the combination of pulsed Doppler flow detection with real time B-mode imaging (Duplex scanning) has provided more precise information which allows the presence of venous thrombi to be detected even more accurately.[133,150] Cranley and his team[148] recently reported an overall accuracy of 94 per cent, a positive test accuracy of 92 per cent, and a negative test accuracy of 96 per cent. These results are extremely good but need to be confirmed by other groups.

Comment Although the capital outlay for this equipment is very large, the prospect of diagnosis by non-invasive means, which is both reproducible and repeatable and does not have the hazard of radiation, is exciting. Ultrasound imaging could become the investigation of first choice for deep vein thrombosis, though we remain sceptical in the light of our initial experience. It will become the investigation of choice in pregnant women if the equipment is available.

Plethysmography (see Chapter 4, pages 85–98)

Various forms of plethysmography have been used to diagnose deep vein thrombosis (see Chapter 4). These include impedance plethysmography,[62,110,111,140,156,157] strain-gauge plethysmography,[26,61] segmental air plethysmography,[29,46] and phleborheography.[34,36]

All these techniques are based on the principal that thrombus interferes with venous blood flow. Photoplethysmography, which measures skin blood volume, cannot be used for the diagnosis of deep vein thrombosis.

Isotope plethysmography is used to test calf pump function not to detect deep vein thrombosis.

Indications

1. Confirmation of the diagnosis of established deep vein thrombosis
2. As a screening test

Contra-indications

None

Advantages

1. It is non-invasive and moderately reproducible
2. All these methods are relatively cheap and easy to learn

Disadvantages

None can detect small calf vein thrombi or non-occlusive axial vein thrombi with certainty

Accuracy

Strain-gauge plethysmography detects venous thrombosis by measuring the maximum venous outflow. It has a sensitivity for axial vein thrombosis of 90 per cent but its sensitivity for calf vein thrombosis is only 60 per cent.[26,61]

Phleborheography measures the changes in calf volume in response to upstream and downstream limb compression and the Valsalva manoeuvre. It has a sensitivity of 90 per cent for axial vein thrombosis, but a sensitivity for calf vein thrombosis of 70–80 per cent.[34,36]

Impedance plethysmography detects thrombosis from the relationship between calf filling during venous congestion and the rate of emptying after congestion. Its sensitivity for detecting axial vein thrombus is 90 per cent, but its sensitivity for calf vein thrombus is only 40 per cent.[110,111,157]

Comment All the plethysmographic techniques are good at detecting axial vein thrombosis that is causing a significant obstruction to blood flow, but they are relatively poor at detecting small haemodynamically insignificant calf vein thrombi. If it is accepted that axial vein thrombosis is the clinically significant form of deep vein thrombus, these tests should be classified as good but if the clinician wishes to detect all forms of thrombus, the plethysmographic techniques are far from ideal because their *overall* accuracy is only 60–70 per cent.

Thermography (see Chapter 4, page 76)

A number of publications have examined the value of thermography for the diagnosis of deep vein thrombosis.[11,12,27,31,32,64,78,99,121,125,130,138] When Bergquist[11] compared the ^{125}I-fibrinogen uptake test with thermography, he found a sensitivity of only 62 per cent but a specificity of 90 per cent. Thermography detected developing thrombi slightly slower than the ^{125}I-fibrinogen uptake test. However, Byström *et al.*[27] found a 94 per cent agreement between phlebography and thermography. Recent studies of Sandler and Martin using liquid crystal contact thermography[138] showed a 97 per cent sensitivity but a specificity of only 62 per cent.

Comment Thermography is a non-specific test but the development of a new portable apparatus has made it more accessible. False-positive results are still a problem but thermography may be a useful method of screening for deep vein thrombosis, as no temperature difference seems to indicate no thrombus.

Blood tests

A number of groups[27,56,66,158] have measured the fibrin degradation products and other coagulation tests to see if any are a marker of thrombosis. The results to date have been disappointing. The new assays of cross-linked fibrin degradation products may be more useful but they need further assessment.

Summary

Despite the plethora of tests that have been discussed above, bipedal ascending phlebography has stood the test of time. B-mode ultrasound imaging is a new and exciting alternative but the equipment required is expensive. The fibrinogen uptake test is the test most often used for screening but combinations of plethysmography with ultrasound flow detection, phleborheography or thermography are valuable alternatives. No test can determine the extent, age and fixity of the thrombus as satisfactorily as phlebography at present but ultrasound techniques may offer an alternative in the future.

Clinical application of tests for deep vein thrombosis

The physical signs of deep vein thrombosis and pulmonary embolism are variable and imprecise but they are the only clinical indication of the presence of thrombosis. Consequently, these signs must be sought by diligent daily examination, especially in the postoperative period when there is a high risk of deep vein thrombosis, and once the signs have been found they should be accepted as an important indication for further investigations to confirm or refute clinical suspicion. No suspicious physical sign should be ignored and no treatment should be given without objective confirmation of the diagnosis.

It is clearly impractical to use phlebography to investigate every patient who has suspicious physical signs. No hospital has the facilities to perform phlebograms on every postoperative patient who has a tender calf and, as more than half of these patients will not have a thrombosis, such an approach would be expensive and impractical.

Patients fall into four distinct *clinical* categories; patients with

1. *definite clinical evidence of pulmonary embolism*, which may or may not be life threatening (i.e. patients with the full clinical picture of pulmonary embolism described in Chapter 20 and in whom there is little doubt about the diagnosis)

2. *symptoms or signs that could be caused by*

pulmonary embolism, which are not life threatening.

(These patients often have one symptom [e.g. chest pain] which could be caused by embolism or could be caused by other conditions, for example pneumonia, myocardial infarction or oesophageal spasm)

3. *definite clinical evidence of deep vein thrombosis*, that is to say, symptoms and signs unlikely to be caused by anything other than deep vein thrombosis (e.g. phlegmasia cerulea dolens, a hard woody calf or a warm leg with mild ankle oedema and tenderness in the calf or along the femoral vein in the thigh)

4. *symptoms or signs that could be caused by deep vein thrombosis*, (e.g. minor calf tenderness)

Our methods of using the above investigations after categorizing the patients into one of these groups are described below. The reason for our preferences, which are italicized, are discussed in the subsequent section.

1. Definite clinical pulmonary embolism

The three objectives of investigation are to confirm the diagnosis of pulmonary embolism, assess its severity and exclude the possibility of further embolism. If the patient is collapsed and hypotensive we resuscitate him/her with oxygen, plasma volume expansion, vasoconstrictor drugs, cardiac massage if indicated, give 12,500 units heparin intravenously and then:

(a) assess the state of the major limb veins from the popliteal to the iliac veins with a *Doppler ultrasound flow detector*, phleborheography or impedance plethysmography;

(b) request *pulmonary angiography* if the clinical signs suggest severe pulmonary artery obstruction with continuing shock and if thrombolysis or embolectomy is contemplated;

(c) request *lung scans* if, or when, the patient's condition becomes more stable.

Pulmonary angiography may have to be performed on the operating table before an emergency embolectomy if the patient's condition is rapidly deteriorating. Embolectomy or thrombolysis should not be attempted without firm objective proof of the diagnosis. Treatment depends upon the severity of the pulmonary artery obstruction. If the obstruction is extensive

and reducing the cardiac output, pulmonary embolectomy or thrombolysis may be indicated (see Chapter 20).

If the embolus is not severe or life threatening, anticoagulants should be given to the patient, the leg veins should be investigated to assess the likelihood of a further embolism, and a ventilation–perfusion scan should be obtained to confirm the diagnosis of pulmonary embolism. Appropriate action can then be taken (see Chapter 18).

2. Possible, non-life threatening pulmonary embolism

The first objective of treatment is the assessment of the possibility of a second, potentially fatal embolism. The second objective is to confirm the diagnosis.

(a) We first assess the patency of the major limb veins (popliteal to iliac) at the bedside with a *Doppler ultrasound flow detector*. Alternatively, impedance plethysmography or phleborheography can be used to test for major axial vein obstruction.

(b) If these tests are abnormal, we give the patient 10,000 units heparin intravenously and request *urgent bilateral ascending phlebography* to assess both the nature and extent of any residual deep vein thrombosis and to plan further treatment. Ventilation–perfusion lung scans are obtained within 24 hours to confirm or refute the clinical diagnosis of pulmonary embolism.

(c) If the bedside tests are normal, we request an urgent *ventilation–perfusion lung scan* followed within 24 hours by *bipedal ascending phlebography*.

If the ventilation–perfusion pulmonary scan is positive but the axial veins are patent on bed-side examination, the risk of further embolism is small, the diagnosis of thromboembolism is recognized and it could be argued that phlebography is not necessary. However, none of the non-invasive tests has a positive test accuracy greater than 90 per cent for non-occlusive axial vein thrombosis, so in these circumstances *we still prefer to perform phlebography* to be quite certain that there is not a large, undetected, non-adherent potential embolus within the leg veins. The phlebogram also helps to decide upon the best form of treatment for the leg vein thrombosis.

3. 'Definite' clinical evidence of deep vein thrombosis without evidence of embolism

The objective of investigating these patients is to confirm the diagnosis and obtain information which may help the clinican to choose the best form of treatment. Any non-invasive investigation which confirms or refutes the diagnosis of thrombosis is helpful.

(a) We assess the axial veins with the *ultrasound flow detector*, other workers prefer phlebography, impedance plethysmography or a combination of ultrasound and plethysmography.

(b) If the non-invasive tests show that there is thrombus confined to the calf, no further urgent investigations are necessary and treatment with heparin can be started. *Phlebograms can be obtained later* to document the features of the thrombus, and to help with future management.

(c) If the non-invasive tests show that there is thrombus in the major axial veins (the popliteal vein or above), we request urgent *bilateral ascending phlebography* in order to assess the possibility of using other forms of treatment (e.g. thrombolysis or thrombectomy) (see Chapter 18). The non-invasive tests are not sufficiently accurate and do not give enough information about the thrombus for management decisions.

For a major vein thrombus we require information about the size, site, age and adherence of the thrombus. Our approach to patients who have these thrombi is therefore similar to our approach to those patients with pulmonary embolism that is not life threatening. We screen the axial veins at the bed-side with an *ultrasound flow detector* and proceed to *phlebography* in all patients in whom the ultrasound test suggests that the thrombosis extends into or above the popliteal vein.

4. Symptoms or signs that could be caused by deep vein thrombosis

This category contains the largest number of patients because non-specific physical signs (e.g. calf tenderness or minor ankle oedema) are very common.

(a) The *non-invasive tests are extremely useful in this group* because they enable the clinician to exclude the possibility of an extensive calf or axial vein thrombosis in most patients and they can be used to screen the patients, daily if necessary, to confirm a negative diagnosis or the absence of thrombus extension. The best approach is to *combine two tests*, for example *ultrasound* with *plethysmography* or *phleborheography* or one of these three tests with the *fibrinogen uptake test*.

(b) *Phlebography* is only indicated if thrombus is found in the axial veins or if the patient develops symptoms which suggest a pulmonary embolism.

Conclusions

It can be seen from the management schemes presented above that before a deep vein thrombosis can be properly managed the following information is required.

1. Is a thrombus present below the knee?
2. Is a thrombus present above the knee?
3. What is the precise extent of the thrombus?
4. Is the thrombus adherent or non-adherent?
5. What is the age of the thrombus?
6. Is the thrombus likely to threaten the life of the patient?
7. Is the thrombus likely to threaten the limb?
8. Will the thrombus cause post-thrombotic symptoms?

The various non-invasive investigations discussed in this chapter and described in Chapter 4 can answer questions 1, 2 and 3 with varying degrees of accuracy, depending upon the site of the thrombus. The relative accuracy of these tests is shown in Table 17.2. These tests provide sufficient information if the clinician is satisfied with approximate answers to questions 1 and 2. If the thrombus is in a major axial vein, we always want to know the answers to questions 3, 4, 5 and 6, and this information is often helpful even if the thrombus is confined to the calf; consequently, we rely heavily upon phlebography.

Table 17.2 does not include the results of greyscale ultrasound venous imaging as venous imaging techniques are still being developed. When this investigation is carried out by an expert it is potentially an accurate method of answering questions 1–5. We await with interest the comparison of this method against phlebography. We suspect that it will be highly 'operator-dependent' and that it will take several months to train the 'operator'. Time will tell whether it will replace phlebography.

Table 17.2   Accuracy of tests used to diagnose deep vein thrombosis

This table gives an indication of the ability of five tests, and two combinations of tests, to answer the clinicians' questions about deep vein thrombosis. A test which examines a whole segment of vein (e.g. the iliac and femoral veins) but which cannot give a precise indication of the exact extent of a thrombus site but can differentiate between above-knee and below-knee thrombosis is scored 60 per cent. Similar estimates have been made to give an approximate score of the ability of each test to answer each question.

Question	Approximate degree of accuracy (%)						
	DU	PRG	IPG	FUT	DU+FUT	DU+IPG	Phlebo
1. Is there thrombus below the knee?	20	60	70	98	98	70	95
2. Is there thrombus above the knee?	85	90	90	30	85	95	99
3. What is the precise extent of the thrombus?	–	60	60	70	75	75	99
4. What is the size (length and width) of the thrombus?	–	–	–	60	50	50	99
5. Is the thrombus adherent or non-adherent?	–	–	–	–	–	–	95
6. What is the state of the upper (cephalad) end of the thrombus?	–	–	–	–	–	–	95

DU = Doppler ultrasound flow detector. PRG = phleborheography. IPG = impedance plethysmography. FUT = fibrinogen uptake test. Phlebo = phlebography.

There is no doubt that the information provided by phlebography is far superior to that provided by the other techniques. Now that non-ionic isosmolar contrast media are available, phlebography is an extremely safe procedure. It requires an X-ray suite and a radiologist's time but is far less expensive than many other radiological investigations. Although phlebography cannot be performed at the bed-side or in the vascular laboratory by a technician, the information it provides cannot be obtained from any of the other methods. This information is invaluable in determining management. In our opinion the use of the non-invasive tests should be restricted to screening. Phlebograms should be requested for any patient who has had a pulmonary embolism, for any patient who has thrombus above the knee and whenever thrombectomy, thrombolysis or caval interruption is contemplated. In our opinion it is acceptable to administer anticoagulants on the evidence of a non-invasive test if the thrombus is confined to the calf and to accept that no significant thrombosis is present on the basis of a negative non-invasive test, provided the test can moderately accurately (70–80 per cent) detect thrombus both in the calf and in axial veins.

It is not acceptable to give anticoagulants solely on the basis of a clinical diagnosis, except to cover the period between making the clinical diagnosis and seeing the results of objective tests.

References

1. Aberg M, Nilsson I M, Hedner U. Antithrombin III after operation. *Lancet* 1973; **2**: 1337.
2. Adolfsson L, Nordenfelt I, Olssen H, Torstensson I. Diagnosis of deep venous thrombosis with ^{99}Tc plasmin. *Acta Med Scand* 1982; **211**: 365.
3. Aird I. *A Companion in Surgical Studies*. London. Churchill Livingstone 1957.
4. Albrechtsoon U, Olsson C G. Thrombosis after phlebography: A comparison of two contrast media. *Cardiovasc Radiol* 1979; **2**: 9.
5. Almen T, Hartel M, Nylander G, Olivercrona N. Effects of metrizamide on silver staining of the aortic endothelium. *Acta Radiol* (Suppl) (Stockh) 1973; **335**: 233.
6. Almen T, Nylander G. False signs of thrombosis in lower leg phlebography. *Acta Radiol* 1964; **2**: 345.
7. Archer G J. Homans' sign. *Lancet* 1985; **1**: 816.
8. Arnoldi C C, Greitz T, Linderholm H. Variations in the cross sectional area and pressure in the veins of the normal human leg during rhythmic muscular exercise. *Acta Chir Scand* 1966; **132**: 507.
9. Belch J J F, McMillan N C, Fogelman I, Capell H, Forbes C D. Combined phlebography and arthrography in patients with painful swollen calf. *Br Med J* 1981; **282**: 949.
10. Bergqvist D, Jaroszewski H. Deep vein thrombosis in patients with superficial thrombophlebitis of the leg. *Br Med J* 1986; **292**: 658.
11. Berquist D, Dahleren S, Efsing H O. Thermographic diagnosis of deep venous thrombosis. *Br Med J* 1975; **4**: 684.
12. Berquist D, Hallböök T. Thermography in screening post-operative deep vein thrombosis: a comparison with the ^{125}I fibrinogen test. *Br J Surg* 1978; **65**: 443.
13. Bertina R M, Broekmans A W, Van Der Linden I K, Mertens K. Protein C deficiency in a Dutch family with thrombotic disease. *Thromb Haemost* 1982; **48**:1.
14. Beswick W, Chmiel R, Booth R, Vellar I, Gilford E, Chesterman C N. Detection of deep venous thrombosis by scanning of ^{99m}Tc labelled red cell venous pool. *Br Med J* 1979; **1**: 82.
15. Blaisdell F W. Low dose heparin prophylaxis of venous thrombosis. *Am Heart J* 1979; **97**: 685.
16. Boey L M, Cloaco C B, Gharavi A E, Elkon K B, Loizou S, Hughes G R V. Thrombosis in systemic lupus erythematosis: striking association with the presence of circulating "lupus anticoagulant". *Br Med J* 1983; **287**: 1021.
17. Brodelius A, Lörinc P, Nylander G. Phlebographic techniques in the diagnosis of acute deep venous thrombosis in the lower limb. *Am J Roentgenol Rad Ther Nucl Med* 1971; **111**: 794.
18. Browse N L, Gray L, Morland M, Jarrett P E M. Blood and vein wall fibrinolytic activity in health and vascular disease. *Br Med J* 1977; **1**: 478.
19. Browse N L, Lea Thomas M, Solan M, Young A E. Prevention of recurrent pulmonary embolism. *Br Med J* 1969; **3**: 382.
20. Browse N L, Lea Thomas M. Source of non-lethal pulmonary emboli. *Lancet* 1974; **1**: 258.
21. Browse N L. *An Introduction to the Symptoms and Signs of Surgical Disease*. London. Edward Arnold 1978.
22. Browse N L. Diagnosis of deep vein thrombosis. *Br Med Bull* 1978; **34**: 163.
23. Browse N L. Diagnosis of deep vein thrombosis. *Br Med J* 1969; **4**: 676.
24. Browse N L. The ^{125}I fibrinogen uptake test. *Arch Surg* 1972; **104**: 160.
25. Browse N L. The value of signs in the diagnosis of

deep vein thrombosis. In: *Venous Disease: Medical and Surgical Management.* Montreux. Foundation International Cooperation in Medical Sciences 1974.

26. Bygdeman S, Aschberg S, Hindmarsch T. Venous plethysmography in the diagnosis of chronic venous insufficiency. *Acta Chir Scand* 1971; **131**: 423.

27. Byström L-G, Larsson T, Lundell L, Abom P-E. The value of thermography and the determination of fibrin–fibrinogen degradation products in the diagnosis of deep venous thrombosis. *Acta Med Scand* 1977; **202**: 319.

28. Carreras L O, Vermylen J G. "Lupus" anticoagulant and thrombosis: possible role of inhibition of prostacyclin formation. *Thromb Haemost* 1982; **48**: 38.

29. Christopoulos D, Nicolaides A N, Malouf G M, Zukowski A, Szendro G, Christodoulou C. Absolute blood volume changes in the lower limb using air-plethysmography. In: Negus D, Jantet G (Eds) *Phlebography '85.* London. Libbey 1986.

30. Conard J, Veuillet-Duval A, Horellou M H, Samama M. Étude de la coagulation et de la fibrinolyse dans 131 cas de thromboses veineuses récidivants. *Nouv Rev Fr Hematol* 1982; **24**: 205.

31. Cooke E D, Pilcher M F. Deep vein thrombosis: preclinical diagnosis by thermography. *Br J Surg* 1974; **61**: 971.

32. Cooke E D, Pilcher M F. Thermography in diagnosis of deep vein thrombosis. *Br Med J* 1973; **2**: 523.

33. Coon W W, Coller F A. Some epidemiological considerations of thrombophlebitis. *Surg Gynec Obstet* 1959; **109**: 487.

34. Cranley J J, Canos A J, Sull W J, Grass A M. Phleborheographic technique for diagnosis of deep vein thrombosis of the lower extremities. *Surg Gynec Obstet* 1975; **141**: 331.

35. Cranley J J, Canos A J, Sull W J. The diagnosis of deep vein thrombosis. *Arch Surg* 1976; **111**: 34.

36. Cranley J J, Gay A Y, Grass A M, Simeone F A. A plethysmographic technique for the diagnosis of deep venous thrombosis of the lower extremities. *Surg Gynec Obstet* 1973; **58**: 111.

37. Culver D, Crawford J S, Gardiner J H, Wiley A M. Venous thrombosis after fractures of the upper end of the femur. A study of incidence and site. *J Bone Joint Surg* 1970; **52**: 61.

38. Day T K, Fish P J, Kakkar V V. Detection of deep vein thrombosis by Doppler angiography. *Br Med J* 1976; **1**: 618.

39. Deacon J M, Ell P J, Anderson P, Khan O. Technitium 99[m] plasmin: a new test for the detection of deep vein thrombosis. *Br J Radiol* 1980; **53**: 673.

40. DeWeese J A, Rogoff S M. Phlebographic patterns of acute deep venous thrombosis of the leg. *Surgery* 1963; **53**: 99.

41. Donati M B, Poggi A. Malignancy and haemostasis. *Br J Haematol* 1980; **44**: 173.

42. Douss T W. The clinical significance of venous thrombosis of the calf. *Br J Surg* 1976; **63**: 377.

43. Dugan M A, Kozar J J, Ganse G. Localization of deep vein thrombosis using radioactive streptokinase. *J Nucl Med* 1973; **14**: 233.

44. Edenbrandt C M, Nilsson J, Oulin P. Diagnosis of deep venous thrombosis by phlebography and 99[Tc] plasmin. *Acta Med Scand* 1982; **211**: 59.

45. Egeberg O. Inherited antithrombin deficiency causing thrombophilia. *Thromb Diath Haemorrh* 1965; **13**: 516.

46. Eiriksson E. Plethysmographic studies of venous disease of the legs. *Acta Chir Scand* (Suppl) 1973; **436**: 1.

47. Evans D S, Cockett F B. Diagnosis of deep venous thrombosis using an ultrasonic Doppler technique. *Br Med J* 1968; **2**: 802.

48. Evans D S. The early diagnosis of venous thrombosis by ultrasound. *Br J Surg* 1970; **57**: 726.

49. Fenech A, Dendy P P, Hussey J K, Bennett B, Douglas A S. Indium[111] labelled platelets in diagnosis of leg vein thrombosis: preliminary findings. *Br Med J* 1980; **280**: 1571.

50. Flanc C, Kakkar V V, Clark M B. The detection of venous thrombosis of the legs using 125[I] labelled fibrinogen. *Br J Surg* 1968; **55**: 742.

51. Forfar J C. A seven year analysis of haemorrhage in patients on long-term anticoagulant treatment. *Br Heart J* 1979; **142**: 128.

52. Gibbs N M. Venous thrombosis of the lower limbs with particular reference to bed rest. *Br J Surg* 1957; **45**: 209.

53. Gregoire R. La phlebite bleue (Phlegmasia cerulea dolens). *Presse Méd* 1938; **2**: 1313.

54. Griffin J H, Evatt B, Zimmerman T S, Kleiss A J, Widemann C. Deficiency of protein C in congenital thrombotic disease. *J Clin Invest* 1981; **68**: 1370.

55. Grimley R P, Slaney G, Hawker R J, Rafiqi E, Drolc Z. Diagnosis of deep vein thrombosis using Indium[111] labelled platelets. *Br Med J* 1981; **282**: 1626.

56. Gurewich V, Hume M, Patrick M. The laboratory diagnosis of venous thromboembolic disease by measurement of fibrinogen/fibrin degradation product and fibrin monomer. *Chest* 1973; **64**: 585.

57. Gyde O H B, Littler W A, Stableforth D E. Fami-

lial antithrombin III deficiency. *Br Med J* 1978; **1**: 508.

58. Gyde O H B, Middleton M D, Vaughan G R, Fletcher D J. Antithrombin III deficiency hypertriglyceridaemia and venous thromboses. *Br Med J* 1978; **1**: 621.

59. Haegar K. Den kliniska thrombusdiagnosens (o) tillforlitlighet. *Svenska Läk Sällsk Förhandl* 1965; **62**: 1067.

60. Haeger K, Nylander G. Acute phlebography. *Triangle* 1967; **8**: 18.

61. Hallbrook T, Gothlin J. Strain gauge plethysmography and phlebography in diagnosis of deep venous thrombosis. *Acta Chir Scand* 1971; **137**: 37.

62. Hanel K C, Abbott W M, Reidy N C, Fulchino D, Miller A, Brewster D C, Athanasolis C A. The role of two noninvasive tests in deep venous thrombosis. *Ann Surg* 1981; **194**: 725.

63. Harwig S S L, Harwig J F, Sherman R, Coleman R E, Welch M J. Radioiodinated plasminogen: an imaging agent for pre-existing thrombi. *J Nucl Med* 1977; **18**: 42.

64. Henderson H P, Cooke E D, Bowcock S A, Hackett M E J. After exercise thermography for predicting postoperative deep vein thrombosis. *Br Med J* 1978; **1**: 1020.

65. Highman J, O'Sullivan E. Isotope venography. *Br J Surg* 1973; **60**: 58.

66. Hirsch J, Gallus A S, Cade J F. Diagnosis of thrombosis. Evaluation of ^{125}I fibrinogen scanning and blood test. *Thromb Diath Haemorrh* 1974; **32**: 11.

67. Hobbs J T, Davies J W L. Detection of venous thrombosis with ^{131}I labelled fibrinogen in the rabbit. *Lancet* 1960; **2**:134.

68. Hobsley M. *Pathways in Surgical Management.* London. Edward Arnold 1979.

69. Homans J. Diseases of the veins. *N Engl J Med* 1944; **231**: 51.

70. Homans J. Thrombophlebitis of the lower extremities. *Ann Surg* 1928; **88**: 641.

71. Horellou M H, Conard J, Bertina R M, Samama M. Congenital protein C deficiency and thrombotic disease in nine French families. *Br Med J* 1984; **289**: 1285.

72. Howe C T. The management of deep vein thrombosis. *Br J Hosp Med* 1970; 348.

73. Hull R, Hirsch J, Sackett D L. Clinical validity of a negative venogram in patients with clinically suspected venous thrombosis. *Circulation* 1981; **64**: 622.

74. Hull R, Hirsch J, Sackett D L, Powers P, Turpie A G G, Walker I. Combined use of leg scanning and impedance plethysmography in suspected venous thrombosis. *N Engl J Med* 1977; **296**: 1497.

75. Hull R, Hirsch J, Sackett D L, Stoddart G. Cost effectiveness of clinical diagnosis, venography and non-invasive testing in patients with symptomatic deep vein thrombosis. *N Engl J Med* 1981; **304**: 1561.

76. Husted S E, Kraemmer Nielsen L, Krusell L, Fasting H, Ostergaard Nielsen B, Bruun Pedersen J, Dalgaard E, Hvid Hansen H. Deep vein thrombosis detection by ^{99m}Tc-plasmin test and phlebography. *Br J Surg* 1984; **71**: 65.

77. Isacson S, Nilsson I M. Defective fibrinolysis in blood and vein walls in recurrent "idiopathic" venous thrombosis. *Acta Chir Scand* 1972; **138**: 313.

78. Jensen C, Knudsen L L, Hecedus V. The role of contact thermography in the diagnosis of deep vein thrombosis. *Eur J Radiol* 1983; **3**: 99.

79. Johansson L, Hedner U, Nilsson I M. A family with thromboembolic disease associated with deficient fibrinolytic activity in vessel wall. *Acta Med Scand* 1978; **208** 477.

80. Jonckheer M H, Abramovici J, Jeghers O, Derume J P, Goldstein M. The interpretation of phlebograms using fibrinogen labelled with ^{99m}Technetium. *Eur J Nucl Med* 1978; **3**: 233.

81. Kakkar V V, Howe C T, Laws J W, Flanc C. Late results of treatment of deep vein thrombosis. *Br Med J* 1969; **1**: 810.

82. Kakkar V V, Sasahara A A. Diagnosis of venous thrombosis and pulmonary embolism. In: Bloom A L, Thomas D P (Eds) *Haemostasis and Thrombosis* Edinburgh. Churchill Livingstone 1981.

83. Kakkar V V. The diagnosis of deep vein thrombosis using fibrinogen test. *Arch Surg* 1972; **104**: 152.

84. Katz R S, Zizic T M, Arnold W P, Stevens M B. The pseudothrombophlebitis syndrome. *Medicine* 1977; **56**: 151.

85. Kempi V, Van der Linden W, Von Schéele C. Diagnosis of deep vein thrombosis with ^{99m}Tc-streptokinase: A clinical comparison with phlebography. *Br Med J* 1974; **4**: 748.

86. Kinmonth J B. Lymphangiography in man. *Clin Sci* 1952; **11**: 13.

87. Knight L C, Primeau J L, Siegel B A, Welch M J. Comparison of ^{111}In labelled platelets and iodinated fibrinogen for the detection of deep vein thrombosis. *J Nucl Med* 1978; **19**: 891.

88. Lambie J M Mahaffey R G, Barber D C, Karmody A M, Scott M M, Matheson N A. Diagnostic accuracy in venous thrombosis. *Br Med J* 1970; **2**: 142.

89. Layfer L F, Jones J V. Calf pain in rheumatoid arthritis. *IMJ* 1979; **155**: 104.

90. Lea Thomas M, Browse N L. Internal iliac vein

thrombosis. *Acta Radiol (Diagn)* (Stockh) 1972; **12**: 660.

91. Lea Thomas M, Carty H. Arteriographic changes in phlegmasia cerulia dolens. *Aust Radiol* 1975; **19**: 57.

92. Lea Thomas M, Carty H. The appearances of artefacts on lower limb phlebograms. *Clin Radiol* 1975; **26**: 527.

93. Lea Thomas M, McAllister V, Tonge K. The radiological appearances of deep vein thrombosis. *Clin Radiol* 1971; **22**: 295.

94. Lea Thomas M, McDonald L M. Complications of phlebography of the leg. *Br Med J* 1978; **2**: 307.

95. Lea Thomas M, McDonald L M. The accuracy of bolus ascending phlebography in demonstrating the ilio-femoral segment. *Clin Radiol* 1977; **28**: 165.

96. Lea Thomas M, O'Dwyer J A. A phlebographic study of the incidence and significance of venous thrombosis in the foot. *AJR* 1978; **130**: 751.

97. Lea Thomas M. Deep vein thrombosis. *Proc R Soc Med* 1970; **63**: 123.

98. Lea .Thomas M. *Phlebography of the Lower Limb.* Edinburgh. Churchill Livingstone 1982.

99. Lindhagen A, Berquist D, Hallböök K, Lindroth B. After-exercise thermography and prevention of deep vein thrombosis. *Br Med J* 1982; **284**: 1825.

100. Loudon J R. ^{125}I-fibrinogen uptake test. *Br Med J* 1976; **1**: 793.

101. Lowe G D O, McKillop J H, Prentice A G. Fatal retroperitoneal haemorrhage complicating anticoagulant treatment. *Postgrad Med J* 1979; **55**: 18.

102. Makin G S. Assessment of a simple test to detect postoperative deep vein thrombosis. *Br J Surg* 1968; **55**: 822.

103. Mant M J, O'Brien B D, Thong K L, Hammond G W, Birtwhistle R V, Grace M G. Haemorrhagic complications of heparin therapy. *Lancet* 1977; **1**: 1113.

104. McFarlane D G, Bacon P A. Popliteal cyst rupture in normal knee joints. *Br Med J* 1980; **281**: 1203.

105. McLachlan M S F, Thomson J G, Taylor D W, Kelly M, Sackett D L. Observer variation in the interpretation of lower leg venograms. *AJR* 1979; **132**: 227.

106. McLachlin J, Richards T, Paterson J C. An evaluation of clinical signs in the diagnosis of venous thrombosis. *Arch Surg* 1962; **85**: 738.

107. Meadway J, Nicolaides A N, Walker C J, O'Connell J D. Value of Doppler ultrasound in diagnosis of clinically suspected deep vein

thrombosis. *Br Med J* 1975; **4**: 552.

108. Moreno-Cabral R, Kistner R L, Mordyka R A. Importance of calf-vein thrombophlebitis. *Surgery* 1976; **80**: 735.

109. Morris G K, Mitchell J R. Evaluation of ^{125}I fibrinogen test for venous thrombosis in patients with hip fractures: a comparison between isotope scanning and autopsy. *Br Med J* 1977; **1**: 254.

110. Moser K M, Brach B B, Dolan G F. Clinically suspected deep venous thrombosis of the lower extremities: a comparison of venography, impedance plethysmography and radio-labelled fibrinogen. *JAMA* 1977; **237**: 2195.

111. Mullick S C, Wheeler H B, Songster G P. Diagnosis of deep venous thrombosis by electrical impedance. *Am J Surg* 1970; **119**: 417.

112. Negus D, Pinto D H, LeQuesne L P, Brown N, Chapman M. [125]I labelled fibrinogen in the diagnosis of deep vein thrombosis and its correlation with phlebography. *Br J Surg* 1968; **55**: 835.

113. Nillius A S, Lindvall R, Nylander G. Dynamic radionucleotide phlebography. A clinical study in patients after total hip replacement. *Eur J Nucl Med* 1978; **3**: 161.

114. Nilsson I M, Krook H, Sternby N-H, Söderberg E, Söderström N. Severe thrombotic disease in a young man with bone marrow and skeletal changes and with a high content of an inhibitor in the fibrinolytic system. *Acta Med Scand* 1961; **169**: 323.

115. Nilsson I M, Ljungner H, Tengborn L. Two different mechanisms in patients with venous thrombosis and defective fibrinolysis: low concentration of plasminogen activator or increased concentration of plasminogen activator inhibitor. *Br Med J* 1985; **290**: 1453.

116. Nylander G. Phlebographic diagnosis of acute deep leg thrombosis. *Acta Chir Scand* (Suppl) 1968; **397**: 30.

117. O'Donnell T F, Abbott W M, Athanasoulis C A, Milan V G, Callow A D. Diagnosis of deep vein thrombosis in the outpatient by venography. *Surg Gynec Obstet* 1980; **150**: 69.

118. Ochsner A, DeBakey M E. Thrombophlebitis: Role of venospasm in the production of the clinical manifestations. *JAMA* 1940; **114**: 117.

119. Ollson P. Variations in antithrombin activity in plasma after major surgery. *Acta Chir Scand* 1963; **126**: 24.

120. Pabinger-Fasching I, Bertina R M, Lechner K, Niessner H, Korininger C H. Protein C deficiency in two Austrian families. *Thromb Haemost* 1983; **50**: 180.

121. Partsch H, Kahn P, Roser-Maass E, Tham B. Telethermography for screening ambulatory

patients with leg vein thrombosis. *Vasa* 1981; **10**: 242.

122. Partsch H, Loefferer O, Mostbeck A. Diagnosis of established deep-vein thrombosis in the leg using ^{131}I fibrinogen. *Angiology* 1974; **25**: 719.

123. Peters A M, Lavender J P, Needham S G, Loutfi I, Snook D, Epentos A A, Lumley P, Keery R J, Hogg N. Imaging thrombus with radiolabelled monoclonal antibody to platelets. *Br Med J* 1986; **293**: 1525.

124. Phillips R S. Prognosis in deep venous thrombosis. *Arch Surg* 1963; **87**: 732.

125. Pochaczevsky R, Pillari G, Feldman F. Liquid crystal contact thermography of deep vein thrombosis. *AJR* 1981; **738**: 717.

126. Poulose K, Kapcar A, Reba R. False positive ^{125}I fibrinogen test. *Angiology* 1976; **27**: 258.

127. Provan J L. Raised skin temperature in the early diagnosis of deep vein thrombosis. *Br Med J* 1965; **3**: 334.

128. Quist G. *Surgical Diagnosis*. London. H K Lewis 1977.

129. Ramsay L E. Impact of venography on the diagnosis and management of deep vein thrombosis. *Br Med J* 1983; **286**: 698.

130. Ritchie W G M, Lapayowker M S, Soulen R L. Thermographic diagnosis of deep venous thrombosis: Anatomically based diagnostic criteria. *Radiology* 1979; **132**: 321.

131. Roberts V C, Cotton L T. Prevention of postoperative deep vein thrombosis in patients with malignant disease. *Br Med J* 1974; **1**: 358.

132. Roberts V C. Fibrinogen uptake scanning for diagnosis of deep vein thrombosis: A plea for standardization. *Br Med J* 1975; **3**: 455.

133. Rollins D, Ryan T J, Semrow C, Buchbinder D. Diagnosis of deep venous thrombosis using real time ultrasound imaging. In: Negus D, Jantet G (Eds) *Phlebology '85*. London. Libbey 1986.

134. Rosenberg R D. Actions and interactions of antithrombin and heparin. *N Engl J Med* 1975; **292**: 146.

135. Rosenthall L. Radionucleotide venography using ^{99m}Tc pertechnetate and the gamma ray scintillation camera. *AJR* 1966; **97**: 874.

136. Rosenthall L. Combined inferior vena cavography, iliac venography and lung imaging with ^{99m}Tc albumin macroaggregates. *Radiology* 1971; **98**: 623.

137. Ruckley C V. [125]I fibrinogen test in the diagnosis of deep vein thrombosis. *Br Med J* 1975; **2**: 498.

138. Sandler D A, Martin J F. Liquid crystal thermography as a screening test for deep vein thrombosis. *Lancet* 1985; **1**: 665.

139. Sandler D A. Homans' sign and medical education. *Lancet* 1985; **1**: 1130.

140. Sandler D, Martin J F, Duncan J S, Blake G M, Ward P, Ramsay L E, Lamont A C, Ross B, Sherriff S, Walton L. Diagnosis of deep vein thrombosis. Comparison of clinical evaluation, ultrasound, plethysmography and venoscan with xray venogram. *Lancet* 1984; **2**: 716.

141. Sas G, Blasko G, Bankegyi D, Jako J, Palos A. Abnormal antithrombin III (antithrombin III "Budapest") as a cause of a familial thrombophilia. *Thromb Diath Haemorrh* 1974; **32**: 105.

142. Seeger W H, Marciniak E. Inhibition of autoprothrombin C activity with plasma. *Nature* 1962; **193**: 1188.

143. Sigel B, Popky G L. Boland J P, Wagner D K, Mapp E McD. Diagnosis of venous disease by ultrasonic flow detection. *Surg Forum* 1967; **18**: 185.

144. Simpson F G, Robinson P J, Bark M, Losowsky M S. Prospective study of thrombophlebitis and "pseudothrombophlebitis". *Lancet* 1980; **1**: 331.

145. Sproull E E. Carcinoma and venous thrombosis: the frequency of association of carcinoma in the body or tail of the pancreas with multiple venous thrombosis. *Am J Cancer* 1938; **34**: 566.

146. Stewart G, Gaunt J I, Croft D N, Browse N L. Isotope lymphography: a new method of investigating the role of the lymphatics in chronic limb oedema. *Br J Surg* 1985; **72**: 906–909.

147. Strandness D E, Sumner D S. Ultrasonic velocity detector in the diagnosis of thrombophlebitis. *Arch Surg* 1972; **104**: 180.

148. Sullivan E D, David J P, Cranley J J. Real time B mode venous ultrasound. J Vasc Surg 1984; **1**: 465.

149. Sumner D S, Baker D W, Strandness D E. The ultrasonic velocity detector in a clinical study of venous disease. *Arch Surg* 1968; **97**: 75.

150. Szendro G, Nicolaides A N, Zukowski A J, Christopoulos D, Malouf G M, Christodoulou C, Myers K. Duplex scanning in the assessment of deep venous incompetence. *J Vasc Surg* 1986; **4**: 237.

151. Tran T H, Marbet G A, Duckert F. Association of heriditary heparin co-factor 2 deficiency with thrombosis. *Lancet* 1985; **2**: 413.

152. Von Kaulla E, Von Kaulla K N. Antithrombin III and diseases. *Am J Clin Pathol* 1967; **48**: 69.

153. Von Kaulla E, Von Kaulla K N. Deficiency of antithrombin III activity associated with hereditary thrombosis tendency. *J Med* 1972; **3**: 349.

154. Warlow C, Ogston D. The ^{125}I-fibrinogen tech-

nique in the diagnosis of venous thrombosis. *Clin Haematol* 1973; **2**: 199.

155. Webber M, Bennet L, Craig M. Thrombophlebitis: demonstration by scintiscanning. *Radiology* 1969; **92**: 620.

156. Wheeler H B, Anderson F A, Cardullo P A, Patwardhan N A, Jian-Ming L, Cutler B S. Suspected deep vein thrombosis. Management by impedance plethysmography. *Arch Surg* 1982; **117**: 1206.

157. Wheeler H B, Mullick S C, Anderson J N, Pearson D. Diagnosis of occult deep vein thrombosis by a non-invasive bedside technique. *Surgery* 1971; **70**: 20.

158. Wood E H, Prentice E R, McNicol G P. Association of fibrinogen–fibrin related antigen (FR antigen) with postoperative deep-vein thrombosis and systemic complications. *Lancet* 1972; **1**: 166.

159. Ygge J. Studies on blood coagulation and fibrinolysis in conditions associated with an increased incidence of thrombosis. Methodological and clinical investigations. *Scand J Haematol* (Suppl) 1970; **11**.

160. Yin E T, Wessler S, Stoll P J. Identity of plasma associated factor X inhibitor with antithrombin III and heparin co-factor. *J Biol Chem* 1971; **246**: 712.

18

Deep vein thrombosis: treatment

Thrombosis in a deep vein occludes its lumen and destroys its valves.[35] If by the term 'treatment' we imply restoration to complete normality, then the treatment of deep vein thrombosis requires either the removal of the thrombus before it has destroyed the valves, or the manipulation of the natural history of the thrombus with measures that will encourage reopening of the lumen and recovery of the valves. The latter approach is not yet possible and therefore the only available treatment is thrombus removal.

If a thrombus cannot be removed, its ultimate effect is, at present, beyond our control. All we can do is prevent further thrombosis, by giving anticoagulants, or stop complications (e.g. pulmonary embolism) by performing surgical venous blockade.

As a result of the inadequacies of the available forms of treatment we tend to seek clinical objectives, often just the relief of symptoms, and call our efforts 'treatment', even though they do not cure.

Our main clinical objectives are:

- prevention of fatal pulmonary embolism. This can be achieved by thrombus removal, venous blockade or the prevention of new thrombosis with anticoagulants.
- reduction of the severity of the post-thrombotic syndrome. This may be achieved by thrombus removal or the prevention of new thrombosis with anticoagulants but is sometimes exacerbated by venous blockade.
- reduction of the severity of the presenting symptoms. This is usually achieved by palliative measures which have no effect on the thrombus.

In clinical terms the first of these three objectives – saving the patient's life – overrides all others, and therefore when the ideal treatment (i.e. the complete removal of a thrombus leaving the veins and the valves intact) is unattainable, the patient may have to accept the post-thrombotic syndrome as the cost of being alive.

There are two methods for removing thrombus – surgical thrombectomy and pharmacological thrombolysis. Both methods are most effective when the thrombus is fresh and non-adherent; a type of thrombus that is often symptomless. By the time that symptoms appear, the thrombus has often become adherent and old, two features which make its removal or dissolution difficult. Both methods of removal have their own contraindications. Whenever possible, pharmacological lysis of thrombus is preferred to surgical thrombectomy because it will affect all the thrombus in a limb, some of which is inaccessible to the surgeon, and it avoids the risks and complications of surgery.

Thrombolysis

The body's fibrinolytic system can be activated to a state in which it will lyse thrombi by two naturally occurring 'activators' – streptokinase (derived from the streptococcus) and urokinase (derived from human urine).[86, 128] Both activators work by activating plasminogen. Streptokinase acts directly by complexing with plasminogen; this exposes the active site on the plasminogen which catalyses the cleavage of plasminogen to plasmin. Urokinase acts directly on plasminogen, coverting it to plasmin. The plasmin produced by these two enzymes breaks fibrin down into a number of soluble products (Table 18.1).

Streptokinase is neutralized in the blood by antibodies which have been produced in response to previous streptococcal infections. These

Table 18.1 Activation of fibrinolysis

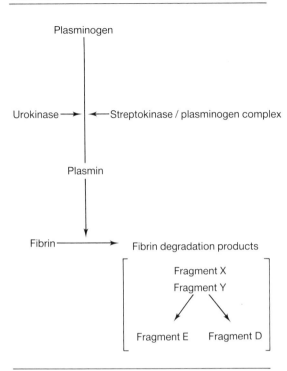

antibodies must be blocked before the streptokinase will begin to complex with plasminogen. Streptokinase is itself highly antigenic, and the level of antistreptococcal antibodies rises and remains very high for 6 months after treatment, making the continuation of treatment beyond 3 weeks ineffective. Urokinase is a human protein and is therefore not antigenic.

Streptokinase

This substance has been more widely used than urokinase (mainly because it is considerably less expensive), though its antigenicity causes more side-effects. In the future it may be replaced by streptokinase analogues and tissue plasminogen activator but the lessons learnt from the use of streptokinase will still be applicable to these new substances because their final common mechanism of action is the conversion of plasminogen to plasmin.

Dose

The blood of the majority of European and American patients has an antistreptokinase titre that can be neutralized by a loading dose of 250,000 units of streptokinase.[4,6,57,58] Most workers do not measure the antibody titre before beginning treatment, unless the patient has a history of a recent streptococcal infection or has had a recent course of streptokinase. The loading dose is given intravenously over 30–60 minutes and is followed by a standard maintenance dose of 100,000 units/hour which is continued for 3–5 days. Other dose regimens have been described but their benefits do not appear to be any greater than those of the regimen described above.[47, 71, 112]

Control

The clinical and haematological effects of streptokinase are monitored in the following ways.
(a) Careful clinical observations to detect any sign of haemorrhage (i.e. blood pressure and pulse rate) or microscopic haematuria (i.e. urinalysis).
(b) Daily or twice daily measurement of the haematocrit.
(c) Measurement of the thrombin clotting time. The thrombin clotting time is prolonged by a reduced plasma fibrinogen and by an excess of fibrin degradation products. If this time is used it should be measured every 4 hours and should be maintained at four to five times longer than the pretreatment control value. A thrombin clotting time which exceeds five times the control value indicates that there is too little streptokinase/plasminogen complex and too much plasminogen being converted to plasmin. This is reversed by increasing the dose of streptokinase. Conversely, a short thrombin clotting time indicates excess streptokinase/plasminogen complex and insufficient plasminogen for conversion to plasmin. This is reversed by *reducing* the dose of streptokinase.
(d) Administration of streptokinase should be stopped if bleeding occurs from wounds, the urinary tract, or the gastrointestinal tract and, if necessary, the effect of streptokinase should be reversed by giving a fibrinolytic inhibitor (e.g. tranexamic acid). Administration of fresh blood and fresh plasma may be

required but this will not always stop the bleeding, as the circulating streptokinase may lyse the infused fibrinogen to produce more fibrinogen degradation products which themselves interfere with the coagulation cascade.

(e) Measurements of fibrin degradation products, plasma fibrinogen, plasmin, antiplasmin, and the bleeding time do not really assist the clinical control of treatment.

Urokinase

Urokinase is extremely expensive when produced by extraction from human urine. Newer methods of production may reduce the cost but both streptokinase and urokinase may eventually be replaced by analogues of streptokinase and genetically engineered tissue plasminogen activator.

Dose

The standard treatment regimen for urokinase is a loading dose of 4000 units/kg given intravenously over 30 minutes followed by 4000 units/kg/hour.[41, 57, 119]

Control

The clinical and haematological effects of urokinase are monitored in the following ways.
(a) Careful clinical observations of blood pressure and pulse rate and urinalysis to detect microscopic haematuria.
(b) Measurement of thrombin clotting time. A thrombin time which is greater than five times the pretreatment control indicates excess activity, and the dose of urokinase should be reduced. A thrombin time which is less than twice the normal value indicates that the dose should be increased. It must be noted that changes in the dose of urokinase based on the thrombin time are the opposite of those needed to correct the effect of streptokinase because the urokinase acts directly on plasminogen whereas streptokinase acts indirectly.
(c) Twice daily haematocrit estimations may reveal occult haemorrhage.
(d) Bleeding is reversed by stopping the administration of urokinase and giving fresh blood or plasma, cryoprecipitates, and fibrinolytic inhibitors.
(e) Measurement of plasma fibrinogen, fibrin degradation products, plasmin, antiplasmin and the bleeding time do not really assist the clinical control of treatment.

Streptokinase analogues

Streptokinase analogues consist of a streptokinase–plasminogen complex with a chemical bond across the active site that is released when the complex is warmed within the bloodstream. A number of these substances are being manufactured. They have a thrombolytic effect which is similar to that of streptokinase,[18] but the effect lasts longer and causes smaller changes of the coagulation tests. These analogues can be given by single or twice daily intravenous injections. In our limited experience these drugs have not been any more effective than streptokinase and they have caused more bleeding complications. Research should be aimed at the development of a safe thrombolytic drug which can be given by a single daily injection.

Tissue plasminogen activators

Streptokinase and urokinase activate the circulating (intrinsic) fibrinolytic system. There is an extrinsic system in tissue fluid which has its own activator – tissue plasminogen activator. It is claimed that the extrinsic system activates only the plasminogen that is bound to fibrin and will therefore only activate plasminogen which is bound to thrombus, not plasminogen which is free in the circulation. If this is true, thrombolysis may be achieved with fewer bleeding complications.

A glycoprotein has been isolated from the culture fluid of a cell-line of human malignant melanoma cells which is almost identical to the glycoprotein of extrinsic plasminogen activator that has been extracted from uterine tissues.[125] In animals this glycoprotein has been shown to have a higher specific thrombolytic activity than urokinase and to produce thrombolysis without systemic fibrinolytic activation. To date there are very few published clinical studies of the effect of tissue plasminogen activator on deep vein thrombosis.

The structure of tissue plasminogen activator

has now been identified by gene probes and the pure compound has been genetically engineered.

A number of studies have been made of the dissolution of the fibrin thrombi found in coronary arteries with a small dose of tissue plasminogen activator given locally or systemically.[122,123] It is claimed that the tissue plasminogen has a beneficial effect but whether it is more effective than streptokinase or really has less risk of haemorrhage remains to be established.[114] Tissue plasminogen activator may replace existing thrombolytic drugs once it can be manufactured cheaply and in large quantities.

Complications of thrombolysis: prevention and treatment

Haemorrhage The incidence of haemorrhagic complications varies in different publications. Minor bruising at venepuncture sites and pressure areas (e.g. the elbows and buttocks) are common (i.e. they occur in up to 50 per cent of patients). Serious bleeding occurs in 5–10 per cent of patients.

Fresh wounds, arterial puncture sites and gastrointestinal ulcers are common sites of serious bleeding, and patients with these abnormalities should not be treated with thrombolytic drugs. Spontaneous urinary tract, gastrointestinal and, occasionally, intracerebral bleeding can occur (Fig. 18.1).

The treatment of haemorrhage is the same irrespective of the type of thrombolytic drug being used. There are no specific antidotes to the thrombolytic drugs themselves, only measures which reverse their effect.

Local pressure on bleeding wounds and vascular puncture sites is important and usually effective. Surgical intervention to stop bleeding should be delayed until the blood fibrinolytic activity returns to normal.

The *systemic* treatment of haemorrhage includes:

- stopping the thrombolytic drug,
- restoring the blood volume with a transfusion of fresh blood (to give platelets and coagulation factors),
- restoring the plasma fibrinogen with fresh blood, fresh plasma or cryoprecipitates,
- reversing the fibrinolysis by giving intravenous tranexamic acid, 1 g imme-

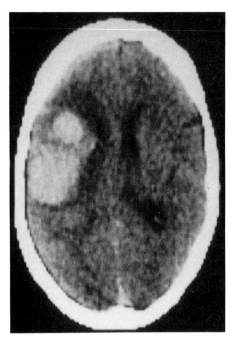

Fig. 18.1 The computerized tomography (CT) scan of a patient treated with a streptokinase analogue showing a large intracerebral haemorrhage which caused a massive stroke and death.

diately and then if necessary 8-hourly, until the bleeding stops.

Allergic reactions These are only a problem with streptokinase; they are the body's response to the injection of a foreign protein.

In our experience fever occurs in 30 per cent of patients, and the more serious reactions (e.g. shivering, rigors, itching, urticarial rashes and loin pain occur in less than 10 per cent of patients.

Treatment should be withdrawn from patients who have rigors, hypotension and loin pain to avoid serious renal damage.

Minor reactions are not an indication to stop treatment, and they can often be prevented by administering antihistamines or hydrocortisone. It is our practice to give 20 mg chlorpheniramine (Piriton) and 25 mg prednisolone intramuscularly 1 hour before giving streptokinase to reduce the incidence of fever, itching and uticaria. Additional corticosteroids can be given during treatment if minor reactions continue.

Major reactions should be treated with intravenous hydrocortisone (100 mg), Piriton

(50 mg) and, if necessary, subcutaneous adrenaline (0.5 ml, 1 in 1000).

Contra-indications to thrombolysis

The principal contra-indication to all forms of thrombolytic therapy is the presence of a site of potential bleeding; these sites are discussed below.

Fresh surgical wounds Some workers have administered thrombolytic therapy within 4 days of surgery but we *never* give thrombolytic drugs within 7 days of any form of surgical operation. Even more caution should be used after ophthalmic, vascular and neurosurgical operations.

Recent arterial puncture wounds It is unlikely that a patient with a deep vein thrombosis will have had a recent arteriogram but it must be remembered that arterial puncture wounds are sealed by thrombus and thrombolytic therapy may lyse the sealing plug of thrombus up to 7 days after the puncture.

Liver and kidney biopsies Lytic therapy is contra-indicated for 7–10 days after a liver or kidney biopsy has been taken.

Known gastrointestinal ulceration A history of peptic ulceration or the presence of an alimentary tract carcinoma are contra-indications to thrombolysis because both conditions can bleed spontaneously and heavily, even when they have caused no previous bleeding problems. A gastrointestinal haemorrhage which begins during thrombolytic therapy may be the first indication of gastrointestinal disease. The first line of treatment is to stop the bleeding by reversing the activation of fibrinolysis; surgical treatment should not be attempted until this has been achieved.

Haemorrhagic diatheses (e.g. thrombocytopenia and haemophilia) These are absolute contra-indications to thrombolysis.

The effect of any previously administered anticoagulant should be reversed before giving a thrombolytic drug because the combination of anticoagulation with plasminogen activation is difficult to control and even more difficult to reverse if bleeding occurs. If anticoagulation is indicated while the need for thrombolysis is being assessed, administer heparin because its action can be rapidly reversed by protamine.

Intracardiac thrombus Thrombolysis softens thrombus before turning it into soluble split products and therefore makes the thrombus more likely to fragment. Emboli from peripheral venous thrombi during thrombolytic therapy are uncommon because these thrombi are not subjected to repeated local trauma, but thrombi in the heart may fragment. A history of a myocardial infarction or the presence of atrial fibrillation should alert the physician to the possibility that thrombolysis could cause an intracardiac thrombus to embolize into the brain or the peripheral vessels. In these patients cardiac thrombus should be excluded by echocardiography before giving thrombolytic drugs.

Duration and termination of treatment

The dissolution of a thrombus by plasmin depends upon the age and accessibility of its contained fibrin.[14] Old fibrin is less susceptible to lysis[22] because of the polymerization and crosslinking between its molecules.

Thrombolysis occurs at the surface of a thrombus and throughout its substance (depending upon the presence of plasminogen trapped within the thrombus). The effect of a thrombolytic agent partly depends upon its ability to diffuse into the thrombus and this in turn depends upon the surface area of thrombus exposed to the bloodstream.

A fresh non-adherent thrombus (i.e. one with young loose-knit fibrin and the majority of its surface exposed to flowing blood) is much more likely to lyse than an old adherent thrombus containing well polymerized fibrin with only 5 per cent of its surface exposed to the blood. It may seem surprising that thrombolytic agents can diffuse into old adherent thrombi, but it must be remembered that thrombi are not inert 'backwaters' of the circulation. Fibrinogen and plasminogen can diffuse into thrombi quite quickly, even when they are 7 or 10 days old.

The symptoms and signs of deep vein thrombosis give little indication of the true age of the thrombus; the phlebogram provides a crude estimate, but in terms of weeks not days (see Chapters 4 and 17). It is rarely worth giving thrombolytic drugs when the thrombus is more than 7–10 days old. We estimate the age of the thrombus from the phlebographic appearance and the history, and only treat patients who have radiologically fresh (less than 7 days old), non-adherent thrombi, or patients who have adherent thrombus but a definite, short clinical history.

As a result of these differences in thrombus behaviour, the response to thrombolytic therapy is unpredictable. Fresh non-adherent thrombus can be expected to lyse more readily than old non-adherent thrombus but the only way to achieve maximum thrombolysis is to monitor the process closely with *repeated phlebography*; no other method is suitable.[50] Non-invasive techniques which measure outflow resistance give no information about the thrombus because a change of outflow resistance is just as likely to have been caused by the development of collateral vessels as by thrombolysis.

Repeated phlebography is undesirable because it causes bleeding and bruising from the venepuncture sites. It is also expensive and not very pleasant. Most clinicians treat their patients for 3 days before performing a check phlebogram and deciding whether to continue treatment. This is a reasonable and acceptable approach because there is usually little change in the thrombus during the first 24–48 hours of treatment.

If there has been worthwhile but incomplete lysis at 72 hours, treatment should be continued for another 48 hours. If there has been no thrombolysis after 72 hours, but there is haematological evidence of adequate activation of the fibrinolytic system, treatment should be abandoned as it is unlikely to have any further effect on the thrombus, and after 5 days the level of antistreptokinase antibodies begins to rise and the patient becomes resistant to treatment.

Treatment can be stopped abruptly because there is no evidence of any rebound phenomenon but the effect of thrombolytic drugs takes at least 4 hours to wear off. If there are no bleeding problems, intravenous heparin can be started 4 hours after stopping treatment. Heparin, 20–40,000 units/24 hours is given; the dose depends upon the coagulation tests used (usually the accelerated partial thromboplastin time). When there have been bleeding complications, the thrombin clotting time should be measured 4 hours after stopping treatment and, if necessary, repeated every 2 hours. Heparin should not be given until the thrombin clotting time is less than twice the pretreatment control value. It may be 12 hours before the test indicates that it is safe to give heparin.

Anticoagulation after thrombolytic therapy is important because any new thrombi that form will contain little plasminogen and will be less susceptible to further attempts at thrombolysis.

Results

The results of thrombolysis can be divided into two categories – the lysis of the thrombi and the long-term clinical results. Lysis of the thrombi has been studied in detail over the past 15 years but the long-term clinical results, which are far more important, have not been fully evaluated.

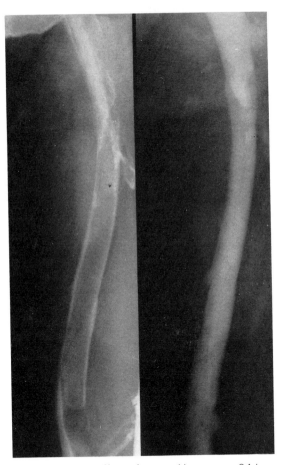

Fig. 18.2 The effect of streptokinase on a 24-hour old thrombus. This patient was being screened daily with a Doppler flow detector. Twenty-four hours before the left-hand phlebogram was performed the superficial femoral vein was patent. On the day of the phlebogram the Doppler flow detector indicated that the vein was occluded, and the X-ray revealed fresh non-adherent thrombus. After 48 hours of streptokinase therapy (right-hand panel) the thrombus was completely lysed.

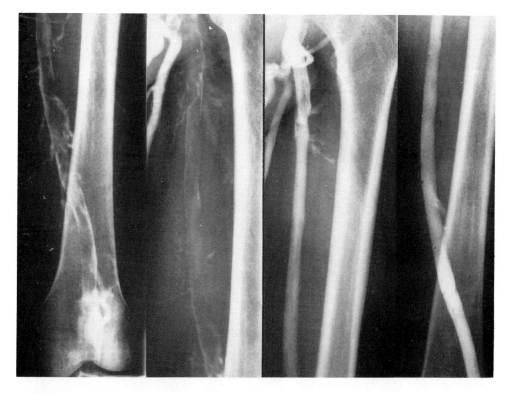

Fig. 18.3 The effect of streptokinase on a 3–4-day old thrombus. This patient had experienced swelling of the leg for 3 days before admission to hospital. The phlebogram (left-hand panels) showed a fresh non-adherent thrombus.

After 3 days of streptokinase therapy (right-hand panels) the thrombus was completely lysed but no valves were visible in the superficial femoral vein.

Factors affecting the success of thrombolysis

Age of thrombus After the early studies of streptokinase, between 1965 and 1970, it became apparent that young thrombus was more susceptible to lysis than old thrombus.[14,22,107] All the subsequent studies make this point but also stress the difficulty of determining the age of a thrombus (Figs 18.2, 18.3, 18.4).

Most patients have thrombi of different ages. A patient may develop a calf pain, indicative of a calf vein thrombosis, 3 weeks before his leg swells, a symptom that indicates that the thrombosis has extended into the popliteal or femoral vein. At that moment he will have thrombus in the calf that is 3 weeks old and thrombus in the thigh that is a few days old. Thrombolytic therapy will lyse the young thrombus but not the old thrombus. Nevertheless, it is better to try treatment than to withhold it, even when the age of the thrombus is in doubt, provided treatment can be given safely.

Adherence of thrombus In our early studies[14] we were impressed by the failure of streptokinase to lyse thrombi that were totally adherent to the vein wall and completely occluding the lumen (Figs 18.5, 18.6). This observation has since been confirmed by some workers and refuted by others.[34,51,68,88,89,95,105,108, 118] This lack of agreement has been caused by two problems. Firstly, the quality of the phlebography affects the number of times that complete occlusion will be diagnosed. A poor phlebogram often shows a non-filled segment which suggests a complete occlusion where an investigation of better quality may show a thin streak of contrast medium outlining the thrombus indicating partial adhesion. Secondly, it is impossible to give a 'phlebographic' age to a thrombus that completely occludes a vein. A completely occluded vein may contain a very old

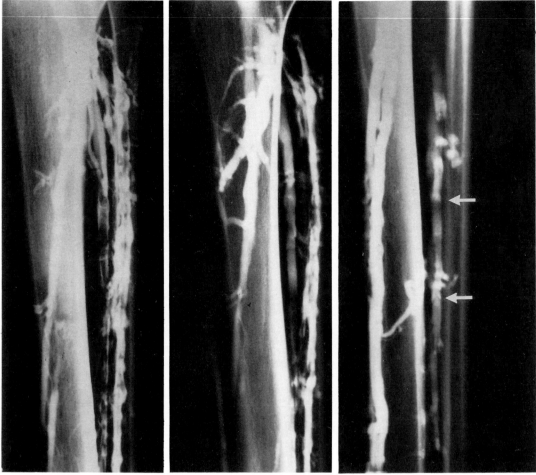

Fig. 18.4 This patient presented with an episode of chest pain. The phlebogram (left-hand panel) showed fresh thrombus in the calf. After 3 days of streptokinase therapy most of the calf thrombus had been lysed (centre panel).

Eighteen months later the calf veins were patent and the veins that had contained thrombus had normal functioning valves (right-hand panel – arrowed).

thrombus, or a young thrombus that has just filled the vein. Complete occlusion and apparent radiological adherence should therefore not be a contra-indication to treatment if the clinical history is distinct and short. Successful lysis is, however, less likely for occlusive thrombosis than for a 'free-floating' thrombus, and until we have a precise method for determining the age of thrombus, the published results of thrombolysis will vary.

Site of thrombosis Most published studies have reported better thrombolysis of axial than of calf vein thrombosis.[34,127] However, when all the

published results are combined there seems to be little difference between the lysis of ilio-femoral and that of superficial femoral vein thrombosis. Between 60 per cent and 80 per cent of fresh thrombi in the major outflow tract veins can be completely or partially lysed, with preservation of valves in less than 33 per cent. A fresh non-adherent thrombus in an axial vein is particularly susceptible to lysis but occasionally this type of thrombus may detach or fragment and become a pulmonary embolus.

Thrombus in the calf is less susceptible to thrombolytic therapy, and phlebography is not

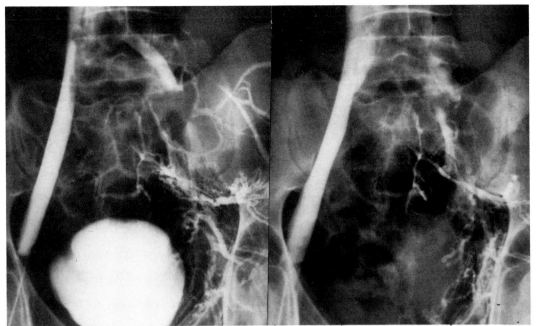

Fig. 18.5 This patient had an adherent thrombus, 7–10-days old, in the left iliac vein (left-hand panel). The phlebogram also showed thrombus jutting into the vena cava.

After 3 days of streptokinase therapy the vena caval thrombus was lysed but the adherent iliac thrombus was unaltered (right-hand panel).

Streptokinase is not effective on ageing adherent thrombus.

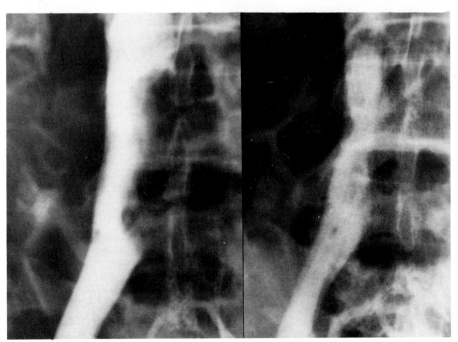

Fig. 18.6 Another example of the failure of streptokinase to lyse adherent iliac vein thrombus while disolving thrombus jutting into the vena cava. (Left-hand panel – pretreatment. Right-hand panel – after treatment.)

the ideal method of assessing calf thrombosis because it cannot display every calf vein (Figs 18.7, 18.8). Studies with the ^{125}I-fibrinogen uptake test show that in some cases radioactivity may fall rapidly during the administration of streptokinase[67] but in other instances it may rise, indicating that thrombi can grow during lytic therapy. This observation suggests that local thrombogenic factors may occasionally override a systemically induced thrombolytic state.

The number of segments of the venous tree that contain thrombus does not seem to effect the response in individual segments. The iliac and calf thrombi of a combined ilio-femoral calf thrombosis will lyse at the same rate as isolated iliac or calf thrombi.

Prevention of pulmonary embolism

There are few published data on the effect of thrombolysis on recurrent pulmonary embolism. Emboli may occur as the result of thrombolytic therapy but when they reach the lungs they are usually lysed by the circulating lytic agent. However, in view of this potential complication thrombolysis cannot be recommended when embolus prevention is the prime objective of treatment.

Long-term value of thrombolysis

The main object of giving a thrombolytic drug is to prevent the development of the calf pump failure syndrome. This will only be achieved if valve function, as well as vein patency, is restored (Fig. 18.4),[14,109] though it is possible that communicating vein valve preservation is more important than axial vein valve preservation (see Chapter 11).

There are few long-term controlled com-

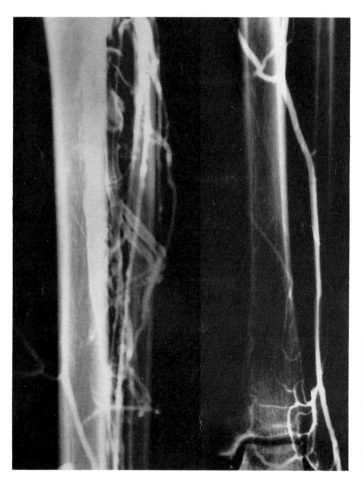

Fig. 18.7 An example of the failure of streptokinase to lyse calf thrombi. The left-hand panel shows the calf veins filled with fresh non-adherent thrombus. After 3 days of streptokinase therapy (right-hand panel) all the calf veins were totally occluded (an os calcis intraosseous phlebogram was needed to confirm this). Nevertheless the patient's pain and swelling had gone, and she was 'clinically' cured. This highlights the inadequacy of physical signs as indicators of the extent of deep vein thrombosis or the success of treatment.

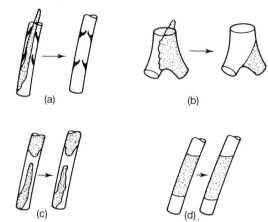

Fig. 18.8 The circumstances in which thrombolysis can be expected to be effective.
(a) Fresh non-adherent thrombus will lyse.
(b) Thrombus jutting into flowing blood will lyse.
(c) Non-adherent thrombus below an occlusion may fail to lyse.
(d) Adherent thrombus which is more than 3 days old is unlikely to lyse.

parisons of the effect of thrombolysis and routine anticoagulation on the post-thrombotic syndrome. Arnesen *et al.*[5] reviewed 35 patients 6 years and 6 months after treatment. Seventeen patients had been treated with streptokinase and 18 had been given heparin.[4] Thirty-four per cent of the group treated with streptokinase and 66 per cent of the group treated with heparin had post-thrombotic symptoms and signs, 3 of the group treated with heparin developed venous ulcers.

Elliot *et al.* followed 51 patients for a mean of 18 months and they found 32 per cent of the group treated with streptokinase had post-thrombotic symptoms compared with 76 per cent of the group treated with heparin.[37]

In contrast Kakkar and Lawrence studied a much larger group (153 patients) for 2 years using clinical and physiological (foot volumetry) assessment; they found *no* difference in the late results between streptokinase and heparin treatment.[70]

It is difficult to compare these three studies. Almost all the patients in the first two studies had axial vein thrombosis, whereas the third study included patients with calf and popliteal vein thrombosis from a number of different trials. It seems logical that the removal of a large thrombus (destined to cause serious obstruction) from an axial vein should reduce the incidence of post-thrombotic sequelae,[97] whereas the partial removal of an extensive thrombosis from the calf is unlikely to restore calf pump function to normal. Ultimately, the risk of developing the post-thrombotic syndrome will depend upon the relative long-term physiological significance of axial vein obstruction and incompetence and communicating vein incompetence. Failure to relieve obstruction might cause early symptoms but these may regress as collateral veins develop. Communicating vein incompetence takes much longer to appear and, as most patients with deep vein thrombosis have some degree of calf vein thrombosis, the short-term improvements derived from the lysis of axial vein thrombus may disappear in the long term as the problems related to the calf vein damage develop. The majority of the long-term haemodynamic studies following thrombolysis report an incidence of moderate or severe dysfunction in 50 per cent of patients, only 25 per cent having returned to normal. *Overall these results suggest that thrombolysis does not significantly reduce the incidence of the post-thrombotic syndrome.*[1, 20, 24, 65, 69, 96, 112, 126]

Indications for thrombolysis

It is customary to state the indications for a treatment before describing either the technique or the results. The proceeding paragraphs reveal that there is considerable doubt about the clinical value of thrombolysis. Furthermore new dose regimens and substances are continually being introduced. When the results of a treatment are uncertain the indications are also in doubt.

Our opinions on the present status and expectations of thrombolytic therapy, based on the conflicting evidence presented above, are given below (Fig. 18.8).

Main axial vein thrombosis, adherent or non-adherent, less than 7 days old, in the absence of contra-indications This should be treated with a thrombolytic drug. The clinical significance of the contra-indications increases with the age and adherence of the thrombus because these factors reduce the chance of successful lysis. For example, we rarely advise thrombolysis of an adherent 7-day-old femoral vein thrombosis in a patient with only moderate symptoms, 14 days after an operation. However, we consider that thrombolysis is the treatment of choice for a young patient who has not had an operation with a fresh, non-adherent, ilio-femoral thrombosis, or a similar but asymptomatic thrombus discovered on Doppler screening after a small pulmonary embolism. We make one exception to this approach. When the phlebogram suggests that the risk of another major embolism is very high, we prefer to prevent further embolism as quickly as possible by removing the thrombus (thrombectomy) or locking it into the limb (vein interruption) rather than rely on thrombolysis.

We expect the lysis of axial vein thrombi to relieve the obstruction to blood flow and perhaps save femoral vein valves in the hope that if there is little or no calf vein thrombus, late sequelae may be reduced.

Combined axial and calf vein thrombosis, adherent or non-adherent, less than 7 days old, in the absence of contra-indications We treat this in a similar manner but have less expectation (probably none) of preventing late sequelae. We consider that limb-threatening phlegmasia cerulea dolens should be treated urgently by thrombectomy but Elliot *et al.* have reported a clinically successful response to streptokinase in two patients with this condition.[38]

Isolated calf vein thrombi These thrombi should not be treated with thrombolytic drugs. They are not a threat to life or limb, whereas thrombolytic drugs can kill. There is a considerable chance that calf thrombi will lyse spontaneously, and there is no evidence that their removal will reduce the incidence of post-thrombotic sequelae.

Thrombectomy

The surgical removal of deep vein thrombi, mainly from the large axial veins, was first practised in the 1920s but was not widely adopted until phlebography improved in the 1940s and 1950s[33, 46, 56, 60, 79, 80, 81] and Fogarty introduced the balloon catheter in 1963.[42, 43, 44]

Technically and radiologically controlled thrombectomy has therefore been practised for approximately as long as thrombolysis, and a similar amount of information is available about its early and late results. Much of this information is anecdotal and almost none of it has been scientifically controlled or prospectively planned. Thrombectomy is used by individual surgeons, in the light of their own interpretation of the significance of the published results, and the indications for its use will therefore be discussed after a description of the technique and a summary of the published results.

Pre-operative preparation

Patients with a deep vein thrombosis should be given the *anticoagulant* heparin once a firm clinical diagnosis has been made. If subsequent investigations show that the clinical diagnosis is wrong, the administration of heparin can always be stopped; its effect will wear-off in 4 hours and no harm will have been done. Failure to give anticoagulants once the clinical diagnosis has been made may allow extension of the thrombus while the patient is awaiting special investigations. A standard loading dose of 5000–10,000 units of heparin followed by a continuous infusion that will provide 20,000–40,000 units/24 hours is sufficient.

Complete bilateral *phlebography* to fully display the lower and upper limits of the thrombus, and the intervening partially occluded veins, and the state of the collateral veins is essential before a thrombectomy can be considered. The decision to perform a thrombectomy is based upon the nature and extent of the thrombus seen on the phlebogram and the severity of the clinical symptoms and signs.

Ascending phlebography usually provides all the information required but it may have to be supplemented with percutaneous femoral vein or trochanteric intraosseous injections to display the upper limits of the thrombus. If the patient has had a pulmonary embolism, a lung scan or pulmonary angiogram may be required to confirm the diagnosis and determine the extent of the pulmonary artery obstruction (see Chapter 20). The bladder should be catheterized so that it does not obscure the intra-operative phlebograms when it fills with radio-opaque urine. As venous thrombectomy is often accompanied by a significant blood loss, 4 units (2 litre) of blood should be crossmatched.

Anaesthesia

We prefer to use general inhalation anaesthesia with muscle relaxation, endotracheal intubation, and positive pressure ventilation. This ensures a positive pressure gradient between the thorax and the groin so that blood flows down the vena cava and iliac veins and out of the femoral venotomy – once the venotomy has been made – thus preventing any loose thrombi moving centrally into the lungs. Controlled positive pressure ventilation plus a steep foot-down position (reversed Trendelenburg) will produce a sustained pressure in the inferior vena cava of 20–30 mmHg and ensure retrograde flow.

Some surgeons prefer to carry out the operation under local, spinal or epidural anaesthesia so that the patient can perform a Valsalva manoeuvre during ballooning but if the operation takes a long time, we have found that the patients co-operation becomes less and less.

The manoeuvres to ensure retrograde blood flow in the vena cava are extremely important because they prevent intra-operative pulmonary embolism and obviate the need for vena cava balloon blockade.[36]

Operating room preparation

The patient is placed supine on an operating table which is suitable for taking intra-operative X-rays of the lower abdomen and both legs. The table is tipped 30° head-up and the patient's legs are abducted to 30°.

The skin of the whole chest, abdomen and both legs is painted with antiseptic. Towels are placed to cover the upper chest, the head and arms, the genitalia and the feet. The abdomen must be prepared in case it is necessary to explore the iliac veins or vena cava, and the chest is prepared in case an emergency pulmonary embolectomy is necessary.

A good intravenous access route should be available, and the central venous pressure should be monitored. The anaesthetist should insert an intra-arterial pressure line and place a Swan–Ganz catheter in the pulmonary artery to monitor pulmonary capillary wedge pressure if the patient has had a pulmonary embolism and has right-sided cardiac embarrassment.

Thrombectomy for ilio-femoral thrombosis[16,17,70]

The common femoral vein below the groin provides access to both the iliac and the superficial femoral veins. An incision is made in the skin of the thigh along the line of the vein,

from the inguinal ligament downwards for about 6 in (15 cm). Subcutaneous oedema may make identification and dissection of the veins difficult. The common femoral vein and its main tributaries (the superficial and deep femoral veins) must be exposed and snared. Minor tributaries should be ligated. The patient should already have been given heparin but if this has been omitted, 5000 units heparin should be administered.

It is essential to handle the veins with great care. They should never be compressed with clamps which could break the thrombus and cause an embolus.

The venotomy should be made before placing clamps on any of the vessels. If the veins are found not to contain thrombus they may then be occluded with soft cushioned clamps of the Fogarty type.

The venotomy must be large enough to allow access to the iliac and superficial femoral vein and the mouths of the deep femoral veins. It should be confined to the common femoral vein and *not* extended down into the superficial femoral vein where the blood flow is less and the risk of post-operative thrombosis is more likely. Thrombus in the common femoral vein will immediately bulge through the venotomy under the influence of the hydrostatic pressure and *the additional positive pressure that the anaesthetist must apply as the venotomy is made*. A non-adherent 'floating' thrombus in the iliac veins may be completely extruded by the positive pressure alone. There is always some bleeding but this can usually be controlled by gentle manipulation of the snares, taking care not to break the thrombus.

A balloon catheter which has a diameter large enough to obstruct the vena cava is then inserted into the venotomy, passed up into the vena cava, inflated and withdrawn until it jams against the end of the common iliac vein to prevent any thrombus in the iliac vein becoming an embolus. This technique replaces the method of inserting a caval blocking balloon through a tributary of the long saphenous vein in the opposite groin. Some surgeons rely solely on the positive pressure ventilation and head-up tilt and use no form of proximal blockade. The only way of ensuring that the balloon catheter is in the vena cava is by watching its passage with an X-ray image intensifier and filling the balloon with a radio-opaque contrast medium instead of saline. A catheter can pass to its full extent but be in the

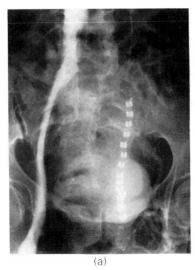
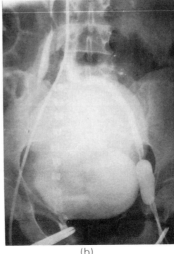
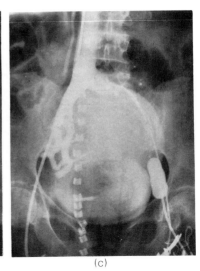

(a)   (b)   (c)

Fig. 18.9 Operative phlebography is an essential part of thrombectomy.

(a) The pre-operative phlebogram of a patient with a complete left iliac vein thrombosis following an hysterectomy.

(b) The thrombectomy has been completed and radio-opaque contrast is being injected into the iliac vein above a balloon catheter which is occluding the common femoral vein. The vena cava is still occluded with a balloon catheter passed via a tributary of the right long saphenous vein. The thrombectomized segment is smooth and patent. There is no residual thrombus.

(c) A second film showing contrast medium in the vena cava confirming the patency of the right iliac vein and vena cava and the clearance of that part of the thrombus that can be seen in (a) spreading up the side wall of the vena cava, from the left iliac vein.

ascending lumbar vein, rather than the vena cava. If an image intensifier is not available, a plain radiograph may be taken. This will demonstrate the position of the catheter in relation to the spine and give some indication of the likelihood of misdirection.

A second balloon catheter is then passed up the iliac vein until it reaches the first balloon, inflated and withdrawn; the pressure in the balloon is carefully controlled by light pressure on the barrel of the syringe to provide a gentle resistance between the balloon and the vein wall to the movement of the balloon. Over-enthusiastic inflation of the balloon can rupture the vein. The procedure is repeated until no more thrombus appears. The blockading balloon is then slowly deflated until it can be withdrawn, bringing with it any small loose pieces of thrombus that have been caught below it.

The iliac segment is then flushed with heparinized saline and an *operative phlebogram* is performed to display the iliac vein and vena cava (Fig. 18.9). If there is residual mural thrombosis or if the upper end of the iliac vein is still

occluded, the ballooning is repeated.

The presence of good back-bleeding from the external iliac vein does not mean that the whole iliac system is patent, because the blood could be coming from the internal iliac vein. Without X-ray control it is not possible to be certain that the veins are clear of thrombus.[83, 91]

If the balloon will not pass into the inferior vena cava or the terminal portion of the common iliac vein cannot be opened, a decision must be made about whether to explore this region through a transperitoneal or retroperitoneal abdominal incision. Unless there is a small spur (see Chapter 9) which can be divided, exploration of the termination of the common iliac vein in the presence of acute thrombosis is unfruitful. Dissection and exposure of the vessels and the liberation of any venous compression by the right common iliac artery is theoretically attractive but rarely helps when there is extensive oedema and inflammation in the vein wall. Occassionally, a retroperitoneal exposure of the iliac vein makes it possible to guide the catheter into the cava in those patients where the catheter persists in entering the ascending lumbar vein. Forcible blind passage of a catheter is extremely dangerous because balloon catheters can pierce the vein wall.[87]

Thrombi are subsequently removed from the distal veins of the leg by elevation, gentle compression with an Esmarch bandage applied from the toes upwards, and the retrograde passage of a balloon catheter. The last option can be difficult because the catheter often impacts in a valve cusp. Partial inflation of the balloon just above a valve sometimes centralizes the tip of the catheter and helps it to pass between the cusps but catheters rarely pass beyond the popliteal vein. The venotomy is closed with a fine monofilament suture.

Thrombus which cannot be removed by these manoeuvres can be attacked in two further ways. Some surgeons expose the upper part of the popliteal vein through an incision on the medial aspect of the lower thigh and make another venotomy for the passage of a balloon catheter in both directions. A few surgeons attempt a more vigorous removal of thrombus from the distal veins with long forceps which are similar to Desjardin's gallstone forceps.

An alternative approach is to pass a guide wire from the posterior tibial vein at the ankle up to the groin with the open end of a balloon catheter attached to the guide wire. This end of the catheter is then pulled up to the groin in an orthograde direction. The balloon is inflated as it enters the vein at the ankle. A special modification to the open end of the catheter is required for this technique.[75]

Although these ingenious techniques sound attractive, no evidence has been published to show that they improve either the immediate or the long-term results.

Compression stockings, passive and active exercises in bed and early activity out of bed encourage venous blood flow and help to reduce the chances of a postoperative thrombosis.

Adjuvant arteriovenous fistulae

There is good experimental evidence which proves that the addition of an arteriovenous fistula below a venous anastomosis improves its chance of staying patent.[36, 54] It may also increase the size of the collateral vessels if the thrombectomy is only partially successful. When non-adherent throm-bus can be extracted from the iliac vein with ease, the vein wall is probably not inflamed and there is no need to form an arteriovenous fistula. The blood flow from the limb combined with anticoagulation should ensure that the vein remains patent. Conversely, an arteriovenous fistula is probably helpful if the vein wall is inflamed, the lumen narrowed, or thrombus has been left on the vein wall. This situation is encountered after an attempt has been made to remove an adherent thrombus when the chance of rethrombosis is high.

The simplest method of making an arterio venous fistula is to use a tributary of the long saphenous vein by sewing it end-to-side to the femoral artery (Fig. 18.10). A loop of ligature material should be left lying loosely around the arteriovenous fistula to help identify it when the decision to ligate it is taken 2–3 months later.

An alternative technique is to divide a branch of the superficial femoral artery in the thigh and sew it end-to-side to the superficial femoral vein. This type of fistula is harder to find and to close, and it does not usually provide such a high blood flow.

Postoperative phlebography

It is important to assess the results of all deep vein operations by confirming vein patency with phlebography. Clinical improvement does not mean that the vein is patent (Fig. 18.11). Most legs

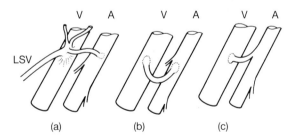

Fig. 18.10 Three simple methods of fashioning an arteriovenous fistula to enhance blood flow after a thrombectomy.

(a) A tributary of the long saphenous vein (LSV) anastomosed to the artery (A).

(b) A segment of superficial vein (a tributary of the long saphenous vein not the main trunk) sewn between the common femoral artery (A) and the vein (V).

(c) A branch of the femoral artery anastomosed to the vein (V).

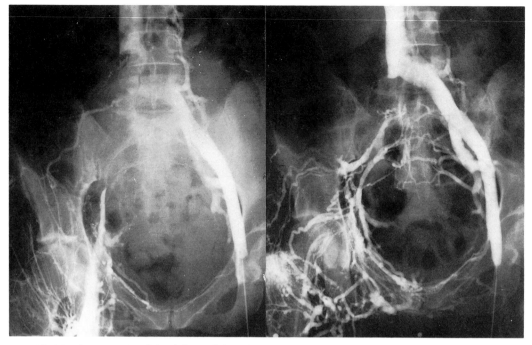

Fig. 18.11   An example of the failure of thrombectomy. The left-hand panel shows an extensive but localized right iliac vein thrombosis with thrombus in the vena cava.

A thrombectomy was performed and the operative phlebogram showed complete clearance of thrombus. Heparin was given to the patient postoperatively.

Five days later the patient's leg was not painful and the swelling had subsided; this was considered a 'clinical' success but the phlebogram (right-hand panel) showed a total rethrombosis. This case, (and Fig. 18.7) emphasizes the inadequacy of using physical signs for the assessment of the results of treatment.

with extensive axial vein thrombosis improve spontaneously without any form of treatment as collateral vessels enlarge and the thrombus retracts. Although the object of thrombectomy is the relief of symptoms, objective evidence must be obtained when claiming that improvement is the direct result of the operation and not simply the result of the natural changes in the thrombus and the collateral vessels.

Complications

Haemorrhage   The main intra-operative complication is blood loss during the passages of the balloon catheter. Rapid loss of blood and a reduction of venous return may precipitate a cardiac arrest if the patient is hypotensive or on the edge of cardiac failure as a result of previous pulmonary embolism.

Pulmonary embolism   Pulmonary embolism is uncommon if positive pressure ventilation and

head-up tilting are used during ballooning. Postoperative pulmonary embolism from residual axial vein mural thrombus or calf vein thrombus occurs in 20 per cent of patients if they are not given anticoagulants.[70,103,129] Anticoagulants must be given postoperatively and, though thrombectomy is an alternative to thrombolysis, when the risk of haemorrhage is high it should not be considered as an alternative to the administration of anticoagulants, except in the most exceptional circumstances.

Rethrombosis   Rethrombosis is the most common postoperative complication. It may occur silently and only be detected by follow-up phlebography or it may be associated with the return of physical signs. Recurrent thrombus is invariably firmly adherent to the vein wall and a repeat thrombectomy is not worthwhile unless the new thrombosis has occurred within 24 hours of the first operation and the repeat operation can be done immediately. Unfortunately, the reappearance of physical signs indicating a rethrombosis tends to occur only when the vein is totally occluded, even though mural thrombus has been building up from the moment of the operation. Such thrombus will be fixed firmly to the vein wall and will be difficult to remove. The best way to avoid recurrent thrombosis is to avoid operating on adherent thrombus.

Rethrombosis is common when the precipitating cause is disseminated malignant disease, presumably because of the hypercoagulable state. It is more prudent to avoid thrombectomy in these circumstances.

Results

There are three objectives of thrombectomy.

- Prevention of pulmonary embolism
- Relief of symptoms in the leg
- Reduction of the incidence of late post-thrombotic sequelae

Prevention of embolism

It is assumed that the removal of a large floating thrombus will reduce the risk of pulmonary embolism because such thrombi do sometimes fragment. There have been no controlled trials to test this hypothesis. Pulmonary emboli do occur after thrombectomy but in the many large series which have been reported there are very few cases of fatal emboli either during or after the operation.

Mavor analysed the incidence of pulmonary embolism (based upon a clinical diagnosis) after thrombectomy in a large series of 260 patients,[70] 127 of whom had had an embolus before operation. Thirty (25 per cent) had postoperative emboli, 7 of which (6 per cent) were fatal. One hundred and thirty-three patients had no clinical evidence of embolism before operation but 6 (5 per cent) of these had postoperative emboli, one (1 per cent) of which was fatal.

In this study only half the thrombectomies were performed with X-ray control. When the incidence of embolism was analysed according to the degree of clearance of the thrombus from the peripheral veins (in those patients who had intra-operative phlebography) the results showed that fatal emboli occurred only when there was incomplete clearance or a failed operation.

These rates of postoperative embolism seem to be high but many of the patients were elderly and 20 per cent had serious medical illness or malignant disease. Other series have reported a lower incidence of postoperative embolism. Mansfield[84] recorded no fatal emboli and five non-fatal emboli after thrombectomy in 62 patients. Eklof studied the incidence of emboli after thrombectomy by performing repeat lung scans. Fifty-six per cent of the 63 patients in a controlled prospective trial had perfusion defects before operation. One week later, 23 per cent of those patients who had been treated surgically had additional defects compared with 15 per cent in the group who had been treated conservatively.[36]

All these studies confirm that thrombectomy does *not* provide complete protection against embolism. Consequently, it is probably safer to combine thrombectomy or replace it with other venous occlusion techniques (see later and Chapter 21) if the intra-operative phlebogram shows residual thrombus or when another embolus might be expected to be fatal. Using this approach in a retrospectively controlled study we reduced an incidence of 14 per cent fatal and 26 per cent non-fatal recurrent emboli to 0 per cent fatal and 12 per cent non-fatal emboli.[13] However, this was not just a comparison of thrombectomy with and without venous blockade but included patients who were given anticoagulants alone if the phlebogram showed no loose thrombus. Van de Berg[121] examined the incidence of pre-operative and postoperative embolism associated with four forms of treatment (Fig. 18.12). Two of the 23 patients who had a thrombectomy alone had fatal postoperative emboli, whereas only 2 of 56 patients who had a thrombectomy and vena caval clip had a non-fatal embolus. In this study the results were weighted against the second (caval occlusion) group as 29 of these patients had had pre-operative emboli whereas none of the first group had had previous emboli.

The result of these studies have been presented in detail to emphasize the paucity of good controlled evidence about thrombectomy and embolism. The results appear to support what would seem obvious, namely that if fresh non-adherent thrombus is completely removed and the patient is given anticoagulants, fatal embolism is eliminated and minor embolism rarely occurs. If the operation fails or is only partially successful

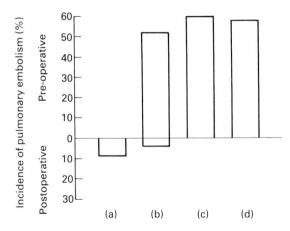

Fig. 18.12 The incidence of postoperative embolism after three types of treatment. (After Van de Berg.[121]

(a) After thrombectomy. (23 patients).

(b) After thrombectomy plus vena cava filter or clip. (56 patients).

(c) After thrombectomy plus vena cava clip plus ateriovenous fistula. (15 patients).

(d) After vena cava clip alone (31 patients).

(leaving either non-adherent thrombus in the calf or mural adherent thrombus in the axial veins), recurrent embolism is not only common but more common than when patients are given anticoagulants alone.

We conclude that, except when it is thought to be the only way to save the life of the limb, thrombectomy should only be performed when the phlebogram indicates that all the thrombus can be removed. If the thrombus cannot be completely removed, a venous blockade procedure should be added or thrombectomy should be avoided.

Relief of symptoms

The massive swelling that may accompany an ilio-femoral thrombosis often disappears as soon as the axial vein patency is restored. Pain and immobility are also relieved and the patient notices the improvement on waking from the anaesthetic. Areas of blue discoloration, which if left untreated may become patches of venous gangrene, may improve in colour and become less painful.[45, 52, 55, 78, 82] This relief persists if the vein does not rethrombose.

Phlebographic clearance, axial vein patency

It must be stressed again that the relief of symptoms must not be interpreted as axial vein patency because symptoms are also relieved by the development of collaterals. The only way to confirm patency is by phlebography. Our interpretation of the many published studies is that approximately 60 per cent of iliac veins can be expected to stay permanently patent after thrombectomy of the ilio-femoral segment. If the patients are divided into those with adherent and those with non-adherent thrombus, the success rate is probably 40 per cent and 80 per cent respectively. In Mavor's series of 75 operations in which he used X-ray control,[70] 27 per cent had either a partial or a complete rethrombosis at 14 days. Five years after operation, 66 per cent of his smaller series, treated without X-ray control, had evidence of rethrombosis. The state of the vein 14 days after operation is not necessarily its final condition.

Mansfield found that 76 per cent of the thrombectomized veins appeared 'normal' at 6 months.[84] Andriopoulos *et al.*[3] had a 60 per cent patency rate when the operation was performed for floating thrombus or phlegmasia cerulea dolens, and Brunner and Wirth[15] reported that 69 per cent of their patients had a complete or partial clearance at 2 years. Ecklof studied 70 patients who had a temporary arteriovenous fistula added to the thrombectomy for 6 months.[36] He found that 38 per cent of iliac veins were normal, 23 per cent had post-thrombotic stenosis and 39 per cent were occluded. In a second study[103] in which 31 patients who had been treated surgically were compared with 32 who had been given anticoagulants, 76 per cent of the surgical group had normal iliac veins at 6 months compared with 35 per cent of the controls. This last observation is very important because iliac veins often recanalize spontaneously and do not have valves. Nevertheless, the difference between the two forms of treatment is highly significant ($P = 0.005$). Unfortunately none of the published studies has described or analysed the results according to the nature of the thrombus and its exact distribution, few studies have a control series for comparison, and the results differ widely between studies.[31, 64, 77]

It appears that thrombectomy has a 60 per cent chance of restoring ilio-femoral vein patency –

sometimes to normal, sometimes with some degree of stenosis. Whether this benefits the patient with respect to the relief of swelling and the development of late post-thrombotic sequelae is not clear. As the ilio-femoral segement has few valves, its main function is that of a conduit; maintaining its patency should therefore be beneficial.

None of the publications quoted say much about superficial femoral vein patency or valve competency. It is therefore impossible to decide whether or not thrombectomy of the superficial femoral vein is worthwhile; in our view it depends upon the presence of popliteal vein thrombosis. It is probably worth removing discontinuous superficial femoral vein thrombus above a normal popliteal vein but a femoral vein thrombus that is continuous, through the popliteal vein, with calf vein thrombus is almost impossible to remove, and we doubt if thrombectomy is clinically beneficial, except in the rare circumstance when *all* the thrombus is fresh and non-adherent and can be extruded easily through the venotomy, without the use of a balloon catheter.

Calf pump failure syndrome

The evidence that thrombectomy affects subsequent calf pump failure is extremely poor and mostly anecdotal. Mavor[70] found a relationship between the state of the ilio-femoral segment and symptoms 6 years after operation. Only 2 of his 13 patients with normal iliac veins had symptoms, whereas 7 of the 9 patients who had recanalized veins, and 13 of the 14 patients with collaterals across the floor of the pelvis had symptoms. The incidence of leg symptoms was lower in the group in which the operation was carried out under X-ray control. Overall, 34 (58 per cent) of Mavor's 59 patients who were studied clinically and venographically between 3 years and 6 years after operation had some problem with their legs.

We suspect that these results are not significantly different from the natural history (see page 307), and this view is supported by the results of non-invasive testing of calf pump function in Ecklof's study. Only 23 per cent of Ecklof's first series of patients[36] had normal calf pump function 6 months after operation; 60 per cent had poor ejection, 17 per cent had reflux, and only 7.5 per cent had a normal venous outflow when measured with strain-gauge plethysmography. In Ecklof's second controlled study[36,102] there were no statistically significant differences in the calf function tests between the group treated with thrombectomy and the group given only anticoagulants, though the phlebographic patency and the absence of ilio-femoral vein obstruction correlated well with femoral vein pressure. Unfortunately, patency was usually associated with reflux. At 6 months all symptoms occurred less frequently in the surgical group, and the difference between the percentage of patients in the control and the percentage of patients in the thrombectomy group that were 'symptom free' (7 per cent vs 42 per cent) was significant; this was also true for ilio-femoral patency (36 per cent vs 76 per cent) and the presence of competent valves (26 per cent vs 52 per cent). Once again the anatomical appearances and the physiological tests failed to correlate, and we suspect that the incidence of the post-thrombotic syndrome will not differ when these two groups of patients are re-examined 5 years later.

Indications for operation

As for thrombolysis the indications for thrombectomy are presented last because they depend upon the reader's interpretation of the significance of the results described above.

It is self-evident that the only circumstance in which thrombectomy can prevent embolism and abolish the incidence of late sequelae is when *all* the thrombus is removed. This can only be achieved when the thrombus is fresh, non-adherent (floating) and limited (i.e. with a clear-cut top and bottom in a large axial vein) (Figs 18.13, 18.14). In these circumstances the balloon catheter can be passed beyond either end of the thrombus and the whole thrombus can be extracted. Thrombus which is adherent cannot be completely removed, and thrombectomy in these circumstances is associated with a significant incidence of minor embolism. This risk would be acceptable if we knew that the reopening of the axial vein would be permanent and beneficial to calf pump function. A proportion of the veins that are successfully opened by thrombectomy, perhaps as many as 50 per cent, will stenose or even occlude during the subsequent 2 years in spite of a course of anticoagulants, and there is little evidence that normal calf pump function can

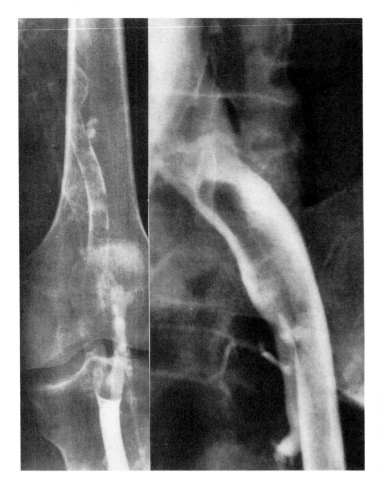

Fig. 18.13 A fresh non-adherent thrombus with clearly defined proximal and distal limits. Thrombectomy is the most suitable method of treatment for this type of thrombus.

be restored in any patient who has extensive calf vein thrombosis.

We therefore believe that there is little justification for performing a thrombectomy on an occluded superficial femoral vein. We would only advise surgery on the ilio-femoral segment when the thrombus is localized to this segment, the clinical history suggests that the thrombus is less than 5 days old, and the clinical signs confirm a significant functional obstruction. In these circumstances we would prefer to use a thrombolytic drug but would operate if these drugs are contra-indicated.

Our attitude to surgical thrombectomy for ilio-femoral thrombosis can be summarized as follows (Fig. 18.15).

- Thrombectomy is only indicated when thrombolysis is contra-indicated.

- Thrombectomy should be used to remove non-adherent thrombus localized to the ilio-femoral or superficial femoral vein, young (less than 3 days old) adherent thrombus localized to the ilio-femoral segment (the iliac and common femoral vein), and recent thrombus in an axial vein threatening the life of the limb (severe phlegmasia cerulea dolens).

- There is no evidence that the *partial removal* of floating or adherent superficial femoral vein thrombus which is continuous with calf vein thrombus reduces the late sequelae, and there is considerable evidence that the risk of pulmonary embolism is increased if the thrombus is not completely removed.

- All patients must be given adequate anticoagulants for 6 months after the operation.

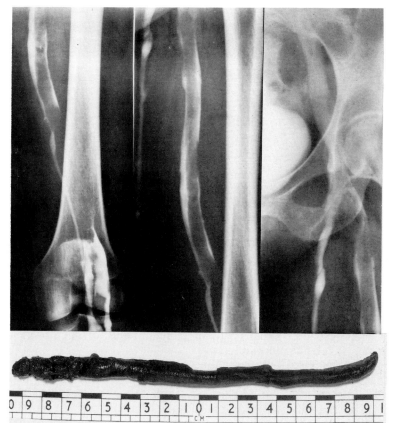

Fig. 18.14 A fresh non-adherent thrombus with clearly defined upper and lower limits that was completely removed with one passage of a balloon catheter.

The patient had had two pulmonary emboli in spite of adequate anticoagulation with heparin, and the thrombus shown was removed from the clinically normal leg.

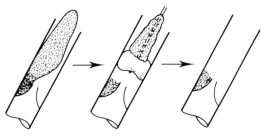

(a)

• An arteriovenous fistula improves patency after thrombectomy but probably only in patients with adherent thrombus. We would fashion an arteriovenous fistula after removing an adherent limited ilio-femoral thrombus, but not after removing a floating non-adherent thrombus.

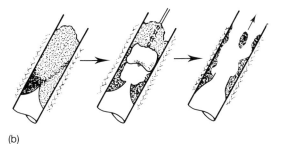

(b)

Fig. 18.15 The type of thrombus which is removable by surgical thrombectomy.

(a) Fresh non-adherent thrombus with clearly defined proximal and distal limits can be completely removed.

(b) Adherent thrombus cannot be completely removed, and the residual mural thrombus gives rise to recurrent pulmonary emboli and causes rethrombosis.

Thrombectomy for phlegmasia cerulea dolens

A total obstruction of the venous outflow from a limb will cause acute ischaemia and rapid death of the tissues. Even when the majority of the limb veins are blocked, the blood usually finds some small vessels to act as collaterals and the limb survives. However, the worse the obstruction the greater the swelling and discoloration and the greater the chance of tissue necrosis.

Phlegmasia cerulea dolens is a swollen, blue painful limb caused by venous obstruction. Its clinical features are described in Chapter 17, page 477 (Colour plate 37).

The skin may blister and become gangrenous (venous gangrene). Treatment in these circumstances is aimed at saving the limb, the risks of minor embolism and late post-thrombotic sequelae become secondary considerations.

- The initial treatment should be full anticoagulation with heparin to try to stop extension of the thrombosis.
- Swelling should be reduced by steep elevation of the leg.
- Analgesics are usually needed.
- Phlebography is essential to define the limits of the thrombosis. It is likely that the deep femoral veins and the internal iliac veins will be occluded as well as the axial veins.
- A general examination is essential to determine a hidden cause of the thrombosis, often malignant disease, because this may influence the management decisions.
- If the skin is ischaemic, blistering and likely to die, an urgent attempt must be made to relieve the outflow tract obstruction. This can only be done surgically. Streptokinase has been used but in our experience it takes too long to work and causes interstitial bleeding from the congested veins within the limb.
- A thrombectomy of the ilio-femoral segment and the superficial and deep femoral veins should be performed to restore some venous drainage from the limb.
- If thrombectomy fails, some surgeons have tried an emergency vein bypass operation to the other limb or the vena cava. These operations are, however, unlikely to work because the veins carrying the blood to the root of the limb are usually blocked and the bypass has an inadequate inflow.
- Do not be in a hurry to amputate tissues

which look ischaemic. It is remarkable how dark blue–black apparently dead skin can recover with time, particularly the skin underneath blisters which always looks purple and dead but often recovers.

Inferior vena cava thrombectomy

The technique of thrombectomy described on pages 512–515 is only applicable to ilio-femoral thrombosis. Thrombus may propagate into the vena cava, and if it is not adherent, it may be a source of potentially lethal emboli (Fig. 18.16). The risk of embolism can be prevented by inserting a vena caval filter (see Chapter 21, page 586) but in the presence of vena caval thrombus there is a considerable risk that this will cause a complete thrombosis of the vena cava. In these circumstances it is better to remove the thrombus. A thrombolytic drug can be used but there is a significant risk of it causing a major embolism and most surgeons prefer to perform a thrombectomy.

Inferior vena caval thrombus can be removed by balloon catheters passed via the femoral veins, but as there is a risk that the passage of the catheter will dislodge thrombus and cause emboli, most surgeons prefer a direct approach to the vena cava.

The vena cava is best exposed through an abdominal transperitoneal incision. A retroperitoneal exposure gives only limited access and cannot be extended. The first manoeuvre should be to place a clamp on the vena cava well above the thrombus to prevent embolism during the subsequent dissection of the cava. The vena cava and common iliac veins are best exposed by reflecting the caecum, ascending colon and duodenum to the left (see Fig. 25.6), and a venotomy is made in the lower part of vena cava. Any contained thrombus can then be extracted with forceps or a balloon. Bleeding from the iliac veins can be controlled by direct pressure or by intraluminal balloons. Once the thrombus has been extracted, bleeding from the lumbar veins can be controlled with direct finger pressure (see Fig. 25.6, page 649). Inferior vena caval thrombosis is often the extension of an iliac vein thrombosis and therefore vena cava thrombectomy may have to be followed by an ilio-femoral thrombectomy. If the thrombectomy is incom-

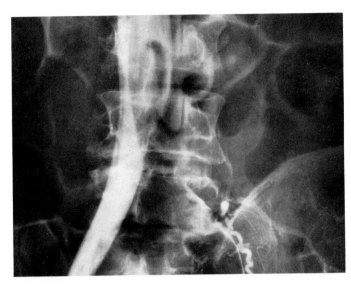

Fig. 18.16 Fresh non-adherent thrombus in the vena cava that might fragment and become a pulmonary embolism if it was treated with streptokinase.

We prefer to remove this type of thrombus surgically or confine it to the vena cava with vena caval blockade.

plete, further embolism can be prevented by plicating or clipping the vena cava just below the renal veins. It is not easy to insert an intraluminal filter when the cava is collapsed.

Combined thrombectomy and thrombolysis

Attempts have been made to improve the results of thrombectomy by infusing streptokinase or urokinase into the thrombectomized segment of vein after the operation.[92,94] A fine catheter is passed into an iliac vein via a small tributary of the long saphenous vein, and a low dose of streptokinase is given in an attempt to produce local thrombolysis without generalized systemic activation of the fibrinolytic system. There is little published evidence to show that this produces better results than thrombectomy alone, and the incidence of complications (e.g. wound haematoma) is increased.

It is only necessary to use thrombolytic drugs in this way if the thrombectomy is incomplete. This usually occurs when the operation has been performed on an ageing adherent thrombus (i.e. in the wrong circumstances). When a thrombectomy is performed in the correct circumstances, postoperative thrombolysis should be unnecessary.

Anticoagulation

Effective anticoagulation should prevent the propagation of existing thrombus by stopping the formation of new thrombus but it has no effect on the behaviour of existing thrombus. Thrombus fragmentation, retraction or adhesion will still occur, and therefore anticoagulants do not prevent embolism or deep vein damage. The most effective anticoagulant is heparin. Heparin should always be given as the initial treatment and should only be replaced by an oral anticoagulant when the circumstances causing the precipitating hypercoagulable state begin to recede. The value of long-term oral anticoagulation is less well documented than the value of heparin.

Heparin

Heparin is a mucopolysaccharide glycosaminoglycan, that inhibits the action of thrombin. Small doses of heparin accelerate the inhibitory effect of antithrombin III on the activation of factor X and can prevent thrombosis if given *before* thrombosis develops. However, much larger doses are required to stop existing thrombus propagating because in these circumstances the heparin has to inhibit thrombin in both the plasma and the thrombus, where it is combined with fibrin. The doses required for the treatment of existing thrombus are therefore 20 times greater than those needed for prophylaxis.

Dose

The precise blood level of heparin that will prevent an existing thrombus growing has not been determined. Studies in animals in which a thrombus has been induced by physical means have shown that thrombosis will not occur if the plasma heparin level is more than 0.3 units/ml or if the accelerated partial thromboplastin time (APPT) is one and one half times longer than the normal.[21]

The circumstances of these animal studies are not the same as those of clinical practice where the patient has a systemic hypercoagulable state, an existing thrombus and possibly local vein wall damage and a reduced venous blood flow.

It is generally accepted that thrombus growth will only be prevented in *man* when the plasma heparin is greater than 0.3 units/ml, the accelerated partial thromboplastin time (APPT) is more than twice normal, or the whole blood clotting time two to three times normal.[57,72] These blood levels are obtained by giving an intravenous loading dose of heparin of 5000 units followed by 20,000–40,000 units/24 hours; the dose should be controlled by a coagulation test. Patients whose APTT level is high before starting treatment will develop an APTT which is twice the laboratory standard plasma normal level with a low level of plasma heparin. Patients with a low APTT level before starting treatment will need more heparin, and therefore have a high blood level, by the time their APTT is doubled (Fig. 18.17).[57] This explains why a small proportion of patients are inadequately anticoagulated and some are over-treated when the dose of heparin is compared with the APTT or other coagulation tests on laboratory control plasma. The correct plasma heparin levels are obtained when *the patient's own pretreatment* APTT (not a laboratory plasma APTT) is doubled (see Fig. 18.17).

Administration

Heparin should be administered *intravenously* and *continuously*.[49,111] It is possible to produce full anticoagulation with subcutaneous injections[2] but we have found that the effect is not so easily controlled or reversed and we have observed a higher incidence of local bruising and haematoma formation.

A number of studies have compared inter-

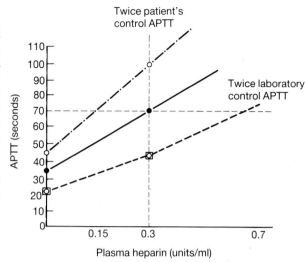

Fig. 18.17 The relationship between the patient's pretreatment APTT (accelerated partial thromboplastin time) and the plasma heparin level during treatment.

A patient with an APTT similar to that of the laboratory control plasma (●—●) will have a plasma heparin of 0.3 units/ml when his APTT is doubled.

A patient with an APTT which is lower than that of the laboratory control plasma (□----□) will have a plasma heparin of 0.7 units/ml when his APTT is prolonged to twice that of the laboratory control plasma, but a plasma heparin level of 0.3 units/ml when his APTT is prolonged to twice that of *his own* pretreatment level. Similarly, a patient with an APTT which is higher than that of the laboratory control plasma (○—·—○) will have a plasma heparin level of 0.15 units/ml when his APTT is prolonged to twice that of the laboratory control plasma, but a plasma heparin level to 0.3 units/ml when his APTT is prolonged to twice that of *his own* pretreatment level. This graph explains why some patients are inadequately anticoagulated and other patients are over-anticoagulated if the APTT ratio is based upon a standard laboratory control plasma. The APTT ratio must be based upon the patient's own pretreatment plasma. If the APTT ratio is based on the patient's pretreatment plasma, doubling the ratio will give a plasma heparin level of 0.3 units/ml.

(Redrawn from Hirsh *et al.*)[57]

mittent with continuous administration. Figure 18.18 shows the blood levels obtained as a result of 6-hourly injections. The half-life of heparin is approximately 1 hour. The anticoagulant effect of a single injection has almost gone within 4 hours. *Patients who are given 6-hourly injec-*

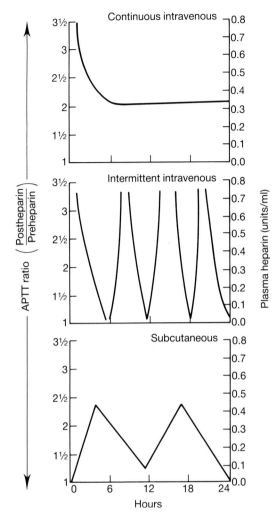

Fig. 18.18 The effect of the route and frequency of administration on the pretreatment and posttreatment APTT ratio and plasma heparin levels. If the pretreatment APTT is doubled, the plasma heparin should be between 0.3 units/ml and 0.4 units/ml–the ideal therapeutic range. It can be seen that neither 6-hourly intravenous injections nor 12-hourly subcutaneous injections produce a sustained therapeutic level of plasma heparin. After 6 hours the effect of an intravenous bolus of heparin has worn off. Four-hourly injections provide a sustained effect but also result in frequent periods of excessive anticoagulation.
(Redrawn from Hirsh *et al.*)[57]

tions are therefore not anticoagulated for 2 of the 6 hours. If, for logistic or clinical reasons, it is decided to give heparin intermittently, it must be given *4-hourly.*

Studies of the incidence of bleeding complications have shown that a continuous infusion causes fewer bleeding complications than intermittent dosage.[49,85,111] This is not surprising in view of the high level of anticoagulation present in the few minutes following each dose. A mathematical compilation of five controlled studies[57] reveals that the incidence of major bleeds was 5 per cent when heparin was administered continuously compared with 12 per cent following intermittent administration.

Laboratory control

The effect of a continuous infusion of heparin should be monitored by measuring the accelerated partial thromboplastin time (APTT) or the clotting time.[10,48,104]

A pretreatment test should be performed and control studies should be repeated 4 hours and 8 hours after beginning treatment. Thereafter the frequency of testing depends upon the variability of the results but a coagulation test should be performed at least once every day.[40,98]

The preceeding paragraph is the counsel of perfection. Many surgeons rely on a standard dose of 40,000 units/24 hours; they reduce this dose if bleeding complications occur, and they measure nothing. This regimen usually succeeds in providing adequate anticoagulation and stops further thrombosis without causing a high incidence of bleeding problems because the relationship between high doses and bleeding is not nearly as clear as that between low doses and recurrent thrombosis.

Intermittent dosage gives such fluctuating levels of coagulation that blood tests are not helpful. It therefore produces an unpredictable effect which cannot readily be controlled.

Duration of treatment

There is no scientific evidence on which to base a decision concerning the duration of heparin therapy. Heparin is given initially because of its instant effect. Oral anticoagulants take 3–5 days to work but the actual anticoagulant effectiveness of these two types of drug has not been compared.

There is a large amount of anecdotal clinical evidence which suggests that heparin prevents new thrombosis and relieves symptoms more effectively than warfarin or phenindione. Most clinicians have seen the sudden return of symptoms with apparent extension of thrombosis when the heparin is replaced by an oral anticoagulant (even when the prothrombin time is within the therapeutic range), followed by the rapid abatement of symptoms and, presumably, the cessation of thrombus growth on reinstituting heparin therapy. This experience is so common that many clinicians give heparin for 7 days before giving the loading dose of an oral anticoagulant. The 7 days of heparin therapy covers the time when it is thought that the hypercoagulable state is maximal and the thrombus is most likely to extend. It allows the thrombus to retract, polymerize and become adherent to the vein wall. After this period the risk of recurrent embolism and thrombosis is less and oral anticoagulants are more likely to be effective. In our opinion heparin therapy should be given for 10 days with a loading dose of an oral anticoagulant being given on the seventh day, if the clinician proposes to institute long-term anticoagulation. *The heparin must not be withdrawn until the prothrombin time is within the therapeutic range.* This means that the heparin should be stopped on the 10th day, and 4 hours later, when its effect has worn off, blood samples should be taken for a prothrombin time estimation. The heparin infusion must then be resumed until the result of the laboratory test is available. If the prothrombin time is two to three times the normal, the heparin infusion can be stopped. If it is less than twice the normal, the heparin infusion must be continued for another 24 hours and the testing process must be repeated.

It is very important to ensure that there is no time when the patient is unprotected. This will happen if the heparin is just stopped on the assumption that the oral anticoagulant is working. Heparin should only be withdrawn after receipt of a satisfactory prothrombin time.

Complications and their treatment

Bleeding Bleeding is the most serious complication.[27] The relationship between overdose and bleeding is unclear. Some studies have shown an increased rate of bleeding when the coagulation time is longer than 60 minutes, some show no relation between APTT and bleeding, and other studies show an increased rate of bleeding with doses greater than 40,000 units/ 24 hours. Some of the variations in these observations are probably caused by the effect of heparin on platelet function.[110]

Bleeding occurs either spontaneously or from wounds. Spontaneous bleeding usually occurs in the subcutaneous tissues beneath pressure areas, or in the retroperitoneum, and it is more common in patients with severe hypertension. Surgical wounds, peptic ulcers and neoplastic ulcers of the gastrointestinal and renal tract may also bleed during heparin therapy. Bleeding is reduced by the following measures.

- Stopping the heparin
- Reversing the effect of the heparin by administering protamine sulphate.[100] Protamine sulphate combines directly with heparin and inactivates it. If a bolus of heparin has just been given, every 100 units of heparin will require 1 mg protamine to neutralize it. If the patient has been having a continuous infusion of heparin it is wise to give 25 mg protamine over 10 minutes and then measure the clotting time or the APTT. Further doses of protamine can be given until the anticoagulation is reversed. During vascular surgery we have found that 25 mg of protamine always reverses the effect of 5000 units heparin given 30–60 minutes previously. *If protamine is given quickly, it can cause hypotension; it should therefore be given slowly and carefully*
- Restoring the blood volume with fresh blood
- Applying local measures as necessary, including surgery to bleeding vessels or ulcers if the blood loss continues after the anticoagulant effect of the heparin has been reversed

Thrombocytopenia Heparin will induce antiplatelet antibodies in approximately 2 per cent of patients. This can cause a thrombocytopenia which may become apparent after 4 or 5 days of treatment. The development of this complication may cause serious bleeding complications and, paradoxically, may also cause thromboembolic complications as a result of platelet aggregation.[73,117]

If arterial platelet emboli occur, the temptation is to continue or increase the heparin but instead heparin administration must be stopped and any problem of tissue ischaemia should be treated surgically. Thrombocytopenic complications (e.g. arterial emboli) are associated with a high morbidity and mortality but fortunately, they are rare. The platelets return to normal when the heparin is stopped.

All patients who have been given therapeutic doses of heparin for more than 5 days, should have a platelet count at the same time as their daily APTT. A rising demand for heparin (i.e. a falling APTT) and a falling platelet count should raise suspicion of heparin-induced thrombocytopenia. The platelet count should be repeated and platelet aggregation studies obtained and, if the number of platelets continues to fall, the heparin must be stopped and replaced with an oral anticoagulant. It has been claimed that low molecular weight heparin does not cause thrombocytopenia.[61]

Sensitivity reactions Heparin occasionally causes an itchy red maculopapular rash. This rash settles quickly when the heparin is stopped, and the itching can be controlled with an antihistamine. Anaphylactic reactions are very rare.

Alopecia Loss of hair is a rare but distressing complication of prolonged heparin therapy. The exact incidence has not been recorded.

Osteoporosis Patients who are given heparin for more than 6 months may become osteoporotic and present with pathological fractures of their vertebrae, ribs and metatarsals.[53,113] This complication is seldom seen, and is said not to occur if the dose of heparin is kept below 10,000 units/day.

In recent years it has become popular to use long-term subcutaneous heparin for the prevention of recurrent deep vein thrombosis and pulmonary embolism when oral anticoagulation is difficult to control or the risks of bleeding are high (e.g. during pregnancy). It is important to restrict the dose of heparin to 5000 units 12-hourly to avoid osteoporosis.

Results

The efficacy of intravenous heparin must be judged against the three objectives of its administration:

- prevention of pulmonary embolism
- prevention of recurrent deep vein thrombosis
- prevention of post-thrombotic sequelae

Prevention of recurrent embolism

Heparin is given to patients with a deep vein thrombosis in the hope that it will prevent existing thrombus fragmenting and embolizing. Evidence that thrombus repeatedly fragments comes from the natural history study of Barker and Priestley[7,8] who showed that 30 per cent of patients who have had one embolus have a further embolus and that 20 per cent of these second emboli are fatal.

The value of heparin in preventing death after the first embolus is based on the study by Barritt and Jordan[9] which is discussed in detail in Chapter 21, page 584. By modern standards this study has many defects but heparin is now established as the accepted initial treatment for pulmonary embolism.[25]

Table 18.2 gives the incidence of recurrent embolism during heparin therapy from 10 studies on 1157 patients, published between 1947 and 1966. It could be argued that knowledge and control of heparin treatment was not as good 20

Table 18.2 Incidence of pulmonary embolism during anticoagulation with heparin*

Reference	No. cases studied	No. fatal emboli	No. non-fatal emboli	Total no. emboli
93	149	0	4	4
29	107	1	3	4
66	346	0	28	28
99	60	7	?	7
30	124	2	12	14
28	152	9	12	21
9	54	0	3	3
19	118	22	?	22
116	20	0	3	3
74	26	0	4	4
Totals	1157	41 (3.5%)	69 (11%)	110 (9.5%)

*Ten studies performed between 1947 and 1966.

years ago as it is now, but nevertheless the incidence of both fatal and non-fatal recurrent emboli (3.5 per cent and 11 per cent respectively) is significant and has not fallen over the years.

Because of our concern about this problem we have developed an approach to the prevention of recurrent embolism based upon phlebography.[13] We reviewed 50 of our patients who had been treated with heparin alone and found that 7 (14 per cent) had had recurrent fatal emboli and 13 (26 per cent) had had recurrent non-fatal emboli. This confirmed our suspicions that heparin did not stop the fragmentation and embolization of existing thrombus, which in 40 per cent of our trial patients was non-adherent (Figs 18.19 and 18.20).

More recent studies have confirmed that emboli occur in spite of heparin, though the incidence of emboli is probably lower than in untreated patients; for example, 21 per cent of the patients with deep vein thrombosis who were given heparin in the control arm of a thrombectomy study had new ventilation–perfusion defects after 7 days of treatment.[103]

There is some evidence that the incidence of recurrent embolism is related to the degree of anticoagulation; Basu *et al.*[10] found a recurrence rate of 25 per cent when the APTT was below 50 s but found no recurrences when it was above 50 s.

We conclude from all this evidence that *heparin therapy does not abolish recurrent embolism.* A definitive comparison of the effect of heparin against no treatment on the mortality and recurrence rate following pulmonary embolism has yet to be performed. As it is logical to prevent new thrombosis in the legs and new thrombus developing around the embolus in the pulmonary artery, a controlled trial with an untreated group will probably never be performed, for ethical and so-called logical reasons. However, the assumption that anticoagulation with heparin always stops further thrombosis in the legs is questioned in the next section, reinforcing our ignorance of the true value of heparin in the treatment of thromboembolism.

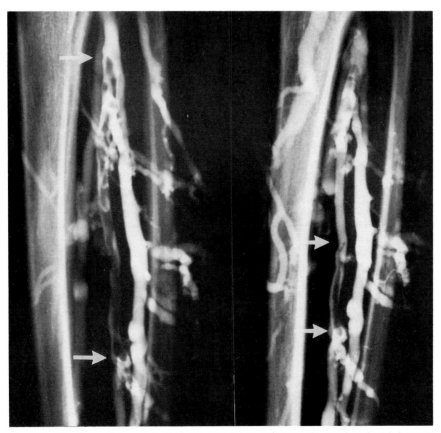

Fig. 18.19   The phlebogram of a patient who was fully anticoagulated with heparin. The day after the first phlebogram the patient experienced an episode of chest pain.
A second phlebogram (right-hand panel) showed that the calf thrombus was 10 cm shorter (arrows).

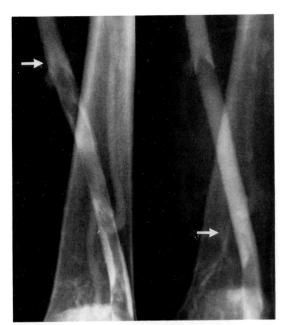

Fig. 18.20 The first phlebogram of this patient (left-hand panel) revealed a non-adherent thrombus showing some signs of ageing, retraction and irregularity. The patient was fully anticoagulated with heparin. Two days later he experienced a severe pleuritic chest pain. A second phlebogram (right-hand panel) showed that part of the thrombus had broken off at a narrow segment to become an embolus.

Prevention of recurrent deep vein thrombosis

The concept that heparin can induce the resorption of thrombus and thus reduce post-thrombotic late sequelae was based upon the belief that it is thrombolytic. This idea was supported by Bauer's claim[11] that 10 years after a thrombosis only 1.3 per cent of a group of patients who had been given anticoagulants had the post-thrombotic syndrome compared to 58 per cent of those patients who had not been given anticoagulants. It was assumed that this difference was caused by thrombolysis but it is unacceptable to make deductions about the effect of heparin from clinical evidence as the physical signs are affected by many different factors. The only way to prove that a drug is thrombolytic is by demonstrating thrombolysis with phlebography. Recently, Vairel *et al.*[120] have suggested that low molecular weight heparin may enhance thrombolysis.

The majority of the phlebographic studies of heparin and deep vein thrombosis are the control arms of studies of thrombolysis. There are no studies comparing the effect of heparin against no treatment. Nevertheless these studies of thrombolysis do describe an effect of heparin, even though the methods of administration, dosage and control vary considerably from study to study.

In 1968 Robertson *et al.*[109] compared heparin with streptokinase. They reported that half of the 23 patients who were given heparin had poor results but unfortunately they did not say whether 'poor' was a worsening or unchanging phlebographic appearance.

In 1969[14] we compared 5 patients treated with heparin for 5 days against 5 patients who were given streptokinase for 3 days and found no change in the phlebographic appearance of the thrombus in those patients given heparin.

In 1969 Kakkar[67] compared heparin with streptokinase and ancrod (Arvin). One of the 10 patients who were given heparin had a fatal pulmonary embolism. Two of the remaining 9 patients showed clearance of the thrombus, in 2 patients the size of the thrombus was slightly reduced and in 5 patients it was unchanged. Fibrinogen uptake tests were also performed. In the two legs in which the thrombus cleared the radioactivity fell quickly, but these legs contained only calf vein thrombi which are known to lyse spontaneously without treatment; it is therefore not known whether the disappearance of the thrombus was the result of spontaneous lysis or fragmentation and embolization. In 2 patients the radioactivity of the thrombus rose suggesting further deposition of thrombosis in spite of adequate anticoagulation.

In 1969 we began a study, based on phlebography, designed to compare the effects of intermittent heparin with those of continuous heparin on deep vein thrombosis. In the pilot study 10 patients with deep vein thrombosis were given 5000 units of heparin 4-hourly for 7 days. When the phlebograms were repeated 5 days later the thrombi of 4 patients had progressed from being non-adherent to adherent thrombus, the thrombi of 4 patients were unchanged and 2 patients showed retraction and shrinkage (Figs 18.21, 18.22, 18.23). The progression to thrombus adhesion and total obliteration of the lumen was most marked in the calf veins. Two

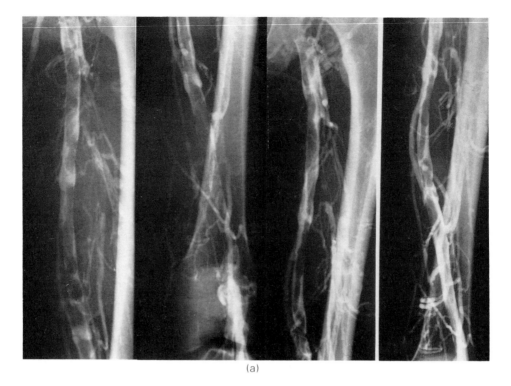

(a)

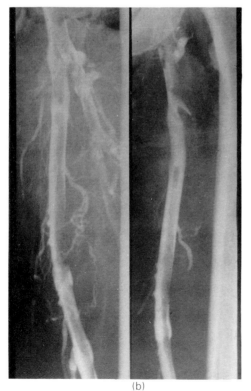

(b)

Fig. 18.21 (a) Retraction of thrombus during anticoagulation with heparin. These phlebograms were obtained before and after 5 days of treatment.

The thrombus in the right-hand panels is smaller, irregular and more clearly defined.

(b) A pair of phlebograms showing similar changes. The thrombus has retracted to half its original width.

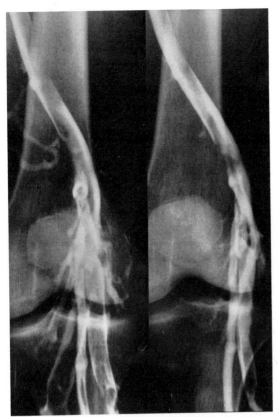

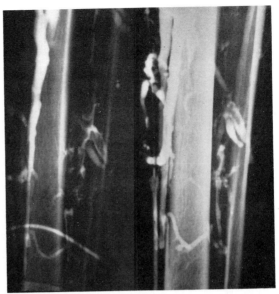

Fig. 18.23 These phlebograms were obtained before and after 5 days of anticoagulation treatment with heparin. They show retraction of the thrombus in a communicating vein but no change in the thrombus in the deep axial vein. The changes in calf vein thrombus during anticoagulation are usually less pronounced than the changes of non-adherent axial vein thrombus.

Fig. 18.22 A phlebogram showing moderate retraction of the thrombus in the upper popliteal vein before and after 5 days of anticoagulation treatment with heparin, and considerable retraction of the thrombus in the lower half of the popliteal vein.

patients had pulmonary emboli during treatment; the source of these emboli was clearly visible on the second phlebogram as a square cut end to a previously long loose thrombus. In the light of these results and the four studies described above the trial was stopped and we were convinced that heparin was not thrombolytic, that it was unethical to treat patients who had non-adherent thrombus with anticoagulants alone, and that though adequate doses of heparin may stop new thrombus forming, they failed to stop emboli or prevent partially occluded vessels becoming totally occluded.

Recent studies have emphasized the failure of heparin to do anything other than maintain the 'status quo'. Elliot[37] has reported that 2 patients out of 25 who were given heparin developed extension of their thrombosis in spite of a clotting time which was 2.5–3 times the normal. Widmer[128] also found no lytic effect with heparin. The phlebograms of 89 per cent of Widmer's 132 patients were unchanged by treatment, 6 per cent had thrombus retraction, 3 per cent were worse with more thrombosis and only 2 per cent showed a significant reduction in the size of the thrombus.

In our opinion there is no clinical evidence that heparin causes or accelerates thrombolysis. Natural thrombolysis is common in small calf vein thrombi but uncommon in the axial veins. The chance of new thrombus forming during adequate anticoagulant therapy is between 5 per cent and 10 per cent and the chance of non-adherent thrombus becoming adherent and totally occluding its containing vein rather than retracting to one side and leaving the lumen open is probably 50 per cent.

Prevention of the calf pump failure syndrome

The possibility that heparin might stop the

progression of thrombosis raised the hope that it might reduce the incidence of the post-thrombotic syndrome. There are, however, no good long-term controlled trials which compare no treatment against a course of heparin. Controls are essential because of the variability of the natural history of thrombosis. Bauer[11] observed that half of his patients had a post-thrombotic syndrome 5 years after a deep vein thrombosis. Many of these patients had been given heparin.

Our own study,[130] comparing anticoagulants alone with anticoagulants combined with embolus-preventing operations (when indicated), showed that 58 per cent of those patients who were given heparin alone had post-thrombotic symptoms at 3 years. The incidence of post-thrombotic symptoms in patients who had had surgical procedures and anticoagulants was similar. We also found that 20 per cent of the legs without phlebographic evidence of thrombosis at the time of presentation had post-thrombotic symptoms.

Widmer studied 34 patients who had been given heparin as part of the control arm of a streptokinase trial 4 years and 7 months after the acute event, and he found that only 35 per cent were normal. The remaining 65 per cent of patients had symptoms and signs of venous insufficiency; 12 per cent had venous ulcers.

These studies do not give any indication that anticoagulants reduce the incidence of the post-thrombotic syndrome, and they confirm the view, repeatedly expressed throughout this book, that all you can expect from anticoagulants is the prevention of further thrombosis. This will save a life or prevent late sequelae in a limb on only a few occasions.

Indications

From the above section the reader might conclude that there is little justification for the use of heparin. A scientifically based argument supporting this view could be produced, and we believe that it would be ethical to restudy the value of heparin in all aspects of the treatment of thromboembolism. Nevertheless, if heparin usually stops new thrombosis, it may be beneficial and we consider its use is justified in the light of our present knowledge.

We give continuous heparin, monitored with APTT, (or occasionally 4-hourly doses of 5000 units of heparin, unmonitored) to *all patients with deep vein thrombosis* provided that there are no contra-indications, as soon as the diagnosis is made on clinical grounds, but the heparin *is never continued without obtaining objective proof of the diagnosis*. Phlebography provides the most complete information about the thrombus. Many of the non-invasive tests can provide proof of the diagnosis but none gives the additional information that we need to help us decide which is the best method of protecting the patient from recurrent embolism or the late sequelae – protection that heparin does not provide.

Oral anticoagulants

The oral anticoagulants, the coumarins (dicoumarol, nicoumalone and warfarin) and the indanediones (anisindione, diphenadione and phenindione), are easily absorbed by the gastro-intestinal tract, and when absorbed they become bound to plasma albumin. The bound drug is inactive; only the small proportion (1–10 per cent) that is unbound is active. These drugs inhibit the action of vitamin K in the synthesis of factors VII, IX and X so that inactive coagulation factors are produced. Only the coumarins are now used as they have fewer side-effects.

The effect of the coumarins is assessed by measuring the prothrombin time. This is usually expressed as the International Normalized Ratio (INR), the ratio between the patient's prothrombin time and the control time obtained with a standardized animal-derived thromboplastin; the thromboplastin is calibrated against an International Reference Preparation. A therapeutic level of anticoagulation is achieved when the INR is 2.5–3.5. This is a new method of calculating the prothrombin time, and was brought about by the withdrawal of the standard human brain thromboplastin because it may contain human immunodeficiency viruses (HIV).

Dose   Warfarin is given as a loading dose of 10 mg followed by 6–10 mg/day, depending upon the prothrombin time. The loading dose of phenindione is 200 mg and the average maintenance dose is 100 mg/day.

Most physicians use warfarin in the first instance because its effect is more predictable, but if the effect of warfarin is difficult to control, it may be necessary to change to phenindione, nicoumalone or dicoumarol.

The half-life of warfarin is 35 hours and a full anticoagulant effect may take 3 or 4 days to develop.

Control The anticoagulant effect is monitored with the prothrombin time using the standardized thromboplastin described above. It must be measured daily until the maintenance dose and the test results are stable. The first measurement should be made 48 hours after the loading dose. Subsequently, the dose is varied by 2 mg amounts until the prothrombin time is between two and three times the normal value.

The prothrombin time cannot be measured accurately in heparinized blood; heparin administration should therefore be stopped 4 hours before taking blood for a prothrombin time test. The heparin should then be resumed until the result of the test is known.

Complications and their treatment

Haemorrhage Bleeding may occur in up to 20 per cent of patients.[57] Haematuria, spontaneous bruising and gastrointestinal bleeding are the common forms of bleeding.

Death as a result of bleeding occurs in less than 0.1 per cent of patients.

Bleeding is stopped by the following measures.

- Administration of vitamin K_1 to reverse the effect on the coagulation factors. Vitamin K_1 can be given orally or intravenously and intravenous administration is usually required when there are bleeding complications. If 5 mg vitamin K_1 are given intravenously (slowly to avoid hypotension and tachycardia), the prothrombin time should return to normal within 4–8 hours[23]
- Infusion of plasma concentrates of factors II, VII, IX and X; this may be required if severe bleeding demands rapid reversal of anticoagulation
- Replacement of blood lost with fresh blood or plasma
- Application of local measures, including surgery, if the bleeding is severe

Interaction with other drugs Many drugs affect the way in which anticoagulants change the action of vitamin K; they are summarized in Table 18.3.

The modes of interaction of these drug vary. Some drugs affect the absorption of vitamin K

Table 18.3 Some of the drugs which affect the effect of oral anticoagulants

Drugs which *increase* anticoagulant effect	Drugs which *decrease* anticoagulant effect
Allopurinol	Alcohol (regular/heavy intake)
Alcohol (occasional intake)	Barbiturates
Anabolic steroids	Cholestyramine
Aspirin	Cimetidine
Cephalosporins	Dichloralphenazone
Chloramphenicol	Diuretics
Cholestyramine	Phenytoin
Clofibrate	Glutethimide
Co-trimoxazole	Griseofulvin
Disulfiram	Rifampicin
Neomycin	
Oxyphenbutazone	
Phenylbutazone	
Quinine	
Quinidine	
Salicylates	
Sulphonamides	
Sulphonylureas	
Tetracyclines	
Tricyclics (imipramine, amitriptyline, nortriptyline)	

or the anticoagulant, others affect metabolic processes in the liver, some alter the plasma albumin binding and some interfere with the metabolism of vitamin K itself. It is important to warn the patient of these interactions and to ask about any drugs they may have taken if a previously stable prothrombin time goes awry. The drugs which most commonly cause problems are the barbiturates, phenylbutazone, aspirin, sulphonamides, steroids and antibiotics.

Sensitivity reactions The indanediones may cause rashes and fever. Fatal renal and liver failure have been reported but these complications are extremely uncommon. Warfarin produces very few sensitivity reactions but occasionally causes skin necrosis.[39] Skin necrosis is more common in females and affects areas which are well covered with fat (e.g. the breasts, buttocks and thighs). The skin turns red and oedematous, blisters and then turns blue–black. A necrotic area of skin may need to be excised and skin grafts may have to be applied.

Pregnancy As warfarin can cross the placental barrier it may cause fetal abnormalities.[115] Chondrodysplasia punctata (skeletal deformities, nasal dysplasia and optic atrophy), mental retardation and blindness have been reported. Oral anticoagulants should not be given in the first trimester of pregnancy and should be given only after careful thought in the second trimester. Fetal abnormalities are unlikely to occur after the first trimester but fetal death may follow placental or maternal haemorrhage. Oral anticoagulants should be avoided in the last 2 months of pregnancy because the trauma of delivery may cause both internal haemorrhage in an anticoagulated fetus and maternal internal haemorrhage.

The simplest solution is to avoid the use of oral anticoagulants at any time during pregnancy or when a woman thinks she might be pregnant.

It is safe to give anticoagulants after pregnancy, and breastfed babies do not become anticoagulated because only a small quantity of the drug is excreted in the milk.

The anticoagulant of choice during pregnancy is heparin because it does not cross the placental barrier. This can be self administered as a subcutaneous injection.

Results

Oral anticoagulants are given to prevent recurrent embolism and recurrent thrombosis and to reduce the incidence of post-thrombotic sequelae.

Prevention of recurrent embolism

There are very few controlled studies of the value of long-term oral anticoagulation in preventing recurrent embolism.

Coon and Willis[27] found a 12.5 per cent incidence of recurrent embolism in patients who had been given a short course of treatment as an inpatient, a 7.2 per cent incidence in patients who had received a full course of treatment as an inpatient, and a 4.6 per cent incidence in patients who had had proper inpatient treatment followed by 3 months of treatment as an outpatient.

The rationale for continuing anticoagulant therapy for 3–6 months is the venographic evidence that thrombus continues to show changes of retraction, vessels recanalize, and collaterals enlarge throughout this time. Furthermore, as we are not usually able to discover the cause of a thrombosis, it is not unreasonable to assume that whatever the cause was, it may take

3–6 months to disappear (i.e. until the patient is fully recovered and active). Our own study[13] showed a reducing incidence of recurrent embolism over several months and few emboli after 6 months, except in those patients who were later found to have had a chronic recurrent thrombotic problem.

Hull *et al.*[63] performed a prospective study of 14 days of heparin therapy followed by the administration of low-dose subcutaneous heparin (5000 units 6-hourly) or full oral anticoagulation therapy for 6 weeks (for calf thrombosis) or 3 months (for axial vein thrombosis). Forty-seven per cent of the patients with axial vein thrombosis (27 per cent of the whole group) who were given uncontrolled long-term heparin developed further thrombosis; there were no recurrences in the group of patients on oral anticoagulants. The incidence of embolism was 3 per cent for the group treated with heparin and 0 per cent for the group given oral anticoagulants. When this study was repeated[62] using a variable dose of heparin, adjusted weekly to prolong the APTT to one and one-half times the normal, the recurrent emboli stopped but bleeding complications increased. The evidence, though sparse, suggests that continuation of anticoagulation therapy with warfarin for 3–6 months after giving heparin for 10 days does reduce the incidence of recurrent embolism.

Prevention of recurrent thrombosis

The study by Hull[63] provides objective evidence that oral anticoagulants reduce the incidence of new thrombosis. No conclusions can be made about the heparin group as some of these patients were not fully anticoagulated. Almost all other published series fail to distinguish between patients who had been given only heparin for 10 days and patients who had been given heparin for 10 days followed by warfarin for 3 or 6 months. The studies quoted on pages 527 and 528 are presented as if they refer to heparin alone but most of the patients were also given oral anticoagulants. Nevertheless, there is much clinical anecdotal experience to support the belief that recurrent thrombosis is more frequent if long-term anticoagulation is not used.[59] Lagerstedt *et al.*[76] compared two groups of 23 and 28 patients with symptomatic calf vein thrombosis. One group was given heparin for 5 days, the other group was given heparin for 5 days and warfarin for 3 months. Both groups wore elastic stockings. The recurrence rate after 3 months was 0 per cent in the group that had been given warfarin and 29 per cent in the group that had not received warfarin ($P = 0.01$). At 1 year the recurrence rates were 4 per cent and 68 per cent respectively.

There is no reason to believe that oral anticoagulants increase the possibility of spontaneous thrombolysis or reduce the likelihood that non-adherent thrombi will become adherent.[32]

Prevention of calf pump failure syndrome

There are no published data on the incidence of post-thrombotic sequelae in patients given long-term anticoagulants compared to patients treated with only a 10-day course of heparin. Although warfarin may reduce the incidence of recurrent axial vein thrombosis, the incidence of post-thrombotic sequelae probably depends upon the extent of the calf vein thrombosis. Unfortunately, we do not know whether warfarin affects the incidence of recurrent calf vein thrombosis, as in the McMaster study[63] neither the adequately treated nor the inadequately treated (heparin) groups had any new calf vein thrombi.

Indications

In the light of our ignorance about the effect of 3–6 months of oral anticoagulation after a deep vein thrombosis, we must ask the question: should this treatment be used at all?

There appears to be enough evidence to support the belief that oral anticoagulants reduce the incidence of recurrent embolism during the 6 months following a thrombosis. There is also some evidence to suggest that oral anticoagulants stop new axial vein thrombosis, and thus may reduce the chance of post-thrombotic calf pump failure but the evidence for this last supposition is extremely weak.

On the basis of these beliefs (not facts) our practice is *to treat all deep vein thrombosis*, in the absence of any strong contra-indication, *with heparin for 7–10 days followed by full anticoagulation with warfarin for 6 months.* Some workers argue that calf vein thrombosis is not a serious problem and treat this for only 6 weeks or 3 months. We think that calf vein

thrombosis is a serious problem; it is a major cause of the post-thrombotic syndrome, and calf thrombi can become emboli. We therefore draw no distinction between the site or the age of the thrombus, or the initial form of treatment (i.e. anticoagulants, surgery or thrombolysis) but prescribe 6 months of anticoagulation therapy for *all* patients after thrombosis.

If the patient remains well during this 6-month treatment period we 'tail-off' the warfarin over a 2-week period (even though there is no evidence of a 'rebound' phenomenon), but ask the patient to return immediately if they experience any leg or chest symptoms. If the patient returns with recurrent symptoms , heparin is reinstated and a phlebogram and ventilation–perfusion scan is performed. If there is any evidence of new thrombosis or embolism, the patient is given warfarin for another 6 months. Recurrence after 1 year of treatment is rare and usually means that the patient has idiopathic recurrent thrombosis (see Chapter 22). Blood coagulation factors (e.g. antithrombin III and protein-C) and tissue fibrinolysis should be measured and the possibility of life long anticoagulation or long-term enhancement of fibrinolysis should be considered. Recurrent thromboembolic disease of this nature occurs in less than 0.5 per cent of patients.

Defibrinogenation

The treatment of venous thromboembolism by defibrinogenation has not developed into a useful form of therapy because it is difficult to control and is of limited value, as antibodies to the defibrinogenating agent develop after 2–3 weeks of administration.[12,101,106]

Summary

Our approach to treatment of deep vein thrombosis based upon phlebography

The treatment options described in this chapter can be used in many ways; the choice of method often depends upon individual preferences and contra-indications rather than on hard scientific evidence of suitability or superiority.

Our approach is as follows (see Fig. 18.24).
1. The pre-treatment investigations used must

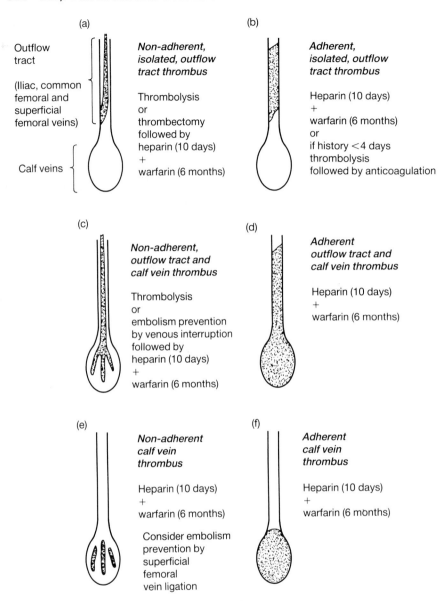

Fig. 18.24   (a – f) Treatment of deep vein thrombosis. A plan of management based upon the phlebographic appearances of the thrombus. (See text p. 537)

provide sufficient information for management. They must:

(a) confirm the presence of thrombosis;

(b) establish the site of the thrombosis;

(c) establish whether the thrombus, particularly its upper limit, is adherent or non-adherent, and indicate its age;

(d) confirm the presence or absence of pulmonary embolism (time and circumstances may only allow this to be done by clinical examination).

2. If the patient has had a pulmonary embolus, the principal object of treatment is the prevention of a second embolus. The ways in which this can be done are described in Chapter 21, (Fig. 21.3).

3. If the patient has not had a pulmonary embolism, the aims of treatment are to abolish the risk of embolism and to minimize the damage to the deep veins.

● *Fresh (less than 5 days old) non-adherent isolated thrombus in the outflow tract (popliteal and above)* This should be removed (Fig. 18.24a). Our preference, in the absence of the risk of bleeding complications, is to use thrombolysis (streptokinase or urokinase).

When there is a risk of bleeding (e.g. postoperatively) and when the thrombus is limited to the ilio-femoral segment we use thrombectomy.

If neither thrombolysis nor thrombectomy can be used, we prevent embolism by a suitably placed vein ligation (preferably at the termination of the superficial femoral vein) or a filter in the inferior vena cava.

All patients are given intravenous heparin before and after their initial treatment for 7–10 days followed by warfarin for 6 months.

● *Adherent isolated thrombus in the outflow tract (popliteal and above)* This should be removed if possible (Fig. 18.24b). The problem is the unknown age of the thrombus. If the clinical picture suggests that the thrombus is less than 4 days old, in spite of its phlebographic adherence, some clinicians would try a course of streptokinase.

If there are contra-indications to thrombolysis and if the history is longer than 3 days, we give heparin to prevent further thrombosis. We do not use thrombectomy in these circumstances because it usually fails and embolism is not a risk.

Heparin is continued for 10 days, followed by warfarin for 6 months.

● *Non-adherent continuous calf and outflow tract thrombus (Fig. 18.24c)* This should be removed by thrombolysis. Thrombectomy is not very effective in these circumstances because it cannot remove the calf vein thrombus.

If thrombolysis is not possible, prevention of embolism should be considered (e.g. a combination of ilio-femoral thrombectomy and vein ligation or vena caval interruption).

● *Adherent continuous calf and outflow tract thrombus (Fig. 18.24d)* This should be treated with anticoagulants unless there is good evidence (a rare circumstance) that the thrombus is less than 3 days old in which case thrombolysis may be tried.

● *Non-adherent calf thrombus (Fig. 18.24e)* This should be treated with anticoagulants.

If the patient has already had a pulmonary embolus which has embarrassed cardiac function, prevention of embolism (superficial femoral vein ligation) should be considered. A few clinicians would consider thrombolysis.

● *Adherent calf vein thrombus (Fig. 18.24f)* This should be treated with anticoagulants.

The calf vein thrombus detected during screening with the fibrinogen uptake test should be monitored daily. Anticoagulants should be given if the thrombus extends towards or into the popliteal vein.

References

1. Albrechtsson U, Anderson J, Einarsson E, Eklöf B, Norgren L. Streptokinase treatment of deep vein thrombosis and the postthrombotic syndrome. Follow-up evaluation of venous function. *Arch Surg* 1981; **116**: 33.

2. Anderson G, Fagrell B, Holmgren K, Johnson H, Ljungberg B, Nilsson E, Wilhelmsson S, Zetterquist S. Subcutaneous administration of heparin. *Thromb Res* 1982; **27**: 631.

3. Andriopoulos A, Wirsing P, Botticher R. Results of iliofemoral venous thrombectomy after acute thrombosis. *J Cardiovasc Surg* 1982; **23**: 123.

4. Arnesen H, Heilo A, Jakobsen E, Ly B, Skaga E. A prospective study of streptokinase and heparin in the treatment of deep vein thrombosis. *Acta Med Scand* 1978; **203**: 457.

5. Arnesen H, Hoiseth A, Ly B. Streptokinase or heparin in the treatment of deep vein thrombosis. *Acta Med Scand* 1982; **211**: 65.

6. Astedt B, Robertson B, Haeger K. Experience with standardized streptokinase therapy of deep vein thrombosis. *Surgery* 1974; **139**: 387.

7. Barker NW, Nygaard KK, Walters W, Priestley JT. A statistical study of postoperative venous thrombosis and pulmonary embolism. III. Time of occurrence during the postoperative period. *Proc Staff Meet Mayo Clin* 1941; **16**: 17.

8. Barker NW, Priestley JT. Postoperative thrombophlebitis and embolism. *Surgery* 1942; **12**: 411.

9. Barritt DW, Jordan SC. Anticoagulant drugs in treatment of pulmonary embolism: controlled trial. *Lancet* 1960; **1**: 1309.

10. Basu, D, Gallus A, Hirsh J, Code J. A prospective study of the value of monitoring heparin treatment with the activated partial thromboplastin time. *N Engl J Med* 1972; **287**: 324.

11. Bauer G. A roentgenological and clinical study of the sequels of thrombosis. *Acta Chir Scand* 1942; **86**: Suppl 74.

12. Bell WR, Pitney WR, Goodwin JF. Therapeutic defibrination in the treatment of thrombotic disease. *Lancet* 1968; **1**: 490.

13. Browse NL, Lea Thomas M, Solan MJ, Young AE. Prevention of recurrent pulmonary embolism. *Br Med J* 1969; **3**: 382.

14. Browse NL, Thomas ML, Pim HP. Streptokinase and deep vein thrombosis. *Br Med J* 1968; **3**: 717.

15. Brunner U, Wirth W. Spätresultate nach thrombecktomie bei iliofemoralvenenthrombose in klinisch-radiologischen vergleich. *Schweiz Med Wschr* 1971; **101**: 1327.

16. Brunner V. Surgery of acute femoro-iliac phlebothrombosis. In: May R (Ed) *Surgery of the Veins of the Leg and Pelvis*. Stuttgart. G Thieme 1979.

17. Brunner V. Thrombektomie bei iliofemoral venenthrombose. *Helv Chir Acta* 1971; **38**: 57.

18. Burnand KG, Sheen J, Lea Thomas M, Browse NL, Feers R, Standing R. Treatment of deep vein thrombosis by slow deacylating streptokinase plasminogen complex (BRL 33575). In: Negus D, Jantet G (Eds) *Phlebology '85*. London. John Libbey 1986; 476.

19. Byrne JJ. Phlebitis. A study of 979 cases at the Boston City Hospital. *JAMA* 1960; **174**: 113.

20. Cairols MA, Marco-Luque MA, Caralt MT, Ballon H, Aced S, Capdevila JM. A phlebographic and ultrasonic evaluation of fibrinolytic therapy. *Vasc Diag Ther* 1983; **3**: 37.

21. Carey LC, Williams RD. Comparative effects of dicoumarol, tromexan and heparin on thrombus propagation. *Ann Surg* 1960; **152**: 919.

22. Chavatzas D, Martin P. A study of streptokinase in deep vein thrombosis of the lower extremities. *Vasa* 1975; **4**: 68.

23. Clagett GP, Salzman E. Prevention of venous thromboembolism. *Prog Cardiovasc Dis* 1975; **17**: 345.

24. Common HH. Seaman AJ, Rosch J, Porter JM, Dotter C. Deep vein thrombosis treated with streptokinase or heparin – Follow up of a randomized study. *Angiology* 1976; **27**: 645.

25. Coon WW, Willis PW, Symons MJ. Assessment of anticoagulant treatment of venous thromboembolism. *Ann Surg* 1969; **170**: 559.

26. Coon WW, Willis PW. Haemorrhagic complications of anticoagulant therapy. *Arch Intern Med* 1974; **133**: 386.

27. Coon WW, Willis PW. Thromboembolic complications during anticoagulant therapy. *Arch Surg* 1972; **105**: 209.

28. Coon W, MacKenzie JW, Hodgson PE. A critical evaluation of anticoagulant therapy in peripheral venous thrombosis and pulmonary embolism. *Surg Gynec Obstet* 1958; **106**: 129.

29. Cosgriff SW, Cross RJ, Habif DV. Management of venous thrombosis and pulmonary embolism. *Surg Clin North Am* 1948; **28**: 324.

30. Crane C. Deep venous thrombosis and pulmonary embolism. *N Engl J Med* 1957; **257**: 147.

31. Cranley JJ, Krause RJ, Stasser ES, Hafner CD. Femoroiliac thrombophlebitis. Immediate and late results after thrombectomy, caval ligation and conservative management. *J Cardiovasc Surg* 1969; **10**: 463.

32. Davies JA, Merrick MV, Sharp AA, Holt JM. Controlled trial of ancrod and heparin in treatment of deep vein thrombosis of lower limb. *Lancet* 1971; **1**: 113.

33. DeWeese JA, Jones TI, Lyon J, Dale W. Evaluation of thrombectomy in the management of iliofemoral venous thrombosis. *Surgery* 1960; **47**: 140.

34. Duckert F, Muller G, Nyman D, Beny A, Prisender S, Madar G, Da Silva MA, Widmer LK, Schmitt HE. Treatment of deep vein thrombosis with streptokinase. *Br Med J* 1975; **1**: 479.

35. Edwards EA, Edwards JE. Effect of thrombophlebitis on venous valves. *Surg Gynec Obstet* 1937; **65**: 310.

36. Eklöf B, Einarsson E, Plate G. Role of thrombectomy and temporary arteriovenous fistula in acute venous thrombosis. In: Bergan JJ, Yao JST (Eds) *Surgery of the Veins*. Orlando. Grune & Stratton 1985.

37. Elliot MS, Immelman EJ, Jeffrey P, Benatar SR, Funston MR, Smith JA, Shepstone BJ, Ferguson AD, Jacobs P, Walker W, Louw J H. A comparative randomized trial of heparin

versus streptokinase in the treatment of acute proximal venous thrombosis. *Br J Surg* 1979; **66**: 838.

38. Elliot MS, Immelman EJ, Jeffrey P, Benatar SR, Funston MR, Smith JA, Shepstone BJ, Ferguson AD, Jacobs P, Walker W, Louw JH. The role of thrombolytic therapy in the management of phlegmasia caerulea dolens. *Br J Surg* 1979; **66**: 422.

39. Faraci P, Deterling R, Stein A, Rheinlander H, Cleveland R. Warfarin induced necrosis of the skin. *Surg Gynec Obstet* 1978; **146**: 695.

40. Fennerty AG, Thomas P, Backhouse G, Bentley P, Campbell IA, Routledge PA. Audit control of heparin treatment. *Br Med J* 1985; **290**: 27.

41. Fletcher AP, Alkjaersig N, Sherry S. The development of urokinase as a thrombolytic agent. Maintenance of a sustained thrombolytic state in man by its intravenous infusion. *J Lab Clin Med* 1965; **65**: 713.

42. Fogarty TJ, Cranley JJ, Krause RJ, Strasser ES, Hafner CD. A method for extraction of arterial emboli and thrombi. *Surg Gynec Obstet* 1963; **116**: 241.

43. Fogarty TJ, Cranley JJ, Krause RJ, Strasser ES, Hafner CD. Surgical management of phlegmasia cerulea dolens. *Arch Surg* 1963; **86**: 256.

44. Fogarty TJ, Krippaehue WW. Catheter technique for venous thrombectomy. *Surg Gynec Obstet* 1965; **121**: 362.

45. Fontaine R, Ruchmann L. The role of thrombectomy in deep venous thrombosis. *J Cardiovasc Surg* 1964; **5**: 298.

46. Fontaine R. Remarks concerning venous thrombosis and its sequelae. *Surgery* 1957; **41**: 6.

47. Gallus AS, Hirsh J, Cade J F, Turpie AGG, Walker IR, Gent M. Thrombolysis with a combination of small doses of streptokinase and full doses of heparin. *Semin Thromb Hemostas* 1975; **2**: 14.

48. Genton E. Guidelines for heparin therapy. *Ann Intern Med* 1974; **80**: 77.

49. Glazier RL, Crowell EB. Randomized prospective trial of continuous or intermittent heparin therapy. *JAMA* 1976; **236**: 1365.

50. Gmelin E, Theiss W. Repeated phlebographic examination during and after fibrinolytic therapy with streptokinase and urokinase. *Cardiovasc Radiol* 1978; **1**: 157.

51. Gormsen J, Laursen B. Treatment of acute phlebothrombosis with streptase. *Acta Med Scand* 1967; **181**: 373.

52. Goto H, Wada T, Matsumoto A, Matsummura H, Souna T. Iliofemoral venous thrombectomy. *J Cardiovasc Surg* 1980; **21**: 341.

53. Griffiths GC, Nichols G, Aster JD. Heparin osteoporosis. *JAMA* 1965; **193**: 85.

54. Gruss JD, Lanbach K. Modifikation der operations technik bei TeiferBecken-und oberschenkel venen thrombose. *Thoraxchirurgie* 1971; **19**: 508.

55. Haller JA, Abrams BL. Use of thrombectomy in the treatment of acute iliofemoral venous thrombosis in forty five patients. *Ann Surg* 1963; **158**: 561.

56. Haller JA. *Deep Thrombophlebitis.* Philadelphia. WB Saunders 1967.

57. Hirsh J, Genton E, Hull R. *Venous Thromboembolism.* New York. Grune & Stratton 1981.

58. Hirsh J, O'Sullivan E F, Martin M. Evaluation of a standard dosage schedule with streptokinase. *Blood* 1970; **35**: 341.

59. Hirsh J. Long term treatment of venous thromboembolism with oral anticoagulants. *Pract Cardiol* 1984; **10**: 235.

60. Homans J. Exploration and division of femoral and iliac veins in treatment of thrombophlebitis of leg. *N Engl J Med* 1941; **224**: 179.

61. Huisse MG, Guillin MC, Bezeaud A, Toulemonde F, Kitsis M, Andreassian B. Heparin associated thrombocytopenia. *In vitro* effects of different molecular weight heparin fractions. *Thromb Res* 1982; **27**: 485.

62. Hull R, Delmore T, Carter C, Hirsh J, Genton E, Gent M, Turpie G, McLaughlin D. Adjusted subcutaneous heparin versus warfarin sodium in the long term treatment of venous thrombosis. *N Engl J Med* 1982; **306**: 189.

63. Hull R, Delmore T, Genton E, Hirsh J, Gent M, Sackett D, McLaughlin D, Armstrong P. Warfarin sodium versus low dose heparin in the long term treatment of venous thrombosis. *N Engl J Med* 1979; **301**: 855.

64. Johansson E, Nordlander S, Zetterquist S. Venous thrombectomy in the lower extremity. Clinical phlebographic and plethysmographic evaluation of early and late results. *Acta Chir Scand* 1973; **139**: 511.

65. Johansson L, Nylander G, Hedner U, Nilsson IM. Comparison of streptokinase with heparin. Late results in the treatment of deep vein thrombosis. *Acta Med Scand* 1979; **206**: 93.

66. Jorpes JE. On the dosage of the anticoagulants, heparin and dicoumarol in the treatment of thrombosis. *Acta Chir Scand* (Suppl) 1950; **149**.

67. Kakkar VV, Flanc C, Howe CT, O'Shea M, Flute PT. Treatment of deep vein thrombosis. A trial of heparin, streptokinase and arvin. *Br Med J* 1969; **1**: 806.

68. Kakkar VV, Flanc C, O'Shea M J, Flute PT, Howe CT, Clarke MB. Treatment of deep vein

thrombosis with streptokinase. *Br J Surg* 1969; **56**: 178.

69. Kakkar VV, Howe CT, Laws JW, Flanc C. Late results of treatment of deep vein thrombosis. *Br Med J* 1969; **1**: 810.

70. Kakkar VV, Lawrence D. Hemodynamic and clinical assessment after therapy for acute deep vein thrombosis: A prospective study. *Am J Surg* 1985; **150**: 54.

71. Kakkar VV, Sagar S, Lewis M. Treatment of deep vein thrombosis with intermittent streptokinase and plasminogen infusion. *Lancet* 1975; **2**: 674.

72. Kapsch DN, Kasulke RJ, Silver D. Anticoagulant therapy. *Vasc Diag Ther* 1981; **19**.

73. Kapsch D, Adelstein E, Rhodes G, Silver D. Heparin induced thrombocytopenia, thrombosis and haemorrhage. *Surgery* 1979; **86**: 148.

74. Kernohan JE, Todd C. Heparin therapy in thromboembolic disease. *Lancet* 1966; **1**: 621.

75. Kiely PE. A new venous thrombectomy technique. *Br J Surg* 1973; **60**: 850.

76. Lagerstedt CI, Olsson CG, Fagher BO, Oqvist BW, Albrechtsson V. Need for long term anticoagulant treatment in symptomatic calf vein thrombosis. *Lancet* 1985; **2**: 515.

77. Lansing A M, Davis W M. Five year follow up study of iliofemoral venous thrombectomy. *Ann Surg* 1968; **168**: 620.

78. Läwen A. Weitere Erfahrungen über operative thromben-entfernung bei Venenthrombose. *Arch Klin Chir* 1938; **193**: 723.

79. Leriche R, Geisendorf W. Resultats d'une thrombectomie precoce avec resection veineuse dans une phlébite grave des deux membres inférieurs. *Presse Méd* 1939; **47**: 1239.

80. Mahorner H, Castleberry JW, Coleman WC. Attempts to restore function in major veins which are the site of massive thrombosis. *Ann Surg* 1957; **146**: 510.

81. Mahorner H. A new method of management for thrombosis of deep veins of the extremities. *Am Surg* 1954; **20**: 487.

82. Mahorner H. Results of surgical operations for venous thrombosis. *Surg Gynec Obstet* 1969; **129**: 66.

83. Mansfield AO, Carmichael JHE, Parry EW. Thrombectomy employing continuous radiographic control. *Br J Surg* 1971; **58**: 119.

84. Mansfield AO. Control of pulmonary embolism. *Ann R Coll Surg Engl* 1972; **51**: 373.

85. Mant MJ, O'Brien BD, Thong KL, Hammond GW, Birtwhistle RJ, Grace MG. Haemorrhagic complications of heparin therapy. *Lancet* 1977; **1**: 1133.

86. Marder VJ. Guidelines for thrombolytic therapy of deep vein thrombosis. *Prog Cardiovasc Dis* 1979; **21**: 327.

87. Masuoka S, Shinomura T, Audo T, Goto K. Complications associated with the use of the Fogarty balloon catheter. *J Cardiovasc Surg* 1980; **21**: 67.

88. Mavor GE, Bennett B, Galloway M, Karmody AM. Streptokinase in iliofemoral venous thrombosis. *Br J Surg* 1969; **56**: 564.

89. Mavor GE, Dhall DP, Dawson AA, Duthie JS, Walker MG, Mahaffy RG, Allardyce M. Streptokinase therapy in deep vein thrombosis. *Br J Surg* 1973; **60**: 468.

90. Mavor GE, Galloway JMD. Iliofemoral venous thrombosis. *Br J Surg* 1969; **56**: 4.

91. Mavor GE, Galloway JMD. Radiographic control of iliofemoral venous thrombectomy. *Br J Surg* 1967; **54**: 1019.

92. Mavor GE, Ogston D, Galloway JMD, Karmody AM. Urokinase in iliofemoral venous thrombosis. *Br J Surg* 1969; **56**: 571.

93. Murray G. Anticoagulants in venous thrombosis and the prevention of pulmonary embolism. *Surg Gynec Obstet* 1947; **84**: 665.

94. Nachbar BB, Beck EA, Senn A. Can the results of treatment of deep venous thrombosis be improved by combining surgical thrombectomy with regional fibrinolysis. *J Cardiovasc Surg* 1980; **21**: 347.

95. Nilsson IM, Olow B. Fibrinolysis induced by streptokinase. *Acta Chir Scand* 1962; **123**: 247.

96. Norgren L, Gjöres JE. Venous function in previously thrombosed legs. *Acta Chir Scand* 1977; **143**: 421.

97. Norgren L, Widmer LK. Venous function evaluated by foot volumetry in patients with a previous deep vein thrombosis treated with streptokinase. *Vasa* 1978; **7**: 412.

98. O'Shea MJ, Flute PT, Pannell GM. Laboratory control of heparin therapy. *J Clin Path* 1971; **24**: 542.

99. Oschner A, DeBakey ME, De Camp PT, De Rocha E. Thrombo-embolism. An analysis of cases at the Charity Hospital in New Orleans over a 12 year period. *Ann Surg* 1951; **134**: 405.

100. Perkins HA, Osborn JJ, Hurt R, Gerbode F. Neutralization of heparin *in vivo* with protamine. A simple method of estimating the required dose. *J Lab Clin Med* 1956; **48**: 223.

101. Pitney WR, Raphael MJ, Webb Peploe MM, Olsen EGJ. Treatment of experimental venous thrombosis with streptokinase and ancrod. *Br J Surg* 1971; **58**: 442.

102. Plate G, Einarsson E, Ohlin P, Jensen R, Clvarfordt P, Eklöf B. Thrombectomy with temporary arteriovenous fistula. The treatment of choice in acute iliofemoral venous thrombosis. *J*

Vasc Surg 1984; **1**: 867.

103. Plate G, Ohlin P, Eklöf B. Pulmonary embolism in acute iliofemoral venous thrombosis. *Br J Surg* 1985; **72**: 912.

104. Pollar L, Thomson JM, Yee KF. Heparin and partial thromboplastin time – an international survey. *Br J Haematol* 1980; **44**: 161.

105. Porter JM, Seamen AJ, Common HH, Rosch J, Eidemiller LR, Calhoun AD. Comparison of heparin and streptokinase in the treatment of venous thrombosis. *Am Surg* 1975; **41**: 511.

106. Rahintoola SH, Raphael MJ, Pitney WR, Olsen EJG, Webb Peploe MM. Therapeutic defibrination and heparin therapy in the prevention and resolution of experimental venous thrombosis. *Circulation* 1970; **42**: 729.

107. Robertson BR, Nilsson IM, Nylander G, Olow B. Effect of streptokinase and heparin on patients with deep venous thrombosis. *Acta Chir Scand* 1967; **133**: 205.

108. Robertson BR, Nilsson IM, Nylander G. Thrombolytic effect of streptokinase as evaluated by phlebography of deep venous thrombi of the leg. *Acta Chir Scand* 1970; **136**: 173.

109. Robertson BR, Nilsson IM, Nylander G. Value of streptokinase and heparin in treatment of acute deep vein thrombosis. *Acta Chir Scand* 1968; **134**: 203.

110. Salzman EW, Rosenberg RD, Smith MH, Lindon JN, Favreau L. Effect of heparin and heparin fractions on platelet aggregation. *J Clin Invest* 1980; **65**: 64.

111. Salzmann EW, Deykin D, Shapiro RM. Management of heparin therapy. *N Engl J Med* 1975; **292**: 1046.

112. Schulman S, Lockner D, Granqvist S, Bratt G, Paul C, Nyman D. A comparative randomized trial of low dose versus high dose streptokinase in deep vein thrombosis of the thigh. *Thromb Haemost* 1984; **51**: 261.

113. Schuster J, Meier-Ruge W, Elgi F. Zur pathologie der osteopathie nach heparinbehandlung. *Dtsch Med Wochenschr* 1969; **94**: 2334.

114. Sherry S. Tissue plasminogen activator. *N Engl J Med* 1985; **313**:1014.

115. Stevenson R, Burton M, Ferlauto G, Taylor H. Hazards of oral anticoagulants during pregnancy. *JAMA* 1980; **243**: 1549.

116. Thompson EN, Hamilton M. Pulmonary embolic disease. *Lancet* 1962; **1**: 1369.

117. Towne JB, Berhard VM, Hussey C, Garancis JC. White clot syndrome peripheral vascular complications of heparin therapy. *Arch Surg* 1979; **114**: 372.

118. Tsapogas MJ, Peabody RA, Wis TK, Karmody AM, Devaraj KT, Eckert C. Controlled study of

119. Urokinase pulmonary embolism trial: Phase 1 results: A cooperative study. *JAMA* 1970; **214**: 2163.

120. Vairel EG, Bonty-Boye H, Toulemonde F, Dontremepuich C, Marsh NA, Gaffney PJ. Heparin and low molecular weight fraction enhances thrombolysis and by this pathway exercises a protective effect against thrombosis. *Thromb Res* 1983; **30**: 219.

121. Van de Berg L. Venous thrombectomies and partial interruption of the vena cava in 125 cases of thrombophlebitis. *J Cardiovasc Surg* 1978; **19**: 143.

122. Verstraete M, Bernand R, Bory M, Brower RW, Collen D, de Bono DP, Erbel R, Huhmann W, Lennane R J, Lubsen J. Randomized trial of intravenous recombinant tissue-type plasminogen activator versus intravenous streptokinase in acute myocardial infarction. *Lancet* 1985; **1**: 842.

123. Verstraete M, Bleifeld W, Brower RW, Charbonnier B, Collen D, de Bono DP, Dunning AJ, Lennane RJ, Lubsen J, Mathey D G. Double blind randomized trial of intravenous tissue-type plasminogen activator versus placebo in acute myocardial infarction. *Lancet* 1985; **2**: 966.

124. Verstraete M, Vermylen J, Amery A, Vermylen C. Thrombolytic therapy with streptokinase using a standard dosage scheme. *Br Med J* 1966; **1**: 454.

125. Weimar W, Stibbe J, Van Seyen AJ, Billan A, de Somer P, Collen D. Specific lysis of an iliofemoral thrombus by administration of extrinsic plasminogen activator. *Lancet* 1981; **2**: 1018.

126. Widmer L K, Brandenberg E, Schmitt H E, Widmer M Th, Voelin R, Zemp E, Madar G. Zum Schicksal des Patienten mit tiefer venenthrombose. *Dtsch Med Wochenschr* 1985; **110**: 993.

127. Widmer L K, Madar G, Duckert F, Müller G, Schmitt H E. Acute deep thrombophlebitis: thrombolytic versus anticoagulant therapy. *Acta Univ Carol (Med Monogr) (Praha)* 1972; **52**: 137.

128. Widmer L K. The treatment of venous thrombosis. Angiological aspects. *Triangle* 1977; **16**: 47.

129. Wilson H, Britt L G. Surgical treatment of iliofemoral thrombosis. *Ann Surg* 1967; **165**: 855.

130. Young A E, Lea Thomas M, Browse N L. Comparison between sequelae of surgical and medical treatment of venous thromboembolism. *Br Med J* 1974; **4**: 127.

19

Deep vein thrombosis: prevention

Deep vein thrombosis in the lower limb causes three clinical problems, *symptoms* (e.g. pain, swelling and difficulty with walking), *the post-thrombotic calf pump failure syndrome* – pain, swelling, pigmentation, dermatitis, lipodermato-sclerosis and ulceration, and *pulmonary embolism*.

The ideal method of prophylaxis would abolish all of these clinical problems by completely eliminating deep vein thrombosis. This objective cannot yet be achieved; our current methods of prophylaxis therefore fall into two categories – those that reduce the incidence of deep vein thrombosis by administering prophylaxis before the causal event and those that prevent pulmonary embolism in the presence of established thrombosis. The first approach (primary prophylaxis) should reduce the incidence of all three clinical problems caused by the thrombosis. The second approach (secondary prophylaxis) is unlikely to affect the initial symptoms or the late sequelae, but it may save the patient's life.

It is often assumed that any form of prophylaxis that reduces the incidence of deep vein thrombosis will *pari passu* reduce the incidence of pulmonary embolism. This assumption is true if deep vein thrombosis is totally abolished but not if the incidence is only reduced. As the evidence concerning the effectiveness of prophylactic regimens at preventing deep vein thrombosis is far better than that concerning pulmonary embolism,[78] these aspects of prevention are discussed separately – deep vein thrombosis prophylaxis in this chapter and pulmonary embolism prophylaxis in Chapter 21.

The aetiology of deep vein thrombosis was summarized by Virchow in 1856[130] as changes in the coagulability of the blood, changes in the blood flow and changes in the vessel wall (see Chapter 16). The two forms of prophylaxis most studied modify the first two of these factors. No method has been devised to change the vessel wall, though attempts to stimulate fibrinolysis might be construed to act in this way, and it is also claimed that dihydroergotamine may have a direct effect on the vein wall. The pharmacological methods mainly alter blood coagulability; the mechanical methods alter blood flow.

Pharmacological methods of prevention

Many pharmacological methods of prevention have been studied but there is no doubt that anti-coagulants, particularly heparin, are the most effective agents for reducing the incidence of deep vein thrombosis.

Oral anticoagulants

In 1959 Sevitt and Gallagher clearly established[115] that oral anticoagulation (they used phenindione) reduces the incidence of deep vein thrombosis and pulmonary embolism.

The two main groups of oral anticoagulants are the coumarins and the indanediones. Both groups work by inhibiting the role of Vitamin K in the synthesis of coagulation factors II, III, IX, and X, so that biologically inactive factors are produced.

The effect of oral anticoagulants is monitored by measuring the activated partial throm-boplastin time or the prothrombin time. The prothrombin time is a reliable test provided standardized tissue thromboplastins are used. For effective anticoagulation, the prothrombin time (using British Standard Thromboplastin) must be between two and four times the control value. Therapeutic prothrombin times measured with

Simplastin (a rabbit brain/lung thromboplastin) should be one and one-half to two times the control value.

Sevitt and Gallagher studied patients with fractures of the neck of femur and showed, at autopsy, a reduction of deep vein thrombosis from 83 per cent to 14 per cent. Other workers[15,40] have confirmed these findings (Table 19.1). The value of oral anticoagulants in the management of hip fractures has also been confirmed with the fibrinogen uptake test by Morris and Mitchell[80,82] who found a reduction in the incidence of thrombosis from 68 per cent to 31 per cent.

There are only a few studies of the value of oral anticoagulants in gynaecological[122] and general surgery but almost all show a beneficial effect.[25]

The four main disadvantages of oral anticoagulants are:

- the time taken to produce an effect (2–4 days)
- the need to perform frequent measurements of the prothrombin time
- the sensitivity of their anticoagulant effect to many other drugs
- the risks of haemorrhage

The risk of haemorrhage involves not only per-operative bleeding and wound haematomata but spontaneous retroperitoneal and intestinal intramural haemorrhage, and bleeding from gastrointestinal ulceration. These problems have inhibited surgeons from using oral anticoagulation for routine prophylaxis in both general and orthopaedic surgery.[81] Nevertheless, it is important to emphasize that an effective form of prophylaxis has been available since 1959, a method proven by a variety of tests, including autopsy, to be effective against venous thrombosis and pulmonary embolism. These drugs have also been shown to reduce the overall mortality rate following hip fractures, an important fact which is discussed in Chapter 21 (page 582).

Heparin

Heparin is a sulphated polysaccharide that accelerates the serine protease neutralizing effects of antithrombin III. Antithrombin III will inhibit those activated clotting factors that have a serine residue at their enzymatically active centre – factors XII, XI, IX, X and thrombin. As the coagulation process is a mutiplying cascade, the amount of heparin required to inhibit one of the factors at the beginning of the cascade (e.g. Xa) is far less than that needed to inhibit thrombin because far less Xa is produced than thrombin. Thus it has been calculated that the inhibition of 32 units of Xa will prevent the formation of 1600 NIH units of thrombin.[134] As inactivation is on a one-to-one basis this means that only one-fiftieth of the amount of heparin required to inactivate thrombin is needed to achieve the same effect if it is given at the beginning of the cascade (at the factor Xa stage) before the thrombin has formed. This is the rationale for giving small doses of heparin *before* the coagulation process that causes a deep vein thrombosis begins. The critical word in the previous sentence is *before*. Prophylactic heparin must be given *before* the operation, *before* the illness or *before* the accident; only the first situation is practical.

Low molecular weight heparin and heparin analogues are said to have a greater inhibitory effect on factor Xa than on thrombin.[5]

In 1950 de Takats[34] suggested that a low dose of heparin given before an operation might prevent thrombosis. Sharnoff[116,117,118] treated a large number of patients in this way, and claimed a reduction in the incidence of fatal pulmonary embolism but had no control patients and no objective evaluation of the incidence of thrombosis in the limbs.

Scientific assessment of the value of low doses

Table 19.1 The effect of oral anticoagulants on the incidence of deep vein thrombosis and pulmonary embolism after hip fractures

Sevitt and Gallagher[115] [Autopsy study]

	Deep vein thrombosis	Fatal embolism	Death
No treatment (150 patients)	83%	10%	28%
Phenindione (150 patients)	14%	0	17%

Morris and Mitchell[80,82] (Autopsy plus isotope scanning)

	Deep vein thrombosis	Fatal embolism	Death
No treatment (74 patients)	100%	8.5%	31%
Warfarin (74 patients)	31%	0	22%

Table 19.2 The effect of low-dose heparin on the incidence of deep vein thrombosis following general surgical operations—a compilation of 24 studies* on 4932 patients

No heparin	30%
Heparin	9%
(5000 units, subcutaneous, 8- or 12-hourly)	

*References 1, 4, 6, 12, 22, 24, 26, 30, 43, 44, 46, 47, 49, 57, 59, 63, 66, 68, 69, 90, 94, 98, 102, 103, 106, 121, 123, 124, 132, 133

Table 19.3 The effect of low-dose heparin on the incidence of deep vein thrombosis following elective hip operations—a compilation of 11 studies* on 979 patients

No heparin	50%
Heparin	19%
(5000 units, subcutaneous, 8- or 12-hourly)	

*References 11, 33, 35, 36, 50, 73, 75, 79, 83, 111, 129

of heparin given subcutaneously followed the validation of the fibrinogen uptake test in 1968. Many studies on the value of low-dose heparin have been published.[13] Provided the heparin has been started at least 2 hours before the operation and continued in doses of 5000 units 12-hourly or 8-hourly, heparin has significantly reduced the incidence of post-operative radioactive fibrinogen detectable calf vein thrombi in almost all studies on general surgical patients. An arithmetical compilation of 24 studies (published between 1971 and 1980) on 4932 patients undergoing general surgical operations who were each given 5000 units heparin 12-hourly or 8-hourly shows that heparin reduces the incidence of deep vein thrombosis from 30 per cent to 9 per cent (Table 19.2).

There is little difference between the clinical effects of sodium and calcium heparin or between the effects of 8-hourly and 12-hourly administration; most surgeons therefore prefer a 12-hourly regimen.

It is important to note that these regimens do not *abolish* thrombosis. In all studies of all forms of prophylaxis there remains a stubborn 5–8 per cent of patients whose thrombi cannot be prevented.

While there is no doubt that subcutaneous heparin effectively reduces the incidence of calf thrombosis in general surgical and urological patients, it is not so effective in orthopaedic patients. Many studies of patients with hip fractures reveal that heparin has no effect, probably because the heparin was started after the trauma occurred, but even the studies of hip replacement, in which heparin is given pre-operatively, show a smaller effect, with a residual thrombosis rate of 20 per cent against a control incidence of 45–60 per cent (Table 19.3). The reason for this failure is not clear but it may be related to the severity of the trauma and local vein wall damage.

Also, phlebographic evidence suggests that heparin is less effective on axial vein than calf vein thrombosis.[12] Unfortunately, some of the studies supporting the opposite view, that heparin has an effect on proximal thrombi, have used the fibrinogen uptake test which is not accurate above mid-thigh level; this important question therefore still needs to be clarified.

Low-dose heparin prophylaxis should be continued while the patient is still at risk of developing a thrombosis (i.e. during continuing bedrest and any debilitating postoperative complications). Once the patient is eating and walking normally, the heparin can be stopped.

There is no doubt that low-dose subcutaneous heparin increases the incidence of bleeding complications.[93] The most common complications are bruising and wound haematomata. It is generally assumed that these are unimportant but if they cause an increase in the incidence of wound infection and incisional hernia then they should be taken into account. Some studies have shown an increase in blood transfusion requirements and operative blood loss but these increases have not always been statistically significant.

The clinical problems caused by bleeding are also related to the nature of the operation. Orthopaedic surgery and open prostatectomy are operations which are bound to cause bleeding but the blood loss rarely causes problems. On the other hand, minor blood loss in ophthalmic or spinal surgery, or bleeding beneath a skin graft can destroy the effect of the operation; any prophylactic regimen that increases the bleeding tendency should therefore be avoided with operations where a small amount of bleeding can cause serious harm. The 8-hourly regimen is generally reported to cause more bleeding than the 12-hourly regimen.[126]

Thrombocytopenia is a well-known complication of intravenous heparin administration[45] but it may also occur with low-dose subcutaneous prophylaxis if the initial platelet count is low or if the prophylaxis is continued for a long period. It is advisable to request a platelet count and test platelet function if heparin is given for more than 10 days.

Intravenous heparin

Negus[89] has shown that the administration of a minute quantity of heparin intravenously (1 unit/kg/hour) can reduce the incidence of deep vein thrombosis to the same level as subcutaneous heparin. In a controlled study of 100 patients the incidence of isotopically diagnosed thrombi in the control group was 22 per cent whereas the incidence in the test group was 4.3 per cent. There was no difference between the effect of intravenous heparin given for 5–7 days and the effect of intravenous heparin given for 2 days followed by subcutaneous heparin but the incidence of wound haematomata in the patients given intravenous heparin was 2 per cent compared to 7.5 per cent in patients given subcutaneous heparin for 5 days after receiving intravenous heparin for 2 days. These studies are interesting because the dose of heparin is so small that the blood levels are not measurable. It is not known whether the mechanism of action is through the inhibition of factor Xa.

Heparin analogues

A number of heparin analogues and low molecular weight heparins are being studied.[61,125] They appear to have a similar or better effect than normal heparin,[85] possibly a lower incidence of bleeding complications,[16] and can be given once a day. Their effect on the incidence of pulmonary embolism has not yet been described. These newer heparins may replace large molecular conventional heparin.

Heparin and dihydroergotamine

Dihydroergotamine (DHE) increases the tone of the peripheral veins by stimulating the α-adrenergic receptors and the smooth muscle cells directly. DHE increases the velocity of venous blood flow by reducing the diameter of the veins but in some patients it also reduces the arterial blood flow. The effect on venous blood flow might be antithrombotic in itself and might increase the effect of the heparin or reduce the dose requirement.

Studies of the effect of dihydroergotamine alone have shown no effect on postoperative calf vein thrombosis but when it is combined with heparin the prophylactic effect of the heparin is enhanced. An arithmetical compilation of four studies[62,65,67,120] on 728 general surgical patients comparing heparin alone (5000 units, 12-hourly) with heparin plus dihydroergotamine (5000 units + 0.5 mg, 12-hourly) shows an incidence of thrombosis of 10 per cent and 6 per cent respectively (Table 19.4). As the number of patients in these trials is relatively small, this difference is not statistically significant; all the studies do, however, show the same trend.

A multicentre study has been published[84] of the effect of heparin alone, two doses of heparin plus DHE, DHE alone, and a placebo. The results suggest that 5000 units heparin plus 0.5 mg DHE given subcutaneously 2 hours pre-operatively, and 12-hourly for 5–7 days, is superior to the other combinations; but the incidence of deep vein thrombosis in the 'DHE 5000 heparin' was no less than the 9 per cent incidence seen in the majority of the other published studies of heparin alone (see Table 19.2). In this study the high incidence of deep vein thrombosis (17.3 per cent) in patients treated with heparin alone is most unusual and difficult to explain. Such results highlight the difficulties that arise when attempting to interpret the meaning of results from multicentre trials. The bleeding complications in the five groups were not significantly different.

In three series[62,111,112] of 390 patients undergoing elective hip surgery the overall incidence of thrombosis in the control and treated groups was 23 per cent and 10 per cent respectively; this difference approaches statistical significance. It is

Table 19.4 The effect of heparin plus dihydroergotamine on the incidence of deep vein thrombosis following general surgical operations—a compilation of four studies* on 728 patients

Heparin alone (5000 units, subcutaneous, 8- or 12-hourly)	10%
Heparin plus dihydroergotamine (5000 units heparin subcutaneous plus 0.5 mg DHE 12- or 8-hourly)	6%

*References 62, 65, 67, 120

possible that the greater effect in orthopaedic patients is related to the higher incidence of axial vein thrombosis in these patients and the possibility that dihydroergotamine increases blood flow more effectively in the axial veins than the calf veins.

It is not advisable to give dihydroergotamine to patients with angina pectoris[96] or peripheral arterial ischaemia. Cases of peripheral gangrene have been reported, the presentation being similar to ergotism.[39,128]

The haemorrhagic complications of heparin are not changed by the addition of dihydroergotamine, unless the dose of heparin is reduced in the belief that the combination of the two drugs enhances the effect of the heparin. This hypothesis has not been fully tested.

Dextran

Dextran 70 or dextran 40, dissolved in 5% dextrose and given intravenously, has an antithrombotic effect by expanding blood volume, coating the formed elements of the blood so preventing their interaction with any damaged areas of vessel wall, inactivating factor VIII and polymerizing with fibrin to make a soft degradable thrombus.[87]

The dose of dextran is usually 500 ml given during the operation, 500 ml given during the next 24 hours and a further 500 ml given the following day. In most controlled studies of deep vein thrombosis after general surgery using the fibrinogen uptake test[2,58,86] for diagnosis, dextran has had little or no effect,[13] but in three studies of hip fractures, involving 246 patients, based on phlebography the incidence of thrombosis was significantly reduced from 41 per cent to 14 per cent. It has therefore been suggested that dextran does not alter the incidence of fibrinogen detectable thrombi in the calf but it does reduce the number of axial vein thrombi detected by phlebography by making the fibrin more susceptible to rapid, spontaneous thrombolysis.

Dextran does appear to have an effect on the incidence of pulmonary embolism (see Chapter 21 page 582) and is given for this reason. This point emphasizes the comment at the beginning of this chapter that there is not necessarily a direct relationship between changes in the incidence of calf vein thrombosis and the incidence of fatal pulmonary embolism; dextran seems to alter the incidence of embolism *without* reducing the incidence of peripheral thrombosis.

Dextran has three adverse side-effects. It may overload the circulation and precipitate heart failure; it should therefore be used with caution in the elderly. It prolongs the bleeding time[32] but none of the clinical studies of its use reports an increase of bleeding complications. It causes anaphylactoid reactions;[95] this is its most serious complication because these reactions can be fatal. However, a fatal reaction probably occurs in less than 0.008 per cent of infusions and in less than 0.01 per cent of patients.[100,113] Fortunately, this problem can be overcome by the preliminary infusion of dextran 1 (molecular weight = 1000) which acts as a hapten and blocks the formation of immune complex.[48,99] In a review of 30,000 patients who were given hapten (dextran 1) before dextran 70, serious immune reactions occurred in 0.0001 per cent.[77]

Anaphylaxis should be treated by intravenous hydrocortisone (100 mg), subcutaneous adrenaline (0.5 ml; 1 : 1000) and anti-histamines.

Aspirin

Aspirin prolongs the bleeding time by inhibiting the ability of platelets to adhere to collagen and to each other. Acetylsalicylic acid inhibits the synthesis of endoperoxides and thromboxane A_2 from the arachidonic acid in platelet membranes by acetylating the platelet enzyme cyclooxygenase which catalyses the oxidation of the arachidonic acid to endoperoxide PGG_2.

The principal effect of aspirin is on the platelets but there is also an effect on prostacyclin production by the vein wall. These two effects are dose dependent, and there is still controversy over the correct therapeutic dose of aspirin. A low dose reduces platelet aggregation by reducing thromboxane A_2 production from the platelets; a high dose inhibits the endothelial cell production of PGI_2 which inhibits platelet aggregation, thus its effect may be thrombogenic.

The doses in the published studies of the value of aspirin as a prophylactic agent vary from 450 mg/day to 4000 mg/day. This makes comparisons difficult. The majority of these studies show no effect on the incidence of fibrinogen detected deep vein thrombosis, and aspirin is therefore not used for prophylaxis.

The gastrointestinal side-effects and increased

bleeding time of aspirin are also considerable disadvantages.

Other platelet inhibiting drugs

Dipyridamole, sulphinpyrazone, hydroxychloroquine, flurbiprofen and ticlopidine have been studied, and none has had a worthwhile effect on deep vein thrombosis.

There are a few studies of the combination of aspirin with dipyridamole which show a significant effect but an equal number of studies do not.

Overall, the evidence that antiplatelet drugs affect the incidence of calf vein thrombosis is equivocal and not sufficient to justify their use.

Stimulation of fibrinolysis

Venous thrombosis is often associated with a reduction of blood and vein wall fibrinolytic activity.[9,55] Attempts to reduce the incidence of thrombosis by stimulating fibrinolysis have failed,[7,17,42] probably for two reasons. Firstly, the few active drugs which will do this take 2–3 weeks to have an effect. Secondly, though resting blood fibrinolytic activity is increased, the fibrinolytic shutdown in response to surgery is not prevented.

Mechanical methods of prevention

Surgeons have long believed that early ambulation prevents venous thrombosis. Unfortunately, early ambulation often means sitting out of bed in a chair, a state which would be better described as 'early stagnation'.

There have been no controlled studies of early ambulation but a number of uncontrolled studies suggest that it is beneficial.[41,70,88,127] Early ambulation is a worthwhile form of physiotherapy for many other reasons and should therefore always be encouraged.

Leg elevation

Elevating the legs during an operation increases the velocity of venous blood flow but does not decrease the incidence of fibrinogen detectable thrombi.[19,108] Nevertheless, it is still a common, and probably sensible, practice to increase venous velocity by elevating the foot of the bed of patients with venous disease and swelling of the lower limb.

Elastic compression

One of the earliest studies of elastic stockings, based upon clinical diagnosis in a large group of patients, indicated that elastic compression might have a worthwhile effect on the incidence of thrombosis and embolism,[131] but when the fibrinogen uptake test became available the studies of the stockings and bandages then available failed to show that they had a beneficial effect.[19,107] However, better stockings were then developed which produced a compression of 20 mmHg at the ankle, gradually reducing along the length of the leg. This pressure is sufficient to produce venous compression and an increased velocity of blood flow *when the patient is supine*, without affecting arterial inflow. These stockings have also been carefully designed so that their tops do not become constriction bands around the thighs.

A number of studies of modern antithromboembolism stockings have shown that they have a significant effect. An arithmetical compilation of four studies[14,54,56,114] on 389 patients shows that stockings reduce the incidence of thrombosis from 43 per cent to 19 per cent (Table 19.5).

The modern stocking is comfortable to wear and can be used throughout the patient's stay in hospital. It has no adverse effects and therefore can and should be used as a routine form of prophylaxis in all patients over the age of 40 years, and in all patients (whatever their age) who have a history of previous deep vein thrombosis.

A major advantage of stockings is that they can be given to all types of patient, medical, surgical, and obstetric without adverse side-effects.

Pneumatic compression

The logical extension of the elastic stocking is a pneumatic compression device that squeezes the leg intermittently, preferably in a graduated, sequential manner, from ankle to groin. The first

Table 19.5 The effect of graduated compression stockings on the incidence of deep vein thrombosis following general surgical operations—a compilation of four studies* on 389 patients

No compression	43%
Compression stocking	19%

*References 14, 54, 56, 114

devices were simple single chamber leggings; the most modern devices have many chambers which can be inflated sequentially to different pressures.

The obvious effect of pneumatic compression is to accelerate venous blood flow.[119] This effect is closely related to the rapidity and duration of the compression.[104,109] Those devices which do not produce a large increase in venous velocity but still reduce the incidence of thrombosis may work by emptying the blood from the valve cusps (the site of origin of thrombi), or by stimulating the release of fibrinolytic activator from the endothelium.[3,64,101] We could not confirm this last suggestion in an unpublished study on 50 patients, and another more recent detailed investigation also suggests that it does not occur.[71]

Two forms of compression have been developed – a rapid short (square wave) compression for 10 s at 50 mmHg followed by a rest for 60 s,[110] and a slowly applied (sine wave) compression taking 30 s to reach a pressure of 50 mmHg followed by a slow reduction with no pressure applied for 60 s.[53] There have been a number of studies of the effect of these different forms of compression on both venous and capillary blood flow. The rapid compression devices have the biggest effect on femoral venous velocity but there is little difference in the clinical effect on calf vein thrombosis of the two types of compression. Some devices have many chambers and produce sequential compression.[91] The slowly compressing single chamber equipment is the cheapest.

A pneumatic legging is a little uncomfortable to wear but not painful. Sweating and irritation of the skin can be reduced by wearing a light stocking of an absorbent material beneath the legging. Without this layer the skin occasionally blisters. The legging has no other adverse effects. In an arithmetical compilation of 11 trials published between 1972 and 1981 studying 902 patients, pneumatic compression reduced the incidence of thrombosis from 20 per cent to 9.6 per cent (Table 19.6).

Pneumatic compression is effective in general, urological and neurological surgery, but its effect in hip surgery is less certain. Only half of the published studies show a significant effect.

Next to elastic stockings the pneumatic legging is the simplest and most acceptable of the mechanical devices. These two methods can be combined by giving the patient stockings on admission to hospital, and applying the pneumatic legging

Table 19.6 The effect of intermittent pneumatic compression on the incidence of deep vein thrombosis following general surgical operations—a compilation of 11 studies* on 902 patients

No compression	20%
Intermittent compression	9.6%

*References 18, 22, 24, 26, 29, 53, 64, 102, 103, 110, 123

over them during the operation, and for as many days after the operation as the patient can tolerate.

Electrical stimulation of the calf muscles

Contractions of the calf muscle not only eject venous blood from the calf but also increase venous blood flow indirectly because they cause an exercise hyperaemia.[37]

A number of studies have been performed to test the effect of electrically induced calf muscle contractions on fibrinogen detectable thrombi in the calf.[8,20,38,92] The variations of method, especially the frequency and strength of the muscle contractions induced, make it unacceptable to consider the results as a single group but the largest group of patients with a similar protocol shows a significant reduction of thrombosis from approximately 25 per cent to 12 per cent.

The disadvantage of electrical stimulation is that it can only be applied to the anaesthetized patient because the stimulus, even when applied gradually rather than as a square wave, is uncomfortable and sometimes painful. In the studies mentioned above the stimulus was applied only during anaesthesia and there was a significant effect. It is, however, well established that many postoperative thrombi begin 2 or 3 days after the operation and therefore electrical stimulation is unlikely to be as effective as methods which can be used after an operation when the patient is conscious.

Other methods The incidence of thrombosis has been shown to be reduced by, for example, the use of a mechanical foot pedal[105] and by a patient-driven pedalling machine[74] – perhaps the best way of getting the patient to exercise *after* an operation.

Commentary

This chapter has been limited to a discussion of

methods for preventing deep vein thrombosis. In surgical patients the main objective of preventing thrombosis is the prevention of pulmonary embolism; any reduction of the incidence of late sequelae is an extra benefit.

There are, however, many patients in whom the prevention of deep vein thrombosis is a worthwhile end in its own right. These are the patients who are put to bed for long periods to help to cure the complications of their venous disease. Patients with venous ulcers often need long periods of bedrest. If the ulcer is the result of previous deep vein thrombosis, the risk of a further thrombosis during the period of bedrest is high. Another thrombosis will add to the calf pump dysfunction and greatly increase the likelihood of recurrent ulceration. These patients should be given an effective form of prophylaxis from the moment they enter hospital. There is no doubt that subcutaneous heparin is the most efficient and safe method for preventing deep vein thrombosis in patients not having an operation. None of the other pharmacological methods approaches its effectiveness, and mechanical methods, even elastic stockings, are often unsuitable for limbs with venous disease and ulcers.

Mechanical methods are suitable for all other categories of patient. As a result of the logistic problems of giving injections of subcutaneous heparin to all patients in hospital, the simplest solution is to use the modern graduated antithromboembolism stocking. Although stockings will not have as great an effect on the incidence of thrombosis as subcutaneous heparin, their effect will be worthwhile. Stockings may also help to prevent those thrombi that begin as a result of admission to hospital, before operation.[52]

A note of caution

Whether any of these methods reduces the incidence of pulmonary embolism or the post-thrombotic syndrome is a question discussed in Chapter 11 and Chapter 21.

When these methods of prophylaxis are being used to prevent pulmonary embolism, the arguments for and against them must be based on the published evidence of their effect on the incidence of embolism, not on their effect on deep vein thrombosis.

Table 19.7 Two methods for calculating the risk of developing a postoperative deep vein thrombosis

Crandon *et al.*, 1980[27,28,31]

$$\text{Index} = -11.3 + 0.009 \times (\text{ELT}) + 0.22 \times (\text{FRAs}) + 0.085 \times (\text{Age}) + 0.043 \times (\% \text{ over weight}) + 2.19 \times (\text{VVs})$$

ELT = Euglobulin Lysis Time; FRA = Fibrin Related Antigen; Age in years; % overweight for height; VVs = Varicose Veins (Present = 1; Absent = 0)

Lowe *et al.*, 1982[72]

$$\text{Index} = \text{Age (years)} + 1.3 \times (\% \text{ weight})$$

Weight as % mean population weight for age, sex and height

Prediction of risk (Table 19.7)

A number of workers have measured every conceivable coagulation factor pre-operatively in an attempt to predict those patients at risk and thus avoid giving a prophylactic drug to those not at risk[97] (see Chapter 17). Crandon *et al.* produced a complex risk index which has been shown in a prospective study to be accurate.[27,28,31] Lowe produced a simplified index.[72] Both these studies showed that the levels of fibrinogen and fibrinolysis are the most useful blood tests for predicting thrombosis (not the coagulation factors), and other investigators have confirmed this. The laboratory tests required to calculate these indices are, however, complex and time consuming, and this approach has not been generally adopted.

Table 19.8 The clinical application of deep vein thrombosis prophylaxis

Risk of thrombosis	Risk of haemorrhage	Prophylaxis
Average	Average	Subcutaneous heparin or dextran, plus stockings
Average	High	Pneumatic compression, plus stockings
High	Average	Oral anticoagulants or subcutaneous heparin, plus stockings
High	High	Weigh the risks of subcutaneous heparin or mechanical methods

Nevertheless, it is the logical way to approach the problem and, if simpler tests can be devised,[51] it may become generally applicable.

In the present state of our knowledge we prefer to make a clinical assessment of the risks of thrombosis and the risks of haemorrhage for each patient and tailor our prophylaxis accordingly.[21] The very high risk patient who is having an operation where bleeding is neither likely nor a risk is given oral anticoagulants; a low risk patient who is having an operation where a small amount of bleeding might jeopardise the operation is given compression stockings. This approach is summarized in Table 19.8.

References

1. A multicentre-controlled trial. Heparin versus dextran in the prevention of deep-vein thrombosis. *Lancet* 1974; **2**: 118.
2. Ahlberg A, Nylander G, Robertson B, Cronberg S, Nilsson IM. Dextran in prophylaxis of thrombosis in fractures of the hip. *Acta Chir Scand* (Suppl) 1968; **387**: 83.
3. Allenby F, Boardman L, Pflug JJ, Calnan JS. Effects of external pneumatic intermittent compression on fibrinolysis in man. *Lancet* 1973; **2**: 412.
4. An International Multicentre Trial. Prevention of fatal postoperative pulmonary embolism by low doses of heparin. *Lancet* 1975; **2**: 45.
5. Anderson LO, Barrowcliffe TW, Holmes E, Johnson EA, Sims GEC. Anticoagulant properties of heparin fractionated by affinity chromatography on matrix bound antithrombin III and by gel filtration. *Thromb Res* 1976; **9**: 573.
6. Ansay J, Fastres R, Kutnowski M, Kraytman M. Prevention des thromboses veineuses profondes post-opératoires par l'héparine sous-cutanée à faible doses. *Ann Chir* 1977; **31**: 263.
7. Atkins P, Brown IK, Downie RJ, Haggart BG, Littler J, Robb PM, Santer GJ, Jones I. The value of phenformin and ethyloestrenol in the prevention of deep venous thrombosis in patients undergoing surgery. *Thromb Haemost* 1978; **39**: 89.
8. Becker J, Schampi B. The incidence of postoperative venous thrombosis of the legs. A comparative study on the prophylactic effect of dextran 70 and electrical calf-muscle stimulation. *Acta Chir Scand* 1973; **139**: 357.
9. Becker J. Fibrinolytic activity of the blood and its relation to postoperative venous thrombosis of the lower limbs. A clinical study. *Acta Chir Scand* 1972; **138**: 787.
10. Bergqvist D, Burmark US, Frisell J, Hallböök T, Lindblad B, Risberg B, Torngren S, Wallis G. Low molecular weight heparin once daily compared with conventional low dose heparin twice daily. *Br J Surg* 1986; **73**: 204.
11. Bergqvist D, Efsing HO, Hallöök T, Hedlund T. Thromboembolism after elective and post-traumatic hip surgery – a controlled prophylactic trial with dextran and low-dose heparin. *Acta Chir Scand* 1979; **145**: 213.
12. Bergqvist D, Hallböök T. Prophylaxis of postoperative venous thrombosis in a controlled trial comparing dextran 70 and low-dose heparin. A study with the ^{125}I-fibrinogen test. *World J Surg* 1980; **4**: 239.
13. Bergqvist D. *Postoperative Thromboembolism*. Berlin. Springer-Verlag 1983; 98.
14. Bolton FJ. The prevention of post-operative deep venous thrombosis by graduated compression stockings. *Scott Med J* 1978; **23**: 333.
15. Borgström S, Greitz T, van der Linden W, Molin J, Rudics I. Anticoagulant prophylaxis of venous thrombosis in patients with fractured neck of the femur. A controlled clinical trial using venous phlebography. *Acta Chir Scand* 1965; **129**: 500.
16. Briel RC. Low dose heparin prophylaxis and post operative wound haematoma. *Int Surg* 1983; **68**: 241.
17. Brown IK, Downie RJ, Haggart B, Litter J, Murray GH, Robb PM, Sauter GJ. Pharmacological stimulation of fibrinolytic activity in the surgical patient. *Lancet* 1971; **1**: 774.
18. Browse NL, Clemenson G, Bateman NT, Gaunt JI, Croft DN. Effect of intravenous dextran 70 and pneumatic leg compression on incidence of postoperative pulmonary embolism. *Br Med J* 1976; **2**: 1281.
19. Browse NL, Jackson BT, Mayo ME, Negus D. The value of mechanical methods of preventing postoperative calf vein thrombosis. *Br J Surg* 1974; **61**: 219.
20. Browse NL, Negus D. Prevention of postoperative leg vein thrombosis by electrical muscle stimulation. An evaluation with ^{125}I-labelled fibrinogen. *Br Med J* 1970; **3**: 615.
21. Browse NL. Personal views on published facts. *Ann R Coll Surg Engl* 1977; **59**: 138.
22. Butson R. Intermittent pneumatic calf compression for prevention of deep venous thrombosis in general abdominal surgery. *Am J Surg* 1981; **142**: 525.
23. Butterman G, Haluszcynski I, Theisenger W, Pabst HW. Postoperative Thromboembolie-

prophylaxe mit reduziertem low-dose-Heparin-Anteil und Dihydroergotamin in fixer Kombination. *MMW* 1981; **123**: 1213.

24. Calnan JS, Allenby F. The prevention of deep vein thrombosis after surgery. *Br J Anaesth* 1975; **47**: 151.

25. Clagett GP, Salzman E. Prevention of venous thromboembolism. *Prog Cardiovasc Dis* 1975; **17**: 345.

26. Clark W B, MacGregor A B, Prescott R J, Ruckley CV. Pneumatic compression of the calf and postoperative deep vein thrombosis. *Lancet* 1974; **2**: 5.

27. Clayton J K, Anderson J A, McNicol GP. Pre-operative prediction of postoperative deep vein thrombosis. *Br Med J* 1976; **2**: 910.

28. Clayton J K, Crandon A J, Peel K R, McNicol GP. Postoperative deep vein thrombosis prophylaxis in high risk patients. *Thrombi Haemost* 1979; **42**: 260.

29. Coe N, Collins R, Klein L, Bettmann M, Skillman J, Shapiro R, Salzman E. Prevention of deep vein thrombosis in urological patients. A controlled, randomized trial of low-dose heparin and external pneumatic compression boots. *Surgery* 1978; **83**: 230.

30. Covey T H, Sherman L, Baue AE. Low-dose heparin in postoperative patients. A prospective coded study. *Arch Surg* 1975; **110**: 1021.

31. Cranden A J, Peel K R, Anderson J A, Thompson V, McNicol GP. Prophylaxis of postoperative deep vein thrombosis. Selective use of low dose heparin in high risk patients. *Br Med J* 1980; **2**: 345.

32. Cronberg S, Robertson B, Nilsson IM, Nilehn J-E. Suppressive effect of dextran on platelet adhesiveness. *Thrombi Diath Haemorrh* 1966; **16**: 384.

33. De Mourgues F, Pagnjer F, Clermont N, Ville D, Moyen B. Etude de l'efficaciteé de l'héparine sous-cutanée utilisée selon deux protocoles dans la prévention de la thrombose veineuse post-opérative aprés prothése totale de hanche. *Rev Chir Orthop* 1979; **65**: 74.

34. de Takats G. Anticoagulants in surgery. *JAMA* 1950; **142**: 527.

35. Dechavanne M, Saudin F, Viala J-J, Kher A, Bertrix L, de Mourgues G. Prévention des thromboses veineuses. Succès de l'heparine à fortes doses lors des coxarthroses. *Nouv Presse Med* 1974; **3**: 1317.

36. Dechavanne M, Ville D, Viala J-J, Kher A, Fairre J, Pousset MB, Dejour H. Controlled trial of platelet anti-aggregating agents and subcutaneous heparin in prevention of postoperative deep vein thrombosis in high risk patients. *Haemostasis* 1975; **4**: 94.

37. Doran FSA, Drury M, Sivyer A. A simple way to combat the venous stasis which occurs in the lower limb during surgical operations. *Br J Surg* 1964; **51**: 486.

38. Doran FSA, White HM. A demonstration that the risk of postoperative deep vein thrombosis is reduced by stimulating the calf muscles electrically during operation. *Br J Surg* 1967; **54**: 686.

39. Echterhoff HM, Kottmann UR, O'Koye XR, Rohner HG. Ergotismus: Eine wichtige Komplikation in der medikamentosen Thromboembolieprophylaxe. *Deutsch Med Wochenschr* 1981; **106**: 1717.

40. Eskeland G. Prevention of venous thrombosis and pulmonary embolism in injured patients. *Lancet* 1962; **1**: 1035.

41. Flanc C, Kakkar VV, Clarke M. Postoperative deep vein thrombosis. Effect of intensive prophylaxis. *Lancet* 1969; **1**: 75.

42. Fossard DP, Field ES, Kakkar VV, Friend J R, Corrigan TP, Flute PT. Fibrinolytic activity and postoperative deep-vein thrombosis. *Lancet* 1974; **1**: 9.

43. Gallus AS, Hirsh J, O'Brien S, McBride J, Tuttle R, Gent M. Prevention of venous thrombosis with small, subcutaneous doses of heparin. *JAMA* 1976; **235**: 1980.

44. Gallus AS, Hirsh J, Tuttle R, Trebilcock R, O'Brien S, Carroll J, Minden J, Hudecki S. Small subcutaneous doses of heparin in prevention of venous thrombosis. *N Engl J Med* 1973; **288**: 545.

45. Godal HC. Report of the international committee on thrombosis and haemostasis. Thrombocytopenia and heparin. *Thrombi Haemost* 1980; **43**: 222.

46. Gordon-Smith IC, Grundy DJ, Le Quesne LP, Newcombe JF, Bramble FJ. Controlled trial of two regimens of subcutaneous heparin in prevention of postoperative deep-vein thrombosis. *Lancet* 1972; **1**: 1134.

47. Groote Schuur Hospital Thromboembolus Study Group. Failure of low-dose heparin to prevent significant thromboembolic complications in high-risk surgical patients. Interim report of a prospective trial. *Br Med J* 1979; **1**: 1447.

48. Gruber UF, Allemann U, Gerber H, Wettler H. Erster direkter Vergleich der allergischen Nebenwirkungen des Dextrans mit und ohne Hapten. *Schweiz Med Wschr* 1982; **112**: 605.

49. Gruber UF, Fridrich R, Duckert F, Torhorst J, Rem J. Prevention of postoperative thromboembolism by dextran 40, low-doses of heparin, or xantinol nicotinate. *Lancet* 1977; **1**: 207.

50. Hampson WG, Harris FC, Lucas HK, Roberts PH, McCall I W, Jackson PC, Powell NL, Standdon GE. Failure of low-dose heparin to prevent deep-vein thrombosis after hip-

replacement arthroplasty. *Lancet* 1974; **2**: 795.

51. Heather B, Jennings S, Greenhalgh R. The saline dilution test – a preoperative predictor of DVT. *Br J Surg* 1980; **67**: 63.

52. Heatley R V, Hughes L E, Morgan A. Pre- or post-operative deep vein thrombosis. *Lancet* 1976; **1**: 437.

53. Hills N H, Pflug J J, Jeyasingh K, Boardman L, Calnan J S. Prevention of deep vein thrombosis by intermittent pneumatic compression of calf. *Br Med J* 1972; **1**: 131.

54. Holford C P. Graded compression for preventing deep venous thrombosis. *Br Med J* 1976; **2**: 969.

55. Isacson S. Low-fibrinolytic activity of blood and vein wall in venous thrombosis. *Scand J Haematol* (Suppl) 1971; **16**.

56. Ishak M, Morley K. Deep venous thrombosis after total hip arthroplasty: a prospective controlled study to determine the prophylactic effect of graded pressure stockings. *Br J Surg* 1981; **68**: 429.

57. Joffe S N. Drug prevention of postoperative deep vein thrombosis. A comparative study of calcium heparinate and sodium pentosan polysulphate. *Arch Surg* 1976; **111**: 37.

58. Johnson S R, Bygdeman S, Eliasson R. Effect of dextran on postoperative thrombosis. *Acta Chir Scand* (Suppl) 1968; **387**: 80.

59. Kakkar V V, Corrigan T, Spindler J, Fossard D P, Flute P T, Crellin R Q, Wessler S, Yin E T. Efficacy of low doses of heparin in prevention of deep-vein thrombosis after major surgery. *Lancet* 1972; **1**: 101.

60. Kakkar V V, Djazari B, Fok J, Fletcher M, Sailly M F, Westwick J. Low-molecular weight heparin and prevention of post-operative deep vein thrombosis. *Br Med J* 1982; **284**: 375.

61. Kakkar V V, Lawrence D, Bentley P G, Detlas H A, Ward V P, Scully M F. A comparative study of low doses of heparin and a heparin analogue in the prevention of post-operative deep vein thrombosis. *Thromb Res* 1978; **13**: 111.

62. Kakkar V V, Stamatakis J, Bentley P, Lawrence D, de Haas H, Ward V. Prophylaxis for postoperative deep-vein thrombosis. Synergistic effect of heparin and dihydroergotamine. *JAMA* 1979; **241**: 39.

63. Kettunen K, Poikolainen E, Karjalainen P, Oksala I, Alhava E, Rehnberg V, Huttunen H, Mattilla M. Low-dose heparin as prophylaxis against postoperative deep vein thrombosis (In Finnish). *Duodecim* 1974; **90**: 834.

64. Knight M T N, Dawson R. Effect of intermittent compression of the arms on deep venous thrombosis in the legs. *Lancet* 1976; **2**: 1265.

65. Koppenhagen K, Wiechmann A, Zuhlke H-V,

Wenig H G, Häring R. Leistungsfähigkeit und Risiko der Thromboembolieprophylaxe in der Chirurgie. Eine vergleichende Untersuchung von Heparin-Dihydergot und "low-dose" Heparin. *Therapiewoche* 1979; **29**: 5920.

66. Kraytman M, Kutnowski M, Ansay J, Fastrez R. Prophylaxie par l'heparine sous-cutanée à faibles doses des thromboses veineuses postopératoires. *Acta Chir Belg* 1976; **5**: 519.

67. Kunz S, Drähne A, Briel R C. Prophylaxe der postoperativen Thromboembolie. Erfahrungen mit Heparin-Dihydergot in der Gynäkologie. In Pabst H W, Maurer G (Eds) *Postoperative Thromboembolieprophylaxe*. Stuttgart, New York. Schattauer 1977; 133.

68. Lahnborg G, Bergström K, Friman L, Lagergren H. Effect of low-dose heparin on incidence of postoperative pulmonary embolism detected by photoscanning. *Lancet* 1974; **1**: 329.

69. Lawrence J C, Xabregas A, Gray L, Ham J M. Seasonal variation in the incidence of deep vein thrombosis. *Br J Surg* 1977; **64**: 777.

70. Leithauser P H, Saraf L, Smyka S, Sheridan M. Prevention of embolic complications from venous thrombosis after surgery; standardized regimen of early ambulation. *JAMA* 1951; **147**: 300.

71. Ljungner H, Bergqvist D, Nilsson I M. Effect of intermittent pneumatic and graded static compression on factor VIII and the fibrinolytic system. *Acta Chir Scand* 1981; **147**: 657.

72. Lowe G D O, Osborne D H, McArdle B M, Smith A, Carter D C, Forbes C D, McLaren D, Prentice C R M. Prediction and selective prophylaxis of venous thrombosis in elective gastrointestinal surgery. *Lancet* 1982; **1**: 409.

73. Lowe L. Venous thrombosis and embolism. *J Bone Joint Surg (Br)* 1981; **63B**: 155.

74. Mühe E. Physikalische Möglichkeiten der Thromboseprophylaxe. *Langenbecks Arch Chir* 1977; **345**: Kongressbericht.

75. Mannucci P M, Citterio L, Panajotopoulos N. Low-dose heparin and deep-vein thrombosis after total hip replacement. *Thromb Haemost* 1976; **36**: 157.

76. Mellbring G, Dahlgren S, Winan B. Prediction of deep vein thrombosis after extensive abdominal operations by the quotient between plasmin and $\alpha2$- antiplasmin complex and fibrinogen concentration in plasma. *Surg Gynec Obstet* 1985; **161**: 339.

77. Messmer K, Ljunstroöm K-G, Gruber U, Richter W, Hedin H. Prevention of dextran-induced anaphylactoid reactions by hapten inhibition. *Lancet* 1980; **1**: 975.

78. Mitchell J R A. Can we really prevent postoperative pulmonary emboli? *Br Med J* 1979; **1**: 1523.

79. Morris GK, Henry APJ, Preston BJ. Prevention of deep-vein thrombosis by low-dose heparin in patients undergoing total hip replacement. *Lancet* 1974; **2**: 797.

80. Morris GK, Mitchell JR. Evaluation of ^{125}I-fibrinogen test for venous thrombosis in patients with hip fractures: comparison between isotope scanning and necropsy findings. *Br Med J* 1977; **1**: 254.

81. Morris GK, Mitchell JR. Prevention and diagnosis of venous thrombosis in patients with hip fractures. A survey of current practice. *Lancet* 1976; **2**: 867.

82. Morris GK, Mitchell JR. Warfarin sodium in prevention of deep venous thrombosis and pulmonary embolism in patients with fractured neck of femur. *Lancet* 1976; **2**: 869.

83. Moskovitz PA, Ellenberg SS, Feffer HL, Kenmore PI, Neviaser RJ, Rubin BE, Varma VM. Low-dose heparin for prevention of venous thromboembolism in total hip arthroplasty and surgical repair of hip fractures. *J Bone Joint Surg (Am)* 1978; **60**: 1065.

84. Multicentre Trial Committee. Prophylactic efficacy of low-dose dihydroergotamine and heparin in postoperative deep venous thrombosis following intra abdominal operation. *J Vasc Surg* 1984; **1**: 608.

85. Murray WJG. MS Thesis 1986. University of London.

86. Myhre H, Holen A. Thrombosis prophylaxis. Dextran or sodium warfarin? A controlled clinical study. *Nord Med* 1969; **82**: 1534.

87. Nair CH, Shah GA, Dhall DP. Operation, dextran and fibrin network structure. *Clin Invest Med* 1985; **8**: A125.

88. Nanson E. Useful measures in the prevention of deep vein thrombosis of the legs. *Can Med Assoc J* 1963; **195**: 88.

89. Negus D. Prevention and treatment of venous ulceration. *Ann R Coll Surg Engl* 1985; **67**: 144.

90. Nicolaides AN, Desai S, Douglas JN, Fourides G, Dupont PA, Lewis JD, Dodsworth H, Luck RJ, Jamieson CW. Small doses of subcutaneous sodium heparin in preventing deep venous thrombosis after major surgery. *Lancet* 1972; **2**: 890.

91. Nicolaides AN, Fernandes F, Pollack AV. Intermittent sequential pneumatic compression of the legs in the prevention of venous stasis and postoperative deep venous thrombosis. *Surgery* 1980; **87**: 69.

92. Nicolaides AN, Kakkar VV, Field ES, Fish P. Optimal electrical stimulus for prevention of deep vein thrombosis. *Br Med J* 1972; **4**: 756.

93. Pachter L, Riles T. Low dose heparin: bleeding and wound complications in the surgical patient. A prospective randomized study. *Ann Surg* 1977; **186**: 669.

94. Plante J, Boneu B, Vaysse C, Barret A, Gouzi M, Bierme R. Dipyridamol – aspirin versus low doses of heparin in the prophylaxis of deep venous thrombosis in abdominal surgery. *Thromb Res* 1979; **14**: 399.

95. Pulsaki EJ. Present status of plasma volume expanders in the treatment of shock. *Arch Surg* 1951; **63**: 745.

96. Raberger G, Schwarz M, Benke T, Kraupp O. Die Wirkung von Dihydroergotamin auf den grossen und kleinen Kreislauf. In Tscherne H, Deutsch E (Eds) *Postoperative Thrombo-embolei-Prophylaxe aus aktueller Sicht.* Stuttgart, New York. Thieme 1981.

97. Rakoczi I, Chamone D, Collen D, Verstraete M. Prediction of postoperative leg-vein thrombosis in gynaecological patients. *Lancet* 1978;**1**: 509.

98. Rem J, Duckert F, Fridrich R, Gruber UF. Subkutane kleine Heparindosen zur Thrombosprophylaxe in der allgemeinen Chirurgie und Urologie. *Schweiz Med Wochenschr* 1975; **105**: 827.

99. Richter W. Hapten inhibition of passive anti-dextran anaphylaxis in guinea pigs. Role of molecular size in anaphylactogenicity and precipitability of dextran fraction. *Int Arch Allergy Appl Immunol* 1971; **41**: 826.

100. Ring J, Messmer K. Incidence and severity of anaphylactoid reactions to colloid volume substitutes. *Lancet* 1977; **1**: 466.

101. Risberg B. Fibrinolysis and tourniquets. *Lancet* 1977; **2**: 360.

102. Roberts VC, Cotton LT. Failure of low-dose heparin to improve efficacy of peroperative intermittent calf compression in preventing postoperative deep vein thrombosis. *Br Med J* 1975; **3**: 458.

103. Roberts VC, Cotton LT. Prevention of postoperative deep vein thrombosis in patients with malignant disease. *Br Med J* 1974; **1**: 358.

104. Roberts VC, Sabri S, Beeley AH, Cotton LT. The effect of intermittently applied external pressure on the haemodynamics of the lower limb in man. *Br J Surg* 1972; **59**: 223.

105. Roberts VC, Sabri S, Pietroni MC, Gurewich V, Cotton LT. Passive flexion and femoral vein flow; a study using a motorized foot mover. *Br Med J* 1971; **3**: 78.

106. Rosenberg IL, Evans M, Pollock AV. Prophylaxis of postoperative leg vein thrombosis by low dose subcutaneous heparin or peroperative calf muscle stimulation: a controlled clinical trial. *Br Med J* 1975; **1**: 649.

107. Rosengarten DS, Laird J, Jeyasingh K, Martin P. The failure of compression stockings (Tubi-

grip) to prevent deep venous thrombosis after operation. *Br J Surg* 1970; **57**: 296.

108. Rosengarten DS, Laird J. The effect of leg elevation on the incidence of deep vein thrombosis after operation. *Br J Surg* 1971; **58**: 182.

109. Sabri S, Roberts VC, Cotton LT. Effects of externally applied pressure on the haemodynamics of the lower limb. *Br Med J* 1971; **3**: 503.

110. Sabri S, Roberts VC, Cotton LT. Prevention of early postoperative deep vein thrombosis by intermittent compression of the leg during surgery. *Br Med J* 1971; **4**: 394.

111. Sagar S, Stamatakis JD, Higgins AF, Nairn D, Maffei FH, Thomas DP, Kakkar VV. Efficacy of low dose heparin in prevention of extensive deep-vein thrombosis in patients undergoing total-hip replacement. *Lancet* 1976; **1**: 151.

112. Schöndorf T, Weber U. Prevention of deep vein thrombosis in orthopaedic surgery with the combination of low dose heparin plus either dihydroergotamine or dextran. *Scand J Haematol* (Suppl) 1980; **36**: 126.

113. Schöning B, Koch H. Pathergiequote verschiedener Plasmasubstitute an Haut und Respirationstractus orthopädischer Patienten. *Anaesthesist* 1975; **24**: 507.

114. Scurr JH, Ibrahim SZ, Faber RG, Le Quesne LP. The efficacy of graduated compression stockings in the prevention of deep vein thrombosis. *Br J Surg* 1977; **64**: 371.

115. Sevitt S, Gallagher NG. Prevention of venous thrombosis and pulmonary embolism in injured patients. *Lancet* 1959; **2**: 981.

116. Sharnoff JG, De Blazio G. Prevention of fatal postoperative thromboembolism by heparin prophylaxis. *Lancet* 1970; **2**: 1006.

117. Sharnoff JG, Kass HH, Mistica BA. A plan of heparinization of the surgical patient to prevent postoperative thromboembolism. *Surg Gynec Obstet* 1962; **115**: 75.

118. Sharnoff JG. Results in the prophylaxis of postoperative thromboembolism. *Surg Gynec Obstet* 1966; **123**: 303.

119. Sigel B, Edelstein A, Felix R, Memhardt C. Compression of the deep venous system of the lower leg during inactive recumbency. *Arch Surg* 1973; **106**: 38.

120. Stamatakis JD, Sagar S, Lawrence D, Kakkar VV. Dihydroergotamine in the prevention of postoperative deep venous thrombosis. *Br J Surg* 1977; **64**: 294.

121. Strand L, Bank-Mikkelsen OK, Lindewald H. Small heparin doses as prophylaxis against deep-vein thrombosis in the major surgery. *Acta Chir Scand* 1975; **141**: 624.

122. Taberner DA, Poller L, Burslem RW, Jones JB. Oral anticoagulants controlled by the British comparative thromboplastin versus low-dose heparin in prophylaxis of deep vein thrombosis. *Br Med J* 1978; **1**: 272.

123. Takkunen O. The effect of different modes of artificial ventilation and of some prophylactic means on the incidence of postoperative deep vein thrombosis. *Ann Chir Gynaecol Fenn* (Suppl) 1975; **191**.

124. Törngren S, Forsberg K. Concentrated or diluted heparin prophylaxis of postoperative deep venous thrombosis. *Acta Chir Scand* 1978; **144**: 283.

125. Törngren S, Kettunen K, Lahtinen J, Koppenhagen K, Brucke P, Hartle P, Hutter O, Haller U, Lahnborg G, Forsskahl B. A randomized study of a semisynthetic heparin analogue and heparin in prophylaxis of deep vein thrombosis. *Br J Surg* 1984; **71**: 817.

126. Törngren S. Optimal regimen of low-dose heparin prophylaxis in gastrointestinal surgery. *Acta Chir Scand* 1979; **145**: 87.

127. Tsapogas MJ, Gousous H, Peadbody RA, Karmody AM, Eckert C. Postoperative venous thrombosis and the effectiveness of prophylactic measures. *Arch Surg* 1971; **103**: 561.

128. Van den Berg E, Walterbusch G, Gotzen L, Rumpf K-D, Otten B, Fröhlich H. Ergotism leading to threatened limb amputation or to death in two patients given heparin-dihydroergotamine prophylaxis. *Lancet* 1982; **1**: 955.

129. Venous Thrombosis Clinical Study Group. Small doses of subcutaneous sodium heparin in the prevention of deep vein thrombosis after elective hip operations. *Br J Surg* 1975; **62**: 348.

130. Virchow R. *Gesammelte Abhandlungen zur wissenschaftlichen Medizin*. Frankfurt. Von Meidlinger Sohn 1856.

131. Wilkins RW, Stanton JR. Elastic stockings in the prevention of pulmonary embolism. *N Engl J Med* 195; **248**: 1087.

132. Williams HT. Prevention of postoperative deep-vein thrombosis with perioperative subcutaneous heparin. *Lancet* 1971; **2**: 950.

133. Wu T, Tsapogas M, Jordan R. Prophylaxis of deep venous thrombosis by hydroxychloroquine sulfate and heparin. *Surg Gynec Obstet* 1977; **145**: 714.

134. Yin ET, Wessler S. Heparin accelerated inhibition of activated factor X by a natural plasma inhibitor. *Biochem Biophys Acta* 1970; **201**: 387.

20

Pulmonary Embolism*

Pulmonary embolism occurs whenever material is carried to, and impacts in, the pulmonary circulation; it occurs when tumour cells, amniotic fluid or parasites are deposited in the lung via the pulmonary circulation. By far the most common source of embolic material is, however, from venous thrombi, and the term 'pulmonary embolism' is generally used to describe emboli caused by venous thrombi which have become detached and have impacted in the pulmonary circulation. This is the definition of pulmonary embolism which will be used here.

Incidence and natural history

It is impossible to estimate accurately the incidence and mortality of a condition, the diagnosis of which depends almost entirely on clinical suspicion and for which there are no generally available confirmatory tests. We know from post-mortem studies that the majority of patients found to have pulmonary emboli at necropsy were not diagnosed in life. Even if there was general agreement about the post-mortem incidence of embolism, this figure would only relate to a selected population of hospital patients. In addition, the figure would not tell us how many patients died from embolism as distinct from those in whom embolism was merely a contributory cause or even an incidental finding. Finally, no post-mortem study will tell us anything about the number of patients who survive pulmonary embolism and therefore nothing about the overall incidence or mortality. At best, estimates of incidence or mortality are just that – estimates.

The Registrar General's figures for England and Wales suggest that some 21,000 patients die as a result of pulmonary embolism each year. There is evidence that the number of cases was increasing year by year.[28] In the United States, Dalen and Alpert[11] have estimated that the total incidence of symptomatic pulmonary embolism is approximately 630,000 cases/year; pulmonary embolism is therefore approximately half as common as acute myocardial infarction and about three times as common as cerebovascular accidents. Of these 630,000 cases, Dalen and Alpert estimate that approximately 200,000 die, and that in 100,000 of these cases pulmonary embolism is the sole cause of death. A number of studies have shown that about a half to two-thirds of patients who die from pulmonary embolism die within 1 hour of onset.[12,15] These deaths may be preventable, in that prophylactic anticoagulant treatment might have prevented preceding deep vein thrombosis, but are unlikely to be preventable in that the diagnosis cannot be established and specific treatment instituted in this short time. According to Dalen and Alpert approximately 67,000 of these 'inevitable' deaths will occur each year in the United States, and a further 133,000 deaths will occur after 1 hour has elapsed. Several studies have shown that the mortality of untreated symptomatic embolism is approximately 30 per cent.[1,19,28] In contrast, the 'Urokinase Pulmonary Embolism Trial' (UPET) found the mortality of diagnosed and treated (heparin or Urokinase) symptomatic embolism accounted for only about 8 per cent.[42] Dalen and Alpert therefore concluded that, in the United States, approximately 120,000 patients die each year, of whom all but 8 per cent die because the diagnosis is not made and treatment is not given. Even if these figures are only approximate, the conclusion is clear: pulmonary embolism is a common disease and a common and largely preventable cause of death – if only clinicians would

*This chapter has been contributed by Graham Miller DM FRCP, Consultant Physician, Brompton Hospital, London.

learn to recognize the condition and treat it energetically.

When pulmonary embolism has occurred, there are a number of possible outcomes. The patient may die immediately, or within a few hours or days, or may recover, either completely or to experience further, possibly fatal (recurrent) embolism. Finally, the patient may go on to develop chronic pulmonary thromboembolism. Each possibility must be examined.

Recovery from pulmonary embolism occurs as a result of natural thrombolysis. The rate of resolution by natural thrombolysis was investigated in the Urokinase Pulmonary Embolism Trial (UPET). As estimated by lung scan, resolution was about 8 per cent at 24 hours and approximately 26 per cent at 2 days. By 2 weeks resolution was about 56 per cent complete but there were still residual abnormalities even at 1 year, when average resolution was still only 77 per cent complete. For the majority of patients resolution is therefore slow after the first few days. All this would suggest that we might find many patients among those who have suffered acute pulmonary embolism who will go on to develop chronic thromboembolic pulmonary hypertension. This is not so. Paraskos *et al.*,[30] studied 60 patients who had originally suffered acute pulmonary embolism of varying degrees of severity and were able to find only one patient who went on to develop chronic thromboembolic pulmonary hypertension. Our own experience has been similar; in 35 patients followed up for 1–8 years, the only patients found to have evidence of pulmonary hypertension at follow-up were those who had first presented as cases of established thromboembolic pulmonary hypertension.[37] None of those patients who originally presented with acute minor or massive pulmonary embolism or even of those with sub-acute massive embolism had any evidence of pulmonary hypertension at late follow-up. It is almost as though chronic thromboembolic pulmonary hypertension has a different aetiology and, as will be seen later, patients with chronic thromboembolic pulmonary hypertension seldom have anything in their history suggesting prior episodes of acute embolism. Perhaps the condition arises as a result of repeated sub-clinical episodes together with some failure of the normal thrombolytic mechanisms.

Recurrent pulmonary embolism is also an infrequent sequel to energetically treated acute embolism; in the study referred to above[37] only 3 out of 35 patients followed up after an episode of acute embolism had symptoms suggesting recurrent embolism. All three patients had originally presented with minor embolism and had one or two further episodes of pleuritic pain which might have represented later recurrence of minor emboli.

Aetiology

Emboli formed of blood clot are the result of venous thrombosis; the aetiology of pulmonary embolism is therefore that of venous thrombosis. Factors which predispose to venous thrombosis may be summarized as 'Virchow's Triad'.

1. Venous stasis
2. Damage to the vessel wall
3. Alteration in the coagulability of the blood.

In practice some, or all, of these factors may be operating together; both damage to the vessel wall and stasis are present during lower limb surgery or trauma, and hormone induced altered coagulability and stasis are present during late pregnancy and following childbirth. It is perhaps more useful to list those clinical situations which commonly precede pulmonary embolism.

Table 20.1 lists only some of the conditions which may predispose to pulmonary embolism but they are those which are most frequently

Table 20.1 Conditions commonly associated with pulmonary embolism

Trauma – particular lower limb or pelvic trauma

Recent (3–14 days) surgery – particularly abdominal or pelvic surgery or lower limb/spinal orthopaedic surgery. Hip replacement

Following childbirth

Prolonged bedrest

Lower limb venous compression/stasis (e.g. during long aeroplane flights)

Steroid therapy

Oestrogen-containing contraceptive 'pill'

Chronic valvular heart disease (plus bedrest)

Neoplastic disease (often occult)

Old age (50 years +)

encountered in practice. It should also be remembered that anyone who has once suffered a pulmonary embolus is at increased risk for further embolism whenever a 'risk situation' is present.

Although deep vein thrombosis with spread of free-floating thrombus is the precursor of pulmonary embolism, the clinical diagnosis of venous thrombosis is too unreliable for this to provide any useful warning of imminent pulmonary embolism. Unfortunately, we probably have to accept that it would be impractical to use more reliable methods for diagnosing venous thrombosis (e.g. phlebography, labelled fibrinogen or plethysmography) in all patients at risk. Preventive measures should therefore be taken in all patients at risk of pulmonary embolism. What these measures should be, and how effective they are, is discussed in Chapters 19 and 21; we are concerned here with indentifying patients at risk. The list of clinical situations associated with risk, given in Table 20.1, indicates those in whom prophylactic measures should be taken. In practice prophylaxis is often neglected in such patients, perhaps because of anxiety about possible bleeding due to anticoagulant therapy. The use of 'mini-dose' subcutaneous heparin is associated with few bleeding problems, and there is evidence that such treatment helps to reduce the incidence of pulmonary embolism.[21,22]

Syndromes of pulmonary embolism

It is often stated that the diagnosis of pulmonary embolism is difficult and that the condition may mimic many other disease states. This is not true. Failure to recognize pulmonary embolism is the result of failure to recognize the fact pulmonary embolism is not one syndrome but the cause of a number of clinically distinct syndromes. Streptococcal tonsillitis and streptococcal septicaemia are both caused by the same organism but no clinician would discuss the two conditions together and expect them to have a uniform clinical presentation. Similarly, the consequences of minor and of massive pulmonary embolism are the causes of completely different clinical syndromes. The clinical presentation of pulmonary embolism is influenced by:

- the size (severity) of embolism,
- the duration of embolism,
- the presence or absence of other, pre-existing cardio-respiratory disease.

A clinically useful classification which takes account of severity and duration is:

1. acute minor pulmonary embolism,
2. acute massive pulmonary embolism,
3. sub-acute massive pulmonary embolism,
4. chronic thromboembolism (chronic thromboembolic pulmonary hypertension).

The differing presentations of these four syndromes of pulmonary embolism will be discussed first; later we will examine how the presence of pre-existing cardio-respiratory disease can modify the presentation.

Acute minor pulmonary embolism

Acute pulmonary embolism does not begin to have a clinically detectable haemodynamic effect until approximately 50 per cent of the pulmonary arterial tree is involved. Minor embolism is defined as involving less than 50 per cent of the pulmonary arterial tree, and the clinically detectable effects are confined to the lungs. There are two symptoms: pleuritic pain and haemoptysis. Haemoptysis, usually seen as blood-streaking of the sputum rather than frank haemorrhage, only occurs when there is a pulmonary 'infarction' (see below) and pleuritic pain only occurs when the pleural surface is involved in the 'infarct'. Most minor pulmonary emboli are therefore clinically silent; this makes it impossible to discuss the incidence of pulmonary embolism. Pulmonary embolism is probably a common event; its incidence will always be under-estimated.

Although the majority of minor pulmonary emboli are silent, overt pulmonary 'infarction' is a common condition. The patient complains of sudden onset chest pain exacerbated by deep inspiration (pleuritic pain) and, some time later, may cough up a little blood-stained sputum. A pleural rub and/or fine crepitations may be heard in the region of the pain. The chest may show a small area of consolidation and this shadow has been described as typically '*wedge-shaped*'. There may be a slight elevation of temperature. There are no other abnormal physical signs, and there is no way to confirm the diagnosis; conventional pulmonary arteriography will not reveal small distal emboli, and lung scintillation scanning will not, with certainty, differentiate the condition from a small area of pneumonic consolidation. The differential diagnosis is from pneumonia /pleurisy of infective origin. It is often assumed that the condition is embolic in origin, if the setting is one in which embolism is common (e.g. a few days after surgery or childbirth). It is important to remember that the physical signs of deep vein thrombosis are very unreliable; the presence of these signs is therefore no more a reliable guide to an embolic cause for pleuritic pain than is their absence a reason for rejecting it. Minor pulmonary embolism resolves spontaneously, and complications (e.g. cavitation or secondary infection) are rare. There is no haemodynamic disturbance and the only treatment required is for pain. The importance of minor pulmonary embolism is that it may herald a further massive, life-threatening, embolus. Management should consist of anticoagulation whenever it is suspected that pleurisy and haemoptysis may be the result of minor embolism.

The concept of pulmonary 'infarction' is not as simple as it may seem. Infarcts follow occlusion of an 'end-artery'. However, the lung has a dual blood supply from the pulmonary and the bronchial circulation. In the experimental model, pulmonary infarction only occurs when there is a pre-existing abnormality of one of these circulations – classically, in mitral valve disease when the pulmonary venous pressure is raised. Haemoptysis and pleurisy are, however, common when minor pulmonary embolism occurs in patients without any previous abnormality of either circulation. The clinical syndrome that we call pulmonary infarction differs from that which follows occlusion of an 'end-artery' elsewhere in the body. Thus the radiological hallmark of pulmonary infarction – the 'infarct shadow' – appears and then resolves in 2–4 days; this occurs more rapidly than would be expected if there was tissue necrosis. These difficulties have lead to the concept of 'incomplete infarction'.[17] Following embolization of the normal lung, there is oedema and red cell infiltration into the alveoli which gives rise to the radiographic opacity and to haemoptysis but this resolves rapidly without tissue necrosis. It should be remembered that a wedge-shaped shadow, being the projected image of a cone whose apex is the occluded vessel and whose base is the pleural surface, will only be seen when the long axis of the cone is at right angles to the x-ray beam. Other infarct shadows will be more nearly circular in shape.

Within the spectrum of minor embolism some emboli are relatively large, though not large enough to cause a haemodynamic disturbance; such emboli may be detected angiographically or by lung scan and may lead to tissue necrosis. The radiological sequel is the development of linear scars and some loss of lung volume, perhaps leading to elevation of a dome of the diaphgragm. Once the volume of embolic material is large enough to occlude more than half of the pulmonary circulation, there is a more or less severe haemodynamic disturbance, and the symptoms and signs of this disturbance predominate giving rise to the second of the syndromes of pulmonary embolism – acute massive pulmonary embolism.

Acute massive pulmonary embolism

There are three haemodynamic consequences of sudden obstruction of more than half of the pulmonary circulation.

1. There is a sudden reduction in cardiac output as the normal flow cannot get past the obstructing embolus; pulmonary venous return falls leading to a fall in left ventricular output. This sudden fall in cardiac output leads to the second most common presenting symptom – syncope; this occurs as a result of a sudden reduction in cerebral blood flow. There may be actual cardiac arrest. On examination there is a (sinus) tachycardia with a sharp upstroke (increased peripheral resistance due to vasoconstriction) and a small volume arterial pulse. If the reduction in cardiac output is severe enough, there is 'shock' involving cold extremities, a low or unrecordable blood pressure, low urine output and mental confusion.

2. Proximal to the obstruction, the thin-walled right ventricle, which is poorly adapted to pump against a high resistance, dilates and 'fails'. At surgery, the dilated right ventricle is seen to contract poorly. This sudden dilatation of the right ventricle may be the cause of central chest pain (indistinguishable from angina) which is a common accompaniment of massive pulmonary embolism. Right ventricular failure is the cause of two of the most important physical signs; the jugular venous pressure is raised and a 'gallop rhythm' is heard at the left sternal edge. A 'gallop rhythm' may be due to a 'stiff', dilated right ventricle which causes an audible filling sound (third heart sound), or it may be due to forceful atrial contraction (fourth heart sound). When there is a tachycardia (a sinus tachycardia is

almost invariable in massive pulmonary embolism) these sounds may fuse and are then referred to as a 'summation gallop'. We have observed two circumstances in which the gallop is lost – when there is atrial fibrillation (loss of fourth heart sound) or when, after a day or more, the patient is recovering and the right ventricular filling pressure has returned to normal (loss of third heart sound).

3. There is a profound disturbance of pulmonary ventilation and perfusion. Sudden onset breathlessness is the most common symptom of massive pulmonary embolism. The mechanism of breathlessness is not well understood but we can assume that a disturbance of pulmonary perfusion and ventilation is in some way responsible. Similarly, some degree of arterial desaturation is almost invariable, though clinically detectable central cyanosis is only present in approximately two-thirds of patients. The cause of arterial desaturation in massive pulmonary embolism is the subject of debate. If a pulmonary artery is blocked, there will be ventilation of a non-perfused segment. This should not cause arterial desaturation unless so much blood is diverted to other segments that oxygenation of this diverted blood is incomplete causing a shunt-like effect. Blood diversion *is* occasionally seen in massive embolism but is unlikely to be enough to explain cyanosis. It has been suggested that partial occlusion of a pulmonary artery leads to an alteration in the surface active properties of the lung supplied by this artery; this results in atelectasis and consequent perfusion of non-aerated lung leading to arterial desaturation.

In some patients the high right atrial pressure may, if there is a patent foramen ovale (present in approximately 25 per cent of adults), lead to right-to-left shunting and provide another mechanism for arterial desaturation. This right-to-left inter-atrial shunting is the mechanism for paradoxical (systemic) embolism which sometimes accompanies pulmonary embolism.

In acute massive embolism the patient is acutely short of breath and is observed to be hyperventilating and tachypnoeic. In a shocked patient who is acutely short of breath and who may be complaining of central chest pain, the differential diagnosis is from myocardial infarction. However, in myocardial infarction involving the left ventricle, breathlessness is the result of left ventricular failure and a high pulmonary venous pressure or even acute pulmonary oedema. Patients with breathlessness from this cause will want to sit upright. In contrast, those patients in whom breathlessness is the result of pulmonary embolism will lie flat in bed and may even lose consciousness if forced to sit up. Generally, myocardial infarction will not result in the signs of right ventricular failure. It is the right ventricular failure which explains the adoption of the supine position; venous return to the right heart, and therefore right ventricular filling pressure, is maximal in the supine position, and the failing right ventricle needs this high filling pressure to maintain its output by the Starling mechanism. Loss of consciousness in the upright position may be due to the loss of filling pressure and therefore due to further reduction in an already critically low cardiac output. In addition, cerebral perfusion is best preserved in the horizontal position. This point has been laboured to emphasize that massive pulmonary embolism does *not* mimic many other conditions; a clear understanding of the physiological disturbance helps to make sense of the symptoms and signs and helps avoid confusion with other possible diagnoses.

In summary, acute massive pulmonary embolism should be suspected whenever the signs of right heart failure are observed in a patient with acute onset dyspnoea and/or syncope.

All the symptoms and signs of acute massive pulmonary embolism can be explained as the result of:

- acute reduction in cardiac output,
- acute right ventricular failure,
- acute disturbance of pulmonary ventilation and perfusion.

These signs and symptoms are summarized in Table 20.2. The frequency with which these symptoms and signs occur as presenting features of massive pulmonary embolism is listed in Table 20.3.

As we have described the symptoms and signs that accompany massive pulmonary embolism, it is now important to discuss those that *do not*. Many clinicians associate pulmonary embolism with pleurisy and haemoptysis. We have seen, however, that these symptoms are associated with minor, peripheral, emboli; there is no *a priori* reason why they need be associated with massive, central embolism. When massive embolism is not associated with these symptoms, the diagnosis is

Table 20.2 Acute massive pulmonary embolism – symptoms and physical signs

	Symptoms	Physical signs	
Acute reduction in cardiac output	Syncope	Small volume, sharp upstroke arterial pulse Sinus tachycardia Low arterial blood pressure Low urine flow Peripheral vasoconstriction Mental confusion	Shock
Acute right ventricular failure	? Central chest pain	Raised JVP Soft or inaudible P2 Gallop Rhythm at left sternal edge	
Acute disturbance or pulmonary ventilation and perfusion	Dyspnoea	Hyperventilation Tachypnoea Central cyanosis	

Table 20.3 Frequency of presenting symptoms and physical signs

Symptoms	
Acute onset dyspnoea	87%
Syncope/'collapse'	70%
Central chest pain	22%
Physical signs	
Sinus tachycardia, small sharp pulse, low blood pressure, low urine flow, peripheral vasoconstriction = 'Shock'	90%
Gallop rhythm LSE	87%
Raised central venous pressure	79%
Central cyanosis	62%
Single second heart sound (S2)	60%
Widely split S2	40%

often, incorrectly rejected. In practice, premonitory minor embolism, with pleuritic pain and/or haemoptysis occurs in approximately 50 per cent of patients up to 7 days before the acute event. At the time of massive pulmonary embolism, pleuritic pain is a feature in only approximately 20 per cent and haemoptysis in only 10 per cent of patients. Pleurisy and haemoptysis, particularly as premonitary events, are therefore useful pointers to the diagnosis but are not necessarily accompaniments.

Similarly, it is often stated that massive pulmonary embolism is associated with the signs of pulmonary hypertension, notably a loud pulmonary valve closure sound (P2). In our experience this is not true. The right ventricle is poorly adapted to generate a high pressure, unless a chronic pressure load has led to hypertrophy. We have seen that the previously normal right ventricle, subjected to a sudden obstruction to outflow, dilates and 'fails' and the right ventricular systolic pressure in massive pulmonary embolism seldom exceeds 50 mmHg (Table 20.4). When the right ventricle fails, its ejection period is prolonged and its end-diastolic pressure rises to almost the same level as the pulmonary diastolic pressure. These changes will lead to wide 'splitting' of the second heart sound (delayed P2) and a soft, not loud, pulmonary component (P2). In practice, a single second heart sound (inaudible pulmonary component) is the most common finding (it occurs in 70 per cent of patients) within 24 hours of the onset of massive embolism, while wide splitting with a soft pulmonary component may be heard after this time and, rarely, earlier. The signs of pulmonary hypertension or a 'heaving' right ventricle should therefore not be expected in massive pulmonary embolism, unless there is pre-existing cardio-respiratory disease which has lead to right ventricular hypertrophy. The fact that these signs have been attributed to massive pulmonary embolism emphasizes the need to distinguish between the various syndromes of pulmonary embolism and the need to consider, separately, the ways in which pre-existing cardiorespiratory disease can modify the presentation.

Sub-acute massive pulmonary embolism

In many ways patients with sub-acute massive pulmonary embolism are only a subgroup of

Table 20.4 Haemodynamic findings in syndromes of pulmonary embolism*

	Pulmonary artery systolic pressure (mmHg)	Pulmonary artery mean pressure (mmHg)	Pulmonary arteriogram: severity index
Minor (n = 17)	28.4 ± 2.1†	19.0 ± 1.5†	9.5 ± 1.0†
Acute massive (n = 42)	41.0 ± 1.2†	28.0 ± 0.75†	24.6 ± 0.4
Sub-acute massive (n = 11)	54.0 ± 5.0†	35.0 ± 3.0†	21.8 ± 1.1
Chronic (n = 8)	85.2 ± 5.7†	48.0 ± 2.2†	20.9 ± 1.0

*Modified from Sutton *et al. Br Heart J* 1977; **39**: 1135.[37]
†Group significantly different ($P > 0.05$) from each of the other groups (unpaired *t*-test)

those patients with massive embolism; those who have survived without treatment for 2 weeks or more. Patients who present as having sub-acute massive embolism are often those in whom failure to recognize and treat the initial massive embolus has led to steady clinical deterioration. Patients with sub-acute massive embolism have, however, a somewhat different presentation than patients with massive embolism; they have slightly different haemodynamic findings and, most importantly, they are much more difficult to treat. It is therefore worthwhile separating these patients in order to retain a clear clinical profile for each of the syndromes of pulmonary embolism.

The most common symptom is of increasing dyspnoea; this is often associated with episodes of pleuritic pain or haemoptysis. A history of cardiovascular 'collapse' is uncommon – perhaps reflecting the fact that, initially at least, these patients had less massive embolism than those in whom collapse demanded immediate recognition and treatment. A history suggestive of deep vein thrombosis is also more common than in those patients with acute massive pulmonary embolism, whereas a clear-cut predisposing cause (e.g. surgery, trauma, etc.) is often absent.[37] The physical signs are those of massive embolism. At cardiac catheterization these patients tend to have significantly higher pulmonary artery pressures (see Table 20.4) and slightly different angiographic appearances.

Chronic thromboembolic pulmonary hypertension

The last of the syndromes of pulmonary embolism is the least common and also that for which the prognosis is poor and treatment unavailing. The patients present with a long history of progressive dyspnoea, exercise intolerance and syncope. A history of a predisposing cause, of pleurisy or haemoptysis, or of a cardiovascular 'collapse' is absent. The only abnormal physical signs are of pulmonary hypertension (a loud pulmonary valve closure sound) and right ventricular hypertrophy. These signs are subtle and easily overlooked; these unfortunate patients are therefore often labelled as 'hysterical'. The diagnosis is confirmed at cardiac catheterization and angiography when the pulmonary artery pressure is found to be much higher than in the other syndromes of pulmonary embolism (see Table 20.4).

Table 20.4 demonstrates that in minor embolism there is no haemodynamic disturbance; pulmonary artery pressure is normal. From the table it would also appear that, for acute massive, subacute massive and chronic embolism, the degree of pulmonary hypertension is related more to the duration of embolism than to the degree of obliteration of the pulmonary vasculature. This may partly be explained by the fact that we would expect cardiac output to increase as the right ventricle adapts to a fixed degree of obstruction. However, the index of severity[26] used is relatively crude; it is derived from the pulmonary arteriogram and almost certainly underestimates small vessel involvement. Increasing obliteration of the pulmonary arterial bed most probably contributes to the higher pulmonary artery pressure observed.

The influence of other cardio-respiratory disease – differential diagnosis

If there is pre-existing cardio-respiratory disease, the clinical presentation and findings may be modified in a number of ways, and the diagnosis is more difficult than when pulmonary embolism is the only disturbance. The inclusion of patients with embolism and other cardio-respiratory disease in descriptions of the clinical profile of pulmonary embolism has contributed to confusion in the past and to assertions that the clinical diagnosis of pulmonary embolism is often difficult. It is true, however, that pulmonary embolism is a common complication of other cardiac and respiratory diseases and that the diagnosis is then much more difficult. In particular, the estimation of severity may be impossible without special investigations (e.g. pulmonary arteriography or lung scanning). In isolated pulmonary embolism severity is assessed from the degree of haemodynamic disturbance. If pre-existing cardiac disease has resulted in right heart failure, or has compromised cardiac output then minor embolism with pleurisy or haemoptysis may mimic massive embolism; the haemodynamic disturbance is, in reality, due to the cardiac disease and not the result of the small embolus. Similarly, if cardiac disease or chronic obstructive airways disease has resulted in pulmonary hypertension, an acute event due to minor embolism may lead to a false diagnosis of chronic thromboembolic pulmonary hypertension.

Radiologically detectable cardiac enlargement is not a feature of isolated pulmonary embolism, and arrhythmias other than a sinus tachycardia are rare. Both cardiac enlargement and arrhythmias may, however, be present as a result of prior cardiac disease. When superadded minor embolism occurs the clinical picture is therefore not that which would be observed if embolism was the only abnormality.

Conditions which may be confused with pulmonary embolism can be grouped as follows.

1. Minor embolism with pre-existing cardio-respiratory disease when the severity of embolism may be overestimated as discussed above
2. Other acute haemodynamic emergencies with 'shock'
   (a) with a raised central venous pressure
   (b) with a normal (or low) central venous pressure

Emergencies with a raised venous pressure include myocardial infarction, acute tamponade (e.g. following aortic dissection), respiratory failure or any condition discussed under (b) in which emergency treatment has included giving a large volume load (intravenous infusion). The differentiating features of myocardial infarction have already been discussed. The presence of a third heart sound will exclude tamponade. (A paradoxical pulse, typical of tamponade, has been described in massive pulmonary embolism, though we have not encountered this.) In acute respiratory failure the arterial $P\text{CO}_2$ will be high; $P\text{CO}_2$ will be low in massive embolism.

Emergencies with a normal venous pressure include the conditions which are most commonly confused with massive pulmonary embolism. Perhaps the most common such 'mimic' is septicaemic shock – gram-negative septicaemia – or any other acute toxic state (e.g. poisoning). Other 'mimics' include concealed haemorrhage and oesophageal rupture. The absence of a raised venous pressure or other signs of right heart failure suggests a cause for 'shock' other than massive embolism. Spontaneous pneumothorax as a cause of acute onset breathlessness is detected by absence of breath sounds on the affected side and by the chest radiograph.

The differential diagnosis of thromboembolic pulmonary hypertension includes so-called 'primary' or 'idiopathic' pulmonary hypertension, heart disease secondary to chronic lung disease – ('Cor pulmonale' and the 'Eisenmenger reaction'), pulmonary vascular disease secondary to a congenital heart defect causing a high pulmonary artery pressure and (originally) left-to-right shunting.

Aids to diagnosis

Electrocardiogram

In minor pulmonary embolism there is no electrocardiographic abnormality, except that which may be due to a pre-existing cardiac abnormality.

In acute or sub-acute massive pulmonary embolism the electrocardiogram (ECG) is abnormal in 85–90 per cent of patients. The abnormalities observed reflect abnormalities of right ventricular depolarization (the QRS complex) and repolarization (the T wave). The most common pattern, present in approximately 40 per cent of patients and often regarded as the 'classical' ECG of massive pulmonary embolism is one in which there is a prominent S wave in standard lead I and a Q wave and inverted T wave in standard lead III, accompanied by T wave inversion in right ventricular leads (leads V1–V3 or V4). This is the so-called 'S1, Q3, T3' pattern (Fig. 20.1). Another commonly found pattern is of right bundle branch block (RBBB), partial (RSR') or complete (Fig. 20.2). It is important to remember that the ECG may be normal despite proven massive embolism. This may be because the changes can be evanescent; we have seen a patient in whom a bundle branch block pattern was present at the time when he suffered a 'collapse' but in whom the ECG had become normal 2 hours later. Very occasionally, the ECG may suggest an inferior myocardial infarct or may even show left-sided (V5–V7) T wave changes – perhaps because the low coronary perfusing pressure has revealed ischaemic changes due to coexisting coronary artery disease.

In chronic thromboembolic pulmonary hypertension the ECG reveals right ventricular hypertrophy. These electrocardiographic findings are summarized in Table 20.5.

Chest radiograph

In minor pulmonary embolism the chest radiograph findings may be completely normal. Abnormal findings that may be observed are:

- infarct shadows – small, ill defined, areas of consolidation which may be 'wedge' shaped,
- linear atalectasis,
- loss of lung volume (raised dome of diaphragm),
- small pleural effusions.

In acute and sub-acute massive embolism it has been stated that the chest radiograph may be normal. This is seldom, if ever, true but the changes are subtle and easily missed. When an embolus occludes a major pulmonary artery the blood flow beyond the occlusion is reduced; this can be recognized as a loss of vascular markings on the chest radiograph – pulmonary 'oligaemia'. As pulmonary emboli affect some, but not all, of the pulmonary arteries, this oligaemia is patchy and confined to affected zones of the lungs. *Patchy oligaemia is the hallmark of massive embolism*, and is almost invariably detectable by the experi-

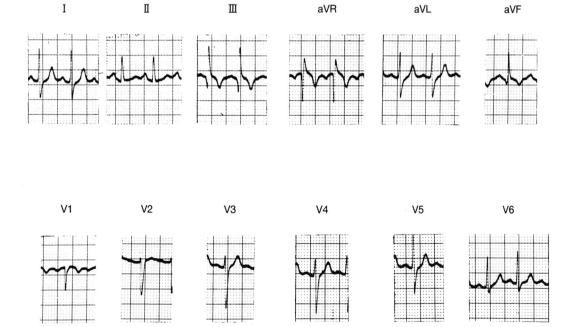

Fig. 20.1 Acute massive pulmonary embolism. Electrocardiogram showing typical 'S1, Q3, T3,' pattern. In this patient there is T wave inversion in lead V1; more typically T wave inversion extends to leads V3 or V4.

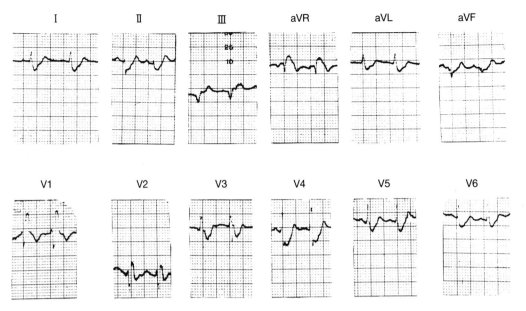

Fig. 20.2 Acute massive pulmonary embolism. Electrocardiogram showing right bundle branch block (RBBB) which is seen in approximately 14 per cent of patients.

Table 20.5 The electrocardiogram

	Pattern	Frequency
Minor embolism	Normal	
Massive embolism	S1, Q3, T3 + T inversion V1– V3 or V4	40%
	S1, Q3, T3	13%
	RBBB	14%
	RSR'V1	16%
	Normal	13%
	Left-sided changes (V5–V7)	4%
Chronic thromboembolic pulmonary hypertension	RVH	

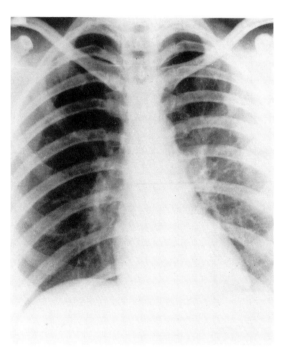

Fig. 20.3 Acute massive pulmonary embolism. Radiograph. The oligaemia of the right lung field is obvious when contrasted with the left lung field where there is 'compensatory hyperaemia' of the upper and mid zones. Note that neither the heart shadow nor the main pulmonary artery is enlarged.

enced observer (Fig. 20.3).[23] Sometimes there is diversion of blood away from affected zones to unaffected zones, and this compensatory blood diversion may be detectable as patchy hyper-aemia. Since significant pulmonary hypertension is not present in isolated acute massive pulmonary embolism the radiological sign of pulmonary hypertension – enlargement of the pulmonary artery – is not a feature of acute embolism. Slight enlargement of the pulmonary arteries can be measured but is not detectable by the naked eye. Failure to appreciate that neither the heart shadow nor the pulmonary artery shadow are enlarged in isolated acute massive pulmonary embolism has lead to wrongful dismissal of pulmonary embolism as the cause of 'collapse'. Although the main pulmonary artery is not noticeably enlarged, slight enlargement of the right or left pulmonary artery with abrupt diminution in calibre at the site of an occluding embolus gives rise to a third radiological sign – the so-called 'plump' or 'pear-shaped' hilar shadow (Fig. 20.4). This shadow is more noticeable on the right than on the left as the left hilum tends to be obscured by the heart shadow. Finally, there may have been minor premonitory emboli before mas-

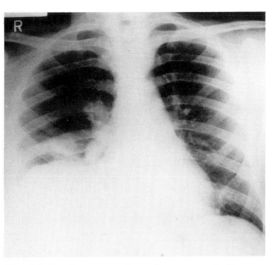

Fig. 20.5 Acute massive pulmonary embolism. Radiograph. Previous 'premonitory' minor emboli have resulted in an 'infarct shadow' at the right base and loss of lung volume with elevation of the right dome of the diaphragm. Subsequent massive embolism has caused oligaemia of the right lung with a prominent right hilum.

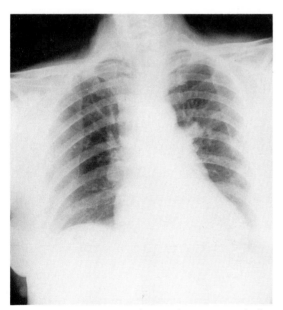

Fig. 20.4 Acute massive pulmonary embolism. Radiograph showing a 'plump' or 'pear-shaped' right hilum due to some enlargement of the right lower lobe artery with a sharp reduction in calibre at the point of occlusion and oligaemia of the right lower zone.

sive embolism occurred, and therefore any of the radiological features described for minor embolism may have had time to develop and may be present in addition to the patchy oligaemia of acute massive embolism (Fig. 20.5).

In chronic pulmonary thromboembolism the same patchy oligaemia may be even more marked but, in addition, there will now be marked enlargement of the main pulmonary artery reflecting the severe pulmonary hypertension that has been present for some time.

Arterial blood gas estimation

There is unlikely to be any disturbance of blood gases in minor embolism but in massive embolism the combination of arterial desaturation and hyperventilation leads to a characteristic abnormality of the blood gases. There is a low arterial Po_2 and a low Pco_2. Values for Po_2 average 48 mmHg and values for Pco_2 average 34 mmHg. Although it is not unique to massive pulmonary embolism, this pattern of a low Po_2 and a low Pco_2 is otherwise uncommon, and it is a helpful confirmatory finding (Fig. 20.6).

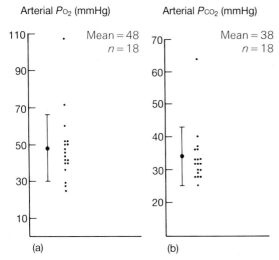

Arterial P_{O_2} (mmHg)   Arterial P_{CO_2} (mmHg)

Fig. 20.6 (a and b)   Values for arterial P_{O_2} and P_{CO_2} in 19 cases of acute massive pulmonary embolism.

Special investigations

Pulmonary arteriography

This is the 'gold standard' for the diagnosis and assessment of pulmonary embolism. Not only does pulmonary arteriography provide a certain diagnosis of all except the smallest emboli but it also provides an estimate of severity and duration of the embolism. Pulmonary arteriography has the disadvantage that it can only be performed in a catheterization laboratory and by experienced operators. An angiographic catheter is passed, under fluroscopic control, into the main pulmonary artery and radio-opaque contrast medium is injected to provide an image of the pulmonary arterial tree. Intravascular contrast medium has a (brief) vasodilator effect. When, as in massive embolism, there is fixed outflow obstruction, the cardiac output cannot increase to compensate and there will be a profound fall in arterial pressure. This could lead to a dangerous fall in coronary perfusion and has lead some investigators to recommend the prior administration of a vaso-constrictor drug. However, very little contrast medium is needed for excellent opacification of the much reduced pulmonary vascular bed of massive embolism. If the dose of contrast medium is reduced to 0.3–0.5 ml/kg bodyweight, there should be no morbidity or mortality, even in the

most desperately sick patients. It may be advisable to use one of the recently introduced non-ionic contrast media, as these have less of a vasodilator effect.

Pulmonary emboli are seen as filling defects within the contrast-filled pulmonary arteries. They may partially or completely occlude a major pulmonary artery or they may be seen as filling defects within an artery giving a 'pipe stem' appearance. Large emboli frequently impact at an arterial bifurcation partially occluding both vessels. A common site for these saddle emboli is the point where the pulmonary artery divides into its upper and lower lobe branches. When emboli are only approximately 1 day old they bulge into the contrast-filled artery thus forming a convex filling defect. Naturally occurring thrombolysis gradually erodes the emboli and organization takes place so that this convex interface is lost. Eventually, thrombolysis erodes the centre of the embolus so that the contrast in the lumen has a convex termination and the filling defect is concave. These last appearances are characteristic of chronic pulmonary embolism. In sub-acute embolism there will be a mixture of appearances; some emboli will appear recent and bulge into the

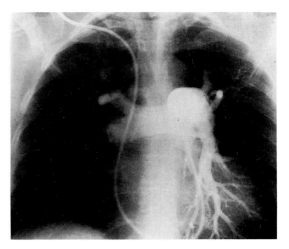

Fig. 20.7   Chronic thromboembolic pulmonary hypertension. Pulmonary arteriogram. The embolic aetiology is inferred from the asymmetrical distribution of occluded vessels with sparing of the left lower lobe artery. There is marked enlargement of the main right and left pulmonary arteries reflecting the severe pulmonary hypertension which is present. Emboli are no longer seen as filling defects, and partial lysis has resulted in a concave interface with the contrast medium in the right lower lobe artery.

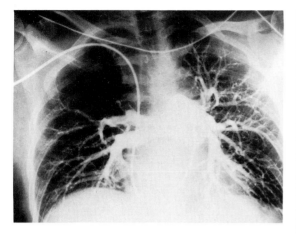

Fig. 20.8 Acute minor pulmonary embolism. Pulmonary arteriogram showing occlusion of the right upper lobe pulmonary artery. There was no haemodynamic disturbance.

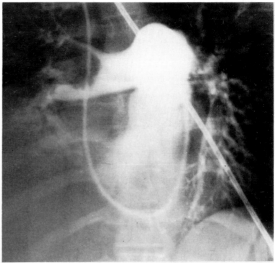

Fig. 20.10 Acute massive pulmonary embolism. Pulmonary arteriogram. There is a 'saddle embolus' astride the bifurcation of the right pulmonary artery causing a convex filling defect typical of acute (recent) embolism.

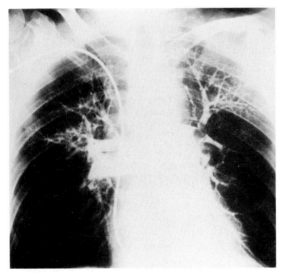

Fig. 20.9 Acute massive pulmonary embolism. Pulmonary arteriogram. There is occlusion of all but the upper lobe arteries, and emboli are seen as filling defects outlined by contrast medium within the pulmonary arteries.

lumen, other emboli will have lost the sharp edge and convex bulge and will be detected because the pulmonary artery beyond is not opacified (Figs. 20.7–20.10).

When pulmonary arteriography is being performed there is an opportunity for measuring right heart pressures. Pressures will be normal in minor embolism but in massive embolism there will be:

- a raised right atrial pressure (mean approximately 9 mmHg), often with a prounounced 'a' wave,
- a right ventricular and pulmonary artery systolic pressure of approximately 40 mmHg,
- a raised right ventricular end-diastolic pressure (12 mmHg) (Fig. 20.11).

If a sample of blood is taken from the pulmonary artery, its saturation will be low, reflecting the low cardiac output; an arterial sample will be approximately 86 per cent saturated. Unfortunately, there is no constant relationship between the height of the pulmonary artery pressure and the severity of acute embolism. This is because as obstruction to outflow increases the right ventricle fails; relatively low pressures may acompany the most massive embolism and herald imminent death. As previously discussed, a high pulmonary artery pressure is a feature of longer standing embolism; the highest pressures are found in patients with chronic embolism.

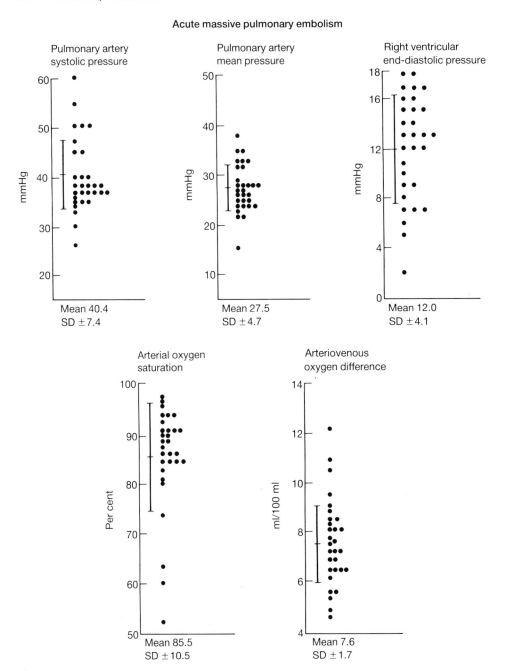

Fig. 20.11   Haemodynamic findings at the time of emergency pulmonary arteriography in 30 patients with angiographically proven isolated acute massive pulmonary embolism.

Lung scanning

Lung scanning for pulmonary embolism has the advantage that it is 'non-invasive' but has the disadvantage that it requires co-operation from the patient and takes some time to prepare and perform. A simple perfusion scan using[131]I-labelled or technetium-labelled macro-aggregates of human albumin will reveal areas of deficient pulmonary blood flow. There are, of course, many other possible causes for deficient blood flow but in the majority of these (*e.g.* space-occupying lesions) there will be an obvious abnormality of the chest radiograph. The finding of areas of deficient blood flow is therefore only suggestive of pulmonary embolism if the chest radiograph is grossly normal. Unfortunately, some patients with bronchial asthma or bronchitis and emphysema may have patchy abnormalities of perfusion with a grossly normal chest radiograph. In a study which compared perfusion scans with pulmonary arteriography Poulouse *et al.*[31] found that of 24 patients who had scans which were highly suggestive of pulmonary embolism only 18 (75 per cent) had angiographically demonstrated emboli. On the other hand, no patients in this study who had clinically suspected embolism and a normal perfusion scan were found to have angiographically detectable emboli. A lung scan seems to be an excellent screening procedure which, if normal, will certainly exclude embolism as a cause of a circulatory emergency. Positive findings should be treated with some caution. The reliability of lung scanning can be significantly increased if the perfusion scan is combined with ventilation scanning. The finding of areas of diminished perfusion without a matching deficiency of ventilation has been claimed to be specific for pulmonary embolism.[3,45] The choice between angiography or lung scanning as a diagnostic procedure will probably be dictated by local circumstances; in an emergency the clinician will use whichever technique is most readily available.

Pulmonary embolism – management

Minor pulmonary embolism

As minor pulmonary embolism causes no important haemodynamic disturbance, there is no need to treat the embolus, though pleuritic pain may require analgesia for symptomatic relief. Whether or not to treat the deep vein thrombosis and whether or not further embolism can be prevented by such treatment is discussed in Chapters 18 and 21.

Acute massive pulmonary embolism

The management of acute massive embolism can be divided as follows

- immediate rescuscitation
- specific treatment
- after care.

Resuscitation

Any patient who has suffered a 'cardiac arrest' is likely to be treated according to a standard protocol. This will include the administration of oxygen by mask or endotracheal intubation, external cardiac massage, correction of acidosis by intravenous administration of sodium bicarbonate and the administration of vasopressor and/or inotropic agents. All these measures are more or less appropriate when cardiac arrest is due to massive pulmonary embolism. External cardiac massage maintains some cardiac output in the presence of a failing left ventricle. In massive pulmonary embolism there is nothing wrong with the left ventricle; the low output state is the result of obstructed right ventricular outflow with a catastrophic fall in pulmonary venous return and left ventricular filling. External massage cannot therefore be expected to have much effect when the arrest is due to massive embolism. There is, however, some evidence that external massage may cause fragmentation and onward propulsion of the embolic material further into the pulmonary arterial tree where its obstructing effect will be less than when it is situated in the main left or right pulmonary arteries.[18] Vigorous massage does, however, involve some danger; one of our patients died not from the embolus (which was removed by pulmonary embolectomy) but from a ruptured liver resulting from over-enthusiastic external massage at the time of the original cardiac arrest.

In addition to conventional rescuscitative measures, it is crucially important that right ventricular filling pressure must be maintained to assist the failing right ventricle by the Starling effect. Systemic venous return is maximal in the supine position; patients with massive pulmonary embolism should therefore be nursed lying flat (in contradistinction to patients with left heart failure and pulmonary oedema). No drug which might have a vasodilator effect should be given; in particular, the administration of morphine can be fatal both by causing vasodilatation and by depressing respiration.

Theoretically, right ventricular filling pressure, and hence right ventricular performance, could be improved by transfusion of a plasma expander (e.g. low molecular weight dextran). This treatment has been used as part of the emergency treatment of massive pulmonary embolism when right atrial pressure is not grossly elevated.[4] In many patients, however, the right ventricle is already grossly distended and these patients may deteriorate further if they are given a transfusion. Isoprenaline may be given to improve right ventricular function and has the advantage of lowering pulmonary arteriolar resistance; it has the disadvantage, however, of causing systemic vasodilatation with consequent lowering of the filling pressure. It is doubtful if vasopressor drugs play any useful part in the emergency treatment of a patient who is probably already maximally vasoconstricted. As a last resort, adrenaline and bolus injections of calcium chloride may sustain the circulation while the patient is being prepared for emergency embolectomy.

Finally, in acute massive pulmonary embolism, the immediate intravenous administration of a large dose of heparin (15,000 units) has been advocated.[2,10,19,29] The theoretical basis for this recommendation lies in the demonstration (in animal experiments) of a serotonin-mediated pulmonary vasoconstrictor effect which accompanies the passage of embolic material to the lungs. This effect can be blocked by large doses of heparin. There is no evidence for this effect in man; the high pulmonary resistance is probably due to the mechanical effect of the occluding emboli. Nonetheless, there is some anecdotal evidence that the immediate administration of a bolus of heparin may be life-saving and cannot, in any case, do harm.

If the cardiac arrest has occurred in a hospital with facilities for emergency femoro-femoral (vein to artery) bypass, this technique can be used to maintain the circulation before the patient is transferred to theatre for embolectomy[32].

The emergency rescuscitation of a patient who

Table 20.6 Massive pulmonary embolism – resuscitation

1. Attempt to maintain oxygenation – 100% oxygen by face mask or endotracheal intubation
2. Correct acidosis – intravenous sodium bicarbonate
3. Maintain venous return at all times – supine position, no vasodilator drugs. Morphine contraindicated
4. A bolus of 15,000 units of heparin, intravenously may be beneficial
5. External cardiac massage may be required but may be ineffective

has suffered a cardiac arrest as a result of massive pulmonary embolism is summarized in Table 20.6.

Specific treatment

The next step in management is to establish the diagnosis by pulmonary angiography or lung scintillation scanning. Only when these techniques are not immediately available should treatment be started on the basis of the physical signs (chest radiograph and ECG) alone. However, the overriding principle of management should be to recognize the urgent need to establish specific treatment. Massive pulmonary embolism is a life-threatening condition; that the patient has survived the initial cardiac arrest or syncopal episode and appears stable is no guarantee of continued survival. Although many patients who die from pulmonary embolism die within minutes or within the first hour,[12,15,28] there remains a significant proportion of patients who will die over the next few hours or days unless something is done to relieve the obstruction to right ventricular outflow and the consequent severe haemodynamic disturbance. There is little or nothing that can be done for those patients who will die soon after the onset of embolism; it is the patients who have survived for an hour or more who deserve our best efforts and who are salvageable.

Conventional treatment for pulmonary embolism is to give heparin by infusion or by repeated doses; however, heparin has no thrombolytic action. It can only be hoped that this treatment will prevent further embolism and that extension by thrombus formation distal to the occluding

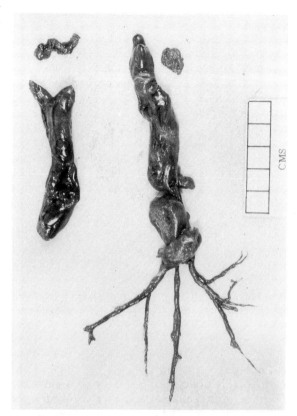

Fig. 20.12 Material removed at emergency pulmonary embolectomy. Note that beyond the embolus 'thrombosis *in situ*' has formed a cast of the branching pulmonary artery.

embolus ('thrombosis *in situ*', Fig. 20.12) will not occur. Resolution of the original embolus is left to the body's natural thrombolytic mechanisms. Naturally occurring thrombolysis is slow and may take weeks to be complete; indeed, there is evidence that such thrombolysis is never truly complete.[36] Two forms of active treatment are available: we may remove the embolus surgically or we may accelerate thrombolysis by giving thrombolytic drugs (e.g. streptokinase or urokinase).

Pulmonary embolectomy as a life-saving operation was first proposed by Trendelenburg.[40] Originally, it was suggested that haemostasis should be achieved by cross-clamping the pulmonary artery while the embolic material was being removed, so-called 'outflow occlusion'. Even today, in the era of cardio-pulmonary bypass, there may sometimes be a place for the (modified)

Trendelenburg operation, though haemostasis is obtained by cross-clamping the cavae ('inflow occlusion') rather than the pulmonary artery. Clark and Abrams have reported a mortality of only 30 per cent in a series of patients treated in this way.[8] Preferably, pulmonary embolectomy is carried out using total cardio-pulmonary bypass. Even in patients with massive embolism and shock the mortality from embolectomy need be no higher than 26 per cent; the majority of deaths result not from failure to re-establish normal haemodynamics but from complications of the initial cardiac arrest or its treatment (e.g. 'brain death').

The alternative to embolectomy is to accelerate thrombolysis by infusing thrombolytic agents. The first thrombolytic agent to be used in the United Kingdom was streptokinase; in the United States urokinase was employed. A number of early reports suggested that resolution of embolism is enhanced when thrombolytic drugs are given.[6,14,20,24,34,35,39] It is now well established that streptokinase or urokinase cause a more rapid[26,38,41-43] and complete[36] resolution of pulmonary emboli than occurs when anticoagulants (e.g. heparin) alone are given. The effect of thrombolytic drugs is most noticeable in those patients who are most in need of urgent treatment – those with massive embolism and shock Figs. 20.13–20.15.

Although thrombolytic drugs will accelerate the resolution of pulmonary emboli, this does not necessarily reduce mortality. In order to demonstrate that thrombolytic treatment or embolectomy improve the prognosis of massive pulmonary embolism it would be necessary to carry out a randomized trial with death as the end-point and a control group who receive either no treatment or heparin alone. We have not felt justified in withholding streptokinase or embolectomy in a patient whose clinical state was deteriorating while on heparin therapy. Instead of using death as an end-point we therefore used 'treatment failure', this was defined as either clinical deterioration leading to a change of treatment or a complication of treatment (e.g. serious bleeding). In this trial the treatment failure rate with heparin was about twice as high as that for streptokinase or embolectomy Fig. 20.16.[25] This experience is the basis for advocating thrombolytic therapy or embolectomy as the proper treatment for massive pulmonary embolism – at least when there is accompanying 'shock'. Thrombolytic therapy

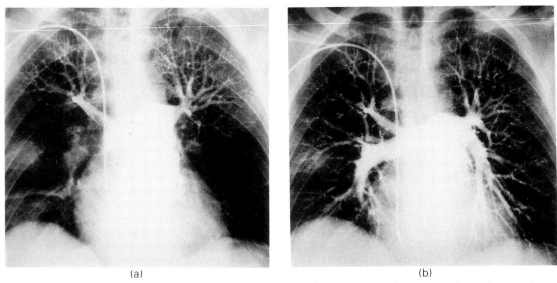

Fig. 20.13 (a and b) Acute massive pulmonary embolism. Pulmonary arteriograms performed at the time of admission to hospital (a) and again (b) 72 hours later following treatment with streptokinase. There is almost complete resolution.

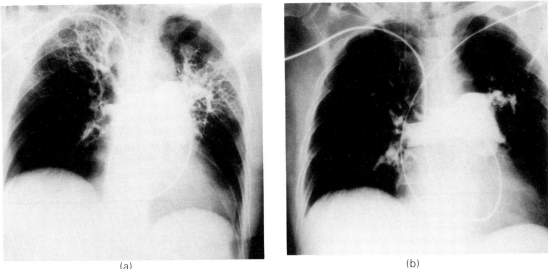

Fig. 20.14 (a and b) Acute massive pulmonary embolism. Pulmonary arteriograms performed at the time of admission and 1 week later following treatment with heparin. There is little, if any, angiographically detectable resolution.

was also advocated as the treatment of choice by a Consensus Development Conference on thrombolysis and thrombolytic therapy sponsored by the National Institutes of Health which reported in 1980.[9] There is now some evidence that, at one year after embolism, patients who received thrombolytic therapy initially have less residual abnormality than those patients who were treated with heparin alone; the latter group have a significantly lower pulmonary capillary blood volume.[36]

Thrombolytic therapy is contraindicated when there is an increased risk of bleeding or when any bleeding would be dangerous. This therapy should therefore not be used when there is a

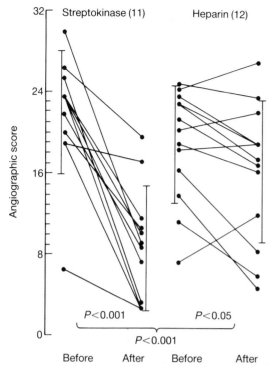

Fig. 20.15 Acute massive pulmonary embolism. Angiographically assessed severity before and 72 hours after treatment with streptokinase (left-hand panel) or heparin (right-hand panel). The vertical bars indicate 1 standard deviation about the mean. (Modified from Tibbutt *et al. Br Med J* 1974; **1**: 343.)

history of active peptic ulceration, when there has been a recent cerebovascular accident, when there is a history of severe hypertension or when there has been recent surgery, trauma or childbirth and bleeding would consititute a serious risk. In practice the risk of bleeding in post-operative patients is the most frequent contraindication. In many patients it is a recent operation which is the cause of the deep vein thrombosis and pulmonary embolism. However, thrombolysis can be used even in these patients provided the operation is one in which bleeding points have been tied and there is no risk of concealed haemorrhage. Thus a patient who has recently had an abdominal operation may be treated safely; however, a patient who has recently had a prostatectomy, for example, or has just been delivered should probably not be given thrombolytic drugs. Other contraindications include previous (within 3 months) streptoccocal infection or streptokinase therapy (strepto-

kinase is contraindicated because of the danger of anaphylaxis; urokinase can still be used), diabetic haemorrhagic retinopathy, coagulation defects (other than those caused by preceding anticoagulant therapy), pregnancy or breast-feeding and infective endocarditis. In all these situations emergency pulmonary embolism under cardio-pulmonary bypass is indicated. There is one other group of patients for whom pulmonary embolectomy is indicated; patients in whom pulmonary embolism is so massive and the clinical state is so precarious that immediate relief of the obstruction is needed if the patient is to survive. Thrombolytic therapy takes several hours for its effect to become apparent, and these patients may not survive that long. These patients have been described by Sasahara[33] who suggests that 'embolectomy is indicated when, after one hour of maximal medical management, (a) the systolic blood pressure is less than 100 mmHg; (b) the urine output is less than 20 cc/hour and (c) the arterial Po_2 is less than 60 mmHg.

The management of acute massive pulmonary embolism following resuscitation can be summarized as follows.

1. Recognize the urgent need to establish diagnosis, and start specific treatment. Massive pulmonary embolism is life threatening, even after recovery from the initial 'arrest'/syncopal attack. Transfer patient to intensive care unit; consider transfer to specialist unit with facilitites for diagnosis and open heart surgery.
2. If possible, establish the diagnosis – by pulmonary arteriography or lung scan.
3. Start thrombolytic therapy (see below), unless this is contraindicated.
4. If thrombolytic therapy is contraindicated transfer patient to operating theatre for embolectomy or consider transfer to a specialist unit if facilitites are not available.

Thrombolytic therapy with streptokinase may be summarized as follow.

0 hours Initial dose, 250,000 IU in 20–100 ml physiological saline by infusion over 30 min. Give hydrocortisone hemisuccinate 100 mg i.v. Reverse previous heparin (if any) with protamine. Obtain initial value for thrombin clotting time and prothrombin time.

30 min Maintenance dose, 100,000 IU/hour by infusion for 24–48 hour (e.g. 750,000 IU in

Early results — massive pulmonary embolism

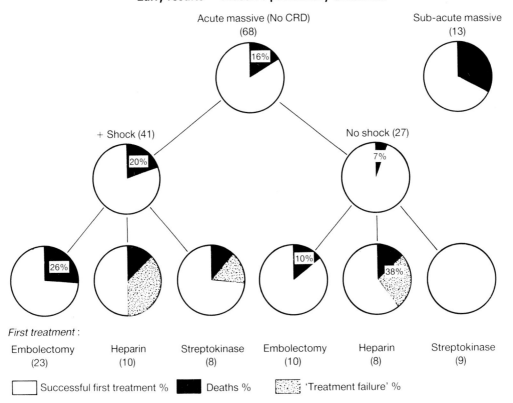

Fig. 20.16 'Pie diagram' summarizing the results of initial treatment with heparin, streptokinase or pulmonary embolectomy in 68 patients with isolated acute massive pulmonary embolism (no other cardio-respiratory disease – CRD). The patients are divided into those with shock (arterial blood pressure less than 100 mmHg systolic) in whom the overall mortality was 20 per cent and those without shock in whom the overall mortality was 7 per cent. The higher overall mortality for 13 patients with sub-acute massive embolism is also illustrated. (Modified from Miller *et al. Am Heart J* 1977; **93**: 568.)

500 ml physiological saline at approximately 20 drops/min to cover next 7.5 hours).

Following thrombolytic therapy the patient is changed to anticoagulant therapy, e.g. at 24–48 hours stop the streptokinase/urokinase, give 7500 IU of heparin by i.v. infusion over 12 hours and then start oral anticoagulants. Over the next 12 hours give 10,000 IU of heparin by infusion and thereafter control dose by monitoring thrombin clotting time (two to four times initial value) over the next 24 hours. Continue oral anticoagulants. At 48 hours, after the end of thrombolytic therapy, stop the heparin infusion and maintain the patient on oral anticoagulants (controlled by prothrombin time) for at least 3 months.

Bleeding is the only important complication of thrombolytic therapy. Sensitivity reactions seldom occur and are, in any case, avoided by giving hydrocortisone at the start of treatment; a mild pyrexia is common but is of no consequence. Bleeding from cut-down or venepuncture sites or from surgical wounds is almost invariable but should not be so severe that it causes problems; it can usually be controlled by local compression. Venepunctures should be reduced to a minimum and arterial puncture or cut-downs should be avoided. It has been our practice to leave a cardiac catheter *in situ* in the pulmonary artery following pulmonary arteriography; this catheter can be used for the infusion of streptokinase and for taking blood samples, thus avoiding more than one cut-down/venepuncture.

Pulmonary embolectomy has the disadvantage of being available in specialist units only and, of course, it requires open heart surgery and a median sternotomy. In all other respects it is a highly effective method of treatment – the abnormal haemodynamic state is rapidly restored to normal following removal of the embolic material. The most hazardous time is during induction of anaesthesia when drug-induced vasodilatation may lead to cardiac arrest, as already described. The anaesthetic should be as light as possible, and its danger may be minimized by the administration of metaraminol to cover induction. Bypass is established using right atrial and aortic cannulation. Following this, a 10–15 min period of ventilatory support will reverse the metabolic disturbance and oxygen debt. The pulmonary artery is then opened, stagnant blood is removed by gentle suction and the emboli are grasped and progressively removed. A final period of supportive bypass precedes closure and return of the patient to the intensive care unit.

It is not possible to make a meaningful comparison between the mortality associated with pulmonary embolectomy (approximately 25 per cent) and that associated with other treatments. Patients referred for pulmonary embolectomy tend to be the most acutely ill and those in whom all other treatment has failed. Many of the deaths are the result of brain damage which occurred at the time of a previous cardiac arrest. There can be little doubt, however, that pulmonary embolectomy can be life-saving.

One other mode of treatment which has been developed[16] is the transfemoral removal of emboli using a specially designed bell-mouthed suction catheter which can be passed, under fluoroscopic control, into the pulmonary artery.

Aftercare

It is general practice to continue oral anticoagulant therapy for 3–6 months following an episode of acute massive embolism. When there has been an obvious predisposing cause, for example surgery, childbirth or prolonged bedrest, it is probably safe to discontinue anticoagulants after this time, though anticoagulant prophylaxis should be re-instituted whenever a patient who has had an embolic episode is at risk again (e.g. when further surgery is planned). When embolism has occurred without a predisposing cause a case can be made for indefinite anticoagulation therapy, though this poses logistical problems and has its own risks. When the use of oral contraceptives was the predisposing factor an alternative method of contraception must be used. There are a very few patients in whom there are continuing episodes of embolism and in whom anticoagulants appear to be ineffective. It is in such patients that the insertion of inferior caval filters has been advocated. Before undertaking a procedure with a significant morbidity and mortality it is essential that repeated embolism should be proven beyond doubt. Patients have been referred to us with a diagnosis of 'repeated embolism unresponsive to anticoagulant therapy' in whom there was no evidence of repeated embolism and in whom pulmonary haemodynamics and pulmonary arteriography were entirely normal.

Sub-acute massive pulmonary embolism

The treatment for patients who have sub-acute massive pulmonary embolism is precisely the same as for patients who have acute massive embolism; unfortunately, the results are less satisfactory. Organized and adherent emboli which are more than a few days old are less readily dissolved by thrombolytic drugs and are less easily removed by embolectomy. Usually, a small improvement is seen following thrombolysis, and a small amount of material is removable at embolectomy (probably representing the most recent emboli). As patients with sub-acute embolism are those who, a week or so before, had acute massive embolism, this gradually worsening prognosis with time emphasizes the need to regard massive embolism as an emergency situation requiring urgent treatment. There is no excuse for prolonged heparin 'treatment' being given to a patient who is slowly deteriorating or who is having repeated episodes of synocope, breathlessness or pleuritic pain.

Chronic thromboembolic pulmonary hypertension

Although most physicians treat patients with chronic thromboembolic pulmonary hypertension with anticoagulants, there is probably no effective treatment for this condition which has a very poor prognosis. Occasional successes have been reported with anticoagulants[44] but the majority of patients will be dead within a few years of diagnosis. Isolated successes have been reported following late embolectomy.[5,27] Recently, Chitwood *et al.* have demonstrated that the chances of successful embolectomy in chronic pulmonary embolism are highest when bronchial arteriography has demonstrated patency of the pulmonary arteries distal to the occluding embolus.[7] Thrombolytic drugs are ineffective but it is possible that proteolytic enzymes (e.g. 'Brinase') may have a role to play, and isolated successes have been reported.[13]

Late results/complications

Apart from rare complications (e.g. necrosis and cavitation of lung) we are concerned with:

- early recurrence,
- late recurrence,

- the development of thromboembolic pulmonary hypertension as a sequel to acute pulmonary embolism.

Early recurrence seldom occurs following energetic treatment of massive pulmonary embolism; the incidence is less than 5 per cent. This may partly be the result of thrombolytic treatment which will promote lysis both of the emboli and of any remaining free-floating deep vein thrombi. It may be the result of anticoagulant treatment which prevents further embolism. Alternatively, it may be that patients who have survived massive embolism developed the condition because most of the venous thrombi became detached, leaving no others to cause recurrence. Whatever the reason, the low incidence of recurrence should prompt a reappraisal of the role of operations on the inferior vena cava (plication, umbrella filters, etc) designed to prevent recurrence. All these

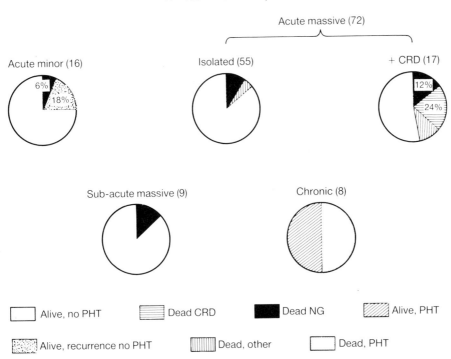

Late prognosis in treated survivors
n = 105   FU = 1–9 years

Acute massive (72)

Acute minor (16)   Isolated (55)   + CRD (17)

6% 18%   12% 24%

Sub-acute massive (9)   Chronic (8)

☐ Alive, no PHT   ▥ Dead CRD   ■ Dead NG   ▨ Alive, PHT

▒ Alive, recurrence no PHT   ▥ Dead, other   ☐ Dead, PHT

Fig. 20.17 'Pie diagram' summarizing the findings at follow up in 105 survivors of treated acute minor, acute massive (with or without associated cardio-respiratory disease) sub-acute and chronic pulmonary embolism.
PHT = pulmonary hypertension. CRD = pre-existing cardio-respiratory disease. NG = neoplastic disease. (Modified from Hall *et al. Br Heart J* 1977; **39**: 1128 and Sutton *et al. Br Heart J* 1977; **39**: 1135.)

procedures have a significant morbidity and a failure rate and mortality which are greater than the incidence of recurrent embolism. They certainly have no place in the management of the acute phase of massive embolism. The patient is in danger from the embolus he already has; caval plication or interruption, by drastically reducing venous return and filling pressure, is likely to prove fatal.

Late recurrence is also rare; in our experience possible further embolic episodes were only seen in patients who initially presented with minor embolism (Fig. 20.17).[37] It is known, however, that patients who have had one embolic episode are at increased risk of suffering another episode if there is a new predisposing factor, for example further surgery at some future date. Patients who give a history of previous embolism should receive heparin prophylatically whenever they are again at risk.

Finally, chronic thromboembolic pulmonary hypertension is a very rare late complication of proven and treated acute or sub-acute pulmonary embolism.[30,37] Patients who present with thromboembolic pulmonary hypertension seldom give a history of any previous condition suggestive of deep vein thrombosis or pulmonary embolism. The most common cause of late mortality is neoplastic disease, undetected at the time of the original embolism but a well-known predisposing factor.

Summary

Pulmonary embolism is a common condition, the incidence of which is, if anything, increasing. Clinical diagnosis is not generally difficult, provided it is recognized that pulmonary embolism is the cause of not one but several, clinically distinct, syndromes. One of these syndromes, acute massive life-threatening embolism requires prompt diagnosis and energetic treatment. Even with expert management, some patients will die, and these patients may well include young, otherwise fit, post-operative patients. Failure to employ prophylactic measures and failure to act promptly and to recognize the urgent need for active treatment must still be responsible for many unnecessary deaths.

References

1. Barritt DW, Jordan SC. Anticoagulant drugs in treatment of pulmonary embolism: controlled trial. *Lancet* 1960; **1**: 1309.
2. Bauer G. Clinical experiences of a surgeon in use of heparin. *Am J Cardiol* 1964; **14**: 29.
3. Bello DR, Mattar AG, McKnight RC, Siegel BA. Ventilation-perfusion studies in suspected pulmonary embolism. *Am J Roentgenol* 1979; **133**: 1033.
4. Bradley RD. *Studies in Acute Heart Failure.* London. Arnold 1977; 62.
5. Brock Lord, Nabil H, Gibson RV. Case of late pulmonary embolectomy. *Br Med J* 1967; **4**: 598.
6. Browse NL, James DCO. Streptokinase and pulmonary embolism. *Lancet* 1964; **2**: 1039.
7. Chitwood WR, Lyerly HK, Sabiston DC. Surgical management of chronic pulmonary embolism. *Ann Surg* 1985; **201**: 11.
8. Clarke DB, Abrams LD. Pulmonary embolectomy with venous inflow-occlusion. *Lancet* 1972; **1**: 767.
9. Consensus Development. Thrombolytic therapy in treatment. Summary of an NIH Consensus Conference. *Br Med J* 1980; **1**: 1585.
10. Crane C, Hartsuck J, Birtch A, Cough NP, Zollinger R, Matloff J, Dalen J, Dexter L. The management of major pulmonary embolism. *Surg Gynec Obstet* 1969; **128**: 27.
11. Dalen JE, Alpert JS. Natural history of pulmonary embolism. *Prog Cardiov Dis* 1975; **17**: 259.
12. Donaldson DA, Linton RR, Rodkey GV. A twenty year survey of thromboembolism at the Massachusetts General Hospital 1939–1959. *N Engl J Med* 1961; **265**: 208.
13. Frisch EP. Personal communication.
14. Genton E, Wolf PS. Urokinase therapy in pulmonary thromboembolism. *Am Heart J* 1968; **76**: 628.
15. Gorham LW. A study of pulmonary embolism. *Arch Int Med* 1961; **108**: 8.
16. Greenfield LJ, Peyton MD, Brown PP, Elkins RC. Transvenous management of pulmonary embolic disease. *Ann Surg* 1974; **180**: 461.
17. Hampton AD, Castleman B. Correlation of postmortem teleroentgenograms with autopsy findings with special reference to pulmonary embolism and infarction. *Am J Roentgenol* 1940; **43**: 305.
18. Heimbecker RD, Keon WJ, Richards KV. Massive pulmonary embolism. A new look at surgical management. *Arch Surg* 1973; **107**: 740.
19. Herman RE, Davis JH, Holden WD. Pulmonary embolism. A clinical and pathologic study with emphasis on the effect of prophylactic therapy with anticoagulants. *Am J Surg* 1961; **102**: 19.
20. Hirsh J, Hale GS, McDonald IG, McCarthy RA,

Pitt A. Streptokinase therapy in acute major pulmonary embolism, effectiveness and problems. *Br Med J* 1968; **4**: 729.

21. International Multicentre Trial. Prevention of fatal post-operative pulmonary embolism by low doses of heparin. *Lancet* 1975; **2**: 45.

22. Kakkar V V. The prevention of acute pulmonary embolism. *Br J Hosp Med* 197; **July**: 32.

23. Kerr IH, Simon G, Sutton GC. The value of the plain radiograph in acute massive pulmonary embolism. *Br J Radiol* 1971; **44**: 751.

24. Miller GAH, Gibson RV, Honey MH, Sutton GC. Treatment of pulmonary embolism with streptokinase; a preliminary report. *Br Med J* 1969; **1**: 812.

25. Miller GAH, Hall RJC, Paneth M. Pulmonary embolectomy, heparin, and streptokinase; their place in the treatment of acute massive pulmonary embolism. *Am Heart J* 1977; **93**: 568.

26. Miller GAH, Sutton GC, Kerr IH, Gibson RV, Honey M. Comparison of streptokinase and heparin in treatment of isolated acute massive pulmonary embolism. *Br Med J* 1971; **2**: 681.

27. Moor GF, Sabiston DC. Embolectomy for chronic pulmonary embolism and hypertension. Case report and review of the problem. *Circulation* 1970; **41**: 701.

28. Morrell MT, Truelove SC, Barr A. Pulmonary embolism. *Br Med J* 1963; **2**: 830.

29. Morris LE, Balk P. The management and mismanagement of acute venous thrombosis of the extremities. *Angiol* 1965; **16**: 339.

30. Paraskos JA, Adelstein SJ, Smith RE, Rickman FD, Grossman W, Dexter L, Dalen JE. Late prognosis of acute pulmonary embolism. *N Engl J Med* 1973; **289**: 55.

31. Poulouse KP, Rebal RC, Gilday DL, Deland FH, Wagner HN. Diagnosis of pulmonary embolism. A correlative study of the clinical, scan and angiographic findings. *Br Med J* 1970; **3**: 671.

32. Reul GJ, Beall AC. Emergency pulmonary embolectomy for massive pulmonary embolism. *Circulation* 1974; **50**; Suppl. 2: 236.

33. Sasahara AA, Barsamian EM. Another look at pulmonary embolectomy. *Ann Thorac Surg* 1973; **16**: 317.

34. Sasahara AA, Cannilla JE, Belko JS, Morse RL, Criss AJ. Urokinase therapy in clinical pulmonary thromboembolism. *N Engl J Med* 1967; **277**: 1168.

35. Sautter RD, Emanuel DA, Fletcher FW, Wenzel FJ, Matson JI. Urokinase for the treatment of acute pulmonary embolism. *JAMA* 1967; **202**: 215.

36. Sharma GVRK, Burleson VA, Sasahara AA. Effect of thrombolytic therapy on pulmonary capillary blood volume in patients with pulmonary embolism. *N Engl J Med* 1980; **303**: 842.

37. Sutton GC, Hall RJC, Kerr IH. Clinical course and late prognosis of treated sub-acute massive, acute minor and chronic thromboembolism. *Br Heart J* 1977; **39**: 1135.

38. Tibutt DA, Davies JA, Anderson JA, Fletcher EWL, Hamill J, Holt JM, Thomas ML, Lee GDJ, Miller GAH, Sharp AA, Sutton GC. Comparison of controlled clinical trial of streptokinase and heparin in treatment of life-threatening pulmonary embolism. *Br Med J* 1974; **1**: 343.

39. Tow DE, Wagner HN, Holmes RA. Urokinase in pulmonary embolism. *N Engl J Med* 1967; **277**: 1161.

40. Trendelenburg F. Uber die operative behandlung der embolie der lungenarterie. *Arch Klin Chir* 1908; **86**: 686.

41. Urokinase Pulmonary Embolism Trial. Phase I results. *JAMA* 1970; **214**: 2163.

42. The Urokinase Pulmonary Embolism Trial. A national co-operative study. *Circulation* 1973; **47**: (suppl. II): 1.

43. Urokinase-streptokinase Pulmonary Embolism Trial. A co-operative study: Phase 2 results. *JAMA* 1974; **229**: 1606.

44. Wilcken DEL, Mackenzie KM, Goodwin JF. Anticoagulant treatment of obliterative pulmonary hypertension. *Lancet* 1960; **2**: 781.

45. Williams O, Lyall J, Vernon M, Croft DN. Ventilation-perfusion lung scanning for pulmonary emboli. *Br Med J* 1974; **1**: 600.

21

Prevention of pulmonary embolism

The prevention of pulmonary embolism falls into two distinct categories: primary prevention – preventing the initiating thrombosis, and secondary prevention – preventing embolism from established thrombosis.

The first approach can only be applied when the time and place of the event that might cause a thrombosis is known (e.g. a surgical operation, parturition, or the beginning of a serious illness).

The second approach is applicable to all patients with a deep vein thrombosis and in particular to those who have already had an embolism. It consists of the therapeutic removal of the thrombus or the confinement of the thrombus to the limbs by some form of venous blockade.

In the late 1960s the development of the fibrinogen uptake test provided a method for testing the efficacy of a number of pharmacological and mechanical methods of prophylaxis against deep vein thrombosis. Although one of the aims of prophylaxis is the prevention of the symptoms of a thrombosis and its post-thrombotic sequelae, the main object is to reduce the incidence of fatal pulmonary embolism. It has been assumed that any method that reduces the incidence of thrombosis will have a similar effect on embolism, but it cannot be assumed that failure to reduce the incidence of thrombosis will mean failure to reduce embolism; and it cannot be assumed that changes in the incidence of the two events (thrombosis and embolism) will move in parallel. For example, it could be that the peripheral thrombi not prevented by a particular form of prophylaxis are the main source of emboli, whereas those thrombi that are prevented by the prophylaxis are the thrombi that would not have become emboli.

These arguments mean that it is essential to test the effectiveness of a prophylactic regimen in a clinical trial that is large enough to show a sig-nificant effect on a relatively uncommon event – fatal pulmonary embolism. Very few trials of this type have been performed. Unfortunately (from a scientific point of view), the results of the early trials were sufficiently suggestive of a positive effect to persuade the organizers of subsequent studies that it was unethical to include an untreated control group. This defect has led to endless discussion and disagreement over the significance of these later trials.

The results of the studies presented in this chapter are discussed in a highly critical manner. This is not meant to be a reflection on the workers who undertook the daunting task of conducting these trials but it is intended to demonstrate the difficulties that these studies present in both their conduct and their interpretation (difficulties which profoundly affect the conduct of our daily surgical practice).

Primary prevention

Oral anticoagulants

The seminal study of Sevitt and Gallagher in 1959[72] showed that the administration of oral anticoagulants to patients who had suffered a hip fracture reduced the incidence of fatal pulmonary embolism from 10 per cent to 1.3 per cent. Although there were only 150 patients in each group, the reduction in overall mortality rate was also significant. In 1966 Eskeland[28] found similar results; fatal embolism was reduced from 7 per cent to 1 per cent.

As so few orthopaedic surgeons used anticoagulants, Morris and Mitchell decided to repeat this study using warfarin.[60] Their groups were smaller (75 patients in each group) but the effect on fatal embolism was the same, 8 per cent in the control group, 0 per cent in the treated group. The difference in total mortality did not reach statistical significance probably because of the small number of patients studied (see Table 19.1, Chapter 19, page 544).

There has, therefore, been a known, proven, effective method of reducing total mortality from fatal pulmonary embolism and deep vein thrombosis after hip fractures since 1959, yet the method has not been adopted by surgeons because of the necessity for laboratory control of the anticoagulation and the high incidence of bleeding complications. Nevertheless, these studies must be the 'gold standard' against which studies of other prophylactic agents should be compared.

Heparin

The International Multicentre Trial published in 1975,[4] organized by Kakkar, studied 4121 patients. Of these patient 2076 were controls, and 2045 were given 5000 units heparin subcutaneously every 8 hours. One hundred of the control patients and 80 of the test patients died. In the control group 16 deaths were caused by fatal embolism compared with 2 deaths in the test group. The difference in overall mortality was not statistically significant. The difference in fatal embolism was statistically significant ($P < 0.005$) (Table 21.1).

Unfortunately, only 72 per cent of the patients who died in the control group and 66 per cent of the patients who died in the test group had an autopsy. Furthermore, the diagnosis of death was made by many different pathologists in different parts of the world. This presents two difficulties:

Table 21.1 The effect of low-dose subcutaneous heparin (5000 units, 8-hourly) on the incidence of postoperative pulmonary embolism[4]

	Controls (2076 patients)	Heparin (2045 patients)
Fatal pulmonary embolism	16	2
Embolism contributing to death	6	3
Other deaths	84	78
Total deaths	100	80

the obvious problem of lack of uniformity between centres but, more importantly, the fact that death from pulmonary embolism is a physiological event, difficult to diagnose at *post mortem*. For every patient who is dead in the autopsy room with a large embolus there is a living patient in the ward with an equally large embolus. The embolus is not the only factor that causes the patient's death; many other properties of the heart and pulmonary circulation are also involved (see Chapter 20). The pathologist cannot take these other factors into account and never sees the patients who survive large emboli.

A smaller study of the effect of low-dose heparin was published by Kiil *et al.* in 1978;[43] it involved 653 controls and 643 treated patients. They found no difference in the incidence of fatal pulmonary embolism, no difference in autopsy-detectable emboli and no difference (in a small subgroup) in the incidence of leg vein thrombosis.[44] Another subgroup was studied with ventilation perfusion scanning and showed no benefit from the heparin.[45] The absence of an effect of heparin on non-fatal lung scan-detectable pulmonary emboli has also been observed in a study from Cape Town.[38]

In a compilation of 28 studies of the effect of low-dose subcutaneous heparin on pulmonary embolism by Bergqvist,[12] the overall mortality rates for controls and treated patients were 4.4 per cent and 3.5 per cent respectively, and the fatal embolism rates 0.8 per cent and 0.3 per cent respectively. In 20 of these studies, however, no patient had a fatal embolism, and in two studies the incidence was not reduced. The overall apparent reduction of fatal embolism is derived solely from two studies, the Multicentre Study already discussed[4] and a smaller study by Sagar[70] which had a 16 per cent mortality rate in the control group. In our opinion and in the opinion of others[55] these figures do not support the widely held view[68] that subcutaneous heparin is a statistically and scientifically proven method for effectively preventing pulmonary embolism in general surgical patients. In our opinion the data is, however, sufficiently suggestive to affect our clinical practice (see page 550); this is a view shared by most surgeons.[13]

Dextran

Dextran was used for the prevention of pulmonary embolism before subcutaneous heparin but has not been studied in any very large randomly allocated controlled clinical trials.

Kline *et al.*[47] studied a group of 435 control patients and 396 patients who were given Dextran 70. They found 14 fatal pulmonary emboli in the control group and 4 in the test group; but there are some diagnostic and logistic defects in this study. Other studies of the effect of dextran on fatal embolism have been based on comparisons with historical controls.[5,46,51] These studies have shown a lower incidence of embolism during the periods of dextran administration but such analyses cannot be considered to be hard scientific evidence because of the lack of randomly selected comparable control studies. In fact, no large study of dextran (against no treatment) has been carried out which is comparable to the quality of the heparin Multicentre International Study. We performed a study[15] in which dextran and pneumatic compression was compared with controls in which the incidence of non-fatal pulmonary embolism was assessed with ventilation perfusion scanning. The test group had a significantly lower incidence of emboli but whether this was caused by the dextran or by the pneumatic compression is open to speculation. Bergqvist did not find that dextran reduced lung scan-detected pulmonary emboli in elective hip surgery.[10]

In a compilation of 23 studies of controls against Dextran 70, Bergqvist[12] found an incidence of fatal embolism of 1.5 per cent and 0.4. per cent respectively, but the statistical validity of such an exercise is open to question.

The data for the effectiveness of dextran, like the data for heparin, do not prove to our scientific satisfaction that dextran is effective against embolism, but the few small controlled studies plus the sequential retrospective analyses all suggest that dextran has an effect which is sufficient to affect our clinical practice.

The workers involved in large multicentre trials felt that the evidence that heparin and dextran reduced the incidence of fatal pulmonary embolism was so good that future studies did not need untreated control groups because they were both unnecessary and ethically unacceptable. Consequently, they embarked upon comparisons of heparin with dextran leaving the vital question of the real effect of both drugs on fatal embolism and total mortality unanswered.

Heparin versus Dextran 70

In 1980 Gruber presented a multicentre comparison of the effect of heparin and dextran in general surgical patients.[39] The dose of heparin was 5000 units, 8-hourly for 6 days; the dose of dextran was 500 ml during operation, 500 ml during the next 24 hours and 500 ml during the subsequent 24 hours. In this study 1991 patients were given heparin and 1993 were given dextran. In the heparin group 37 patients died; 38 patients given dextran died. Eighty per cent of the patients had autopsies. In the heparin group 3 patients were thought to have died of pulmonary embolism compared with 5 patients in the dextran group. Gruber concludes that both regimens have the same effect but this study does *not* show that either treatment is better than nothing at all. The main difference between Gruber's groups was the increased incidence of haemorrhage in those patients treated with heparin.

It is not valid to compare these results with the control group of a study performed 5 years previously. In the 1975 Multicentre Trial[4] the mortality rate of the control group, excluding the fatal emboli, was 4.0 per cent. In the heparin group, excluding the fatal emboli, the mortality rate was 3.8 per cent. In Gruber's 1980 study[39] mortality rate in the heparin group, excluding the fatal emboli, was 1.8 per cent. The patients studied in the first trial must therefore have been considerably different, as their mortality rate was twice that reported in the second study. It is quite unacceptable to equate the heparin arm of a 1975 trial with the heparin arm of a 1980 trial. This means that there is no way of deciding whether the 1980 heparin and dextran comparison trial had any effect on the incidence of pulmonary embolism whatsoever.

Mechanical methods

There are no studies of the effect of mechanical methods of prophylaxis on fatal pulmonary embolism, except an early clinical study of Wilkins *et al* in 1950 which was, unsupported by autopsy. The Wilkins' study showed a reduction of the incidence of fatal embolism in patients who wore elastic stockings.[77,78]

Clinical comment

The preceding paragraphs have discussed the evidence provided in the published clinical studies of the prevention of pulmonary embolism from a critical scientific point of view. Clinical medicine is rarely guided by hard scientific facts. Clinicians must make up their minds on the basis of evidence which they know will never be perfect because of the biological nature of disease and the patients it affects.

Although we have expressed grave doubts about the scientific validity of much of the evidence concerning the current methods used for preventing pulmonary embolism, this does not mean that we ignore it, rather it makes us wish to stimulate others to perform better studies, including untreated controls, and it affects our clinical practice as given below. It may never be unequivocally shown that these methods of prophylaxis truly cause a reduction in the incidence of thromboembolism because of the logistic problems of performing large clinical trials and because the incidence of the disease appears to be declining.[26,48,69] Our clinical policy is as follows.

Our primary prevention regimen

We believe that the circumstantial evidence is sufficient to justify the use of prophylactic agents against pulmonary embolism.

Patients less than 40 years old, who have no history of deep vein thrombosis, are given antithromboembolism stockings. If pneumatic compression is available, it can be used during and after operation. This attitude is based on the sound evidence that these methods reduce the incidence of deep vein thrombosis (see Chapter 19) and the knowledge that fatal pulmonary embolism is a rare complication in patients under 40 years of age.[11]

Patients over the age of 40 years who are having major operations are given antithromboembolism stockings on admission and either subcutaneous heparin (5000 units 12-hourly for 5 days) or Dextran 70 (500 ml × 3 in 48 hours). We prefer dextran because it is easier to give and causes fewer bleeding problems. Anaphylaxis can be almost abolished by the preliminary injection of hapten.

We advise orthopaedic surgeons performing hip surgery to use dextran or heparin plus dihydroergotamine (DHE) as this latter combination has a greater effect on the peripheral thrombosis of these patients than heparin alone and consequently may be more effective in reducing embolism.

For patients undergoing operations where a minor haemorrhage might jeopardize the result (ophthalmic, plastic, and neurological surgery) we prefer to use mechanical methods of preventing pulmonary embolism.

We protect patients at high risk (e.g. those with a known previous episode of pulmonary embolism) by administering oral anticoagulants or intravenous heparin starting before surgery.

If the current trials of low molecular weight heparin and heparin analogues find that these substances are as effective against embolism in a single daily dose as standard 12-hourly heparin, with a lower incidence of haemorrhage, we would consider adopting them and giving up dextran.

Secondary prevention (prevention of embolism from established thrombosis)

Thirty per cent of patients who survive a pulmonary embolism are known to have a second embolus, and 20 per cent of these second emboli will prove to be fatal.[6]

There will always be patients who have sporadic deep vein thrombosis because initiating incidents (e.g. an illness or an accident) often begin before prophylaxis can be started, and no form of prophylaxis is perfect. It is therefore important to ensure that a patient who has a deep vein thrombosis does not have a pulmonary embolus. It is even more important to ensure that a patient who has already had one pulmonary embolism does not have a second one which may be fatal.

There are three ways in which peripheral thrombi can be prevented from becoming emboli.

- The thrombus can be removed.
- The thrombus can be 'locked-in' in the limbs.
- The growth of new fresh thrombus can be prevented with anticoagulants.

It is common practice to treat a patient who has a deep vein thrombosis or pulmonary embolism with anticoagulants and hope that no further emboli occur. Table 21.2 gives the incidence of fatal and non-fatal emboli that occur if this approach is followed. The incidence of recurrent fatal emboli during and after treatment with heparin and/or oral anticoagulants can be as high as 10 per cent and non-fatal embolism can occur in 10–15 per cent. A compilation of 14 studies on 2196 patients (Table 21.2) reveals an average inci-

Table 21.2 The incidence of recurrent pulmonary embolism during and after treatment with heparin. A compilation of 14 studies* on 2196 patients, performed between 1947 and 1966

Incidence of recurrent fatal embolism = 2.5% (Range 0–18.6)
Incidence of recurrent non-fatal embolism = 8.5% (Range 1.0–19.1)
Total recurrence rate = 11% (Range 2–20)

*References 2, 7, 8, 19, 22, 23, 24, 29, 30, 41, 42, 50, 62, 64

dence of recurrent fatal embolism of 2.5 per cent and non-fatal embolism of 8.5 per cent – a total recurrence rate of 11 per cent. The studies of Table 21.2 were performed in the 1950s and 1960s but many recent studies have confirmed that the treatment of deep vein thrombosis with anti-coagulants does *not* abolish recurrent pulmonary embolism[16].

Phlebography

A rational approach to the problem requires its definition. The size, state, and age of a thrombus can only be determined by phlebography. In our opinion phlebography is the best investigation to guide the management of deep vein thrombosis and a mandatory investigation for all patients who have suffered a pulmonary embolus.[17]

The object of phlebography is to determine the nature of the thrombus and to assess the likelihood of further embolism. Treatment can then be conducted on a rational basis.[16] The phlebographs should show all the main veins in *both* legs from the ankle to the vena cava. Unilateral phlebography dictated by the side of the symptoms is not acceptable because the asymptomatic leg often contains a large non-adherent thrombus. Ascending phlebography which fails to delineate the iliac veins and lower vena cava is also inadequate. Further radiographs must be taken using femoral vein, or intra-osseous injections if necessary.

A sensible form of treatment cannot be planned without displaying the whole venous tree and the bottom and top of the thrombus.

The source of emboli

In a radiological study of the leg veins of 201 patients who had suffered a pulmonary embo-

lism,[18] we found residual thrombus in the calf of 26 per cent, in the thigh of 23 per cent and in the pelvis of 13 per cent. No thrombus was seen in 28 per cent, and 9 per cent were excluded from the calculations because they had asymmetrical bilateral thrombi. Forty-one per cent of the legs containing thrombus *had no physical signs*. These findings agree with the post-mortem studies of Gibbs[33] and show that, though the calf is the most common site for thrombosis, patients with pulmonary emboli frequently have thrombi in larger veins.

In another analysis of the phlebograms of a group of 50 patients who had had one clinical episode of pulmonary embolism,[16] we found residual thrombus present in 39 patients. In 17 patients it was below the level of the knee joint, in 15 patients it was in the superficial femoral vein, in 6 patients it was in the common femoral and iliac veins and 1 patient had residual thrombus in the vena cava. This distribution of thrombi is similar to that found in the larger series mentioned above. In this study, however, particular attention was paid to the nature of the thrombus. The thrombus was a fresh, non-adherent and considered to be a potential embolus in 19 of the 39 patients (38 per cent) with residual thrombus. In 1 patient the embolus was thought to have come from the calf. Fourteen (out of 15) of the patients had residual non-adherent femoral vein thrombi, and 4 (out of the 7) patients had residual iliac/vena caval non-adherent thrombi. Thus phlebography not only detected the presence of thrombus but indicated the likelihood of further embolism and the need for active treatment to prevent further embolism in 19 of 50 patients.

Thrombectomy or thrombolysis

Removing a thrombus stops it becoming an embolus. It may also relieve any venous obstruction and possibly save the valves. These two methods of treating deep vein thrombosis are discussed in detail in Chapter 18.

Surgical removal can only be complete if the thrombus has clearly defined limits which are accessible to a balloon catheter. A thrombus confined to the femoral vein can be completely removed. A thrombus in the femoral vein that extends into many small venous tributaries in the calf cannot be completely removed, even with repeated manual compression and calf bandaging during thrombectomy. In these circumstances thrombectomy may have to be combined with a surgical 'locking-in' procedure to prevent recurrent embolism, followed by anticoagulants to prevent new thrombosis.

Pharmacological thrombolysis with streptokinase or urokinase can lyse thrombi beyond the reach of the balloon catheter, but by causing thrombi to fragment these drugs occasionally cause emboli; this is rarely a serious complication. Thrombolysis successfully prevents embolism only if it dissolves all the thrombus, which is only possible if the thrombus is very fresh. `

Venous interruption

Pulmonary embolism cannot occur if the veins between the thrombus and the heart are occluded.

There are two ways of deciding where to occlude the veins. The first is to ignore the site of the thrombus and occlude the outflow tract of both limbs and the pelvis, in the vena cava below the renal veins. The second is to select the site of venous occlusion or partial interruption according to the site of the thrombus revealed by a phlebogram.

If a patient is having multiple small almost microscopic emboli, the vena cava must be ligated.[61,71]

Caval interruption[73]

This must be carried out with care in a patient with a raised pulmonary artery pressure and right heart failure because the sudden reduction of venous return may precipitate a cardiac arrest. We ligate the vena cava below the renal veins through a right flank extraperitoneal approach, while monitoring the cardiac output. A trial clamping of the vena cava before the ligation will confirm that it is safe to proceed.

All except very small emboli can be prevented from reaching the lungs by a partial occlusion of the vena cava. The many ways of achieving this occlusion are shown in Fig. 21.1. Surgical plication with multiple stitches, a grid of stitches and pericaval clips have been largely replaced by the development of filters that can be inserted transluminally, but surgeons should be aware of the earlier methods because they are still needed on special occasions.

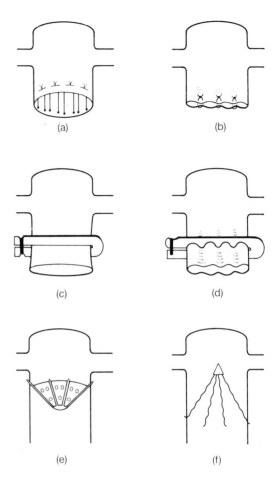

Fig. 21.1 Methods of partial inferior vena cava interruptation. (a) The DeWeese filter.[25] (b) The Spencer plication.[74] (c) The Moretz clip.[58] (d) The Miles clip.[54] (e) The Mobin-Uddin umbrella.[57] (f) The Greenfield filter.[35]

The filters which have been most studied are the Mobin-Uddin[56,57] and the Greenfield[35] devices. The Greenfield device appears to have the lowest incidence of complications (e.g. misplacement, migration, and thrombosis). It is inserted, under local anaesthesia, retrogradely through a venotomy in the internal jugular vein, guided into place under radiographic control and fixed in the vena cava just below (upstream) to the entry of the renal veins (Fig. 21.2).[34] Greenfield has reported a series of 303 filter insertions,[37] 30 per cent were inserted because anticoagulation had failed to prevent recurrent embolism and 37 per cent were inserted because the patient had

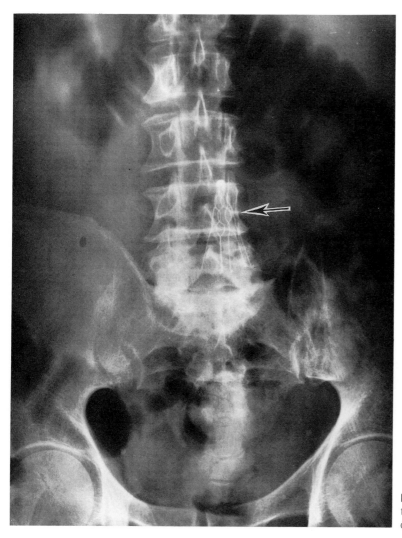

Fig. 21.2 A Greenfield filter in the lower part of the inferior vena cava.

a contraindication to anticoagulation. The filter was misplaced (usually in the iliac or renal veins) in 3 per cent of cases. No patient died as a result of the insertion of the filter.

One hundred and ten patients have been reviewed up to 7 years after filter insertion.[36,37] 44 per cent were still taking anticoagulants. Twelve per cent had had recurrent episodes of venous thrombosis and 4.5 per cent had had recurrent emboli. However, 45 per cent needed elastic stockings to control oedema and 9 per cent had venous ulcers. The long-term patency rate of those vena cavae that were normal and patent at the time of filter insertion was 97 per cent. The Greenfield filter can be placed above the renal veins.

There is little doubt that the Greenfield filter is better than the previously described devices in its facility of placement, prevention of embolism and ability to preserve vena caval patency. However, 45 per cent of patients subsequently need elastic stockings and 9 per cent get venous ulcers. Although the vena cava was patent in most of these patients, it is not clear whether the complications are caused by the original thrombosis or the filter.

No venous interruption procedure is 100 per cent effective,[27,65] and new devices continue to be invented.[52,66]

The use of vena caval interruption as a prophy-

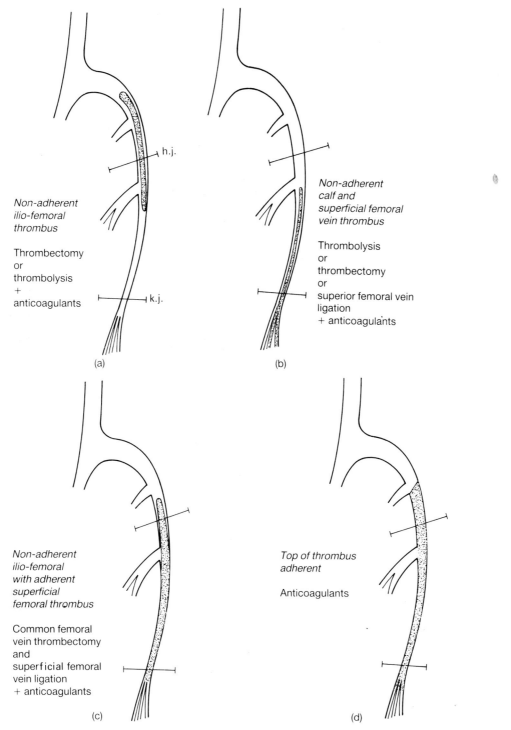

Fig. 21.3 Our scheme of treatment for the prevention of pulmonary embolism based upon the phlebographic features of the thrombus.

h.j. = hip joint; k.j. = knee joint. (All patients are given heparin for 7–10 days followed by warfarin for 6 months.

lactic measure has been advocated but not widely adopted.[20,31,49,67,71]

As the complications of any form of vena caval interruption affect both legs,[14,76] we prefer to select the level of our venous interruption procedures according to the phlebographic appearances, occluding the vein as close to the upper end of the thrombus as possible.

Phlebographically-based venous interruption

The results of phlebography in patients with both deep vein thrombosis and pulmonary emboli have been described earlier in this chapter. In a series of 50 patients, 19 legs contained non-adherent thrombus[16], in 11 patients the thrombus was below the inguinal ligament (in the superficial femoral or calf veins) and in another 3 patients the thrombus was below the inguinal ligament but extended into the common femoral vein. The thrombi in these 14 patients were all 'locked-in' by ligating the superficial femoral vein below the groin. This is a simple procedure that can be performed under local anaesthesia. Only 4 patients had thrombi in their iliac veins or vena cava with a propagating non-adherent tail that could not be removed through a common femoral venotomy because it was adherent; they all had a vena caval interruption. None of the 19 patients had emboli after their 'locking-in' procedure.

It is our experience that most loose residual thrombi in patients who have had a 'herald' embolus are below the groin. When the thrombus cannot be removed it can be 'locked-in' by ligating the superficial femoral vein just below its junction with the deep femoral vein.

This approach was suggested many years ago by Homans[40] and was practised extensively by his surgical service and others[1,21] but fell into disrepute because some patients had further emboli. We believe that further emboli occurred because the ligation was not preceded by a phlebogram but was carried out blindly. In some cases the ligature was probably tied around a thrombus in the femoral vein, not above the thrombus, thus making further embolism highly likely.

The ligation of the superficial femoral vein, in the presence of a pre-existing thrombosis, does not cause any additional symptoms in the legs. In a comparison[80] between patients with thrombus of a similar extent, but adherent at its upper end, treated with anticoagulants, and patients with non-adherent thrombus treated with femoral vein ligation, ligation did not increase the incidence of post-thrombotic symptoms. The symptoms score of patients with femoral vein thrombosis treated medically or surgically was the same. The percentage of patients in both groups developing the post-thrombotic syndrome 3 years later was quite high (50 per cent), and 10 per cent had venous ulceration. This incidence of complications is almost identical to that observed following the insertion of a Greenfield filter which suggests that the complications are caused by the initial thrombosis, not by the filter or the ligation.

The plan of treatment which we adopt is shown in Fig. 21.3. It is a combination of removal, locking-in or anticoagulation based upon the phlebographic findings. Our early studies convinced us that this policy reduced the incidence of pulmonary embolism without increasing the incidence of post-thrombotic symptoms in the legs.

Anticoagulants

Table 21.2 shows clearly that anticoagulants will not stop recurrent embolism; the explanation for this is shown in Fig. 21.4. Loose non-adherent thrombus will still fragment and embolize inspite of heparin. Provided anticoagulants are used as the main form of treatment only when there is adherent thrombus, recurrent embolism will not occur. In a comparison between a group of 50 patients treated with anticoagulants and a group of 31 patients who had phlebograms and anticoagulants alone only when there was no non-adherent thrombus in the veins above the calf, we found 20 recurrent emboli (7 fatal and 13 not fatal) in the first group and 4 small non-fatal emboli in the control group whose treatment was based on the phlebographic findings.[16] Only one of the emboli in the second group occurred within 1 month of treatment.

Our view of the significance of non-adherent thrombus has been confirmed in a study by Norris et al.[63] of 78 patients with deep vein thrombosis. Three of the 5 patients with non-adherent thrombus (60 per cent) had pulmonary emboli compared to 4 of the 73 patients with adherent thrombus (5.5 per cent).

Treatment based on phlebography therefore allows the rational use of anticoagulants alone in 60 per cent of patients and avoids the risk of recurrent embolism. Anticoagulants should be

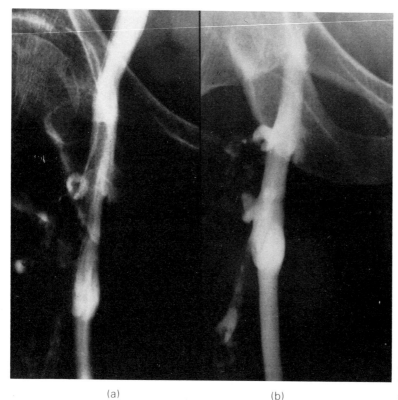

(a)   (b)

Fig. 21.4 (a) The phlebogram of a patient who presented with a small pulmonary embolus. The top of the residual thrombus is 'square cut' indicating that it has recently fractured at this site.

(b) The phlebogram of the same patient after 4 days of full anticoagulation with heparin, 1 day after a new episode of pleuritic chest pain. The thrombus has moved to the lungs. Heparin does not stop residual non-adherent thrombus from fragmenting and becoming a pulmonary embolus.

given to all patients who have a venous thrombosis or pulmonary embolism but will only prevent recurrent embolism in those patients with adherent or calf vein thrombosis. The effect of anticoagulants in these circumstances lies in their ability to prevent *new* fresh non-adherent thrombus forming.

Commentary

The studies discussed in the preceding section reinforce our view that no treatment of deep vein thrombosis should be undertaken without having a detailed knowledge of the state of the thrombus. Immediate anticoagulation is always indicated to prevent new thrombosis but in up to 20 per cent of patients additional surgical measures may be required to prevent a recurrent fatal embolism.

It has been suggested that to perform phlebograms on all patients who have had an embolus, however small, to pick up the 20 per cent that need more than anticoagulants is not cost effective, but amongst the patients with non-adherent thrombus will be that group (4 per cent of the total) who

will have a fatal recurrent embolism. A mandatory phlebogram on 100 patients, with adequate surgical action (if indicated) on 20 patients to save 4 lives seems to us to be worthwhile – until the day when deep vein thrombosis is completely abolished. Furthermore, the confirmation of the diagnosis and the subsequent avoidance of bleeding complications and death from *unnecessary* anticoagulation is undoubtedly worthwhile.

References

1. Allen A W. Interruption of the deep veins of the lower extremities in the prevention and treatment of thrombosis and embolism. *Surg Gynec Obstet* 1947; **84**: 529.
2. Allen E V, Hines E A, Kvate W F, Barker N W. The use of dicoumarol as an anticoagulant, experience in 2307 cases. *Ann Intern Med* 1947; **27**: 371.
3. Amador E, Li T K, Crane A. Ligation of inferior vena cava for thromboembolism. Clinical and autopsy correlations in 119 cases. *JAMA* 1968; **206**: 1758.
4. An International Multicentre Trial. Prevention of

fatal postoperative pulmonary embolism by low doses of heparin. *Lancet* 1975; **2**: 45.

5. Atik M, Broghamer W. The impact of prophylactic measures in fatal pulmonary embolism. *Arch Surg* 1979; **114**: 366.

6. Barker NW, Priestley JT. Postoperative thrombophlebitis and embolism. *Surgery* 1942; **12**: 411.

7. Barker NW. Anticoagulant therapy in thrombosis and embolism. *Postgrad Med J* 1947; **1**: 265.

8. Barritt DW, Jordan SC. Anticoagulant drugs in treatment of pulmonary embolism, controlled trial. *Lancet* 1960; **1**: 1309.

9. Benavides J, Noon R. Experimental evaluation of inferior vena cava procedures to prevent pulmonary embolism. *Ann Surg* 1967; **166**: 195.

10. Bergqvist D, Efsing HO, Hallböök T, Hedlund T. Thromboembolism after elective and post traumatic hip surgery – a controlled prophylactic trial with dextran and low dose heparin. *Acta Chir Scand* 1979; **145**: 213.

11. Bergqvist D, Lindblad B. A 30 year survey of pulmonary embolism verified at autopsy, an analysis of 1274 surgical patients. *Br J Surg* 1985; **72**: 105.

12. Bergqvist D. *Postoperative Thromboembolism*. Berlin. Springer-Verlag 1983; 102 & 138.

13. Bergqvist D. The prevention of postoperative embolism in Sweden. *Thromb Haemost* 1985; **53**: 239.

14. Blumenberg RM, Gelfland ML. Long term follow up of vena caval clips and umbrellas. *Am J Surg* 1977; **134**: 205.

15. Browse NL, Clemenson G, Bateman NT, Gaunt JI, Croft DN. Effect of intravenous Dextran 70 and pneumatic leg compression on the incidence of postoperative pulmonary embolism. *Br Med J* 1976; **2**: 1281.

16. Browse NL, Lea Thomas M, Solan MJ, Young AE. Prevention of recurrent pulmonary embolism. *Br Med J* 1969; **3**: 282.

17. Browse NL, Lea Thomas M, Solan MJ. The management of the source of pulmonary emboli. The value of phlebography. *Br Med J* 1967; **4**: 596.

18. Browse NL, Lea Thomas M. Source of non-lethal pulmonary emboli. *Lancet* 1974; **1**: 258.

19. Byrne JJ. Phlebitis. A study of 979 cases at the Boston City Hospital. *JAMA* 1960, **174**: 113.

20. Carmichael D, Edwards S. Prophylactic inferior vena caval plication. *Surg Gynec Obstet* 1967; **124**: 785.

21. Colby F. The prevention of fatal pulmonary emboli after prostatectomy. *J Urol* 1948; **59**: 920.

22. Coon WW, Mackenzie JW, Hodgson PE. A critical evaluation of anticoagulant therapy in peripheral venous thrombosis and pulmonary embolism. *Surg Gynec Obstet* 1958; **106**: 129.

23. Cosgriff SW, Cross RJ, Habif DV. Management of venous thrombosis and pulmonary embolism. *Surg Clin North Am* 1948; **28**: 324.

24. Crane C. Deep venous thrombosis and pulmonary embolism. *N Engl J Med* 1957; **257**: 147.

25. De Weese MS, Hunter DC. A vena cava filter for the prevention of pulmonary emboli. *Bull Soc Int Chir* 1958; **17**: 17.

26. Dismuke SE. Declining mortality from pulmonary embolism in surgical patients. *Thromb Haemost* 1981; **46**: 17.

27. Donaldson M, Wirthlin L, Donaldson G. Thirty year experience with surgical interruption of the inferior vena cava prevention of pulmonary embolism. *Ann Surg* 1980; **191**: 367.

28. Eskeland G, Solheim K, Skjörten F. Anticoagulant prophylaxis, thromboembolism and mortality in elderly patients with hip fractures. A controlled clinical trial. *Acta Chir Scand* 1966; **131**: 16.

29. Fontaine R, Kiény R, Tuchmann L, Suhler A, Babin S. Quelques réflexions sur les embolies pulmonaries d'après une statistique personnelle de 409 thromboses veineuses récentes. *Ann Chir Thorac Cardiovasc* 1965; **4**: 1296.

30. Fuller CH, Robertson CW, Smithwick RH. Management of thromboembolic disease. *N Engl J Med* 1960; **263**: 983.

31. Fuller C, Willbanks O. Incidental prophylactic inferior vena cava clipping. *Arch Surg* 1971; **102**: 440.

32. Gazzaniga AG, Cahill JL, Replogle RL, Tilney NL. Changes in blood volume and renal function following ligation of the inferior vena cava. *Surgery* 1967; **62**: 417.

33. Gibbs NM. Venous thrombosis of the lower limbs with particular reference to bed rest. *Br J Surg* 1957; **45**: 209.

34. Greenfield LJ, Langham MR. Surgical approaches to thromboembolism. *Br J Surg* 1984; **71**: 468.

35. Greenfield LJ, McCurdy JR, Brown PHP, Elkins RC. A new intracaval filter permitting continued flow and resolution of emboli. *Surgery* 1973; **73**: 599.

36. Greenfield LJ, Peyton R, Crute S, Barnes R. Greenfield vena caval filter experience: Late results in 156 patients. *Arch Surg* 1981; **116**: 1451.

37. Greenfield LJ. Results of catheter embolectomy and Greenfield filter insertion. In Bergan JJ, Yao JS (Eds) *Surgery of the Veins*. Orlando. Grune and Stratton 1985; 479.

38. Groote Schuur Hospital Thromboembolus Study Group. Failure of low dose heparin to prevent significant thromboembolic complications in

high risk surgical patients. *Br Med J* 1979; **1**: 1447.

39. Gruber UF, Saldeen T, Brokop T, Eklöf B, Eriksson I, Goldie I, Gran L, Hohl M, Jonsson T, Kristerson S, Ljungström KG, Lund T, Maartman Moe H, Svensjö E, Thomson D, Torhorst J, Trippestad A, Ulstein M. Incidences of fatal postoperative pulmonary embolism with dextran 70 and low dose heparin. An International Medicine Multicentre Trial. *Br Med J* 1980; **280**: 69.

40. Homans J. Thrombosis of the deep veins of the lower leg causing pulmonary embolism. *N Engl J Med* 1934; **211**: 993.

41. Jorpes JE. On the dosage of the anticoagulants, heparin and dicumarol, in the treatment of thrombosis. *Acta Chir Scand* (Suppl) 1950; **149**.

42. Kernohan RJ, Todd C. Heparin therapy in thromboembolic disease. *Lancet* 1966; **1**: 621.

43. Kiil J, Kiil J, Axelsen F, Andersen D. Prophylaxis against postoperative pulmonary embolism and deep-vein thrombosis by low-dose heparin. *Lancet* 1978; **1**: 1115.

44. Kiil J, Moller JC. Postoperative deep vein thrombosis of the lower limb and prophylactic value of heparin evaluated by phlebography. *Acta Radiol (Diagn) (Stockh)* 1979; **20**: 507.

45. Kiil J, Taagehoj-Jensen F. Pulmonary embolism associated with elective surgery, detected by ventilation–perfusion scintigraphy. *Acta Chir Scand* 1978; **144**: 427.

46. King R, Daly A. The prevention of postoperative pulmonary emboli with low-molecular-weight dextran. *Am J Obstet Gynecol* 1975; **123**: 46.

47. Kline A, Hughes LE, Campbell H, Williams A, Zlosnick J, Leach KG. Dextran 70 in prophylaxis of thromboembolic disease after surgery: a clinically oriented randomized double-blind trial. *Br Med J* 1975; **2**: 109.

48. Knight B, Zaini MR. Pulmonary embolism and venous thrombosis. A pattern of incidence and predisposing factors over 70 years. *Am J Forensic Med Pathol* 1980; **1**: 227.

49. Korwin SM, Callow AD, Rosenthal D, Ledig B, Deterling RA, O'Donnell TF. Prophylactic interruption of the inferior vena cava. *Arch Surg* 1979; **114**: 1037.

50. Little JM, Loewenthal J, Mills FH. Venous thrombo-embolic disease. *Br J Surg* 1966; **53**: 657.

51. Ljungström KG. Dextran 70 as prophylaxis against lethal postoperative pulmonary embolism. *Läkartidningen* 1975; **72**: 2284.

52. Maas D, Demierre D, Wallsten H, Senning A. A new vena caval filter for the prevention of pulmonary embolism. *J Cardiovasc Surg* 1985; **26**: 116.

53. Maraan B, Taber R. The effects of inferior vena caval ligation on cardiac output, an experimental study. *Surgery* 1968; **63**: 996.

54. Miles RM, Chappell F, Renner O. A partially occluding vena cava clip for the prevention of pulmonary embolism. *Am Surg* 1964; **30**: 40.

55. Mitchell JRA. Can we really prevent postoperative pulmonary emboli. *Br Med J* 1979; **1**: 1523.

56. Mobin-Uddin K, McLean R, Bolooki H. Caval interruption for prevention of pulmonary embolism. *Arch Surg* 1969; **99**: 711.

57. Mobin-Uddin K, Smith PE, Martinez LD, Lombardo CR, Jude JR. A venacaval filter for the prevention of pulmonary embolism. *Surg Forum* 1967; **18**: 209.

58. Moretz WH, Rhode CM, Shepherd MH. Prevention of pulmonary emboli by partial occlusion of the inferior vena cava. *Am Surg* 1959; **25**: 617.

59. Moretz W, Naisbitt P, Stevenson G. Experimental studies of temporary occlusion of the inferior vena cava. *Surgery* 1954; **36**: 384.

60. Morris GK, Mitchell JRA. Warfarin sodium in prevention of deep venous thrombosis and pulmonary embolism in patients with fractured neck of femur. *Lancet* 1976; **2**: 869.

61. Mozes M, Bogokowsky H, Antebi E, Tzur N, Penchas S. IVC ligation for pulmonary embolism. Review of 118 cases. *Surgery* 1966; **60**: 790.

62. Murray G. Anticoagulants in venous thrombosis and the prevention of pulmonary embolism. *Surg Gynec Obstet* 1947; **84**: 665.

63. Norris CS, Greenfield LJ, Herrmann JB. Free floating iliofemoral thrombus. *Arch Surg* 1985; **120**: 806.

64. Oschner A, DeBakey ME, De Camp PT, Da Rocha E. Thrombo-embolism. An analysis of cases at the Charity Hospital in New Orleans over a 12 year period. *Ann Surg* 1951; **134**: 405.

65. Parrish EH, Adams JT, Pories WJ, Burget DE, De Weese JA. Pulmonary emboli following vena cava ligation. *Arch Surg* 1968; **97**: 899.

66. Roehm JO, Gianturco C, Barth MH. Percutaneous interruption of the inferior vena cava. In Bergan JJ, Yao JS (Eds) *Surgery of the Veins*. Orlando. Grune and Stratton 1985; 487.

67. Rosenthal D, Cossman D, Matsumoto G, Callow A. Prophylactic interruption of the inferior vena cava. A retrospective evaluation. *Am J Surg* 1979; **137**: 389.

68. Ruckley CV. Protection against thromboembolism. *Br J Surg* 1985; **72**: 421.

69. Ruckley CV. Pulmonary embolism in the Edinburgh surgical audit. *Thromb Haemost* 1981; **46**: 18.

70. Sagar S, Massey J, Sanderson JM. Low-dose heparin prophylaxis against fatal pulmonary

embolism. *Br Med J* 1975; **4**: 257.

71. Schauble JF, Stickel DL, Anlyan WG. Vena caval ligation for thromboembolic disease. *Arch Surg* 1962; **84**: 17.

72. Sevitt S, Gallagher NG. Prevention of venous thrombosis and pulmonary embolism in injured patients. *Lancet* 1959; **2**: 981.

73. Silver D, Sabiston DC. The role of vena caval interruption in the mangement of pulmonary embolism. *Surgery* 1975; **77**: 1.

74. Spencer FC. Experimental evaluation of partitioning of the inferior vena cava to prevent pulmonary embolism. *Surg Forum* 1960; **10**: 680.

75. Stewart JR, Peyton JWR, Crute SL, Greenfield LJ. Clinical results of suprarenal placement of the Greenfield vena cava filter. *Surgery* 1982; **92**: 1.

76. Wheeler CG, Thompson JE, Austin DJ, Patman DR, Stockton RL. Interruption of the inferior vena cava for thromboembolism. *Ann Surg* 1966; **163**: 199.

77. Wilkins RW, Mixter G, Stanton JR, Litter J. Elastic stockings in the prevention of pulmonary embolism. *N Engl J Med* 1952; **246**: 360.

78. Wilkins RW, Stanton JR. Elastic stockings in the prevention of pulmonary embolism. II. A progress report. *N Engl J Med* 1953; **248**: 1087.

79. Williams BT, Roding B, Schenk WG. Experimental evaluation of haemodynamic effects of inferior vena cava ligation. *J Cardiovasc Surg* 1970; **11**: 454.

80. Young AE, Lea Thomas M, Browse NL. Comparison between sequelae of surgical and medical treatment of thromboembolism. *Br Med J* 1974; **4**: 127.

22

Superficial thrombophlebitis

Many words have been used over the past 100 years to describe venous thrombosis. 'Thrombophlebitis' and 'phlebothrombosis' were the terms in common use until 30 years ago; the former was used to describe a thrombus which was adherent to an inflamed vein wall, the latter was used to describe fresh thrombus free from or just loosely adherent to a normal noninflamed vein wall. Both words were used for thrombosis in any vein.

As our understanding of postoperative deep vein thrombosis grew, it became apparent that neither of these terms should be used, as neither of them described the precise pathology and, even if they did, we were unable to determine the pathology *in vivo* and apply the correct word.

The generally accepted solution is to use a simple term, that does not imply a pathological mechanism, for all forms of thrombosis in the deep veins, *deep vein thrombosis*, and reserve the term 'thrombophlebitis' for superficial thrombosis, secondary in most cases, but always associated with inflammatory changes in the vein wall.

Pathology

Superficial thrombophlebitis is the combination of thrombosis and phlebitis in a superficial vein in any part of the body. In most cases the thrombosis is secondary to the phlebitis but in some circumstances changes in the blood cause spontaneous thrombosis with a secondary phlebitis.

Aetiology

The common causes of an inflammatory response in the vein wall are as follows.

External trauma

A blow or prolonged pressure from the edge of a tight bandage can injure a superficial vein, particularly its endothelium. The resulting oedema, leucocytic infiltration and exposure of subintimal collagen following the shedding of damaged endothelial cells stimulates thrombosis.[16,46]

Thrombophlebitis is a common complication of varicose veins probably because their prominence makes them more vulnerable to local trauma.[11,20]

Superficial thrombophlebitis in pregnancy probably occurs because pregnancy causes varicose veins.[1] Whether venous stasis in varicose veins can cause a thrombophlebitis in the absence of a coagulation defect is extremely doubtful.[45] Thrombosis in varicose veins rarely extends into the deep veins but it can occur.

Internal trauma

A direct injury to the endothelium causing loss of endothelial cells initiates a progression of events which is the same as that initiated by external trauma.

Physicians are the common cause of intravenous injuries.[4,17,41] Simple venepuncture and indwelling catheters often cause phlebitis. The chemical composition of the infusion set and cannula also effect the incidence of phlebitis. The longer the catheter is in place, the higher the incidence of thrombophlebitis. Any injected substance which is not iso-osmolar and non-cytotoxic will destroy endothelium.[13,43] Many intravenous infusion fluids are both hypertonic and extremely noxious. Many drugs damage the endothelium. Common substances (e.g. pentobarbitone and diazepam) often cause a painful chemical thrombophlebitis, and the older contrast media used for phlebography sometimes caused superficial and deep phlebitis.

The slower the venous blood flow, the higher the incidence of thrombosis. Thus an injection into a vein on the dorsum of the hand is more likely to cause a thrombophlebitis than an injection into a vein in the cubital fossa. Many hypertonic phlebitis-promoting substances must be given directly into a large central vein where the blood flow is high, the catheter is in the centre of the bloodstream away from the vein wall and the injectate is quickly diluted.

The thrombus which forms around an intravenous catheter may become infected if organisms enter the vein through the skin puncture wound. This can give rise to an abscess and septicaemia.[8,27,34,40]

Post-infusion and injection phlebitis is a common cause of annoying and sometimes painful symptoms in all hospital patients and can cause pulmonary embolism.[47]

Primary vein wall inflammation

Inflammatory changes may arise spontaneously in the vein wall and cause thrombosis. The best example of this is the superficial thrombophlebitis which often precedes or accompanies thromboangiitis obliterans (Buerger's disease).[7] Although this condition is primarily an arteritis of unknown cause (but inextricably linked with smoking), many authorities will not diagnose it without clinical evidence of venous as well as arterial thromboses. The cause of the histological changes seen in the vein wall of patients with Buerger's disease has not been elucidated. In a neurovascular bundle the inflammatory process may simply spread directly from the artery to the vein, but in the superficial veins this cannot be the case.

Inflammatory changes adjacent to a vein, whether they be caused by trauma, infection, chemical or physical processes, can spread into the vein wall and cause thrombophlebitis. Infection may also spread into a vein and cause a septic thrombophlebitis.

Vein wall infiltration

Nearby disease, particularly malignant disease, may spread into a vein, replace the endothelium and cause a thrombophlebitis. Some tumours, notably carcinoma of the kidney and primary vascular tumours, actually spread along the lumen of their draining veins and cause it to thrombose. Carcinoma of the breast can cause superficial thrombophlebitis in the breast (Mondor's sign) and in the arm.

Vein wall fibrinolytic activator deficiency (idiopathic superficial thrombophlebitis)

A small group of patients present with recurrent episodes of superficial thrombophlebitis, but no evidence of occult malignant disease, collagen disease or vascular problems such as Buerger's disease. Some patients also have recurrent deep vein thrombosis.

The search to find a coagulation defect in these patients is usually unsuccessful,[19] except for the very rare coagulation abnormality of antithrombin III deficiency, but abnormalities of fibrinolysis have been found (Table 22.1). These patients may have a reduced resting level of blood fibrinolytic activity, a raised plasma fibrinogen, a reduced increase in blood fibrinolytic activity following venous congestion and a reduced vein wall activator production in both leg and arm veins.[5,21,31,33]

It is reasonable to assume that 'idiopathic' superficial thrombophlebitis is a primary abnormality of vein wall fibrinolytic activator production, the cause of which remains unknown.

Table 22.1 Mean blood and tissue fibrinolytic activity and plasma fibrinogen concentration in 16 patients with vein wall fibrinolytic activator deficiency (idiopathic superficial thrombophlebitis) and 48 normal subjects[23]

Test	Normal subjects (Mean)	Patients with superficial thrombophlebitis (Mean)	Significance of difference (*t*-test)
Dilute blood clot lysis time (min)	256	608	$P < 0.0001$
Fibrin plate lysis area (mm^2)	453	240	$P < 0.0001$
Plasma fibrinogen (g/litre)	2.75	4.13	$P < 0.0001$
Vein wall activator activity (units)	24	11.6	$P < 0.009$

Primary blood changes

Thrombosis following injury is clearly caused by the vein wall damage. The superficial thrombophlebitis associated with changes in the blood may also be a primary vein wall abnormality if the blood changes are the result of a failure of the venous endothelium to produce coagulation factors or fibrinolytic activators because the production of these substances by the vein wall is not only of importance to the coagulability of the blood as a whole but is also an important local protective mechanism.

A number of diseases which alter blood coagulability are associated with superficial thrombophlebitis.

The attacks of superficial thrombophlebitis caused by *occult malignant disease* are usually transient and migratory. The fault appears to be primarily in the blood.[10,36,37] Coagulation changes include an increase of factor VIII.

The vein wall fibrinolytic activity of patients with advanced carcinoma has not been studied extensively but the normal decrease of blood fibrinolytic activity that follows surgical operations is greater in patients with malignant disease.[6]

Primary blood diseases such as polycythaemia,[25] thrombocythaemia and sickle cell disease[26] can cause superficial thrombophlebitis.

What initiates an episode of thrombophlebitis migrans is not clear. It may be minor unnoticed local trauma, or a blood change plus a local change such as stasis, or a local loss of the vein wall antithrombosis protective mechanism. Whatever the order of events, there is ultimately a thrombosis and a phlebitis which lasts for a few days and then resolves, sometimes with venous recanalization.

Diagnosis

Clinical presentation

Local The patient presents with a tender 'sausage-shaped' mass which is deep to the skin. The surrounding tissues may be oedematous and the overlying skin may be red and hot. The mass corresponds to the line of a vein which may be visible and slightly distended upstream from the thrombosis.

There may be evidence of previous attacks of thrombophlebitis, for example pigmented areas of skin over thickened cord-like veins, and evidence of primary venous disease (e.g. varicose veins).

The pain and tenderness develops in a few hours and can be severe. The symptoms may extend along the whole length of a vein. Long saphenous vein thrombophlebitis may spread from the ankle to the sapheno-femoral junction and cause iliac vein thrombosis.

There is often a history of local trauma – a blow or prolonged pressure. The patient may have had an intravenous injection for the induction of anaesthesia or the administration of drug therapy.

General It is important to ask all the normal systematic questions, as these may reveal loss of appetite, loss of weight, backache, intermittent claudication or other symptoms of an underlying problem (e.g. an occult carcinoma or thrombo-angiitis obliterans).

Care must be taken to examine the calf muscles and the local lymph glands because the differential diagnoses include deep vein thrombosis, erysipelas, lymphangitis and acute lipodermatosclerosis.

Investigations

The initial investigations are directed towards finding a cause for the thrombosis (if it is not an obvious superficial thrombophlebitis in a large varicose vein) and excluding deep vein thrombosis.

Deep vein thrombosis is rare when the superficial thrombophlebitis is in a varicose vein (3 per cent) but it is present in 40 per cent of patients with superficial thrombophlebitis in clinically 'normal' veins.[3] The absence of varicose veins on clinical examination is therefore an indication for phlebography which occasionally reveals a non-adherent thrombus which is capable of becoming an embolus (Fig. 22.1).

Full blood investigations should be performed, especially coagulation factors, platelet count and platelet function studies, plasma fibrinogen and euglobulin lysis time. Blood studies may reveal a lymphoma or there may be polycythaemia, thrombocythaemia or sickle cell disease.

It may be necessary to perform X-ray contrast studies of the stomach, colon and kidney, gastro-intestinal endoscopy, chest X-ray and liver and pancreas computerized tomography (CT) scans to discover clinically occult malignant disease.

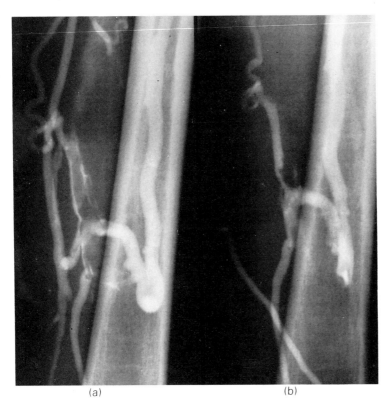

(a)   (b)

Fig. 22.1 (a) Non-adherent mural thrombus in a superficial vein.

(b) Adherent mural thrombus in a superficial vein.

Arteriography may be required to exclude thrombo-angiitis obliterans.

If all these investigations are negative, a histochemical study of vein wall fibrinolysis is indicated.

Treatment

The vigour of treatment depends upon the severity of the symptoms and the underlying cause.

Thrombophlebitis in varicose veins This is best treated with a firm compression bandage and by urging the patient to walk. Sitting still or lying in bed encourages the thrombus to spread. Firm support and mild analgesia (e.g. aspirin) usually relieves the pain sufficiently to allow walking. Many physicians give stronger anti-inflammatory drugs (e.g. indomethacin) but these drugs can have serious adverse effects and should not be used for a benign self-limiting, though painful, condition. An old-fashioned treatment is to apply a bandage impregnated with glycerine and icthyol. This makes the skin of the leg hot and acts as a counter irritant. It also sets into a firm good quality compression bandage. Apart from the fishy smell and grey colour this treatment has much to commend it.

Very occasionally, the pain is so severe that the patient has to rest in bed for a few days. If this happens, it is wise to give the patient intravenous or subcutaneous heparin until the pain has subsided and walking can begin because superficial thrombophlebitis can spread into the deep veins through the communicating veins.

Occasionally, a large varix thromboses and causes a large tender mass that does not subside within a few days. The pain and swelling can be relieved immediately by expressing the thrombus from the vein through a small venotomy made under local anaesthesia. An incision 0.5 cm long into the vein allows the surgeon to express the soft red-black thrombus which reduces the tension and instantly relieves the pain. One stitch and a pressure dressing controls any tendency to bleed.

Ascending long saphenous vein thrombophlebitis This is usually a complication of varicose veins but can accompany phlebitis of other origins. Once the thrombus passes the mid-point of the thigh, there is a risk that it will extend into the femoral and iliac veins and surgical treatment is urgently required.[15,28] The saphenous vein should be ligated at its termination and separated from the femoral vein. Before tying the vein, feel it carefully and open it to make sure that there is no intraluminal free-floating thrombus which a ligature might divide and turn into an embolus.

Infusion phlebitis

Most intravenous injection or infusion phlebitides resolve quickly if the injection or infusion is stopped. Although the vein is painful, it should be compressed with a firm bandage and the pain should relieved by mild analgesia. The arm should not be kept in a sling.

Infusion phlebitis should not be seen in the leg because intravenous infusions should never be given into leg veins, except in extreme emergencies.

The addition of heparin to the infusion fluid does not reduce the incidence of phlebitis[39] but the application of a heparinoid cream over the inflamed vein may produce symptomatic relief.[30]

Infusion phlebitis can be avoided by using non-irritant cannulae, iso-osmolar infusion fluids, changing the site of infusion after 24–48 hours, using large central veins for the infusion of phlebotoxic substances and taking careful antiseptic precautions.[12]

Infected superficial thrombophlebitis

If a thrombus becomes infected, the vein may have to be opened through a long longitudinal venotomy and the infected clot removed.[38] It is sometimes easier to remove the whole vein. Septicaemia caused by fragments of infected thrombus breaking free into the circulation is stopped by ligating the vein above the area of septic phlebitis and, if the thrombus in the vein is purulent, excising the vein.

Secondary thrombophlebitis migrans

Management of secondary thrombophlebitis involves treatment of the underlying cause plus palliation for the local symptoms – compression, mild support and exercise.

When thrombophlebitis migrans is associated with malignant disease this is usually advanced and inoperable; the underlying cause must, however, be sought and treated if possible.

If thrombophlebitis is caused by blood abnormalities (e.g. thrombocythaemia and polycythaemia) correction of the blood abnormality will stop the attacks of thrombophlebitis.

If a phlebogram reveals the presence of a deep vein thrombosis, the patient should be fully anticoagulated.

Vein wall fibrinolytic activator deficiency

If all investigations, except the tests of blood fibrinolysis and vein wall activator activity, are negative then it is reasonable to assume that vein wall fibrinolytic activator deficiency is the cause of the recurrent thrombophlebitis, and the patient should be treated by enhancing blood fibrinolysis.

Many drugs stimulate natural fibrinolysis in the short term but only two substances produce a sustained long-term effect. The drug we have used is stanozolol;[9] Nilsson has used ethyloestranol.[14,22,32] Both drugs are mild anabolic sex hormones. They both take between 3 weeks and 3 months to work but will return the tests of blood fibrinolytic activity to normal (Table 22.2). Both drugs cause mild water retention, and stanozolol has mild androgenic effects (oligomenorrhoea, acne and, very rarely, hirsutism).

In a group of 16 patients who had pure superficial thrombophlebitis, we found that stanozolol stopped the attacks in 13 patients and reduced their frequency in the other 3 patients.[23] The Malmo group treated 49 patients, who had a mix-

Table 22.2 The effect of stanozolol (5 mg b.d.) on the mean blood fibrinolytic activity and plasma fibrinogen of 12 patients with vein wall fibrinolytic activator deficiency (idiopathic superficial thrombophlebitis)[23]

Test	Before treatment	After treatment	Significance of difference (t-test)
Dilute blood clot lysis time (min)	578	172	$P < 0.003$
Fibrin plate lysis area (mm^2)	247	409	$P < 0.01$
Plasma fibrinogen (g/litre)	3.4	2.9	$P < 0.03$

ture of recurrent superficial and deep vein thrombosis, with ethyloestranol. They saw no recurrent attacks over a 16-month period in the 45 patients whose blood fibrinolytic activity returned to normal levels.[18] In both these studies the close correlation between the cessation of attacks and the return of blood fibrinolytic activity to normal adds weight to the belief that the cause of the thrombophlebitis was a deficiency of fibrinolysis.

References

1. Aaro LA, Johnson TR, Juergens JL. Acute superficial venous thrombophlebitis associated with pregnancy. *Am J Obstet Gynecol* 1967; **97**: 514.

2. Albrechtsson V, Olsson CB. Thrombotic side effects of lower limb phlebography. *Lancet* 1976; **1**: 723.

3. Bergqvist D, Jaroszewski H. Deep vein thrombosis in patients with superficial thrombophlebitis of the leg. *Br Med J* 1986; **292**: 658.

4. Brown GA. Infusion thrombophlebitis. *Br J Clin Pract* 1970; **24**: 197.

5. Browse NL, Gray L, Jarrett PEM, Morland M. Blood and vein wall fibrinolytic activity in health and disease. *Br Med J* 1977; **1**: 478.

6. Browse NL, Gray L, Morland M. Changes in the blood fibrinolytic activity after surgery. The effect of deep vein thrombosis and malignant disease. *Br J Surg* 1977; **64**: 23.

7. Buerger L. The association of migrating thrombophlebitis with thromboangitis obliterans. *Int Clin* 1909; **3**: 84.

8. Collin J, Collin C, Costable FL, Johnston IDA. Infusion thrombophlebitis and infection with various cannulas. *Lancet* 1975; **2**: 150.

9. Davidson JF, Lockhead M, McDonald GA, McNichol GP. Fibrinolytic enhancement by stanozolol. A double blind trial. *Br J Haematol* 1972; **22**: 543.

10. Edwards EA. Migrating thrombophlebitis associated with carcinoma. *N Engl J Med* 1949; **240**: 1031.

11. Edwards EA. Thrombophlebitis in varicose veins. *Surg Gynec Obstet* 1938; **66**: 236.

12. Elfring G, Hastbacka J, Tammisto T. Infusion thrombophlebitis and its prevention. *Am Heart J* 1967; **73**: 717.

13. Elfring G, Saikkn K. Effect of pH on the incidence of infusion thrombophlebitis. *Lancet* 1966; **1**: 953.

14. Fearnley GR, Chakrabarti R, Evans JF. Mode of action of phenformin plus ethyloestranol on fibrinolysis. *Lancet* 1971; **1**: 723.

15. Galloway JMD, Karmody AM, Mavor GE. Thrombophlebitis of the long saphenous vein complicated by pulmonary embolism. *Br J Surg* 1969; **56**: 360.

16. Ghildyal SK, Pande RC, Mistra TR. Histopathology and bacteriology of postinfusion phlebitis. *Int Surg* 1975; **60**: 341.

17. Hastabacka J, Tammisto T, Elfving G, Tiitinen P. Infusion thrombophlebitis. *Acta Anaesthesiol Scand* 1965; **10**: 9.

18. Hedner V, Nilsson IM, Isacson S. Effect of ethyloestranol on fibrinolysis in the vessel wall. *Br Med J* 1976; **2**: 729.

19. Hume M. Blood coagulation in deep and superficial thrombophlebitis. *Arch Surg* 1966; **92**: 934.

20. Husni EA, Williams WA. Superficial thrombophlebitis of lower limbs. *Surgery* 1982; **91**: 70.

21. Isacson S, Nilsson IM. Defective fibrinolysis in blood and vein walls in recurrent "idiopathic" venous thrombosis. *Acta Chir Scand* 1972; **138**: 313.

22. Isacson S, Nilsson IM. Effect of treatment with combined phenformin and ethyloestranol on the coagulation and fibrinolytic systems. *Scand J Haematol* 1970; **7**: 404.

23. Jarrett PEM, Morland M, Browse NL. Idiopathic recurrent superficial thrombophlebitis, treatment with fibrinolytic enhancement. *Br Med J* 1977; **1**: 933.

24. Jones MV, Craig DB. Venous reaction to plastic intravenous cannulae, influence of cannula composition. *Can Anaesth Soc J* 1972; **19**: 491.

25. Kwaan HC, Suwanwela N. Inhibitors of fibrinolysis in platelets in polycythaemia vera and thrombocytosis. *Br J Haematol* 1971; **21**: 313.

26. Kwaan HC. Inhibitors of fibrinolysis. *Thromb Res* 1972; **2**: 31.

27. Leading Article. Septic thrombophlebitis and venous cannulas. *Lancet* 1970; **2**: 406.

28. Martin P, Lynn RC, Dibble JM, Aird I. *Peripheral Vascular Disorders*. Edinburgh. Livingstone 1954.

29. Medical Research Council Trial. Thrombophlebitis following intravenous infusion. A trial of plastic and red rubber giving sets. *Lancet* 1957; **1**: 595.

30. Mehta PP, Sagar S, Kakkar VV. Treatment of superficial thrombophlebitis. A randomized double-blind trial of heparinoid cream. *Br Med J* 1975; **3**: 614.

31. Nilsson IM. In Davidson JF, Samama MM, Desnoyes PC (Eds). *Progress in Chemical Fibrinolysis and Thrombosis*. New York. Raven Press. 1975.

32. Nilsson IM, Hedner V, Isacson S. Phenformin and ethyloestranol in recurrent venous thrombosis. *Acta Med Scand* 1975; **198**: 107.

33. Pandolfi M, Isacson S, Nilsson IM. Low fibrinolytic activity in the walls of veins in patients with thrombosis. *Acta Med Scand* 1969; **186**: 1.

34. Pruitt B A Jr, Stein JM, Foley FD, Moncrief JA, O'Neill JA. Intravenous therapy in burn patients. Suppurative thrombophlebitis and other life-threatening complications. *Arch Surg* 1970; **100**: 399.

35. Ritchie WMG, Lynch PR, Stewart GJ. Effects of contrast media on normal and inflamed canine veins. *Invest Radiol* 1974; **9**: 444.

36. Soong BCF, Miller SP. Coagulation disorders in cancer. III Fibrinolysis and inhibitors. *Cancer* 1970; **25**: 867.

37. Stein JM, Pruitt BA. Suppurative thrombophlebitis, a lethal iatrogenic disease. *N Engl J Med* 1970; **282**: 1452.

38. Stradling JR. Heparin and infusion phlebitis. *Br Med J* 1978; **4**: 1195.

39. Thomas ET, Evers W, Racz GB. Post infusion phlebitis. *Anesth Analg (Cleve)* 1970; **49**: 150.

40. Thomas ML, Briggs GM, Kuan BB. Contrast agent induced thrombophlebitis following leg phlebography: meglumine ioxaglate versus meglumine othalamate. *Radiology* 1983; **147**: 399.

41. Vere D, Sykes C, Armitage P. Venous thrombosis during dextrose infusion. *Lancet* 1960; **2**: 627.

42. Welch GW, McKeel DW, Silverstein P, Walker HL. The role of catheter composition in the development of thrombophlebitis. *Surg Gynec Obstet* 1974; **138**: 421.

43. Wessler S. Thrombosis in the presence of vascular stasis. *Am J Med* 1962; **33**: 648.

44. Woodhouse CRJ. Infusion thrombophlebitis, the histological and clinical features. *Ann R Coll Surg Engl* 1980; **62**: 364.

45. Zollinger RW, Williams RD, Briggs DO. Problems in the diagnosis and treatment of thrombophlebitis. *Arch Surg* 1962; **85**: 18.

23

Congenital venous abnormalities

The blood vessels develop into their mature organized and remarkably constant pattern from a sponge-like collection of capillaries.[55] It is an extraordinary achievement of organization and growth, controlled by factors of which we have no knowledge or understanding. The end result is billions of humans with a remarkably similar venous anatomy. It is hardly surprising that this development occasionally falters leaving isolated individuals with abnormal veins. These congenital abnormalities are rare but must be recognized if only because they are often best treated conservatively. The unsightliness of these abnormalities combined with ignorance of their natural history tempts surgeons to treat them surgically but as they have been present since birth, any physiological abnormality that they might cause is usually well compensated, and direct surgical treatment may make it worse.

Pathology

There are four main forms of congenital abnormality of the veins: aplasia, hypoplasia, reduplication and the persistence of vestigial vessels. Each may be associated with other abnormalities of the cardiovascular and musculoskeletal systems. The valves may, independantly, be absent or abnormal. One group of abnormalities is sufficiently common to justify an eponym – the Klippel–Trenaunay syndrome.

Aplasia

Aplasia is a total absence of a vein. Failure of a segment of a vein to develop tends to occur when that vein has a complicated embryological derivation involving the union of a number of more primitive veins. For example, the vena cava has a

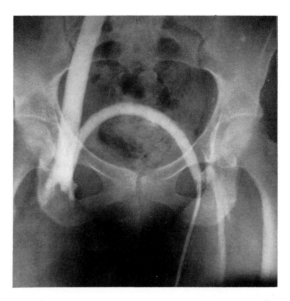

Fig. 23.1 Aplasia of the left external iliac vein.
X-ray contrast medium injected into the foot has ascended in the superficial femoral and saphenous veins as far as the common femoral vein. Thereafter it flowed across to the right common femoral vein. No iliac vein is visible. The patient had had a large vein across the abdomen since childhood and had never had a clinical event suggestive of deep vein thrombosis.

complex derivation (see Chapter 2) and is the most common site of venous aplasia.[13,40] Inferior vena caval aplasia usually affects the hepatic portion so that its *renal* segment has to connect with the right atrium via collaterals.

Aplasia of the iliac vein (Fig. 23.1)[24,29] and the deep veins in the leg is uncommon, except in association with the other abnormalities that form the Klippel–Trenaunay syndrome (see later). One-third of the patients with this syndrome have aplasia of the iliac, common superficial and deep femoral or popliteal veins.

The prevalence of venous aplasia has not been well documented.

Membranous occlusion

Membranes are sometimes left across a vein at the site where two primitive vessels should have connected.

Membranes are commonly found just below the diaphragm at the embryological junction of the subcardinal and the intersubcardinal anastomoses close to the point where the ductus venosus joins the left hepatic vein (Fig. 23.2).[18,41]

It is not known whether the membrane is a failure of fetal development or an extension of the obliteration of the ductus venosus. As the membrane is sometimes small, the stenosis extensive and the histological appearance variable, it has been suggested that it might be an acquired lesion superimposed upon congenital predisposition.[6] The membrane may be complete or perforated and consists of collagen, endothelium and elastic

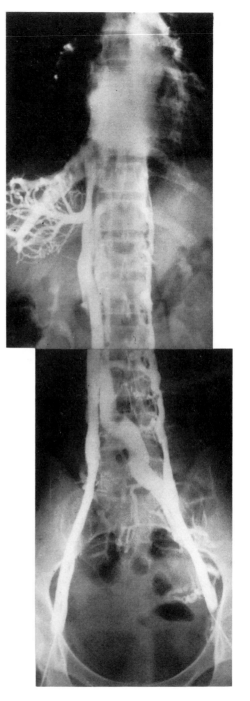

Fig. 23.3 Congenital hypoplasia of the inferior vena cava.

The right common iliac vein continues as a narrow hypoplastic vena cava. The left common iliac vein drains into the right and left lumbar azygos veins.

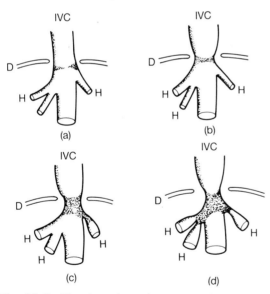

Fig. 23.2 The sites of membranous occlusion of the inferior vena cava.

Congenital stenosis or occlusion of the suprarenal inferior vena cava may take the form of a partial membrane (a), a complete membrane (b) or a membrane and thrombosis which may involve one or all of the hepatic veins (c and d).

IVC = Inferior Vena Cava; D = Diaphragm; H = Hepatic Vein.

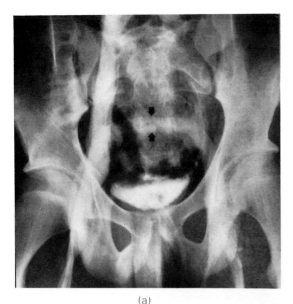

(a)

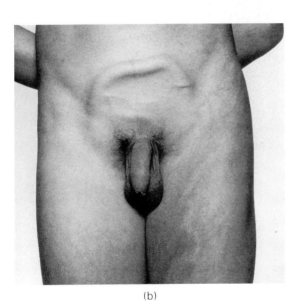

(b)

Fig. 23.4 Iliac vein hypoplasia in a patient with the Klippel–Trenaunay syndrome.

(a) This phlebogram shows a large collateral vessel crossing from the left to the right common femoral vein below a hypoplastic left external and common iliac vein.

(b) The large collateral vein shown in the phlebogram (a) was clearly visible in the subcutaneous tissues. The patient asked for the vein to be removed. He was told that it should never be removed or ligated because it was the main venous outflow tract of his left leg.

tissue but no muscle. The majority of reports about this abnormality have come from the eastern hemisphere. The prevalence of this condition is not known.

Hypoplasia

Patients presenting with the symptoms of aplasia of the inferior vena cava or iliac veins may be shown, with phlebography, to have a very narrow channel in the correct anatomical site suggesting that the vessel is hypoplastic not aplastic. Without direct examination of the vessel by surgical exposure and histological analysis, it is not possible to know whether such a phlebographic appearance is truly hypoplasia or an acquired abnormality secondary to an event such as thrombosis. Nevertheless, if veins can be aplastic, they must occasionally be hypoplastic. Figure 23.3 shows a patient who appears to have a hypoplasia of the inferior vena cava.

Hypoplastic veins are often associated with other abnormalities, for example the Klippel–Trenaunay syndrome (Fig. 23.4a and b).

The prevalence of venous hypoplasia is not known.

Reduplication

Reduplication of veins is common (see Chapter 2). Double inferior vena cavae, double renal veins passing in front, or behind the aorta, double superficial femoral and double saphenous veins are all well recognized (Figs. 23.5, 23.6).

Reduplication of the vena cava results from persistence of both lumbar supracardinal veins in their entirety. The two cavae may be of equal size, or the right vena cava may be larger. The mechanism that causes reduplication of lower limb veins is unknown but it is presumably a minor failure of fetal organization, as the structure of the second vein is alway identical to that of its partner.

Persistent fetal veins

This has already been identified as a cause of reduplication but sometimes veins that are present in the fetus in areas distant from the normal main veins may persist into adult life. The best example of this is the persistent lateral limb bud vein seen on the outer side of the leg of many patients with the Klippel–Trenaunay syndrome (see Fig.

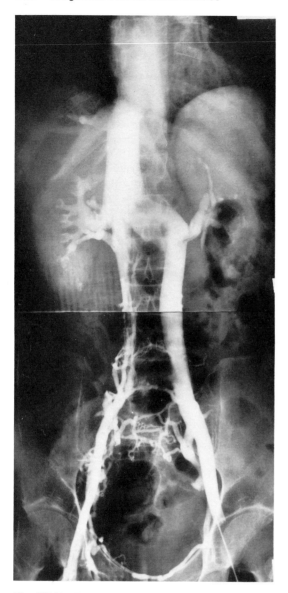

Fig. 23.5 Double (right and left) inferior vena cavae. The patient presented with swelling of the right leg caused by thrombosis of the right-sided vena cava following plication of this vessel to prevent recurrent pulmonary emboli. A phlebogram had not been performed before the plication. This phlebogram was obtained when the patient had further emboli via the left-sided vena cava.

23.12a). Some venous haemangioma should be included in this category. Many of these vascular malformations are not true tumours but are hamartomas or simply areas of disorganized

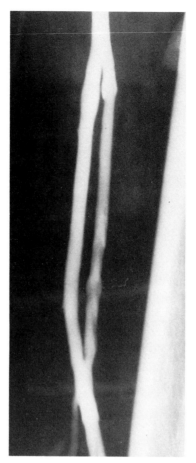

Fig. 23.6 A double superficial femoral vein. This is a common anatomical variant.

persistent fetal veins (see Chapter 26). These veins have the same histological structure as normal veins but are often dilated and without valves.

Valve abnormalities

Congenital absence of the valves is extremely rare.[5,27,36] It can affect only the lower limb veins or the whole body. We have seen three patients who had congenital absence of valves in 30 years experience, and less than 50 cases have been reported in the literature (Fig. 23.7).

Kistner has described a group of patients with *floppy valves*.[21] This abnormality is an enlarged valve cusp with a long, free edge that allows the cusp to prolapse when subjected to retrograde flow. Whether this is a congenital or an acquired abnormality is not known.

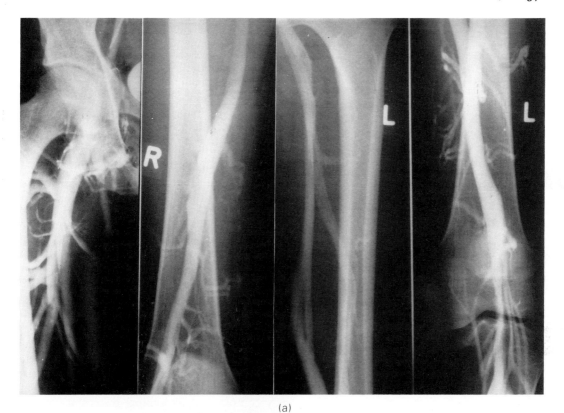

(a)

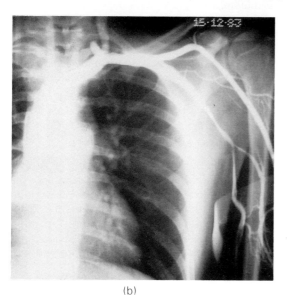

(b)

Fig. 23.7 Congenital absence of the valves.
(a) The descending phlebograms of a patient who had had swollen legs and recurrent ulceration since adolescence. The valve aplasia allows the contrast medium to reflux into all the tributaries. The absence of valves and valve sinuses gives the phlebogram an 'arteriogram-like' appearance.
(b) There were no valves in the arm veins.

Vein wall deficiencies

The walls of varicose veins and of veins taken from relatives of patients with varicose veins but without varicose veins themselves have been found to contain more of the tissue lysosomal enzymes that control mucopolysaccharide metabolism.[38] This may be the congenital abnormality that is responsible for the abnormal collagen and polysaccharide content of varicose veins and for their tendency to be a family trait.

Varicose veins are discussed in detail in Chapters 5, 6, 7 but are mentioned here to emphasize the fact that the primary (non-thrombotic) variety may be a congenital abnormality.

Major venous abnormalities are rarely found in association with other conditions which affect the collagen composition of the blood vessels to cause aneurysms and spontaneous rupture of arteries (e.g. Marfan's syndrome and Ehlers–Danlos syndrome), though varicose veins are said to be more common in patients with Type I Ehlers–Danlos syndrome. The veins are probably affected in the same way as the arteries but the intraluminal pressure may not be sufficient to cause fatigue and distention.

Congenital vena caval obstruction

Clinical presentation

Aplasia

The majority of patients with aplasias or hypoplasias have few symptoms and the clinical signs of a well compensated venous obstruction, because the abnormality has been present since birth and collateral vessels have had time to develop.

The most common complaint is of *visible varicose veins* in the subcutaneous tissues of the abdominal wall (Fig. 10.1, page 290). These are collateral veins which run across the abdomen and chest wall to connect the veins of the lower limbs with the veins of the axilla and neck.

Iliac vein aplasia may present with large suprapubic collateral vessels (Fig. 23.4b). Provided these collaterals are large enough to carry the increased blood flow that occurs during muscle exercise, the patient may have no other symptoms. If the collaterals are inadequate, the secondary changes in the upstream veins may cause aching pain, venous claudication, varicose veins, oedema, lipodermatosclerosis and ulceration. The symptoms of venous outflow obstruction are discussed in detail in Chapters 9, 11 and 12.

Subdiaphragmatic vena caval occlusion

The symptoms and signs of subdiaphragmatic vena caval occlusion are a mixture of the effects on the systemic venous return and hepatic blood flow.

The obstruction to blood flow from the limbs may cause oedema and venous distension. Collateral veins may be visible on the abdomen and chest wall.

If the condition is longstanding, skin changes develop in the lower leg, (pigmentation, eczema, lipodermatosclerosis and even ulceration may be present). The ulceration is often widespread and in sites other than the medial side of the lower leg.

The effect on hepatic venous drainage is similar to that of the Budd–Chiari syndrome, namely ascites, hepato-splenomegaly and portal hypertension with oesophageal varices. The patient may complain of abdominal distension and/or haematemesis.

Although the obstruction is above the level of the renal veins, uraemia and renal failure are uncommon.

As this is a congenital abnormality, the collateral venous circulation for the limbs and liver is often adequate for many years and patients do not develop symptoms until they are 20–30 years old.

Investigations

The most important investigation is a careful phlebographic anatomical delineation of the problem. Injections are needed from below (bilateral femoral phlebography) and sometimes from above (retrograde percutaneous catheterization via an arm vein) so that the extent of the occlusion and its relation to the hepatic and renal veins are displayed.

It is also essential to assess liver function (biochemically and by biopsy) and renal function. Liver function is usually normal, but there may be hypoproteinaemia if ascites and portal hypertension have been present for a long time. The liver biopsy will show centrilobular venous congestion, and possibly centrilobular cellular damage and fibrosis.

Blood coagulation should be studied if an operation involving a vascular prosthesis is contemplated.

Patients with complete aplasia of the hepatic portion of the inferior vena cava develop a large azygos vein. This usually provides an adequate outflow tract and the patient is therefore symptomless but the enlarged azygos vein may be visible on a routine chest X-ray (see Fig. 10.7, page 296).

Treatment

Aplasia of the vena cava rarely requires treatment. Symptoms in the lower limbs can usually be controlled with elastic stockings. If the patient has severe symptoms (e.g. venous claudication), the occlusion can be treated by *a bypass operation* between the highest part of the iliac system that is patent and the right atrium.[32,53]

The bypass (made of externally supported PTFE, 12–18 mm in diameter) is attached to the lower vena cava using an oblique retroperitoneal approach and is passed up behind the liver, through the diaphragm, before being attached to the right atrium which is exposed through a right anterolateral thoracotomy. The blood flow is normally sufficient to maintain patency, and an arteriovenous fistula is not required. It is wise to maintain the patient on antiocoagulants for 3–6 months while the lining of the graft becomes established and stable.

The same operation can be used for subdiaphragmatic membranous occlusions, provided the hepatic veins are patent and can drain retrogradely down the vena cava into the bypass.

If the hepatic veins are aplastic or obstructed by the aplasia or the membrane, the subdiaphragmatic vena cava must be exposed, the *membrane excised* and, if necessary, the *vena cava widened* with a patch graft of vein or PTFE.[54]

Sometimes the membrane can be split by direct pressure from a finger inserted into the vena cava via the right atrium[19] but this gives less satisfactory results than membrane excision.

A note of caution The large azygos vein carrying blood around an aplastic or occluded inferior vena cava may be discovered during a pulmonary or cardiac operation. We, and others,[12] have seen patients in whom this vein was ligated during the performance of the thoracic part of an oesophagectomy die as a result of hepatic and renal failure. Thus although vena caval atresia seldom requires surgical correction, the natural collaterals can confuse interpretation of the chest X-ray and cause technical problems during the surgical exposure of other intrathoracic structures. All surgical trainees should be told that if they meet a large collateral vein within the thorax, they should never ligate it.

Klippel–Trenaunay syndrome

Definition

This syndrome was first described in 1900 by Klippel and Trenaunay in the *Archives of General Medicine of Paris*[22] when they recorded the combination of a cutaneous naevus, varicose veins and bone and soft tissue hypertrophy affecting one or more limbs. Trelat and Monod[48] had previously noted an association between tissue hypertrophy and varicose veins.

In 1907 Parkes Weber[33] described a group of patients with limb hypertrophy associated with large arteries, an increased blood flow, and varicose veins.

For a number of years many investigators considered that these two publications described two variations of the same abnormality, and many classifications have grouped them together. The main cause of confusion was the mistaken belief that tissue overgrowth was always caused by arteriovenous fistulae but when Lindenauer[26] showed that venous obstruction without a change in blood flow may cause tissue overgrowth these two syndromes became disentangled.

Klippel–Trenaunay syndrome (KTS) This is an abnormality of the veins, skin capillaries, soft tissues and bones of the limb, *without any pathological arteriovenous fistulae.*

Parkes Weber syndrome This is the congenital persistence of multiple diffuse microscopic arteriovenous fistula. All the other features of the syndrome (e.g. limb overgrowth and varicose veins) are secondary effects of the fistulae.

The KTS is therefore a diffuse mesodermal abnormality, often associated with lymphatic dysfunction and other congenital abnormalities; whereas the Parkes Weber syndrome is a pure abnormality of the arteriolar microcirculation.

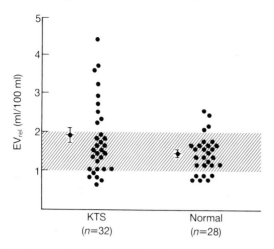

Fig. 23.8   The volume of blood (E V rel) expelled from the foot veins during knee bending exercise in 28 normal limbs and 32 limbs with the Klippel–Trenaunay syndrome (KTS). The shaded area is the normal range.

The difference between the mean values is not statistically significant.

Modified from Baskerville *et al.*, 1985.[3]

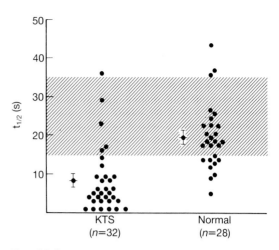

Fig. 23.9   The rate of refilling ($t_{\frac{1}{2}}$) of the leg veins, after exercise, in 28 normal limbs and in 32 limbs with Klippel–Trenaunay syndrome (KTS); the shaded area is the normal range. The difference between the means is statistically significant. $P < 0.0005$ (Mann–Whitney U test).

Modified from Baskerville *et al.*, 1985.[3]

The prevalence of these two congenital vascular abnormalities is not known.

Pathophysiology

The symptoms of KTS are related to disordered calf pump function and tissue hypertrophy.

Calf pump efficiency

Most patients with KTS have good calf muscles which can pump the venous blood out of the affected limb but the abnormal veins usually have incompetent valves which increase refilling time.[3] Figure 23.8 shows the relative expelled foot volume of 32 patients with KTS compared to that of 28 normal limbs. The variation of results amongst the patients is larger than in the normal limbs, but the number of patients who have expelled volumes below the 'normal' limit is no greater than in the normal group. The very large quantities of blood expelled from the foot in some patients is a reflection of the gross distention of the veins and the strong calf muscles of young adults.

Figure 23.9 shows the 50 per cent refilling time of the same group of 32 patients. The mean refilling time for the normal limbs was 21 s, and that

for the KTS limbs was 8.7 s. The refilling time was improved but not corrected by a mid-thigh tourniquet which occluded the superficial veins. There is no doubt that the abnormal subcutaneous and deep veins in limbs with KTS are grossly incompetent, yet the calf pumps of this group of patients (who had a mean age of 28 years) were able to deal with the reflux.

Calf blood flow

The mean resting calf blood flow of KTS limbs, measured by venous occlusion strain-gauge plethysmography, is approximately 50 per cent greater than that of normal limbs (Fig. 23.10). The range of blood flow is wide but even the highest rates of flow are still within the normal range.[2] There is therefore no haemodynamic evidence of arteriovenous fistulae. Multiple arteriovenous fistulae would cause blood flows 10–20 times greater than normal. Nevertheless, the increased blood flow does suggest a reduced peripheral resistance. It may be that this reduced resistance resides within the naevus because the mean blood flow of the KTS limbs with small or no naevi was 2.2 ml/min/100 ml, whereas the flow in the limbs with large naevi was 3.8 ml/min/100 ml; this is a statistically significant difference.

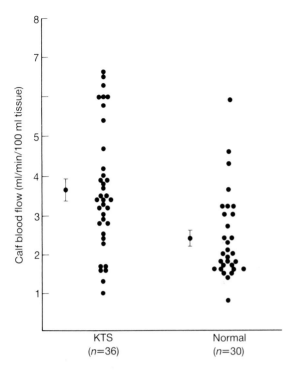

Fig. 23.10 The resting calf blood flow in 30 normal limbs and 36 limbs with the Klippel–Trenaunay syndrome (KTS). All the values for the two groups lie within the normal range but the difference between the mean values is statistically significant. *P* < 0.001 (Mann–Whitney U test).
Modified from Baskerville *et al.*, 1985.[3]

The blood flow is not related to the degree of hypertrophy.

These studies suggest that the subcutaneous venous abnormality and the naevus are congenital defects; the naevus allows an increased but not an abnormal resting blood flow. The tissue hypertrophy does not appear to be caused by either the increased blood flow (because it occurs in limbs without naevi and with normal blood flow) or the venous abnormality (because the calf pump function is usually normal). We believe it is a primary congenital abnormality of the mesoderm.

Bones and soft tissues

The bones and the soft tissues may overgrow, in some cases to a size justifying the term 'gigantism'.[49,52] Histological examination of these hypertrophic tissues reveals no abnormality.

All the constituents of normal tissues are present in normal amounts.

Many believe that the bony overgrowth is related to the changes in capillary and venous blood flow but the precise causal mechanism is not known.[17,46]

Veins

The walls of the abnormal veins are thickened and contain more muscle fibres which suggests an hypertrophic and hyperplastic response to the increased venous pressure.[2,25] The production of fibrinolytic activator by the walls of these veins, assessed by incubation on a fibrin plate, is reduced but the clinical significance of this observation is uncertain.

Blood

A careful study of the clotting factors in the blood of patients with KTS has revealed an increase of thrombin activation.[4] It is not known whether this is a primary or secondary abnormality.

Clinical presentation

Patients usually present soon after birth with one or a combination of the three main features – the naevus, tissue hypertrophy or varicose veins.[3,15,28,37,44,50,51,56] The naevus is usually the first abnormality to be noticed by the child's parents. Hypertrophy may not become obvious for years, and varicose veins are often not noticed until the child begins to walk or even many years later.

The degree and extent of each abnormality varies from patient to patient. Some patients have extensive naevi, a moderate number of varicose veins and little tissue hypertrophy. Other patients have gigantism, a few varicose veins and little or no visible naevi. In the 49 patients we have studied in detail[3] 47 had naevi, 49 had varicose veins and 36 had noticeable hypertrophy.

The majority of patients have KTS abnormalities in one leg, either leg being equally affected. In approximately 15 per cent of patients both legs are affected and in 5 per cent both legs and one arm are affected. In a few patients (5 per cent) the abnormality is confined to the arm.[9] KTS in all four limbs is very rare.

The naevus

At birth the naevus is usually pale purple. It may be a few patches on one limb, or it may involve the whole limb or the whole body (Fig. 23.11a–d). Approximately 25 per cent of patients have naevi which extend beyond the affected limb. In 50 per cent of patients the naevus tends to fade as the years pass, and in some patients it is almost invisible by adulthood. Sometimes the surface of the naevus is rough and verrucose. Prominent nodules are susceptible to injury and may bleed freely (Colour plate 34).

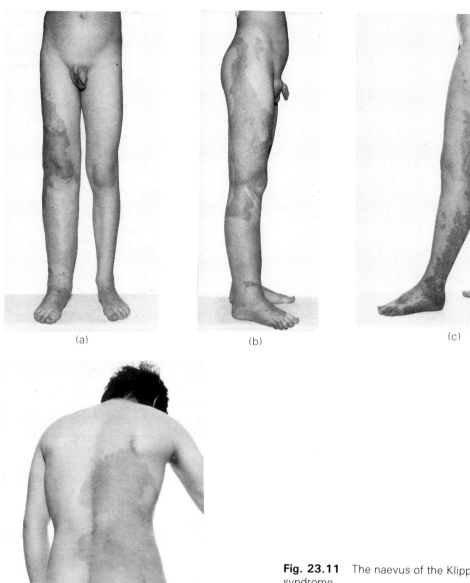

(a)   (b)   (c)

(d)

Fig. 23.11   The naevus of the Klippel–Trenaunay syndrome.
(a) and (b) Anterior and lateral views showing a 'metameric' appearance of the naevus. The subcutaneous veins are not prominent.
(c) A 'patchy' naevus.
(d) A naevus extending onto the buttock and trunk.

Varicose veins

The varicose veins are cosmetically disfiguring and cause discomfort and swelling in 90 per cent of patients. The pain is an aching sensation that is exacerbated by standing and gets worse as the day passes. The pain is relieved by elevating the leg and a night's rest.

The veins are often large and extensive and their appearance is a common reason for referral to a surgeon. Men often ignore the disfigurement as it develops slowly over many years but the combination of the prominent veins, naevus and hypertrophy leads most young women to seek treatment at an earlier stage.

The unusual distribution of the veins should alert the clinician to the possibility that they are not simple varicose veins, even if the patient presents in adult life. Although the common type of varicose vein can appear all over the leg, the larger dilated subcutaneous veins tend to run towards the line of the saphenous veins. The veins of patients with KTS are often in unusual positions, the most common being a large vein running down the *lateral side of the limb* (Fig. 23.12a and b, Colour plate 33). This is probably the fetal lateral limb bud vein which has failed to regress (the long saphenous vein is derived from the fetal medial limb bud vein). It may begin at the ankle, have many dilated tributaries and run the whole length of the limb to the upper thigh where it penetrates the deep fascia to connect with the deep femoral vein or disappears beneath the gluteus maximus muscle to join a tributary of the internal iliac vein. There are always many communicating veins between such a vein and the deep calf veins (see Fig. 23.19 and 23.21).

Sometimes the long saphenous vein is dilated (Fig. 23.12c) but it is often small and competent. Occasionally, both the lateral and medial subcutaneous veins are abnormal.

Varicosities may be present in the pelvis and be the cause of rectal and submucosal venous congestion and haemorrhage. In our own series of patients *20 per cent had rectal bleeding* and *10 per cent had haematuria*; 33 per cent had phlebographic evidence of abnormal intrapelvic veins.

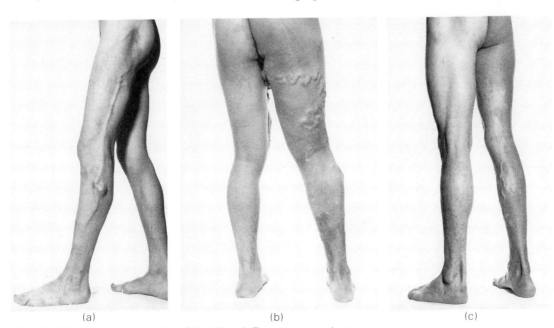

(a)   (b)   (c)

Fig. 23.12 The varicose veins of the Klippel–Trenaunay syndrome.

(a) The typical lateral vein. This vein passed beneath the gluteus maximus muscle to drain into the internal iliac vein.

The 'blow-out' in the mid-calf lay over a large incompetent communicating vein.

(b) A lateral vein which ran across the back of the thigh to drain into the postero-medial tributary of the saphenous vein.

(c) A dilated abnormal long saphenous vein. This patient also had abnormal veins on the lateral side of the leg.

Attacks of *superficial thrombophlebitis* are uncommon (6 per cent) but a history of chest pain, haemoptysis and collapse should be sought, as 20 per cent of our patients had clinical evidence of *pulmonary embolism*.

Swelling

Most legs with KTS are slightly oedematous but it is not always easy to distinguish a mild oedema from soft tissue hypertrophy until the patient has been in bed for 24 hours and the oedema has reabsorbed.

Gross oedema is rare except when there is extensive aplasia or hypoplasia of the deep veins or associated lymphatic obliteration (Fig. 23.13).

Oedema caused by these abnormalities will be made worse if the superficial veins are removed.

Skin changes

Pigmentation, eczema, lipodermatosclerosis and ulceration are uncommon (10 per cent) while the calf pump remains efficient; as the years pass the incidence of these complications increases (Fig. 23.14a and b). It is, however, unusual to find an elderly patient who has KTS with a venous ulcer.

Bone hypertrophy

Any or all of the bones in the limb may overgrow. A discrepancy between the length of the limbs is

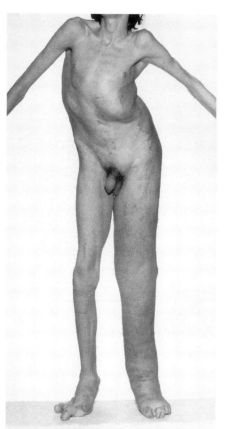

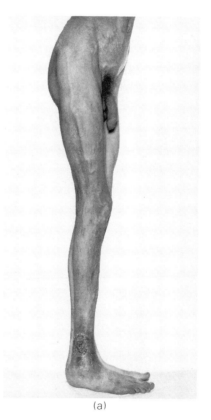

(a)

Fig. 23.13 Oedema of the leg. This patient, who had an elongated, hypertrophic limb with a naevus extending onto the trunk and a congenital deformity of the spine, had marked lymphoedema. A lymphangiogram showed peripheral lymphatic obliteration. Some parts of the naevus were covered with lymphatic vesicles (see Fig. 23.17a).

Fig. 23.14 The ulcers of the Klippel–Trenaunay syndrome.

Ulcers are relatively uncommon and often appear in unusual sites.

(a) This patient had an ulcer just above the lateral malleolus at the bottom of a long incompetent lateral vein.

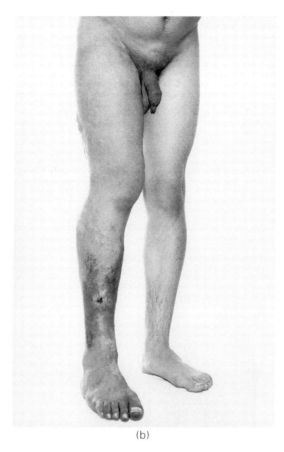

(b)

Fig. 23.14 (b) This patient had an active ulcer over the centre of the tibia and a healed ulcer above the lateral malleolus. His veins are shown in Fig. 23.12b.

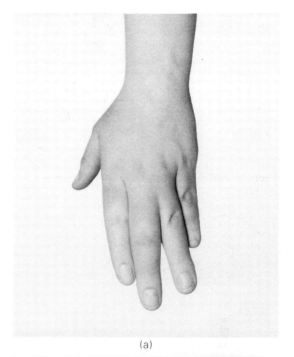

(a)

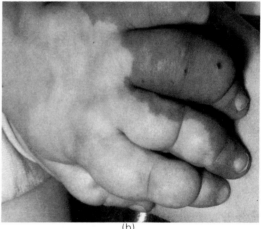

(b)

Fig. 23.15 Bony hypertrophy of the fingers.
(a) This patient had marked overgrowth of the middle and ring fingers of the left hand. A naevus and varicose veins were present in the forearm and upper arm.
(b) The bones of the thumb, index and little fingers are the same size as those of the right hand.

often present at birth. This may increase during the first few years but then tends to remain static; we have not seen the leg length disparity increase after the age of 10 years. This is an important difference from the Parkes Weber syndrome in which the overgrowth gets progressively worse throughout childhood until the epiphyses fuse.

There is no pattern to the bony hypertrophy. Sometimes all the bones of a limb are involved; less commonly, hypertrophy may affect the phalanges of one toe, or the bones of the lower leg but not those of the upper leg (Fig. 23.15a and b, Colour plate 35).

The difference in leg lengths may cause a lumbar scoliosis and flexion deformities of the joints of the hypertrophic limb.

Soft tissue hypertrophy

The majority of patients with KTS have some soft tissue hypertrophy, but the skin over the hypertrophied subcutaneous tissues and bone usually

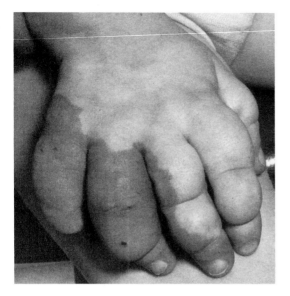

Fig. 23.16 Soft tissue hypertrophy.
This is the hand of a 30-year-old man with
Klippel–Trenaunay syndrome in both legs and in the
right arm. The enlargement is caused by soft tissue
hypertrophy. Sometimes there is plexiform
neurofibromatosis. The naevus is obvious. The hand
functioned normally.

looks quite normal. In two-thirds of our patients
with unilateral KTS the volume of the affected
foot was 5–50 per cent greater than that of the
normal foot. Some of this swelling was oedema,
some was caused by the dilated veins and some
was hypertrophy. It is often difficult to separate
these three different causes of swelling clinically,
except when the soft tissue overgrowth is localized
to a digit, or part of the foot (Fig. 23.16).

Other abnormalities

Lymphatics

The KTS is often associated with lymphatic
abnormalities.[31,56] Twenty per cent of patients
have cutaneous vesicles which leak lymph.
The groups of vesicles have the same clinical
appearance as the vesicles of lymphangioma circumscriptum but the underlying abnormality – multiple subcutaneous lymph cysts not
connected to the main lymphatics – is much more
diffuse than the lesion of lymphangioma circumscriptum (Fig. 23.17a and b).

Lymphangiography revealed peripheral lymphatic obliteration in 8 out of 14 of our patients,
the other patients were normal.[3] The lymphatic
defect is probably part of the general mesodermal
abnormality but it may be an acquired abnormality secondary to the prolonged venous hypertension and high lymph flow.

Bony abnormalities

Bony abnormalities such as spina bifida, pelvic
non-fusion, syndactyly and coxa vara, have each
been observed in our own series of patients.
Others investigators have reported digital
agenesis, atresia of the ear canal, and
clinodactyly.

Other congenital malformations do not seem to
occur. This is surprising as cardiac abnormalities
are reported in association with some forms of
congenital lymphoedema.[20]

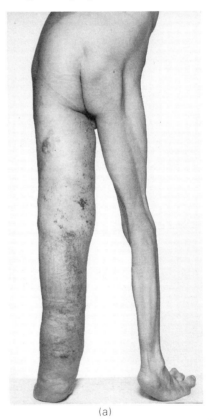

(a)

Fig. 23.17 Lymphangiomatous vesicles.
(a) This patient had a pale naevus but multiple
lymphangiomatous vesicles all over the skin; and
lymphoedema.

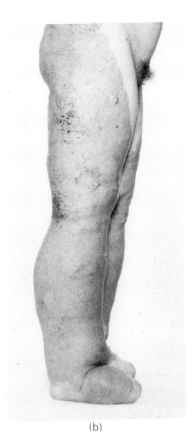

(b)

Fig. 23.17 (b) The enlargement of this patient's leg was caused by soft tissue hypertrophy not by lymphoedema but the skin was covered with lymphatic vesicles. The toes of both feet were amputated to allow the patient to wear ordinary shoes, and some years later she had a Charles' type reducing operation.

Investigations

The diagnosis of KTS is made at the bedside on the basis of the three diagnostic abnormalities together with a history that began at birth and the absence of any evidence of arteriovenous fistulae. Any doubt about the presence of arteriovenous fistulae, should be excluded by measuring the limb blood flow and, on rare occasions, by arteriography.

Foot volumetry This investigation is useful when deciding whether the reflux is embarassing the calf pump. Most patients can reduce their foot volume to the normal range during exercise,[3] but have an increased rate of refilling (see Fig. 23.8 and 23.9).

Venous outflow Plethysmography may define the degree of outflow obstruction in patients with deep vein atresia but the results are usually normal.

Phlebography This is difficult but *essential*.[23,42,45,47]

Standard ascending phlebography should be the first investigation, because it is essential that the state of the deep veins is known. The course and destination of the large subcutaneous veins is often best displayed by direct injection into an abnormal vein (Fig. 23.18).

If the radio-opaque contrast medium is injected into the large veins at various points along the limb, the many sites of superficial-to-deep connections can be demonstrated (Fig. 23.19).

The delineation of pelvic vein abnormalities may require direct percutaneous common femoral vein phlebography. In the rare patient whose femoral vein is absent, abnormal veins around the bladder and rectum can be demonstrated with percutaneous intraosseus trochanteric phlebography.

In our series[3] all of the 49 KTS limbs had an abnormal lateral limb bud vein (see Fig. 23.12a). This vein was connected to the deep calf veins by large communicating veins in over 50 per cent of limbs. The lateral vein drained into the deep thigh veins in 50 per cent of the limbs (Fig. 23.21a and b), into the gluteal veins in 33 per cent (Fig. 23.20a and b) and into the long saphenous vein in 15 per cent.

Most limbs (80 per cent) had normal, slightly dilated or reduplicated deep veins. Twenty per cent of limbs had deep vein atresia or hypoplasia affecting the superficial femoral vein (see Fig. 23.21b), which in a few limbs also affected the common femoral and iliac veins (see Fig. 23.4a).

Deep vein aplasia (Fig. 23.22) is not a common finding[43], and clearly cannot be the cause of either the superficial venous abnormality or the soft tissue and bony hypertrophy.

Arteriography Arteriography and measurements of blood flow may be necessary to exclude the presence of arteriovenous fistulae.[8,34]

Scannograms These are X-rays of the bones of the limbs taken at a fixed distance against a background graticule. A scannogram allows the exact measurement of bone length (Fig. 23.23).[1] Simple bedside measurements are difficult and inaccurate when there is soft tissue hypertrophy. If these measurements are repeated over the years,

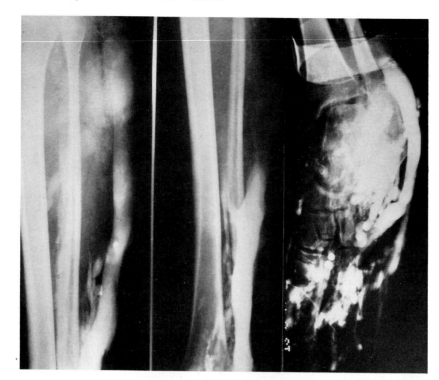

Fig. 23.18 A phlebogram showing a large incompetent lateral vein.

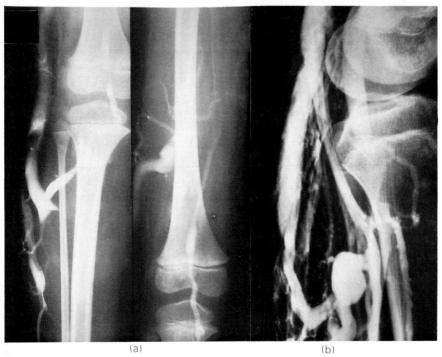

(a)   (b)

Fig. 23.19 Examples of communications between the abnormal superficial veins and the deep veins.
(a) An ascending phlebogram showing a communication between the lateral vein and a hypoplastic popliteal vein (left-hand panel) and the lateral vein draining into the deep femoral vein. The superficial femoral vein is also hypoplastic. (b) A large lateral mid calf communicating vein.

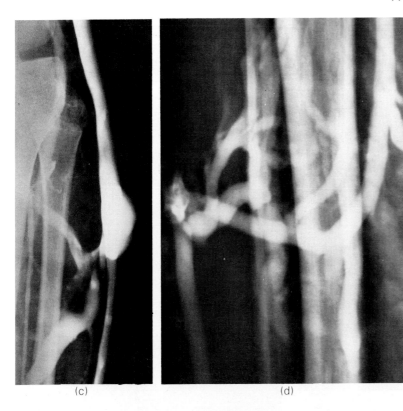

Fig. 23.19 (c) A large posterior mid calf communicating vein. (d) A large lateral vein crossing the back of the calf to communicate with the deep veins on both sides of the calf.

(c)

(d)

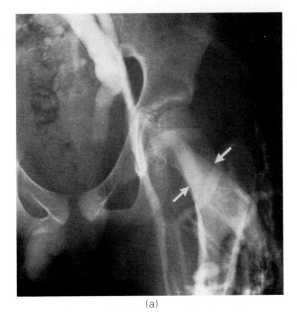

(a)

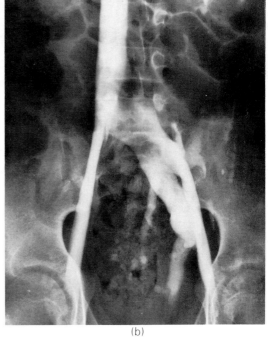

(b)

Fig. 23.20 (a) A phlebogram showing a large lateral vein draining into the internal iliac vein.

(b) The internal iliac vein of the same patient. Its stem and its superior gluteal tributaries are dilated and abnormal. There are phleboliths in the pelvis.

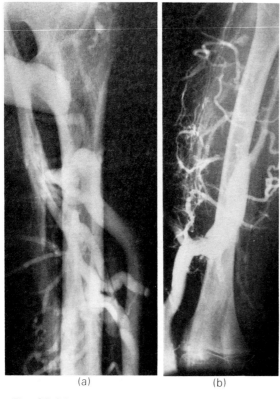

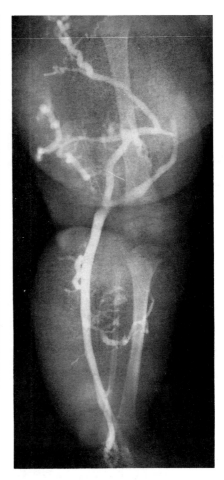

Fig. 23.21 (a) A phlebogram showing a large lateral vein draining into the deep femoral vein.

(b) A large lateral vein draining into the superficial femoral vein, which is hypoplastic.

the change in limb length discrepancy can be noted and orthopaedic correction can be advised if necessary.

Chest and abdominal X-rays   A chest X-ray is an important initial investigation to exclude other congenital abnormalities and detect cardiomegaly caused by arteriovenous fistulation. An abdominal X-ray may reveal pelvic phleboliths if the veins of the pelvis are abnormal (Fig. 23.24).

CT and NMR   Scans with and without radio-opaque contrast injections can outline the exact anatomical distribution of the clusters of abnormal veins in the limbs and, more particularly, in the pelvis.

Endoscopy   Symptoms such as haematuria or rectal bleeding must be fully investigated by cystoscopy, proctoscopy and sigmoidoscopy and by the usual X-ray studies. Other causes of bleeding must be excluded before attributing it to the venous malformation.

Fig. 23.22   Deep vein aplasia.
The ascending phlebogram of a 6-month-old child with an enlarged leg and a naevus showing a large lateral vein and no deep veins. The arteriogram and calf blood flow were normal.

Blood investigations   In view of the increased incidence of thromboembolic complications, it is wise to perform a full study of circulating coagulation and fibrinolytic factors.

Differential diagnosis   The investigations outlined above will reveal the nature of other abnormalities often confused with the KTS (e.g. venous angiomata, gigantism, multiple arteriovenous fistulae, the post-thrombotic syndrome and lymphoedema).

Treatment

Many patients need no treatment for the KTS but

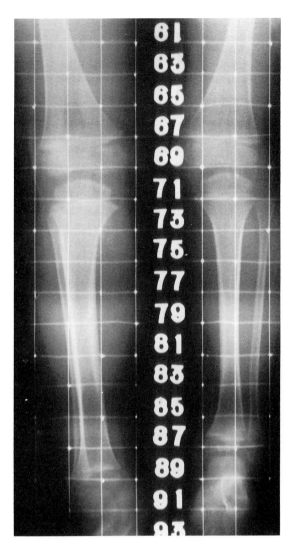

Fig. 23.23   A scannogram.

Clinical measurement of leg length is sufficient for the adjustment of the heel of the shoe but precise measurements of bone length are required when choosing the optimum time for epiphysiodesis.

The graticules are 2 cm wide. The tibia of the right leg is 1.75 cm longer than the left tibia.

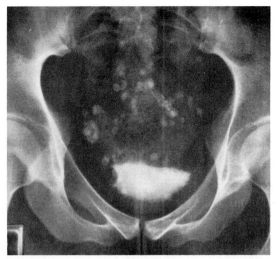

Fig. 23.24   Phleboliths in the pelvis. This patient had many abnormal veins in the pelvis and had had recurrent episodes of haematuria.

even when the condition is symptomless we advise patients to wear elastic stockings.

Elastic stockings

The principal complaints of aching, mild swelling and visible veins are best treated by *elastic compression*. This treatment has brought consi-derable relief to all our patients. Patients must be told that they will have to wear the stockings at all times, for the rest of their lives. A full-length stocking is preferable as it compresses the vessels in the upper thigh and prevents reflux from the gluteal or deep thigh veins. A below-knee stocking is, however, easier to put on and is adequate if the major abnormalities are below the knee.

Superficial vein surgery

Superficial veins should not be removed when there is aplasia of the deep veins.

Surgery to the superficial veins should only be advised when skin changes (e.g. pigmentation, eczema or ulceration) are present.

Patients who insist on surgical removal of the large visible veins for cosmetic reasons should be told that recurrences are inevitable because of the diffuse nature of the abnormality, unless extensive excisions are performed.

If the deep veins are normal, the large subcutaneous trunks can be removed by stripping, and at the same time the incompetent communicating veins between the abnormal surface veins and the deep veins can be ligated and divided. This is a major rather than a minor procedure but it usually alleviates the aching pains and gives a temporary cosmetic improvement. All patients must continue to wear elastic stockings after the operation. Localized subcutaneous angiomatous collections of veins, particularly those involving the skin, can be excised without complications.

Deep vein surgery The deep vein aplasia rarely needs to be treated because the large superficial veins provide an adequate outflow tract. A total common femoral and iliac aplasia may be helped by a vein bypass once the patient is fully grown, if the aplasia is causing severe swelling and venous claudication. We have not seen a patient with these symptoms because all our patients have had adequate collateral vessels.

The naevus Many patients ask for treatment of the naevus. It is best to reassure them that it is likely to fade and to avoid any surgical treatment.

Cosmetic creams and paints often provide good camouflage. Laser coagulation may be used for particularly dark areas but is not a practical treatment for a naevus that covers the whole limb and it may leave unsightly white scars.

Verrucose patches, caused by protruding dilated intradermal venules sometimes bleed and may become infected. These patches are best treated by local excision. Suture lines in the naevus heal normally but dilated venules often develop in the scar. Excision and skin grafting may be required for large areas of abnormal skin.

Reducing operations Patients who have concomitant lymphatic obliteration or diffuse lymphangiomatosis sometimes develop severe swelling of the leg. If the skin vesicles become chronically infected, they may be replaced with hypertrophic bleeding granulation tissue. These patients may benefit from either a Homans' or a Charles' type of reducing operation.

The venous abnormality makes the operation difficult and bloody. Wound healing is often slow but once healing has occurred the combination of the subcutaneous excision and the ligation of the abnormal veins can reduce the limb to an acceptable size.

Amputations Gigantism of the toes or forefoot is often best treated by local amputation because it enables the patient to wear a shoe of a normal size and to walk properly (see Fig. 23.17b). Normal walking is important because it means that the calf muscles contract properly and venous calf pump function improves.

Control of limb growth Careful measurements of limb length will indicate whether any length discrepancy is stable or is increasing. Mild stable differences in leg length can be treated by raising the heel of the shoe of the normal leg.

An increasing discrepancy should be treated by retarding growth by epiphyseal stapling or epiphysiodesis (Fig. 23.25a and b).[7,14,35] The time at which this procedure is performed must be carefully calculated from age–growth charts in consultation with an orthopaedic surgeon. The operation itself is not difficult as the venous abnormality does not extend into the bones.

Prevention of bleeding Haematuria and rectal bleeding from submucosal vesicles and rectal veins are difficult to control. Local sclerosing injections may be helpful. We have not had to excise bowel or bladder to stop bleeding and would hesitate to do so because of the problem of defining the source of bleeding from a pelvic abnormality which is so diffuse.

Ancillary procedures Table 23.1 lists the operations that we have performed on our patients. Many of the operations on our patients are simply 'tidying up' procedures. Although 50 per cent of our patients have had some form of

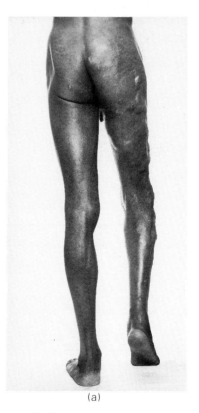

(a)

Fig. 23.25 (a) This patient had developed fixed flexion of the knee and ankle joints because his leg length had not been corrected.

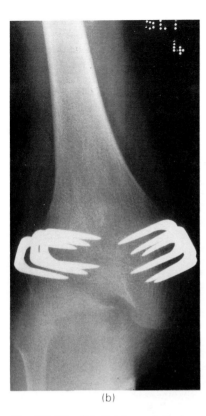

Fig. 23.25 (b) Epiphyseal staples, inserted to retard the growth of the leg.

Table 23.1 The 88 procedures performed on 38 patients with Klippel-Trenaunay syndrome[3]

Procedure	Number (%)
Vein ligation and stripping	49 (56)
Excision of angioma	11 (13)
Excision of Ulcer and Skin Graft	8 (9)
Excision of lymphatic vesicles	4 (4.5)
Amputation of digits	4 (4.5)
Epiphyseal stapling	4 (4.5)
Reducing operations	2
Excision of fibroma	2
Evacuation of spontaneous haematoma	2
Injection of subcutaneous varices	1
Injection of rectal varices	1
Total	88

phlebography or the abnormal muscle on CT scanning.[56] If the vein is not thrombosed, the symptoms can be relieved by dividing the abnormal strand of muscle.

operation on the veins, the mainstay of treatment has been good elastic support.

Thrombosis prophylaxis As patients with KTS are at increased risk of thromboembolism, they should be given *prophylatic subcutaneous heparin whenever they are admitted to hospital.* Once these patients have had a thrombosis, serious consideration should be given to the administration of oral anticoagulants for the rest of their lives.

Popliteal vein entrapment

Abnormalities of the insertion of the gastrocnemius muscle into the femur may cause compression of the popliteal vein in a similar fashion to the better known popliteal artery entrapment syndrome.[10,11,39] The patient complains of intermittent swelling and discomfort brought on by exercise or presents with an acute popliteal vein thrombosis. The diagnosis depends upon seeing a localized compression of the popliteal vein on

References

1. Anderson M, Green WT, Messner MB. Growth and predictions of growth in the lower extremities. *J Bone Joint Surg* 1963; **45**: 1.
2. Baskerville PA, Ackroyd JS, Browse NL. The aetiology of the Klippel Trenaunay syndrome. *Ann Surg* 1985; **202**: 624.
3. Baskerville PA, Ackroyd JS, Thomas ML, Browse NL. The Klippel Trenaunay syndrome: clinical and haemodynamic features and management. *Br J Surg* 1985; **72**: 232.
4. Baskerville PA, Browse NL. Coagulation factors in patients with the Klippel Trenaunay syndrome. In Press.
5. Basmajian JW. The distribution of valves in the femoral, external iliac and common iliac vein and their relationship to varicose veins. *Surg Gynec Obstet* 1952; **95**: 537.
6. Benbow EW. Idiopathic obstruction of the inferior vena cava, a review. *J R Soc Med* 1986; **79**: 105.
7. Blount WP, Clarke GR. Control of bone growth by epiphyseal stapling: a preliminary report. *J Bone Joint Surg* 1949; **31A**: 464.
8. Bourde C. Classification des syndrome de Klippel–Trenaunay, et de Parkes Weber d'apres des donnees angiographiques. *Ann Radiol (Paris)* 1974; **17**: 153.
9. Coget JM, Merlen JF, Arnolstan M, Klippel Trenaunay syndrome of the upper extremity. *Phlebologie* 1983; **36**: 271.

10. Connell J. Popliteal vein entrapment. *Br J Surg* 1978; **65**: 351.

11. Edmonson HT, Crowe JA. Popliteal artery and venous entrapment. *Am J Surg* 1972; **38**: 657.

12. Effler DB, Greer AE, Sifers EC. Anomaly of the vena cava inferior, report of a fatality after ligation. *JAMA* 1951; **146**: 1321.

13. Elke M, Ludin H. Drainage der unteren Korperhalfte bei Agenesie und erworbenem verschluss der vena cava candalis. *Fortschr Roentgenstr* 1965; **103**: 665.

14. Green WT. Equalization of leg length. *Surg Gynec Obstet* 1950; **90**: 119.

15. Hollier LH. Surgical treatment of congenital venous malformations. In Bergan JJ, Yao JST (Eds) *Surgery of the Vein*. New York. Grune & Stratton 1985; 275.

16. Hunter GC, Malone JM, Moore WS, Misiorowski RL, Chvapil M. Vascular manifestations in patients with Ehlers–Danlos syndrome. *Arch Surg* 1982; **117**: 495.

17. Hutchinson WJ, Burdeaux BD. The influence of stasis on bone growth. *Surg Gynec Obstet* 1954; **99**: 413.

18. Kimwa C, Shirotani H, Hirooka M, Terada M, Iwahashi K, Maetani S. Membranous obliteration of the inferior vena cava in the hepatic portion. *Cardiovasc Surg* 1963; **4**: 87.

19. Kimwa C, Shirotani H, Kuma T, Hirooka M, Havashi K, Tsunekawa K, Matsuda S. Transcardiac membranotomy for obliteration of the vena cava in the hepatic portion. *J Cardiovasc Surg* 1962; **3**: 393.

20. Kinmonth JB. *The Lymphatics* 2nd edition London. Edward Arnold 1982.

21. Kistner RL. Surgical repair of the incompetent femoral vein valve. *Arch Surg* 1975; **110**: 1336.

22. Klippel M, Trenaunay P. Du noevus variqueux osteo-hypertrophique. *Arch Gen Med (Paris)* 1900; **185**: 641.

23. Lea Thomas M, Andress MR. Angiography in venous dysplasias of the limbs. *Am J Roentgenol* 1971; **113**: 722.

24. Lea Thomas M. Agenesis of the iliac veins. *J Cardiovasc Surg* 1984; **25**: 64.

25. Leu HJ, Wenner A, Spycher MA, Brunner V. Ultrastrukturelle Veranderungen bei venoser Angiodysplasie von Typ Klippel Trenaunay. *Vasa* 1980; **9**: 147.

26. Lindenauer SM. The Klippel Trenaunay syndrome: varicosity, hypertrophy and haemangioma with no arteriovenous fistula. *Ann Surg* 1965; **162**: 303.

27. Lodin A, Lindvall N, Gentele H. Congenital absence of venous valves as a cause of leg ulcers. *Acta Chir Scand* 1958; **116**: 256.

28. Malan E, Puglionisi A. Congenital angiodysplasias of the extremities. I: Generalities and classification, venous dysplasias. *J Cardiovasc Surg* 1964; **5**: 87.

29. Martorell F. Aplasia of the iliac vein. *Angiologia* 1971; **23**: 117.

30. Muller N, Morris DC, Nichols DM. Popliteal artery entrapment demonstrated by CT. *Radiology* 1984; **151**: 157.

31. O'Donnell TF. Congenital mixed vascular deformities of the lower limbs. *Ann Surg* 1977; **185**: 162.

32. Ohara I, Ouchi H, Takahashi K. A bypass operation for occlusion of the hepatic inferior vena cava. *Surg Gynec Obstet* 1963; **117**: 151.

33. Parkes-Weber F. Angioma formation in connection with hypertrophy of limbs and hemihypertrophy. *Br J Dermatol* 1907; **19**: 231.

34. Partsch H, Lofferer O, Mostbeck A. Zur Diagnostik von arteriovenosen Fisteln bei Angiodysplasien der Extremitaten. *Vasa* 1975; **4**: 288.

35. Phemister DB. Operative arrestment of longitudinal growth of bones in the treatment of deformities. *J Bone Joint Surg* 1933; **15**: 1.

36. Plate G, Brudin L, Eklof B, Jensen R, Ohlin P. Physiologic and therapeutic aspects in congenital vein valve aplasia of the lower limb. *Ann Surg* 1983; **198**: 229.

37. Poulet J, Ruff F. Les dysplasies veineuses congenitales des membres. *Presse Med* 1969; **77**: 163.

38. Prerovsky I, Linholt J, Dejdar R, Svejcar J, Kruw J, Vavrejn B. Research on primary varicose veins and chronic venous insufficiency. *Rev Czech Med* 1962; **8**: 171.

39. Rich NM, Hughes CW. Popliteal artery and vein entrapment. *Am J Surg* 1967; **113**: 696.

40. Sarma KP. Anomalous inferior vena cava. Anatomical and clinical features. *Br J Surg* 1966; **53**: 600.

41. Sen PK, Kinare SG, Kelkar MD, Paralkar GB, Mehta JM. Congenital membranous obliteration of the inferior vena cava. *J Cardiovasc Surg* 1967; **8**: 344.

42. Servelle M, Babillot J. Les malformations des veines profondes dans le syndrome de Klippel et Trenaunay. *Phlebologie* 1980; **33**: 31.

43. Servelle M, Zolotas E, Soulie J, Andrieux J, Cornu C. Syndrome de Klippel et Trenaunay: malformations iliaques et poplitee. *Arch Mal Coeur* 1965; **68**: 1187.

44. Servelle M, Klippel Trenaunay's syndrome. *Ann Surg* 1985; **201**: 365.

45. Servelle M. La phlebographie va-t-elle nous permettre de demembrer le syndrome de Klippel et Trenaunay et l'hemangiectasie hypertrophique de Parkes-Weber. *Presse Med* 1945; **53**: 353.

46. Servelle M. Stase veineuse et croissance osseuse. *Bull Acad Nat Med* 1948; **132**: 472.

47. Thomas ML, MacFie GB. Phlebography in the

Klippel Trenaunay syndrome. *Acta Radiol (Diagn) (Stockh)* 1974; **15**: 43.

48. Trelat U, Monad A. De L'hypertrophie unilaterale partielle ou totale du corps. *Arch Gen Med* 1869; **2**: 536.

49. Van der Molen HR. Maladie de Klippel Trenaunay et grosses jambes. *Societe Francaise Phlebologie* 1968; **2**: 187.

50. Van der Molen HR. Quelques remarques cliniques au sujet des dysplasies vasculaires. *Phlebologie* 1980; **33**: 43.

51. Van der Stricht J. Syndrome de Klippel et Trenaunay et Phacomatoses. *Phlebologie* 1980; **33**: 21.

52. Vollmar J, Vogt K. Angiodysplasie und Skeletsystem. *Chirurg* 1976; **47**: 205.

53. Vollmar J. Malformations of the leg and pelvic veins. In May R (Ed) *Surgery of the Veins of the Leg and Pelvis*. Stuttgart. Georg Theime 1974; 200.

54. Watkins E, Fortin CL. Surgical correction of a congenital coarctation of the inferior vena cava. *Ann Surg* 1964; **159**: 536.

55. Woollard HH. The development of the principal arterial stems in the forelimb of the pig. *Contributions to Embryology* (Carnegie Inst) 1922; **22**: 139.

56. Young AE. Congenital mixed vascular deformities of the limbs and their associated lesions. In *Birth Defects: Original Article Series*. 1978; **14**: 289.

24

Occlusion of the veins of the upper arm and neck

The two major problems that affect the veins of the upper arm and neck are axillary and subclavian vein thrombosis and obstruction of the superior vena cava. Primary varicose veins are never found in the upper limb, but congenital and acquired arteriovenous fistulae can cause secondary varicose veins which can be treated by eradicating the underlying cause.

The valves may be congenitally absent from the upper limb veins but this does not cause any clinical problems. Injuries to the great veins in the upper limb, supraclavicular region and thorax do occur, and these are discussed in Chapter 25. Superficial thrombophlebitis is discussed in Chapter 22 and angiomata, which may also affect the upper limb, are discussed in Chapter 26.

Axillary/subclavian vein thrombosis

Thrombosis of the axillary/subclavian vein was originally described by Sir James Paget in 1875[25] and by von Schroetter in 1884;[42] it is therefore frequently called Paget–Von Schroetter's syndrome. It is a rare condition, accounting for 1 or 2 per cent of all cases of venous thrombosis.[1,6,7,13,15,28]

Aetiology

Thrombosis of the axillary vein may be a primary or secondary event, though some investigators doubt a primary aetiology and try to find a cause for all cases.

It often follows excessive or unusual physical exercise and has consequently been called 'effort thrombosis'.[20] The greater incidence of axillary vein thrombosis in men compared with that in women, and the greater incidence in the right arm,[4,20,41] are indicative of the relevance of physi-cal exertion to its development.

Many workers consider that external compression of the axillary vein as it enters the thoracic inlet is a major aetiological factor[1,11,24] and some investigators have implied that thoracic inlet/outlet compression is the cause of all axillary vein thromboses.[10,12,36] There is, however, considerable disagreement over the anatomical structure that causes the obstruction. A cervical rib (Fig. 24.1), a congenital web (Fig. 24.2), the first rib, the subclavius and scalenus anterior muscles, an anteriorly placed phrenic or accessory phrenic nerve, the pectoralis minor muscle, the clavicle or a malunited fracture of the clavicle, and a persistent axillo-pectoral muscle (Fig. 24.3) have all been incriminated.[1,41,16,8,5,9,31,45]

A number of large reviews of axillary vein thrombosis have suggested that it is more likely that several factors, acting in combination, are responsible for its development.

Tilney and his colleagues[41] recognized the role of 'effort' in the development of primary axillary vein thrombosis but also reported that secondary thrombosis caused by local inflammation from intravenous catheters and irritant solutions was an important cause.

In 1977 Campbell et al.,[6] described 8 patients with 'effort' thrombosis; 10 with internal injury (e.g. an intravenous cathether or infusion), 6 with extrinsic compression and 1 with a hypercoagulable state.

Sundqvist et al.,[38] examined the blood for evidence of an abnormality of systemic fibrinolysis in 60 patients with axillary vein thrombosis and found it to be present in nearly 50 per cent of these patients, though it is possible that this was an effect rather than a cause of the condition. Within this group of patients they also found:

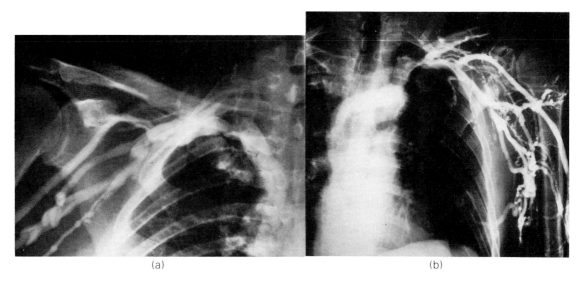

(a)   (b)

Fig. 24.1   (a and b) Two examples of narrowing of the axillary/subclavian vein associated with a cervical rib.

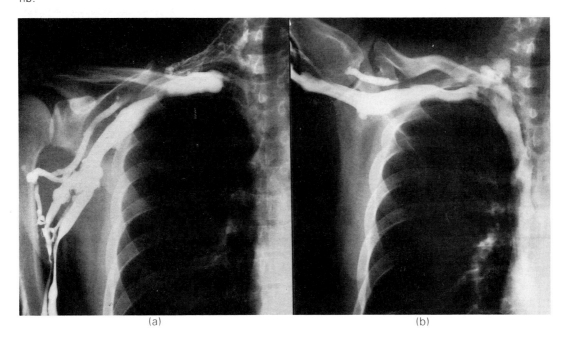

(a)   (b)

Fig. 24.2   (a) An intraluminal congenital septum producing almost complete obstruction of the subclavian vein, with the arm by the side.
   (b) The obstruction was less when the arm was elevated.

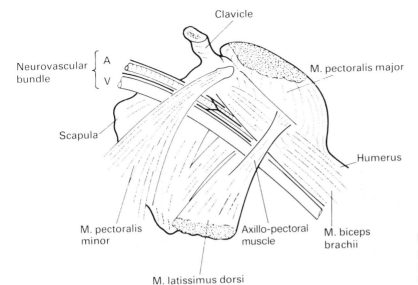

Fig. 24.3 The anatomical position of a persistent axillo-pectoral muscle, a rare cause of axillary vein occlusion.[5,8]

- evidence of coincidental leg vein thrombosis in 6 patients;
- a family history of leg vein thrombosis in 8 patients;
- a history of trauma to the shoulder in 2 patients (one had a fracture of clavicle);
- excessive 'effort' in 5 patients (including long-distance swimming and chopping down trees);
- cervical ribs in 2 patients;
- contraceptive pill ingestion in 10 patients;
- pregnancy in 2 patients;
- cancer of the breast in 1 patient (Fig. 24.4);
- cancer of the prostate in 1 patient;
- 2 patients who were severely ill in the intensive care unit;
- 2 patients who had recently suffered a myocardial infarct (one developed pneumonia);
- 2 patients who were alcoholic.

This particular series of patients, which highlights the multiplicity of causes, was unusual in several respects. There was a high incidence of women with the condition, only 12 per cent gave a history of trauma and only 5 per cent had clear-cut clinical evidence of thoracic outlet/inlet syndrome.

Martin *et al.*,[22] reported that half of their 20 patients with an axillary vein thrombosis had a demonstrable cause for the condition. The causes which they reported included breast carcinoma (Fig. 24.4), a central venous pressure catheter,

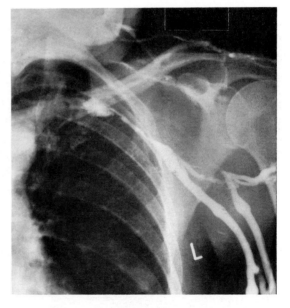

Fig. 24.4 An axillary vein occlusion which developed after a mastectomy followed by radiotherapy given to treat a Stage II carcinoma of the breast. The axillary vein is narrow and irregular.

heroin addiction, and cervical ribs (see Fig. 24.1).

In 3 patients presenting with venous gangrene of the hand the initiating factors were reduced tissue perfusion, hypercoagulability and venous injury.[35]

Recently, 2 patients have been reported in

whom thrombosis developed after the creation of an arteriovenous fistula for haemodialysis.[23]

The association of axillary vein thrombosis with both malignancy and intravenous infusions, particularly long central catheters, is common to most of these studies. The operation of axillary clearance of lymph glands or radiotherapy to the axilla are known to carry a risk of axillary vein thrombosis. This is an important cause of swelling of the arm in patients who have had treatment for carcinoma of the breast (see Fig. 24.4).

Comment   As for deep vein thrombosis of the leg, the aetiology of axillary vein thrombosis is almost certainly multifactorial, and thoracic outlet compression is rarely the sole cause of 'primary' or idiopathic thrombosis. Thoracic outlet compression does, however, appear to be an important factor and should always be considered in patients presenting with this condition.

Stevenson and Parry[36] have suggested that a compression abnormality can always be detected in the opposite normal limb of patients presenting with 'idiopathic' axillary vein thrombosis, if axillary phlebograms are obtained during differing degrees of shoulder abduction (Fig. 24.5). This study was inevitably open to observer bias and requires confirmation by other investigators before it can be fully accepted. In our experience,

bilateral axillary vein thrombosis is extremely rare, except in patients with terminal malignant disease. This observation suggests that bilateral anatomical abnormalities are rare or their presence is insignificant.

Clinical features

Most series,[4,6,41] with one exception,[38] show a male to female preponderance of approximately three to two. The majority of patients are between the ages of 35 years and 45 years, and the thrombosis commonly involves the dominant right arm.

Patients complain of discomfort and weakness developing within 24 hours of excessive or unusual exercise.[4] The discomfort varies between a dull ache with a feeling of tightness to a severe pain. The hand and forearm become cold and hand and finger movements are diminished. The arm then gradually becomes swollen and blue from the fingertips to the shoulder. Enlargement of the female breast has been reported to occur on the side of the occlusion[7] if the pectoral and scapular regions become oedematous.

On examination there is usually evidence of pitting oedema of the fingers, hand and forearm, and a variable amount of oedema of the upper arm.[41] The oedema is most obvious over the dorsum of the hand. The skin has a diffuse blue

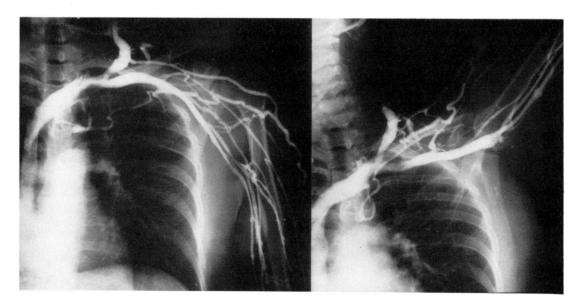

Fig. 24.5 An axillary vein obstruction at the thoracic inlet (left-hand panel) which was more apparent when the arm was elevated (right-hand panel).

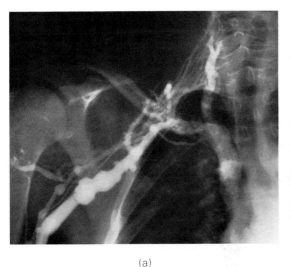 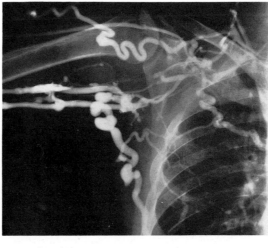

(a)   (b)

Fig. 24.6 (a and b) Two axillary phlebograms showing supraclavicular and cervical collaterals (a) and chest wall collaterals (b). Both sets of collaterals provide alternative pathways past an axillary vein occlusion.

tinge and is cool to the touch; there is often a clear line of demarcation between these changes and normal skin over the upper arm or shoulder. The main subcutaneous veins, the basilic and cephalic, are the first to distend but later there is a generalized distension of all the veins and venules.[3] The distended veins feel tense and do not collapse when the arm is elevated above the level of the right atrium. Collateral veins develop over the chest wall and shoulder in the weeks succeeding a thrombosis as anastomoses open up between the tributaries of the axillary and cephalic veins and the intercostal veins (Fig. 24.6).

In approximately 50 per cent of patients the axillary vein may be palpable as a thickened tender cord high up on the lateral side of the axilla.[4] If there is extension of the thrombosis into the subclavian vein (a common event), there may be supraclavicular tenderness. The supraclavicular hollow and the subclavian dimple may also be filled in, and the face and neck may become swollen if the thrombus extends into the jugular vein or superior vena cava.[41]

Late sequelae and complications in the arm

The majority of patients develop an adequate collateral circulation and have no late sequelae but if this does not occur, patients may complain of recurrent swelling and pain during arm exercise[4] or severe fatigue and discomfort after exercise.[6] At worst, they may develop disabling venous claudication of the arm.

The late sequelae described above appear to be dependent upon the aetiology of the thrombosis[6] and the success of the treatment.[4]

Venous gangrene of the hand is a rare complication Colour plate 39 but at least four cases have been reported,[1,26,35] and we have seen three patients with this complication all in the terminal stages of advanced disseminated malignant disease; it may therefore not be quite so uncommon.

Differential diagnosis

In the early stages, symptoms of weakness, coldness and skin discoloration may suggest arterial ischaemia but the presence of normal pulses and the development of oedema, cyanosis and distended veins usually make the correct diagnosis apparent. External compression of the veins by malignant lymph nodes, Pancoast's tumour or soft tissue sarcomata (Fig. 24.7) must always be excluded, and computerized tomography (CT) and lymphography may be required if this is suspected. Lymphoedema and cellulitis are other rare causes of a painful and swollen arm.

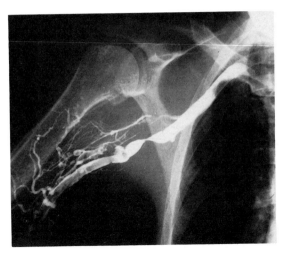

Fig. 24.7 A stricture of the axillary vein caused by a myosarcoma with fresh thrombus in the brachial veins.

Pulmonary embolism

Although some studies have suggested that pulmonary embolism is uncommon in association with axillary vein thrombosis,[14,41] other workers have shown that this complication occurs in 5–10 per cent of patients.[1,6,43] A small group of patients have repeated pulmonary emboli and develop pulmonary hypertension. Massive or fatal pulmonary embolism from an axillary vein thrombosis is, however, extremely rare (Fig. 24.8).

Diagnosis and investigations

A careful history and general examination are essential to detect or exclude any of the many causes of axillary vein thrombosis outlined in the section on aetiology. Particular attention should be paid to a history of unusual exercise and recent intravenous injection or catheterizations. Careful questioning may reveal evidence of a known hypercoagulable state or a family history of thrombosis. Exposure to the contraceptive pill may also be relevant.

During the examination, it is important to look for evidence of malignant disease, particularly of the breast, prostate and lung and also lymphoma. There may be clinical evidence of cervical ribs or thoracic outlet syndrome, for example disappearance of the radial pulse when the arm is elevated to 180° (Adson's test).[2]

A full red and white cell count should be

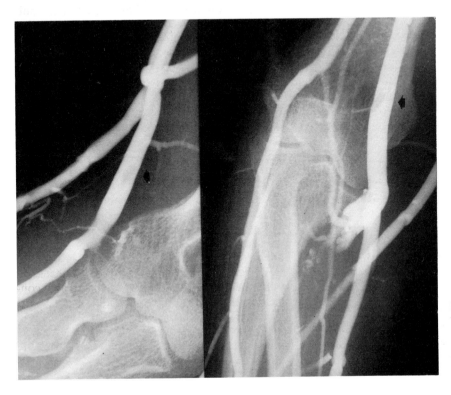

Fig. 24.8 A small fresh loose thrombus (arrowed) within the basilic vein which has the potential to embolize to the lung.

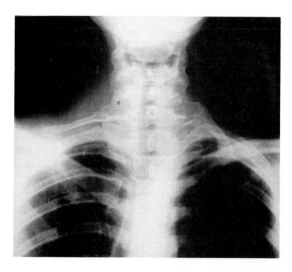

Fig. 24.9 Cervical ribs are usually easy to see on a plain radiograph of the thoracic inlet.

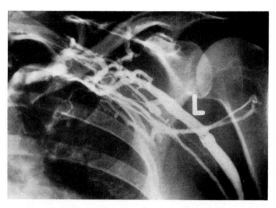

Fig. 24.10 An example of a 'short' occlusion of the axillary vein.

performed to exclude polycythaemia and leukaemia, and a platelet count should be carried out to exclude thrombocytosis (thrombocythaemia).

A chest X-ray may reveal a carcinoma of bronchus or secondary deposits from a distant malignancy. Cervical ribs may also be seen on a chest X-ray but thoracic inlet and cervical spine films should always be requested (Fig. 24.9).

Screening for hypercoagulation should include measurement of the common coagulation factors and antithrombin-III and protein-C levels, together with tests of fibrinolysis.[38] These tests take time to organize and obtain; they do not affect the initial management but may affect later care.

Non-invasive investigations with arterial and venous Doppler flow detectors should show a normal arterial pressure at the wrist but proximal venous occlusion and loss of the Valsalva response in the peripheral arm veins. Grey-scale ultrasound imaging with Duplex high resolution ultrasound scanning may localize the occlusion and show the extent of the thrombosis.

Impedence plethysmography has been reported to have good sensitivity and specificity (over 90 per cent) when compared with phlebography in the diagnosis of axillary vein thrombosis.[27,26]

Ascending brachial venograms are the best means of diagnosis and provide the information required for proper management. Two main phlebographic patterns have been described.[4] The first pattern is a short, localized obstruction at the junction of the subclavian vein with the axillary vein (between the first rib and the clavicle) (Fig. 24.10). The second pattern is a long obstruction extending distally down the axillary vein into the brachial vein (Fig. 24.11). Martin *et al.*,[22] reported that in over 70 per cent of their cases the thrombosis extended into the subclavian vein, but the innominate vein was rarely involved. It is often quite difficult to determine the proximal extent of the thrombosis.

Ventilation–perfusion lung scans and pulmonary angiography may be indicated if there is a suspicion of pulmonary embolism.

Digital subtraction arteriography of the subclavian and axillary arteries in different degrees of shoulder abduction may help to confirm the presence of a thoracic outlet obstruction (Fig. 24.12).

Treatment

Many patients present days or weeks after the onset of symptoms. By this time, conservative treatment, plus careful follow-up, is the only practical method of management[45] with a view to some form of delayed venous reconstruction if severe post-thrombotic symptoms develop later.[18] Conservative treatment consists of bedrest, administration of anticoagulants and, very rarely, a stellate ganglion block when this is indicated.[4]

In one study, 21 out of 24 patients treated conservatively, half with anticoagulants, developed symptoms of chronic venous insufficiency,[39] and persistent symptoms were present in 8 of the 31 patients reported by Tilney *et al.*,[41] who were available for long-term follow-up. Tilney concluded that new forms of treatment should be

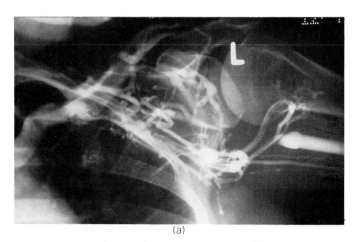

(a)

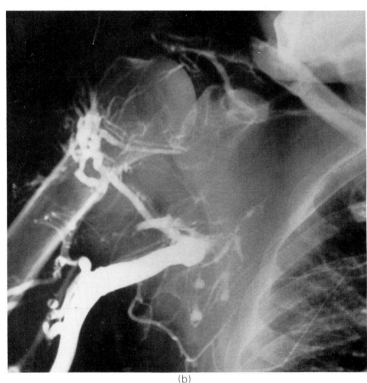

(b)

Fig. 24.11 (a and b) Two examples of 'long' occlusions of the axillary and subclavian veins. In both cases the occlusion begins at the level of the axillary skin fold.

considered but our own clinical experience has not been so depressing. Two-thirds of our patients have recovered to such a degree that they have had very minor symptoms which are not incapacitating.

The active measures that have been tried include thrombolysis[4] and thrombectomy,[21] alone or in combination with decompression of the axillary vein or thoracic inlet.[10] Delayed venous reconstruction or bypass can be tried in patients treated conservatively who continue to have disabling symptoms.

Venous thrombectomy alone has been only moderately successful (Table 24.1),[10,21] and the addition of first rib resection has not appreciably improved results.

Thrombolysis using either streptokinase[10] or urokinase[4] in combination with thoracic outlet

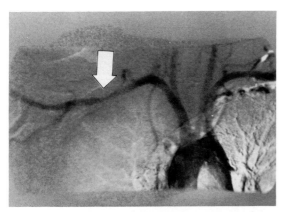

Fig. 24.12 A digital subtraction angiogram showing kinking and narrowing of the axillary artery which is only apparent when the arm is elevated.

exploration (where this is indicated by phlebography) appears to be more successful, and this is now probably the treatment of choice, if the thrombosis is less than 3 days old.

After confirming the diagnosis of an acute thrombosis with phlebography, (Fig. 24.13), a course of streptokinase or urokinase is given through a catheter which is advanced up the arm until it is in apposition to the thrombus. Denck *et al.*,[10] claimed favourable results with streptokinase (250,000 units given in 30 min, followed by 100,000 units / hour for 5 days) combined with intravenous heparin from the third day. Fibrinolysis was controlled by thrombin times and fibrinogen levels. Dunant[12] also reported good results in 17 out of 25 patients when fibrinolysis was combined with outlet decompression. Other workers have claimed more success with urokinase than with streptokinase.[4,45]

All these studies reported additional benefit from exploration and decompression of the axillary vein after successful thrombolysis, but exploration was not beneficial if thrombolysis was unsuccessful.

If early management of the acute thrombosis is unsuccessful, or the patient presents too late for thrombolysis and develops persistent symptoms, venous reconstruction can be considered. Autogenous vein[29] or the ipsilateral internal jugular vein[18,44] usually combined with a temporary arteriovenous fistula[19] have both been used to bypass late occlusions. There are only a few isolated reports of the results of this type of surgery but they are encouraging; the internal jugular vein appears to be the bypass of choice. We recommend that such operations should only be performed when the patient is severely disabled and by surgeons who are skilled in the techniques of direct major vein surgery and that the operation should preferably be part of a properly controlled clinical study.

Prognosis

Aggressive early treatment appears to give better results than conservative management. If the degree of residual disability after axillary vein thrombosis has been underestimated, late venous reconstruction by bypass may offer hope for the chronic sufferer. It is, however, surprising that there are so few complications when the brachial vein is resected for a valve transfer operation.[40] This makes us think that it is the local abnormality, the extent of the initial thrombosis and the effectiveness of the collaterals (Fig. 24.14) that determine the late sequelae. We need to know much more about these factors so that we can decide which patients need early agressive treatment and which patients can be treated conservatively before we become too attracted to the surgical appeal of venous reconstruction.

Table 24.1 Results of treatment of acute axillary thrombosis[12]

Treatment	Number of arms treated	Recanalization			Persisting symptoms	
		Complete	Partial	Nil	None	Present
Anticoagulants	42	2	8	32	13	29
Thrombectomy	9	2	4	3	3	6
Thrombectomy plus 1st rib resection	6	2	2	2	2	4
Thrombolysis	12	8	2	2	6	6
Thrombolysis plus 1st rib resection	12	10	2	0	10	2

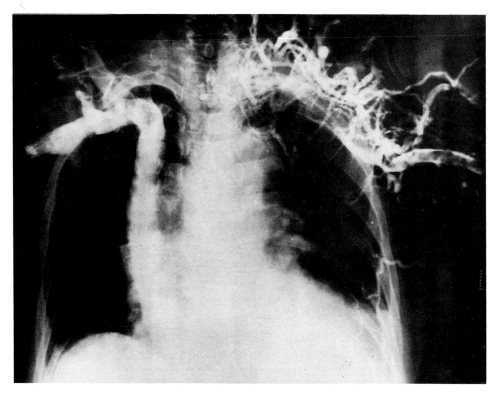

Fig. 24.13   An acute axillary thrombosis. This phlebogram shows fresh non-adherent thrombus within the axillary, subclavian and brachiocephalic veins of the left side. The right-sided vessels and superior vena cava are normal.

Superior vena caval occlusion and thrombosis

Thrombosis of the superior vena cava is commonly an acute event, usually caused by a rapidly growing intra-thoracic neoplasm (80–95 per cent). This neoplasm is most often a carcinoma of the bronchus (75 per cent, Fig. 24.15) but lymphomas (25 per cent, Fig. 24.16), thymomas and carcinoma of the thyroid may also lead to occlusion (Fig. 24.17). Retrosternal goitres (see Fig. 24.20), rarer mediastinal tumours and secondary deposits can also produce obstruction. In the past, syphilitic thoracic aneurysms were an important cause of thrombosis; this was the cause of the superior vena cava obstruction in the first description of this syndrome, published by William Hunter in 1747.[17] Constrictive pericarditis and mediastinal fibrosis (Fig. 24.18), a condition similar to retroperitoneal fibrosis, are also recognized as rare but important conditions which may lead to thrombosis.

Spontaneous thrombosis of the superior vena cava can occur but it is rare (Fig. 24.19). The increasing use of intravenous cannulation and the injection of hyperosmolar fluids into the neck veins may cause thrombosis. Thrombosis may also follow local injuries and iatrogenic injuries occurring during surgery to the heart and pericardium.

Normally, when the superior vena cava becomes obstructed the azygos, the hemiazygos, the internal mammary, the lateral thoracic and vertebral veins act as collateral channels (see Fig. 24.18 and 24.19).

Clinical features

Patients with superior vena caval obstruction usually present with swelling of the face and neck, and shortness of breath, which is often acute in onset. Very occasionally, patients may complain of tinnitus and deafness, epistaxis, a dry cough and dysphagia. The skin of the face is hyperaemic

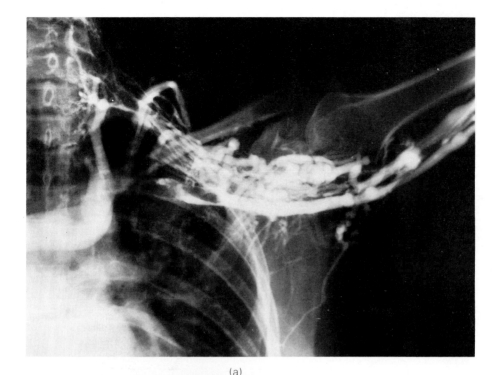

(a)

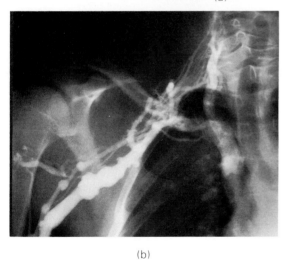

(b)

Fig. 24.14 (a and b) Two examples of adequate collaterals around a longstanding axillary vein thrombosis. These patients had few symptoms.

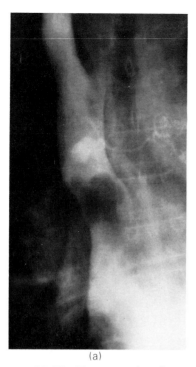

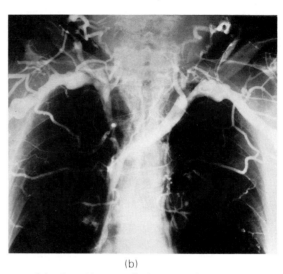

(a)   (b)

Fig. 24.15 Two examples of a carcinoma of the bronchus producing superior vena cava obstruction.
(a) This phlebogram shows a localized filling defect caused by a small mass of tumour protruding into the vena cava.
(b) This phlebogram shows the innominate veins and the superior vena cava compressed by surrounding tumour.

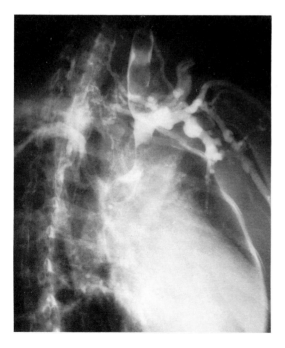

Fig. 24.16 Superior vena cava obstruction caused by Hodgkins disease. Fresh thrombus is present in the brachiocephalic and jugular veins.

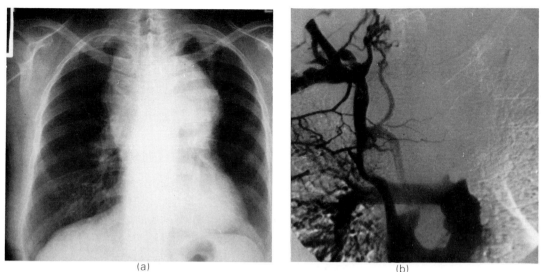

(a)   (b)

Fig. 24.17 An enlarged retrosternal thyroid gland obstructing the superior vena cava.
   (a) The mediastinal mass.
   (b) A digital subtraction angiogram showing compression and displacement of the right innominate vein and the vena cava with obstruction of the left pulmonary artery.

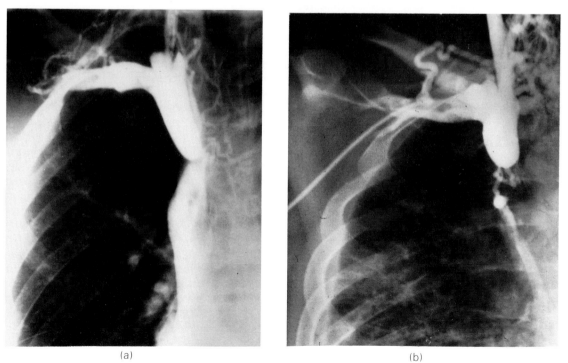

(a)   (b)

Fig. 24.18 Two examples of mediastinal fibrosis causing superior vena cava obstruction. (a) A partial obstruction.
   (b) Total occlusion.

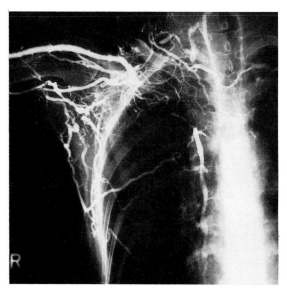

Fig. 24.19   An acute idiopathic total obstruction of the superior vena cava. Note the collateral pathways through the intercostal veins into the azygos vein.

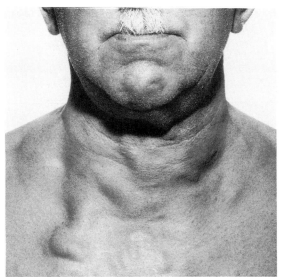

Fig. 24.20   A patient with a retrosternal goitre causing obstruction of the superior vena cava. The neck veins are distended, and a large collateral vein can be seen crossing in front of the clavicle carrying blood down to the tributaries of the inferior vena cava.

and cyanotic, and the jugular veins which are visibly distended do not alter in size with respiration or when the patient sits upright (Fig. 24.20). If there is no hepatomegaly or ankle oedema heart failure is unlikely; but exophthalmos may occasionally be present. In the late stages patients may complain of a feeling of congestion of the head, marked confusion, restlessness, dizziness, syncope and somnolence.

Investigations

A chest X-ray commonly reveals the cause of the problem, if this is not clinically apparent. Computerized tomography (CT) may provide better evidence of the presence and extent of mediastinal tumours. A tissue diagnosis should be obtained before any treatment is begun. Non-invasive tests (e.g. ultrasonography and plethysmography) may be used in screening but phlebography is required to confirm the diagnosis of a spontaneous or primary superior vena caval thrombosis (see Fig. 24.15–24.20). This can usually be obtained by bilateral brachial vein injections of contrast medium. The technique is described in greater detail in Chapter 4, page 126.

Treatment

An extensive carcinoma of the bronchus (see Fig. 24.15) occluding the superior vena cava is best treated by irradiation. If there has been no thrombosis, irradiation often alleviates the caval obstruction and produces marked symptomatic improvement.

Individual cases have been reported where the occluded vena cava has been successfully bypassed but this operation is rarely indicated when the condition is secondary to malignant disease. A venous reconstruction can be performed with a graft fashioned from panels of long saphenous vein[30] or an externally supported synthetic polytetrafluoroethylene (PTFE) prosthesis.[32,33] The bypass usually has to reach from a patent neck vein to the right atrium, superior vena cava or azygos vein. The number of patients who have been treated by these procedures provide an insufficient basis on which to base an opinion on their long-term effectiveness.[34]

References

1. Adams JT, McEvoy RK, DeWeese JA. Primary deep venous thrombosis of the upper extremity. *Arch Surg* 1965; **91**: 29.
2. Adson AW, Coffey JR. Cervical rib. *Ann Surg* 1927; **85**: 839.
3. Aird I. In *A Companion in Surgical Studies.* London. Churchill Livingstone 1957.
4. Becker GJ, Holden RW, Rabe FE, Castaneda-Zuniga WR, Sears N, Dilley RS, Glover JL. Local thrombolytic therapy for subclavian and axillary vein thrombosis. *Radiology* 1983; **149**: 419.
5. Boontje AH. Axillary vein entrapment. *Br J Surg* 1979; **66**: 331.
6. Campbell CB, Chandler JG, Tegtmeyer CJ, Berstein EF. Axillary, subclavian and brachiocephalic vein obstruction. *Surgery* 1977; **82**: 816.
7. Coon WW, Willis PW. Thrombosis of the axillary and subclavian veins. *Arch Surg* 1967; **94**: 657.
8. Corning HK. *Lehrbuch der topographischen Anatomie* 24th edition. Munich. Bergmann 1949; 635.
9. Daskalakis E, Bouhoutsos J. Subclavian and axillary vein compression of musculo skeletal origin. *Br J Surg* 1980; **67**: 573.
10. Denck H, Fischer M, Kasprzak P. Thrombolysis in acute axillary vein thrombosis. *Int Angiol* 1984; **3**: 161.
11. De Weese JA, Adams JT, Gaiser DL. Subclavian venous thrombectomy. *Circulation* 1970; **42**: 158.
12. Dunant JH. Subclavian vein obstruction in thoracic outlet syndrome. *Int Angiol* 1984; **3**: 157.
13. French GE. Spontaneous thrombosis of the axillary vein. *Br Med J* 1944; **2**: 277.
14. Gillmer DJ, Mitha AS. Primary (stress) thrombosis of the upper arm associated with multiple pulmonary embolism. *S Afr Med J* 1980; **57**: 251.
15. Hughes ESR. Venous obstruction in the upper extremity (Paget–Schroetter's Syndrome). *Int Abstr Surg* 1949; **88**: 89.
16. Hughes ESR. Venous obstruction of the upper extremity. *Br J Surg* 1948; **36**: 155.
17. Hunter W. History of aneurysms of aorta with some remarks on aneurysms in general. *Med Observ Inquiries* 1747; **1**: 323.
18. Jacobson JH, Haimov M. Venous revascularisation of the arm. Report of three cases. *Surgery* 1977; **81**: 599.
19. Johnson V, Eiseman B. Evaluation of arterio-venous shunt to maintain patency of venous autograft. *Am J Surg* 1969; **118**: 915.
20. Kleinsasser LJ. "Effort" thrombosis of the axillary and subclavian veins. *Arch Surg* 1949; **59**: 258.
21. Mahorner H, Castleberry JW, Coleman WO. Attempts to restore function in major veins which are the site of massive thrombosis. *Ann Surg* 1957; **146**: 510.
22. Martin EC, Koser N, Gordon DH. Venography in axillary–subclavian vein thrombosis. *Cardiovasc Radiol* 1979; **2**: 261.
23. Mashiah A, Liebergall M, Pasik S, David A, Barkhayim Y. Axillary vein thrombosis: A rare complication following creation of arteriovenous fistula for haemodialysis. *J Cardiovasc Surg* 1986; **27**: 291.
24. McLeer RS, Kesterson JE, Kirtley JA, Love RB. Subclavian and anterior scalene muscle compression as a cause of intermittent obstruction of the subclavian vein. *Ann Surg* 1951; **133**: 588.
25. Paget J. *Clinical Lectures and Essays.* London. Longman's Green 1875.
26. Paletta FX. Venous gangrene of the hand. *Plast Reconstr Surg* 1981; **67**: 67.
27. Patwardhan NA, Anderson FA Jr, Cutler BS, Wheeler HB. Non-invasive detection of axillary and subclavian venous thrombosis by impedence plethysmography. *J Cardiovasc Surg* 1983; **24**: 250.
28. Prescott SM, Tikoff G. Deep venous thrombosis of the upper extremity, a reappraisal. *Circulation* 1979; **59**: 350.
29. Rabinowitz AR, Goldfarb D. Surgical treatment of axillo-subclavian venous thrombosis; A case report. *Surgery* 1971; **70**: 703.
30. Rheinlander HF. Superior vena cava replacement; Report of a successful autogenous composite graft. *J Thorac Cardiovasc Surg* 1969; **57**: 774.
31. Sachatello CR. The axillopectoral muscle (Langer's axillary arch): A cause of axillary vein obstruction. *Surgery* 1977; **81**: 610.
32. Sauvage LR, Gross RE. Evaluation of venous autografts and aortic homografts in canine intrathoracic venae cavae for periods of up to eight years. *J Thorac Cardiovasc Surg* 1967; **53**: 549.
33. Sauvage LR, Gross RE. Observations on experimental grafts in intrathoracic vena cavae. *Surg Gynec Obstet* 1960; **110**: 569.
34. Skinner DB, Saltzman EW, Scannell JG. The challenge of superior vena caval obstruction. *J Thorac Cardiovasc Surg* 1965; **49**: 824.
35. Smith BM, Shield GW, Riddell DH, Snell JD. Venous gangrene of the upper extremity. *Ann Surg* 1985; **201**: 511.
36. Stevenson IM, Parry EW. Radiological study of the aetiological factor in venous obstruction of the upper limb. *J Cardiovasc Surg* 1975; **16**: 580.
37. Sullivan ED, Reece CI, Cranley JJ. Phleborheo-

graphy of the upper extremity. *Arch Surg* 1983; **119**: 1134.

38. Sundqvist SB, Hedner U, Kullenberg HKE, Bergentz SE. Deep venous thrombosis of the arm: A study in coagulation and fibrinolysis. *Br Med J* 1981; **283**: 265.

39. Swinton NW, Edgett JW, Hall RJ. Primary subclavian–axillary vein thrombosis. *Circulation* 1968; **38**: 737.

40. Taheri SA, Lazar L, Elias S, Marchand P. Vein valve transplant. *Surgery* 1982; **91**: 28.

41. Tilney NL, Griffith HJG, Edwards EA. Natural history of major venous thrombosis of the upper extremity. *Arch Surg* 1970; **101**: 792.

42. Von Schroetter L. Erkrankungen der Gefasse. In Nothnagel CNH (Ed) *Handbuch der Pathologie und Therapie*. Vienna. Holder 1884.

43. Weinberg G, Pasternack BM. Upper extremity suppurative thrombophlebitis and septic pulmonary emboli. *JAMA* 1978; **240**: 1519.

44. Witte LC, Smith AC. Single anastomosis vein bypass for subclavian vein obstruction. *Arch Surg* 1966; **93**: 664.

45. Zimmerman R, Morl H, Harenberg J, Gerhardt P, Kuhn HM, Wahl P. Urokinase therapy of subclavian–axillary vein thrombosis. *Klin Wochenschr* 1981; **59**: 851.

25

Venous injury

The veins are frequently injured when there is soft tissue or bony trauma and during many surgical operations. The small and medium sized veins which are most commonly damaged can usually be ignored or ligated without causing any ill-effects. Problems arise when large deep limb veins are damaged, as ligation of these vessels (which was commonly practiced before the Second World War) can have disasterous consequences. It is now recognized that restoration of the continuity of the large veins of the limbs, abdomen and thorax can reduce late morbidity and preserve limbs. Unfortunately, many venous injuries pass unnoticed at the time of trauma and are only suspected later when the post-thrombotic syndrome develops. This is particularly common after fracture of the tibia (Fig. 25.1), which often causes a deep vein thrombosis days or weeks after the injury and the post-thrombotic syndrome many years later.[26,39]

Incidence

For the reasons outlined above, it is very difficult to obtain an accurate assessment of the incidence of venous injuries. Many injuries pass undetected and others are recognized but not recorded. Few patients with lower limb fractures have a phlebogram on admission to hospital because the care of the fracture predominates, and it is only many years later when post-thrombotic symptoms develop that a phlebogram indicates that a concomitant venous injury has passed unrecognized.

Veins are frequently damaged when their accompanying artery is injured, and large series of vascular injuries during both peace and war have shown that the incidence of major venous injury appears to be increasing.[16,30,46,50,58,59,66,74]

In the First World War, surgeons advocated

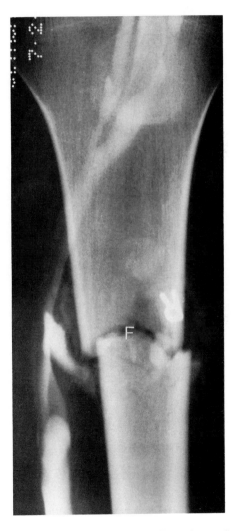

Fig. 25.1 (a) An example of the deep vein damage caused by fractures of the tibia. (F = fracture)
The deep veins are distorted and partially occluded.

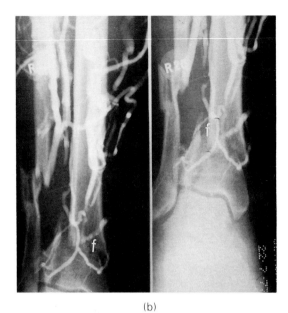

(b)

Fig. 25.1 (b) Another example of the deep vein damage caused by fractures of the tibia. (F = fracture)
The deep veins are distorted and partially occluded.

Table 25.1 Incidence of venous and arterial injuries in the Korean War[32]

	Number	Percentage
Major arterial injury	79	44
Major venous injury	71	40
Minor arterial injury	30	16

Table 25.2 Incidence of venous and arterial injuries in 500 combat casualties of the Vietnam War[58]

Total number of vascular injuries	718
Total number of venous injuries	194
Number of isolated venous injuries	28
Number of combined venous and arterial injuries	166

Table 25.3 Incidence of combined arterial and venous injuries in the Vietnam War[54]

Artery injured	Number of arterial injuries	Number of concomitant venous injuries (%)
Axillary	59	20 (33.8)
Brachial	283	54 (19.0)
Iliac	26	11 (42.3)
Common femoral	46	17 (36.9)
Superficial femoral	305	139 (45.5)
Popliteal	217	116 (53.5)
Total	936	357 (37.9)

ligation of injured arteries and veins to save life,[7] and some even suggested that ligation of undamaged limb veins might be beneficial if the artery had to be tied off.[42] Other surgeons had observed that the chances of limb survival were reduced if the major artery and vein of the limb had both been divided.[37,43] The incidence of venous injuries was not recorded in the First World War.

In a review of vascular injuries in the Second World War DeBakey and Simeone[14] concluded that concomitant vein ligation did *not* increase the chance of limb survival. No mention was made of the harmful effects of venous ligation, and the number of servicemen with venous injuries was not recorded.

In the Korean War, Hughes[33,34] reported that there were nearly as many injuries to major veins as injuries to the major arteries (Table 25.1), but in the Vietnam War the number of venous injuries had dropped to nearly a third of the number of arterial injuries (Table 25.2).[54,59,63] Only 38 per cent of the 936 arterial injuries which made up the Vietnam vascular registry[54] had an associated major venous injury (Table 25.3). Eighty per cent of the venous injuries were associated with arterial injuries, and more than 50 per cent of the popliteal artery injuries were associated with a concomitant venous injury. In the Yom Kippur War of 1973 there were only 15 severe venous injuries out of 82 vascular injuries.[66]

The vessels most frequently injured in the early years of the 'troubles' in Northern Ireland were the popliteal artery and vein; this was a result of the practice called 'knee-capping' – a particularly unpleasant and disabling form of penalty in which the popliteal fossa is deliberately shot through by a bullet.[50]

The incidence of venous injuries occurring in the civilian population has been steadily rising. In 1960 Gaspar and Trieman[20] reported that of 228 civilian patients with arterial injuries only just over 20 per cent had concomitant venous injuries. In 1966[74] the same group of workers reported 92

Table 25.4 Site of venous injuries

Traumatic (3 series)

	Vollmar[77]	Caspar and Treiman[20]	Rich *et al.*[58]
Inferior vena cava	2	8	—
Superior vena cava	0	1	—
Common iliac vein	2	1	11
Brachiocephalic vein	1	1	—
Brachial vein	10	7	54
Axillary vein	1	1	20
Femoral vein	5	9	156
Popliteal vein	2	4	116
Internal jugular	0	8	—
Portal	0	1	—

Iatrogenic[77]

Inferior vena cava (nephrectomy)	1
Inferior vena cava (aorto-iliac)	2
External iliac vein (ureterostomy)	1
External iliac vein (hernia)	1
Common femoral vein (varicose veins)	1
Common iliac vein (catheterization)	1

venous injuries but the proportion of venous to arterial injuries had not increased significantly. Four years later, Drapanas *et al.*[16] found a 41 per cent incidence of concomitant venous injury in their series of civilian arterial injuries.

By 1979 Vollmar[76] reported that 66 per cent of arterial injuries were associated with an injury to the accompanying veins, though not all the venous injuries required reconstruction. Vollmar observed that arterial injury occurred in 0.3–0.5 per cent of patients with major trauma, and he suggested that major venous injury was probably more common because the veins were more vulnerable. Conversely, Vollmar found that 75 per cent of the patients presenting with venous injuries had associated arterial injuries. During an 8-year period he reconstructed 30 venous injuries; seven of these injuries were iatrogenic. The distribution and site of the injuries is shown in Table 25.4; the series reported by Gasper and Trieman[20] and Rich *et al.*[58] are shown for comparison.

Since 1980, four further series of civilian venous injuries have been reported from the United States[3,23,30,46] where a rising incidence of civilian violence has been mirrored by an increase in the number of serious venous injuries.

Classification

A vein may be injured in one of five ways (Table 25.5).

Table 25.5 Type and cause of vein injuries

Injury	Cause
Incision	Direct external and internal forces
Laceration (tear)	Direct external and internal forces or avulsion of tributaries
Contusion	Direct blunt injury
Intramural tear	Stretching (indirect force)
Complete division	Direct or indirect external or internal force

Incision or laceration

This type of injury is usually caused by an external force (e.g. a cut or stab from a knife, bullet, shell or bomb fragment). Iatrogenic penetrating venous injuries are also becoming more common, as vascular surgery and invasive radiology increase. The resulting laceration can be subdivided into three main types (Fig. 25.2):

1. a clean cut into the lumen of the vein, often on two surfaces if the knife or bullet traverses the vein; (Fig. 25.2(a))
2. an irregular laceration caused by a rough penetrating agent (e.g. a spicule of bone) or by the avulsion of a tributary; (Fig. 25.2(c))
3. complete venous transection. This is really a form of incision or laceration but is classi-

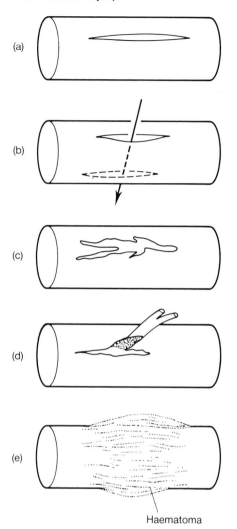

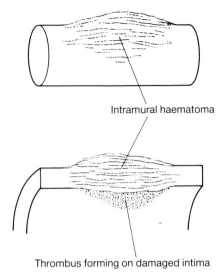

Intramural haematoma

Thrombus forming on damaged intima

Fig. 25.3 Venous contusion. All layers of the vein wall may be involved with thrombus forming on damaged intima or exposed collagen.

Haematoma

Fig. 25.2 Types of venous laceration (see Table 25.5). (a) Incision. (b) Transfixion. (c) Irregular laceration. (d) Avulsion of a tributary. (e) Complete transection.

fied separately in Table 25.5 because it presents special technical problems. (Fig. 25.2(e)).

Contusion

This type of injury results from a blow or crushing injury which does not disrupt the wall of the vein. The main damage is usually on the internal surface, with bruising extending through the media towards the adventitia.

The endothelial cells of the intima may be damaged or shed with no obvious external signs of injury but this can initiate mural thrombosis (Fig. 25.3). The medial muscle cells may also be damaged without external signs of injury and, in the most severe injury, cells in all layers of the vessel wall can be severely crushed and killed. If the vein wall is heavily contused and the intima is damaged, secondary thrombosis usually follows. A vein may become bruised simply by being involved in a large fracture haematoma.

Stretching

When a vein lies close to a bone or joint which has fractured or dislocated it may be damaged by being overstretched. Dislocations of the hip, knee, and shoulder are the most common causes of this type of injury. A severe stretch may completely disrupt one or more layers of the vein wall, usually the intima and media, leaving the vessel held together by the adventitia (Fig. 25.4). A less severe stretch may only damage the intima.

The exposed collagen makes thrombosis likely and, occasionally, 'false aneurysms' develop.

A severe deceleration injury can tear the inferior vena cava as it passes through the diaphragm. This injury is similar to the tear of the aortic arch that occurs in aeroplane and motor car crashes. If the vena cava is completely divided, the patient usually dies rapidly of exsanguination.

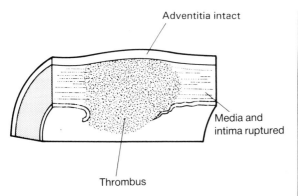

Adventitia intact

Media and
intima ruptured

Thrombus

Fig. 25.4 The effect of a venous stretching injury. The adventitia remains intact, but the media and intima may disrupt. Intramural haematoma distorts the lumen, damages the endothelium and causes intralumenal thrombosis.

Iatrogenic injuries

These have become an important group of venous injuries with the growth and extension of vascular surgery and the increase in interventional radiology (see Table 25.4). There is a high risk of venous injury whenever a structure is being dissected off a major vein. Operative venous injuries are particularly common in the pelvis where tumours of the bowel or aortic aneurysms may be closely applied to the iliac veins or to the inferior vena cava. Dissection of the common iliac artery from the underlying vein can be extremely difficult, and if a small tear is made in the vein because the vein wall is adherent to the artery, further traction on the artery simply enlarges the tear. Forceps should never be pushed behind the iliac artery without first dissecting a clear passage between the artery and the vein. Other common sites of surgical venous damage are in the femoral triangle and the popliteal fossa where the femoral and popliteal veins are often adherent to the adjacent artery and are joined by many small tributaries.

Inadvertent ligature of a major vein is another important and, unfortunately, not uncommon iatrogenic venous injury. The femoral and popliteal veins have often been tied during varicose vein operations by inexperienced surgeons (Fig. 25.5), usually because they have not fully displayed the anatomy of the sapheno-femoral or sapheno-popliteal junctions (see Chapter 7).

Major veins should not be ligated after inadvertent injury unless the haemorrhage is of

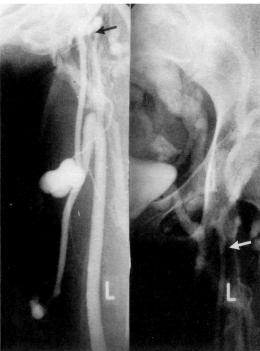

Fig. 25.5 An iatrogenic venous injury. This phlebogram shows the result of inadvertently ligating the femoral vein during a varicose vein operation. The occlusion has extended below the site of the ligature (arrowed) to the entry of a large tributary and proximally to the beginning of the common iliac vein.

such life-threatening proportions that vein ligation is the only hope for the patient's survival.

Another increasingly common form of venous injury is that which results from catheters inserted into veins by radiologists or physicians. Tears occur if the catheter happens to enter the vein in the angle between it and a tributary. Even small injuries carry an increased risk of intraluminal thrombosis with embolization of the thrombus, and if veins such as the vena cava are ruptured, severe haemorrhage may result.

Arteriovenous fistulae may develop if a penetrating injury traverses both a vein and an artery.[16] Arteriovenous fistulae may also complicate lumbar disc surgery if adjacent walls of the iliac artery and vein are inadvertently damaged.[24,40,45]

Badly placed sutures at an inguinal or femoral hernia repair may occlude or damage the external iliac or femoral vein as it passes beneath the inguinal ligament.

Toxic substances injected into a vein may damage the endothelium and cause thrombosis. This type of venous injury is discussed in Chapter 22 page 595.

Clinical presentation

Most venous injuries are associated with other injuries to soft tissues, arteries and bones, the symptoms of which often overshadow those of the venous injury. Massive haemorrhage can, however, occur from a penetrating wound in a vein, especially if it is associated with an open wound, and during an operation, haemorrhage from a venous injury may be more frightening and difficult to control than arterial haemorrhage because there is very little spontaneous reduction in bleeding from venous spasm. Blood escapes rapidly and continually until thrombus occludes the wound or the blood pressure falls.

Even if the connective tissues around a venous injury remain intact, a massive haematoma can occur around the lacerated vessel. The patient rapidly develops hypovolaemic shock with faintness, pallor, tachycardia and hypotension progressing to cardiac arrest, if no remedial action is taken.

Blunt trauma or stretching causing intramural bruising and oedema and intraluminal thrombosis may result in venous obstruction. The veins in the limb then become congested, the skin becomes cyanotic and the soft tissues swell. Surface veins become engorged and fail to collapse when the limb is elevated above heart level. If there is an associated injury to the artery (this occurs in 80 per cent of patients), there may also be signs of distal ischaemia, and these signs may predominate.

Investigation

Phlebography is the only investigation that may be helpful in making a diagnosis of the site and nature of a venous injury (see Fig. 25.5),[21] but if the injury is severe and the patient is shocked, surgical exploration is the quickest way of making the diagnosis and applying effective treatment, provided the surgeon is skilled in vascular surgical techniques.

Treatment; general considerations

Venous injuries present two main clinical problems, blood loss and vein repair.

Major blood loss

Venous bleeding from an open wound should be suspected if the blood is dark and rapidly rises from the base of the wound without evidence of pulsation. The first aid treatment is to apply local pressure to the wound and, if possible, elevate the affected part. Pressure and elevation should be maintained while the patient is being transferred rapidly to hospital. Blood is cross-matched and intravenous catheters are inserted for resuscitation.

The catheters should be put into the normal arm if there is an upper limb injury, and they should be placed in the internal jugular vein or an arm vein if the injury is in the lower limb or abdomen. In patients with major vein injuries in the superior mediastinum, a central venous catheter may have to be inserted via a femoral vein. A central venous catheter allows blood to be rapidly infused and may also be used to measure central venous pressure; it is therefore an invaluable adjunct to the management of all major venous injuries.

The patient should be anaesthetized in the operating room and the wound gently inspected. If this inspection is accompanied by further profuse haemorrhage, pressure should be reapplied to control the bleeding until an appropriate level of resuscitation has been achieved and adequate quantities of cross-matched blood are available for surgery to be commenced. Bleeding from a wound in the limb can be controlled with a pneumatic tourniquet and surgical exploration can be carried out in a bloodless field but tourniquets should not be applied indiscriminately before the patient enters hospital. A loose, badly applied tourniquet may cause venous engorgement and increase, rather than reduce blood loss.

Wounds should be extended to allow easy access to the injured vein. Bleeding can usually be controlled by gentle direct 'finger' pressure (Fig. 25.6) on or on either side of the bleeding point until the vein has been dissected and can be clamped above and below the injury (Fig. 25.6). If this cannot be done, bleeding can be controlled by inserting two Fogarty balloon catheters into the vessel through the tear (Fig. 25.7).

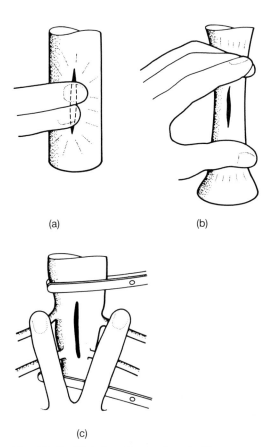

(a)　　　　　　　　　(b)

(c)

Fig. 25.6 Digital methods of controlling venous haemorrhage. (a) Direct finger pressure. (b) Proximal and distal finger pressure. (c) Proximal and distal venous occlusion by clamps with finger control of the tributaries.

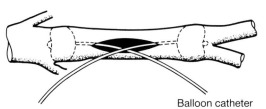

Balloon catheter

Fig. 25.7 Control of venous haemorrhage by intralumenal balloon tamponade. Fogarty balloon catheters are inserted proximally and distally through the venotomy and are inflated until they stop the blood flow.

Once the damaged vein has been dissected free from its surrounding tissues, the venous injury and any associated injuries to nearby arteries and nerves should be assessed. A decision can then be made about the best method of repair. It is preferable to repair the venous injury first, even if there are other vascular injuries, though it is of course important to gain control of any arterial bleeding before beginning the venous repair.

Anticoagulation

Systemic heparin has not been shown to improve the long-term patency of venous repair[1,27,79] but we give heparin, 5000 units intravenously, as soon as we are ready to apply vascular clamps to the vein, except when there is extensive soft tissue contusion and uncontrolled bleeding. Heparin should always be given if there is an associated arterial injury requiring arterial occlusion and reconstruction. Some workers have advocated the use of dextran in addition to heparin[17,27] but we find that this combination increases capillary oozing which makes the surgery more difficult and increases the risk of postoperative haematomata.

History of vein repair

Travers and Cooper[73] reputedly performed the first venous repair in 1816. In 1877 Eck[19] performed the first veno-venous anastomosis when he anastomosed the portal vein to the inferior vena cava, and Schede (1882)[64] was credited by Murphy[47] with the first successful venous repair by lateral suture. Kümmel in 1899[38] performed the first end-to-end venous anastomosis, and Clermont (1901)[11] successfully joined a divided inferior vena cava, but Carrel and Guthrie (1906)[8] provided the necessary experimental background for consistent and successful venous repair. Rich *et al.*[54,55,59] popularized venous repair in battle injuries and showed that this reduced limb loss and subsequent morbidity from chronic venous obstruction.

Techniques of vein repair

Lateral suture

A simple side-hole in a vein can be sutured with a carefully placed single or continuous vascular

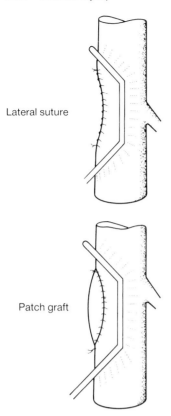

Lateral suture

Patch graft

Fig. 25.8   The lateral suture and patch repair of venous injuries. These repairs can often be performed with the lumen partially occluded with a Satinsky clamp.

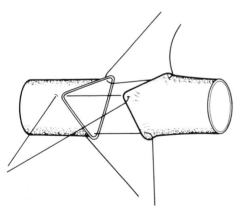

Carrel triangulation sutures

Fig. 25.9   The Carrel triangulation technique of venous anastomosis. Stretching each segment of vein with the stay sutures stops the intervening continuous suture causing a stenosis.

suture (prolene, 5/0 or 6/0 is ideal), while the vein is occluded either side of the tear by gentle finger pressure or by a Satinsky clamp (Fig. 25.8). Although this procedure may cause a little narrowing of the vein (Fig. 25.8), the narrowing is unlikely to be significant if a segment of vein wall has not been lost.[20,34,67]

Vein patch

If a segment of vein wall has been lost, or if the vessel is small (e.g. the popliteal vein), it is probably better to close the defect with a vein patch to prevent narrowing (see Fig. 25.8).[8,58,75] The patch should be fashioned from a nearby tributary or a subcutaneous vein from the opposite limb. *It should not be taken from a major subcutaneous vein of the injured limb* (e.g. the saphenous vein) because this may later serve as an important collateral vessel if the damaged vein becomes occluded.

End-to-end anastomosis

When the vein wall is extensively damaged, transected, or a complete segment is destroyed, it usually has to be replaced by a graft. Veins can rarely be mobilized and stretched so that they can be sutured end-to-end, except when there is a clear incised wound.[62] In these circumstances ligation of the tributaries may be needed in order to mobilize the vein, and the anastomosis is best performed using the Carrel triangulation technique (Fig. 25.9).[9]

Vein replacement

Autogenous vein is the material of choice for vein replacement.[22,50,55,58] The veins commonly used as grafts include the long and short saphenous veins, the cephalic vein and the internal jugular vein. The internal jugular vein was first used for meso-caval bypass grafts[29] but has also been used to bypass axillary vein obstruction.[36,72] It has the advantage of being of similar size to the iliac and femoral veins. The subcutaneous veins are usually too small for a simple end-to-end anastomosis, and if the saphenous or cephalic veins are used, a composite graft must be made in order to produce a tube whose diameter is equal to that of the damaged vein (Fig. 25.10). This is achieved by

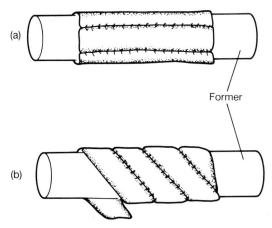

Fig. 25.10 Two forms of composite grafts which can be used to bridge complete deficiencies in large veins. (a) A panel graft, (b) a spiral graft.

splitting two or three segments of vein longitudinally and sewing them together along their lateral margins.[2,18,50] The resulting wide-bore tube can then be anastomosed, end-to-end, to the damaged vein after excising the damaged segment.

An alternative method of producing a wide-bore tube is to split the vein and sew it as a spiral (see Fig. 25.10); this has proved satisfactory in some circumstances.[15,30] End-to-end anastomoses are preferred to end-to-side anastomoses for the reconstruction.

Flow-enhancing arteriovenous fistulae

There is good experimental evidence that venous anastomoses have better patency rates when there is a high rate of blood flow passing through the anastomosis.[39,65,68]

The increased rate of blood flow can be achieved by forming a temporary arteriovenous fistula up-stream to the anastomosis (Fig. 25.11). Most authorities[66,68,77] suggest that a temporary arteriovenous fistula should be kept open for 3 months after reconstructive venous surgery. Fashioning a fistula adds time to the procedure; this is a factor that must be considered if there are other severe injuries needing treatment. Intermittent pneumatic compression applied to the distal part of the limb is an alternative method of enhancing venous flow and reducing the incidence of postoperative thrombosis.[28]

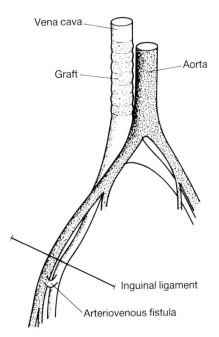

Fig. 25.11 A flow enhancing arteriovenous fistula which should be used to increase venous blood flow after a venous repair. (See Fig. 9.12, page 281.)

Manoeuvres to remove propagated thrombosis

Before the vascular clamps are removed and venous blood flow is released, the vein should be washed out with heparinized saline and, if there is any suspicion of poor blood flow from either side of the anastomosis, a Fogarty balloon catheter should be passed as far as possible in both directions.[62] If distal thrombus is suspected and the balloon will not pass beyond the nearest competent valve, an Esmarch bandage applied from the foot to the wound may be used to express thrombus. These precautions should always be taken if there has been a long interval between the injury and the operation.

Repair of concomitant injuries

When the veins have been reconstructed, the arterial injuries can be repaired, followed by internal or external fixation of fractures, suturing of torn tendons and repair of nerves. When manipulating and fixing fractures great care must be taken not to disrupt the vascular anastomoses.[50,56] All ischaemic tissue should be widely excised.

Repair of one large vein probably guarantees a sufficient outflow tract, even if there are, for example, two large popliteal veins that have been damaged. Care should be taken at all times to preserve the superficial veins in the injured limb.[60,62] If all the subcutaneous veins draining a digit, hand or foot are severed some must be repaired as the deep veins at the wrist and ankle are often small and an insufficient outflow tract. Small veins (e.g. digital veins) may be repaired with end-to-end anastomoses or interposition vein grafts using an operating microscope.

Drainage and antibiotics

Suture lines in veins bleed more than suture lines in arteries; all wounds should therefore be closed over suction drainage. Broad-spectrum antibiotics which are effective against staphylococci and anaerobic organisms (especially clostridia) should be given for 5 days if the wound is contaminated or the tissues are extensively damaged.

Fasciotomy

The fascia enclosing the anterior and the posterior compartments of the lower limb should be divided if there has been a prolonged period of arterial ischaemia or severe venous congestion.[50,55] It is always better to err towards unnecessary fasciotomy than to risk loss of the limb.

Special problems

Inferior vena caval injuries

These injuries are usually the result of stab or gunshot wounds of the abdomen.[44,51,53,69,78] The injured segment of vein must be fully exposed, either by reflecting the root of the mesentery and fourth part of the duodenum to the patient's right (as when exposing the aorta) or by reflecting the caecum and ascending colon to the patient's left.[44] This later, almost retroperitoneal, approach gives better access to the vena cava above the right renal vein (Fig. 25.12). If an abdominal incision is extended above the right costal margin and through the diaphragm to open the thorax, the liver can be turned to the patient's left and the whole of the upper abdominal and the thoracic inferior vena cava exposed.[44]

The lumbar veins drain into the postero-lateral aspect of the inferior vena cava. Access to this surface of the vein is difficult because it lies

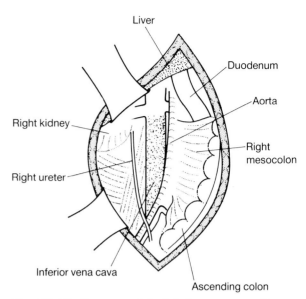

Fig. 25.12 Exposure of the inferior vena cava. The duodenum and ascending colon are freed along their lateral border and are reflected to the left to expose the sub-hepatic inferior vena cava.

directly on the vertebral column. This makes control of haemorrhage through a caval tear difficult and finger control (see Fig. 25.6) or pressure with pledgets[53,69] around the tear may be all that is initially possible. With better exposure it may be possible to apply a Satinsky type of partially occluding clamp (see Fig. 25.8).[78]

If the tear is a simple anterior laceration, it may be closed with a continuous 5/0 prolene suture. If both the anterior and posterior surfaces of the vein have been injured, the anterior tear may have to be extended after the bleeding has been fully controlled and the posterior tear may have to be closed from within, before the anterior defect is closed. If the vessel wall has been severely damaged or disrupted, the injured segment should be replaced with an end-to-end interposition graft. An externally supported PTFE graft is the material of choice for replacement of the vena cava,[13] and a high blood flow in the postoperative period is ensured by the formation of a distal arteriovenous fistula between the iliac or femoral vein and a small branch of the corresponding artery or by anastomosing a small tributary of the vein to the artery (see Fig. 18.10, page 515).

Blood loss from the retrohepatic portion of the vena cava or the hepatic veins can be controlled by

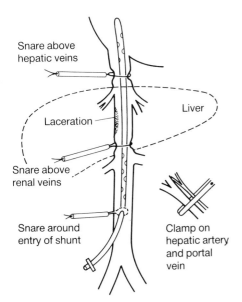

Snare above
hepatic veins

Liver

Laceration

Snare above
renal veins

Snare around
entry of shunt

Clamp on
hepatic artery
and portal
vein

Fig. 25.13 Isolation of the liver blood supply.
A plastic 'shunt' containing side holes at either
end is positioned across the liver and held in place by
'snares' around the supra- and sub-hepatic
segments of the vena cava to prevent venous blood
flowing up beside the shunt. If the portal vein and
hepatic artery are also occluded, all blood flow to the
liver is stopped.

isolating the liver from its blood supply. An intraluminal shunt may be inserted through the
femoral vein, iliac vein or lower part of the cava
and held in place by tapes placed above and below
the liver and tightened to occlude venous flow
other than through the shunt (Fig. 25.13). Double
balloon catheters have been produced to allow
rapid liver and caval isolation through a femoral
venous cut-down before the cava is exposed.

Iliac vein injuries

When there is extensive damage to the iliac veins
consideration must be given to direct replacement
or bypass. A bypass may be placed end-to-side
across the damaged vein, or the opposite long saphenous vein may be used as a bypass from the
femoral vein below the ligated vein to the normal
femoral vein (The Palma operation – see Chapter
9, page 281).[52] Both these procedures should be
combined with a distal arteriovenous fistula. It is
much easier to perform a Palma operation than to
carry out an orthotopic replacement or bypass.

Internal iliac vein injuries

A damaged internal iliac vein should be ligated.
There is no need to repair it as there are many
veins that cross the floor of the pelvis that can act
as collaterals.

Left renal vein injuries

If the left renal vein is damaged between the
inferior vena cava and its suprarenal tributaries it
may be tied without affecting renal blood flow or
renal function. Damage to the veins in the hilum
of the kidney should be repaired if possible but
injuries in this area are often associated with
arterial and pelvi-ureteric damage which may
necessitate nephrectomy.

Subclavian and axillary vein injuries

The axillary and subclavian veins may be injured
by penetrating wounds above and below the
clavicle and by fractures of the clavicle and first
rib.

As these veins lie behind the clavicle, they may
be difficult to expose, especially if they are bleeding profusely.[5,6,25,35,70] Some of the bleeding can be
reduced by inflating a tourniquet high on the arm
to above systolic pressure to prevent arterial
inflow to the arm and so reduce venous outflow.
If the vein is not totally divided but cannot be
seen, the bleeding can be controlled by passing
balloon catheters proximally through an upper
arm vein so that a balloon can be inflated on either
side of the tear. In a desperate life-saving situation, which usually means that there is massive
bleeding from the central end of a totally divided
subclavian vein, the clavicle should be divided or
the mediastium should be opened through a
sternal splitting incision to gain control of the
jugular and innominate veins or superior vena
cava (Fig. 25.14).[78]

The subclavian and axillary veins can be ligated
without risk to the viability of the limb. Tears can
be sutured but it is probably not wise to attempt a
resection and interposition or bypass graft in the
emergency situation. Reconstructions can be considered later if the ligation causes disabling symptoms – an unusual event (see Chapter 24).

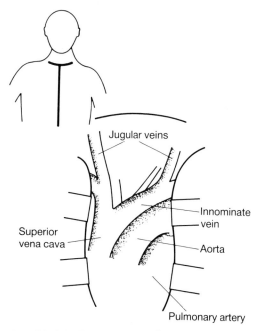

Fig. 25.14 The exposure of the large veins in the root of the neck.

Iatrogenic injuries

Minor tears in veins that occur during an operation can usually be controlled by one or two carefully places sutures across the tear while the bleeding is controlled with pressure and suction. Sometimes the tear may be difficult to see (e.g. when an iliac vein is torn during the dissection of the iliac artery). To avoid this complication many surgeons advocate simply mobilizing an artery on either side and applying clamps without putting a snare around the artery. In difficult circumstances access may be improved by transecting the artery to reveal the anterior surface of the vein.

Venous occlusion by accidental ligation or secondary thrombosis

This is another form of venous injury most often caused by an inexperienced surgeon mistakenly ligating a deep vein or accidentally including a deep vein in a mass ligature (see Chapter 7, page 212). The presence of a major vein obstruction is indicated by swelling of the limb, distention of the veins and generalized tightness and pain in the muscles. If this complication is suspected, its presence can be confirmed by a non-invasive test, for example Doppler flow detection, impedance plethysmography or phleborheography (see Chapter 4) but the precise site of the occlusion must be demonstrated by ascending phlebography before surgical exploration is undertaken (see Fig. 25.5).[21]

The occluded vein is explored through an appropriately sited incision which is usually the incision of the previous operation. The vein is inspected and palpated to determine the level of the occlusion and the presence of distal thrombosis.

Heparin is administered systemically, tapes are placed around the vessel above and below the damaged area and vascular clamps are applied. Any obstructing ligatures are removed and a venotomy is made in the contused or thrombosed vein. Thrombus can be gently removed with a Fogarty catheter, and the presence of intact intima can be confirmed before the venotomy is closed. If there is intimal damage with loss of endothelium, the segment should be replaced by one of the techniques described above. Consideration should also be given to forming a distal arteriovenous fistula to try to maintain patency. Flow may also be encouraged by applying intermittent pneumatic compression to the legs. Systemic anticoagulants (heparin followed by warfarin) should be given for 4–6 weeks.

Postoperative monitoring

In the early postoperative stages flow through the vein may be assessed with a Doppler flow detector. Phlebograms should be performed if there is any indication that the vein has re-occluded, a complication which may be treated by venous thrombectomy if a thrombosis is confirmed. Phlebography should be performed at some stage in the early postoperative period to confirm patency, and it should be repeated a few months later to document long-term success. The venous phase of a digital subtraction arteriogram may provide useful information about the patency of large vein repairs.

Results

The simultaneous repair of a venous injury associated with an arterial injury has been shown to improve limb survival.[10,32,59,60,63,67,71] Although vein ligation is known to be followed by a significant incidence of chronic venous insufficiency,[33,56,60] the long-term patency rates following vein repair are not well documented. Hobson et al.[29] claimed that approximately one-third of their venous reconstructions were 'successful'. More recently, Hobson[30] has claimed better results for femoral venous reconstructions with 74 per cent 'judged' patent postoperatively. The extent and site of the initial injury may have considerable bearing on the outcome because a simple lateral suture is unlikely to cause thrombosis or occlusion whereas a long graft, especially if a composite graft or an artificial prosthesis is used, has a high chance of failure. The reason for our lack of knowledge lies in the relative scarcity of these injuries. It is difficult for one surgeon to obtain a large series of these injuries, except during times of war.

Complications of venous injuries and their repair

The common complications of venous injuries are: air embolism, arteriovenous fistula, pulmonary embolism, post-thrombotic limb, secondary infection and bleeding.

Air embolism

This is usually a complication of injuries of the veins of the head, neck and upper limb. It may also be seen in association with a tension pneumothorax combined with an intrathoracic venous injury. The most common cause is careless manipulation of the vein during exploration of a venous injury. Air must always be prevented from entering the vein by downstream compression, lowering the level of the damaged vein beneath that of the right atrium, and asking the anaesthetist to apply strong positive pressure ventilation. Since the introduction of positive pressure ventilation, air embolism is a rare occurrence.[76]

Arteriovenous fistula

This is usually caused by a penetrating injury that passes through an adjacent artery and vein. A fistula develops immediately through the incisions or through a haematoma between the two vessels.

Traumatic arteriovenous fistulae have been

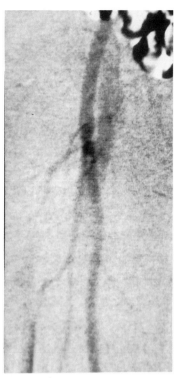

Fig. 25.15 A traumatic arteriovenous fistula. This is a digital subtraction arteriogram showing contrast medium passing down the femoral artery and entering the femoral vein rather than passing distally down the limb. It followed a femoral artery puncture for cardiac catheterization.

reported after lumbar disc surgery if the rongeur passes through the anterior longitudinal ligament into the iliac vessels.[24,40,45] Fistulae may also follow penetrating injuries in the groin (e.g. knife wounds or cardiac catheterization) (Fig. 25.15) if both the femoral artery and femoral vein are inadvertently punctured.[57] Ligation of the renal artery and vein or of both the splenic vessels in a mass ligature is a reported cause of traumatic arteriovenous fistulae.[31]

The diagnosis of an arteriovenous fistula is made by finding distended pulsating veins, a palpable thrill and loud bruit and a positive Branham's sign.[4] There may be signs of right-sided congestive heart failure or high output left heart failure with engorged neck veins, crepitations in the lungs and ankle oedema.[48]

The site of the fistula should be localized by arteriography (see Fig. 25.15) and then closed by surgical suture. The artery should be controlled above the fistula before the vein and the artery are dissected. The vessels can then be separated and the communication closed. It may be necessary to open the artery and close the hole into the vein from the lumenal side of the artery or even replace the involved segment of artery.[31]

Pulmonary embolism

Cook and Haller[12] suggested that pulmonary embolism was likely to be a common complication of vein repair, because if the repair was unsuccessful, it would thrombose and the thrombus might propagate proximally from the site of the repair before breaking off and embolizing to the lungs. This has not been borne out by clinical experience,[16,54] and the incidence of thromboembolism is said to be higher after popliteal ligation than after vein repair.[56] Nevertheless, pulmonary emboli will inevitably occasionally follow any form of direct deep vein surgery.

Post-thrombotic syndrome

Despite the early enthusiastic reports of improved limb salvage by combining venous and arterial repair, the success of venous repair may be as low as 30 per cent,[29] though this figure may have increased with improvements in technique.[30]

The long-term results of venous repair are not known. Many of the 'successful repairs' probably thrombose in the postoperative period. A proportion will then recanalize giving the patient a better outlook than if the vein had been ligated[61] but it is not unreasonable to expect that almost half of the patients who have had a venous reconstruction will develop a post-thrombotic syndrome. No reliable figures are available to confirm or refute this prediction.

Secondary infection

The use of autogenous tissues for grafts, careful excision of devitalized tissue, antibiotic prophylaxis, and the use of delayed primary suture should reduce secondary infection to a minimum.[41] Delayed primary suture is a vital part of the management of gunshot wounds but major arteries and veins must not be left uncovered in the base of a wound.[14] The skin should not be closed but some tissue, preferably muscle, should be mobilized to cover the vessels, especially if they contain suture lines closed with non-absorbable materials.

Limb loss

Gangrene only follows a major vein injury when there is an associated arterial occlusion or when all the veins of the limb have been transected or occluded. The latter situation occurs with traumatic amputations, usually at the level of the knee where the popliteal vein is the only effective outflow when even multiple venous anastomoses can be insufficient to allow an adequate circulation. If arterial insufficiency can be corrected, a limb should survive even if its main axial vein is occluded. The limb may become swollen and discoloured,[34] and oedema of muscles enclosed within tight compartments may make them and their adjacent nerves ischaemic.[16,50,54] The importance of careful clinical observation of the anterior and posterior deep compartments of the leg and the flexor compartments of the forearm cannot be over-emphasized. Any swelling, tenderness, induration, pain or loss of function should be treated by immediate and extensive fasciotomy.[16,50] An adequate vein repair should reduce the incidence of compartment compression syndromes when there is extensive soft tissue and major vein damage, and should also reduce the incidence of distal gangrene.

Comment

Venous damage to small vessels is common and unimportant. Major vein damage from trauma fortunately seldom occurs except in armed conflicts or insurrections. Careful venous repair or reconstruction is important, especially following injury to the popliteal vein. It is important to try to keep the blood flow through a repaired vein as high as possible, but collateral veins, however small, must not be sacrificed. The incidence of long-term sequelae after venous injuries and reconstruction is not known but basic principles[62] insist that it is preferable to repair rather than to ligate a major vein.[23,30,46]

The surgeons of North America, Israel and Northern Ireland[34,50,62] have shown the value of successful venous repair in avoiding amputation and severe venous congestion. Although many of the initial reports were mainly on missile injuries, more recent studies have shown that military prin-

Table 25.6 Success of venous repair[50]

	Number	Success	Amputation
Lateral suture	12	9	2
Panel grafts	6	6	0
Vein graft (delayed)	5	2	1
Vein patch (delayed)	7	6	0
End-to-end anastomosis	3	1	1
Ligation	3	0	1

ciples can be translated to civilian practice.[23,30,46] The technique of lateral suture should be used whenever possible, but when there is extensive vein wall damage, the panel-graft or spiral graft techniques are valuable, using the contralateral long saphenous vein to make the composite grafts.

Venous injuries rarely occur in isolation, and it is difficult to assess the results of treatment without taking into consideration the scale and extent of the other injuries, both their management and an appraisal of their results.

References

1. Baird RJ, Lipton IH, Miyagishima RT, Labrosse CJ. Replacement of the deep veins of the leg. *Arch Surg* 1964; **89**: 797.
2. Benvenuto R, Rodman FSB, Gilmour J, Phillips AF, Callagham JC. Composite venous graft for replacement of the superior vena cava. *Arch Surg* 1962; **89**: 100.
3. Blumoff RL, Powell T, Johnson G. Femoral venous trauma in a university referral center. *J Trauma* 1982; **22**: 703.
4. Branham HH. Das arteriellvenöse Aneurysma. *Arch Klin Chir* 1896; **33**: 1.
5. Brawley RK, Murray GF, Crisler C, Cameron JL. Management of wounds of the innominate, subclavian and axillary blood vessels. *Surg Gynec Obstet* 1970; **131**: 1130.
6. Bricker DL, Noon GP, Beall AC, DeBakey ME. Vascular injuries of the thoracic outlet. *J Trauma* 1970; **10**: 1.
7. Brooke B. Surgical applications of therapeutic venous obstruction. *Arch Surg* 1929; **9**: 1.
8. Carrel A, Guthrie CC. Uniterminal and biterminal venous transplantation. *Surg Gynec Obstet* 1906; **2**: 266.
9. Carrel A. La technique opératoire des anastomoses vasculaires et la transplantation des viscères. *Lyon Méd* 1902; **98**: 859.
10. Chandler JG, Knapp RW. Early definitive treatment of vascular injuries in the Vietnam conflict. *JAMA* 1967; **202**: 960.
11. Clermont G. Suture latérale et circulaire des veins. *Presse Méd* 1901; **1**: 229.
12. Cook FW, Haller JA. Penetrating injuries of the subclavian vessels with associated venous complications. *Ann Surg* 1962; **155**: 370.
13. Dale WA. Peripheral venous reconstruction. In Dale WA (Ed) *Management of Vascular Surgical Problems*. New York. McGraw-Hill 1985.
14. DeBakey ME, Simeone FA. Battle injuries of the arteries in World War II: An analysis of 2471 cases. *Ann Surg* 1946; **123**: 534.
15. Doty DB, Baker WH. Bypass of the superior vena cava with a spiral vein graft. *Ann Thorac Surg* 1976; **22**: 490.
16. Drapanas T, Hewitt RL, Weichert RF, Smith AD. Civilian vascular injuries: A critical appraisal of three decades of management. *Ann Surg* 1970; **172**: 351.
17. Eadie DGA, de Takats G. The early fate of autogenous vein grafts in the canine femoral vein. *J Cardiovasc Surg* 1966; **7**: 148.
18. Earle AS, Horsley JS, Villavicencio JL, Warren R. Replacement of venous defects by venous autografts. *Arch Surg* 1960; **80**: 119.
19. Eck NVK. Voprosu o perevyazke vorotnois veni. Predvaritelnoye soobshtshjenye. *Voen Med J* 1877; **130**: 1.
20. Gaspar MR, Treiman RL. The management of injuries to major veins. *Am J Surg* 1960; **100**: 171.
21. Gerlock AJ, Muhletaler CA. Venography of peripheral venous injuries. *Radiology* 1979; **133**: 77.
22. Haimovici H, Hoffert PW, Zinicola N, Steinman C. An experimental and clinical evaluation of grafts in the venous system. *Surg Gynec Obstet* 1970; **131**: 1173.
23. Hardin WD, Adinolfi MF, O'Connell RL, Kerstein MD. Management of traumatic peripheral vein injuries. *Am J Surg* 1982; **144**: 235.
24. Hernando FJS, Paredero VM, Solis JV, Rio AD, Parra JJL, Orgaz A, Aroca M, Tovar A, Delbosque VP. Iliac arteriovenous fistula as a complication of lumbar disc surgery. *J Cardiovasc Surg* 1986; **27**: 180.
25. Hewitt RL, Smith AD, Becker ML, Lindsey ES, Dowling JB, Drapanas T. Penetrating vascular injuries of the thoracic inlet. *Surgery* 1974; **76**: 715.
26. Hjelmstedt AU, Bergvall S. Phlebographic study of the incidence of thrombosis in the injured and uninjured limb in 55 cases of tibial fracture. *Acta Chir Scand* 1968; **134**: 229.
27. Hobson RW, Croom RD, Rich NM. Influence of heparin and low molecular weight dextran on the patency of vein grafts in the venous system.

Ann Surg 1973; **178**: 773.

28. Hobson RW, Lee BC, Lynch TG, Jain K, Yeager RA, Jamil Z, Padberg FT. Use of intermittent pneumatic calf compression in femoral venous reconstruction. *Surg Gynec Obstet* 1984; **159**: 284.

29. Hobson RW, Wright CB, Swann KG, Rich NM. Current status of venous injury and reconstruction in the lower extremity. In *Venous Problems*. Bergan JJ, Yao JST (Eds) Chicago. Year Book Medical Publishers 1978.

30. Hobson RW, Yeager RA, Lynch TG, Lee BC, Jain K, Jamil Z, Padberg FT. Femoral venous trauma: Techniques for surgical management and early results. *Am J Surg* 1983; **146**: 220.

31. Hollman E. *Abnormal Arteriovenous Communications* 2nd edition. Illinois. Thomas 1937.

32. Hughes CW. Acute vascular trauma in Korean casualties. *Surg Gynec Obstet* 1954; **99**: 91.

33. Hughes CW. Arterial repair during the Korean war. *Ann Surg* 1958; **157**: 155.

34. Hughes CW. Vascular surgery in the armed forces. *Milit Med* 1959; **124**: 30.

35. Hunt TK, Blaisdell FW, Okimoto J. Vascular injuries of the base of the neck. *Arch Surg* 1969; **98**: 586.

36. Jacobson JH, Haimov M. Venous revascularization of the arm. Report of three cases. *Surgery* 1977; **81**: 599.

37. Jacobson WHA. In Rowlands RP, Turner P (Eds) *The Operations of Surgery* 6th edition. London. J & A Churchill 1915; 843.

38. Kümmel 'H. Abkürzung des Heilungsverlaufs Laparatomierter durch frühzeitiges Aufstehen. *Verh Dtsch Ges Chir* 1908; **37**: 1.

39. Kunlin J, Kunlin A, Richard S, Tregovet T. Le rétablissment de la circulation veineuse par greffe en cas d'oblitération traumatique ou thrombophlebitique. *Mem Acad Clin* 1953; **79**: 109.

40. Linton RR, White PD. Arteriovenous fistula between the right common iliac artery and inferior vena cava: A report of its occurrence following operation for ruptured intervertebral disc with cure by operation. *Arch Surg* 1945; **50**: 6.

41. Livingstone RH, Wilson R. Gunshot wounds of the limbs. *Br Med J* 1975; **1**: 667.

42. Makins GH. *On Gunshot Injuries to the Blood Vessels*. Bristol. John Wright 1919.

43. Matas R. Surgery of the vascular system. In Keen WW (Ed) *Surgery, its Principles and Practice by Various Authors*. Philadelphia. WB Saunders 1921.

44. Mattox KL. Abdominal venous injuries. *Surgery* 1982; **91**: 497.

45. May ARL. Brewster DC, Darling RC, Browse NL. Arteriovenous fistula following lumbar disc surgery. *Br J Surg* 1981; **68**: 41.

46. Mullins RJ, Lucas CE, Ledgerwood AM. The natural history following venous ligation for civilian injuries. *J Trauma* 1980; **20**: 737.

47. Murphy JB. Resection of arteries and veins injured in continuity: end to end suture. Experimental and clinical research. *Med Rec* 1897; **51**: 73.

48. Nicalodoni C. Phlebarteriectasie der rechten oberen extremität. *Arch Klin Chir* 1875; **18**: 252.

49. Nylander GH, Semb C. Veins of the lower part of the leg after tibial fractures. *Surg Gynec Obstet* 1972; **134**: 974.

50. O'Reilly NJG, Hood JM, Livingston RH, Irwin JWS. Penetrating injuries of the popliteal vein: a report on 34 cases. *Br J Surg* 1980; **67**: 337.

51. Ochsner JL, Crawford ES, DeBakey ME. Injuries of the vena cava caused by external trauma. *Surgery* 1961; **49**: 397.

52. Palma EC, Esperon R. Vein transplants and grafts in the surgical treatment of the post phlebitic syndrome. *J Cardiovasc Surg* 1950; **1**: 94.

53. Quast DC, Shirkey AL, Fitzgerald JB, Beall AC, DeBakey ME. Surgical correction of injuries of the vena cava: an analysis of 61 cases. *J Trauma* 1965; **5**: 3.

54. Rich NM, Baugh JH, Hughes CW. Acute arterial injuries in Vietnam: 1000 cases. *J Trauma* 1970; **10**: 359.

55. Rich NM, Collins GV, Anderson CA, McDonald PT. Autogenous venous interposition grafts in repair of major venous injuries. *J Trauma* 1977; **17**: 512.

56. Rich NM, Hobson RW, Collins GJ, Anderson CA. The effect of acute popliteal venous interruption. *Ann Surg* 1976; **183**: 365.

57. Rich NM, Hobson RW, Collins GJ. Traumatic arteriovenous fistulas and false aneurysm: A review of 558 lesions. *Surgery* 1975; **78**: 817.

58. Rich NM, Hughes CW, Baugh JH. Management of venous injuries. *Ann Surg* 1970; **171**: 724.

59. Rich NM, Hughes CW. Vietnam vascular registry: a preliminary report. *Surgery* 1969; **65**: 218.

60. Rich NM, Jarstfer BS, Greer TM. Popliteal artery repair: causes and possible prevention. *J Cardiovasc Surg* 1974; **15**: 340.

61. Rich NM, Sullivan WG. Clinical recanalization of an autogenous vein graft in the popliteal vein. *J Trauma* 1972; **12**: 919.

62. Rich NM. Principles and indications for primary venous repair. *Surgery* 1982; **91**: 492.

63. Rich NM. Vascular trauma in Vietnam. *J Cardiovasc Surg* 1970; **11**: 368.

64. Schede M. Einige Bemerkungen über die Naht von Venenwunden, nebst Mittheilung eines Falles von geheilter Naht der Vena cava inferior. *Arch Klin Chir* 1892; **43**: 338.

65. Scheinin TM, Jude JR. Experimental replacement of the superior vena cava: effect of a temporary

increase in blood flow. *J Cardiovasc Surg* 1964; **48**: 781.

66. Schramek A, Hashmonai M. Vascular injuries in the extremities in battle casualties. *Br J Surg* 1977; **64**: 644.

67. Spencer FC, Grewe RV. The management of acute arterial injuries in battle casualties. *Ann Surg* 1955; **141**: 304.

68. Stansel HC Jr. Synthetic inferior vena cava grafts. Influence of increased flow. *Arch Surg* 1964; **89**: 1096.

69. Starzl TE, Kaupp HA, Beheler EM, Freeark RJ. The treatment of penetrating wounds of the inferior vena cava. *Surgery* 1962; **51**: 195.

70. Steenberg RW, Ravitch MM. Cervico-thoracic approach for subclavian vessel injury from compound fracture of the clavicle: considerations of subclavian–axillary exposures. *Ann Surg* 1963; **157**: 839.

71. Sullivan WG, Thornton FH, Baker LH, La Plante ES, Cohen A. Early influence of popliteal vein repair in the treatment of popliteal vessel injuries. *Am J Surg* 1971; **122**: 528.

72. Thompson BW, Read RC, Casali RE. Interposition grafting for portal hypertension. *Am J Surg* 1975; **130**: 733.

73. Travers B, Cooper A. *On Wounds and Ligature of Veins. Surgical Essays.* London. 1818; **1**: 243.

74. Treiman RL, Doty D, Caspar MR. Acute vascular trauma. A fifteen year study. *Am J Surg* 1966; **111**: 469.

75. Vollmar J. Plastiche eingriffe an den tiefen Venen. In Kappert A, May R (Eds) *Das postthrombotische Zustandsbild der extremitäten.* Bern. Hueber 1968.

76. Vollmar J. Venous trauma. In May R (Ed) *Surgery of the Veins of the Leg and Pelvis.* Stuttgart. Georg Thieme 1979.

77. Vollmar J. Venous trauma. *Maj Prob Clin Surg* 1977; **134**: 25.

78. Wood M. Penetrating wounds of the vena cava, recommendations for treatment. *Surgery* 1966; **60**: 311.

79. Zincola N, Hoffert PW, Haimovici H. Autogenous vein bypass grafts in the venous system; an experimental evaluation. *Bull Soc Int Chir* 1962; **21**: 265.

26

Venous tumours

In this chapter the word 'tumour' is interpreted literally as *a mass* so that three rare conditions of the veins can be discussed – cystic mucoid degeneration of the vein wall, cavernous haemangioma and leiomyoma/leiomyosarcoma. All these conditions may present as a palpable mass or with the sequelae of major vein obstruction. Only leiomyoma/leiomyosarcoma is a true neoplasm.

Cystic degeneration of the vein wall

Cystic degeneration in the wall of an artery was first reported in 1947[6] in the external iliac artery and has since been observed in the popliteal, radial, ulnar and other small arteries. It was first described in a vein in 1963.[35]

Pathology

All reports describe this lesion as a cystic swelling in the wall of a vein containing a transparent gelatinous material which is similar to that found in a subcutaneous ganglion.

The cyst lies between the media and adventitia and has a collagenous wall. Collections of acid mucin-like material are also found between the fibromuscular tissues as well as in the cavity of the cyst. The wall on the luminal side of the cyst retains an endothelial covering (Fig. 26.1).

No analyses of vein cyst contents have been reported but the analysis of the contents of popliteal artery adventitial cysts shows the material to be a mucoprotein with little or no hydroxyproline; this finding suggests that it is not derived from collagen.[28] The true origin and nature of these cysts is yet to be determined. The veins reported to have been affected are the iliac veins,[17] the common femoral vein,[4,19,22] and the subcutaneous veins at the ankle and wrist.[38] All these sites are close to joints; this is a feature of subcutaneous ganglions, and it has been suggested that the common subcutaneous ganglion may begin in a very small blood vessel.[20]

Clinical presentation

The patient presents with a lump or with the symptoms of venous obstruction. The lump itself is not usually painful or tender. It is often impalpable and is usually too deep for fluctuation to be felt. Cysts on subcutaneous veins may be single or multiple and cause few problems other than mild aching pain and disfigurement. Cysts on the femoral vein tend to present with venous obstruction (swelling, superficial venous distention and venous claudication) before the patient notices a lump.

Investigation

The diagnosis of venous compression or obstruction is made by phlebography. The vein may be stenosed or totally occluded. Occlusion or compression indicates the site of the problem but gives no hint of the diagnosis. A stenosis, especially if it is asymmetrical, suggests an external lesion and should raise the suspicion of a vein wall cyst, even though extrinsic lesions (e.g. lymphadenopathy) are far more likely causes of venous compression.

The presence of a cystic mass can sometimes be confirmed with ultrasound but is best seen with computerized tomography (CT) scanning. The combination of a CT scan and phlebogram should pinpoint the size and position of the lesion, and its radiodensity gives a clue to its nature.

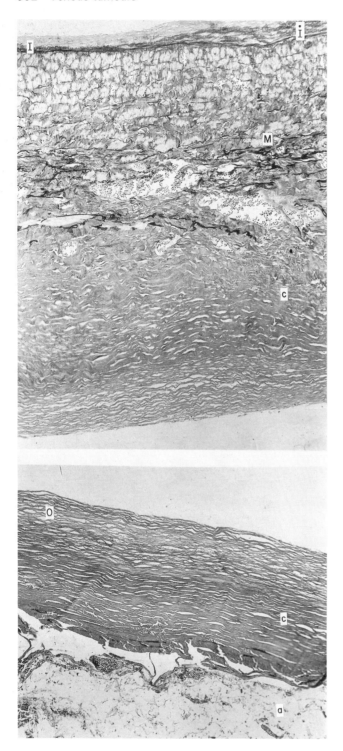

Fig. 26.1 Photomicrographs of the inner
(I) and outer (O) walls of a femoral vein wall
cyst. The inner wall consists of intima (i)
and medial smooth muscle (M); the outer
wall consists of adventitia (A) and laminae
of collagen (C) suggesting that the cyst
developed between the adventitial and
medial layers.

Lymphangiography may be required to exclude compression by enlarged lymph nodes. These tumours must be differentiated from leiomyosarcomata and extrinsic compression because their treatment is so different.

Treatment

The lesion should be explored and fully exposed. Two methods of treatment are possible, total excision of the whole vein and vein replacement or evacuation and partial excision of the cyst. At operation these cysts feel cystic and look bluish in colour. If the CT scan shows a mass with a radiolucent fluid-like content, it is safe to confirm the diagnosis at operation by aspiration or frozen section. If jelly-like material is obtained, the lumen can be restored by removing either the outer wall of the cyst, without opening the vein, or the inner wall of the cyst, through a venotomy. The latter approach is advisable if there is any suggestion of intraluminal thrombus at the site of the venous constriction. If the outer wall can be removed without opening the vein, the risk of postoperative thrombosis is almost certainly reduced. The patient should be given a course of heparin after the operation.

There is a small chance of recurrence if only one wall of the cyst, inner or outer, is removed because the mucoid degeneration has usually spread into the tissues around the cyst (see Fig. 26.1).

If there is any doubt about the pathology of the lesion, it should be treated as if it was a neoplasm and should be completely excised together with a segment of vein. The vein may then have to be reconstructed with a vein graft or prosthesis.

Venous (cavernous) haemangioma

Venous haemangiomata are formed from venular capillaries, venules and large veins. Those derived from venules form skin lesions (e.g. the port wine stain). Malformations of large veins often occur in association with other congenital abnormalities, for example the Klippel-Trenaunay syndrome, but they are commonly connected to other abnormal veins in the limb and are not usually an independant abnormality (see Chapter 23).

Venous haemangioma which occur in an otherwise normal limb present a distinct clinical problem.

Pathology

The blood vessels in early fetal life form a network of undifferentiated tubes. Between the fifth and tenth week of intra-uterine life the vessels begin to organize into the system which we recognize in adult life.[42] It is believed that most vascular abnormalities begin as a failure of organization in this period. A venous haemangioma is a collection of large dilated disorganized veins which drain into a normal venous system. They are not true neoplasms and would be better described as hamartomata than as angiomata. They do not undergo malignant change. We are not aware of any reports of malignant venous haemangiosarcomas. They commonly occur in the subcutaneous tissues and between the muscles of the limbs but often extend into adjacent skin, muscle, and, occasionally, into bone. The upper and lower limbs are equally affected. They fluctuate in size but tend to progressively distend and enlarge. Thrombophlebitis and calcification of the thrombus to produce 'phleboliths' are common complications. It is unusual for these tumours to seriously affect the function of adjacent or even extensively involved muscles but muscular exercise may damage the veins and precipitate thrombosis or haemorrhage. Joint movements may be affected, and flexion deformities may develop if the veins protrude into the joint cavity and cause recurrent haemarthroses. The overall size of the limb is not affected, as it is in the Klippel-Trenaunay syndrome.

The arteries of the limb are normal. Some venous angiomata are associated with lymphatic dilatation and lymph reflux.

Clinical presentation

Most patients present in their early years when they or their parents notice a *variable swelling* in the limb with dilated veins in or under the skin or a bluish discoloration of the skin (Fig. 26.2a and b, Colour plate 36).[5]

When a venous haemangioma is deep within the limb, there may be no visible mass and the only complaint is of pain.

The nature of the pain varies. It is usually a dull

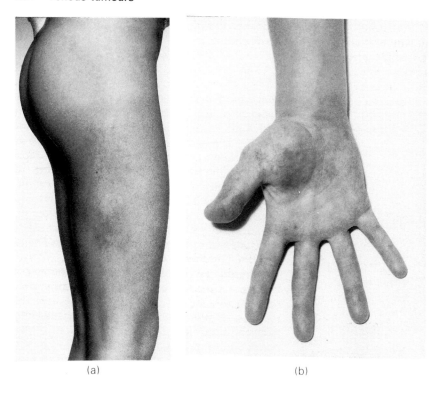

(a)

(b)

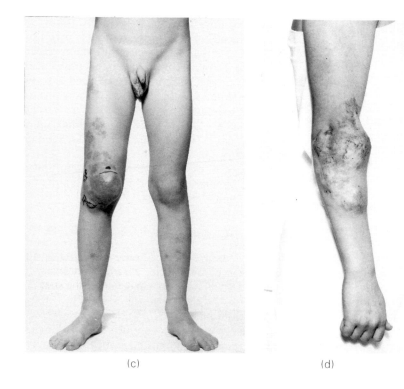

(c)

(d)

Fig. 26.2 Four examples of venous angiomata.

(a) A soft variable swelling on the lateral aspect of the thigh. This angioma is in the subcutaneous tissues, and there are only minor changes in the overlying skin.

(b) A venous angioma involving the skin, subcutaneous tissues and muscles of the thenar eminence and the thumb.

(c) A venous angioma involving the skin and subcutaneous tissues over the right knee but not extending into the knee joint or quadriceps femoris muscle.

(d) A venous angioma involving the skin and subcutaneous tissues over the lateral and posterior aspects of the right elbow joint. The joint was not involved but the lesion extended deep into the extensor muscles of the forearm.

ache which may be present at all times, but worse when the limb is dependent and relieved by elevation. This type of pain is probably caused by the tension of venous distention.

Sharp tingling sensations or areas of cutaneous sensory loss may occur if a haemangioma involves a nerve.

Episodes of haemorrhage or thrombophlebitis, which are usually related to local trauma, can cause severe pain. Haematomata and bruising may appear, and tender masses of venous thrombosis may be palpable. These painful episodes usually subside within 5–10 days.

The pain may be exacerbated by exercise if the haemangioma is infiltrating a muscle or bulging into a joint. An extensive haemangioma in the quadriceps femoris muscle can cause so much pain on walking that a child may develop a fixed flexion deformity of the knee.

Sudden swelling and stiffness of a joint, commonly the knee joint, may be caused by an acute serous effusion or bleeding into the joint.

Repeated knee or hip joint irritation may cause muscle spasm, deformity, limping, and secondary scoliosis and back pain; all these complications are severely disabling (Fig. 26.3).

Examination reveals a soft *compressible* mass which collapses when raised above the level of the heart but becomes tight and distended when dependent or if the downstream veins are occluded with a tourniquet. There may be a venular naevus in the overlying skin (Fig. 26.2c and d). If the lesion is in the subcutaneous tissues, it will give the skin a dark blue tinge. Although the mass is compressible, there may be hard nodules within it – the remnants of episodes of thrombosis.

The muscles and arteries of the limb are usually normal but nearby joints may contain an effusion and joint movements may be limited. Venous angiomata may involve nerves and cause motor and sensory neurological defects. Multiple venous haemangiomata are uncommon in contrast to multiple capillary haemangiomata (strawberry naevi) which are common.

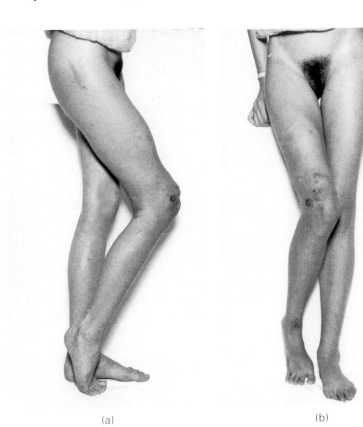

(a)

(b)

Fig. 26.3 This patient has an extensive venous angioma involving the knee joint and quadriceps femoris muscle. Recurrent episodes of pain and haemarthroses have caused a fixed flexion deformity of the knee and ankle joints. The knee joint had to be arthrodesed and the Achilles tendon had to be lengthened to restore walking to normal.

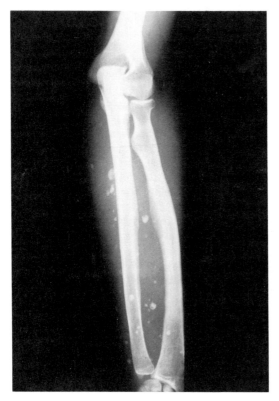

Fig. 26.4 A plain X-ray of a forearm with an extensive deep venous angioma containing many phleboliths.

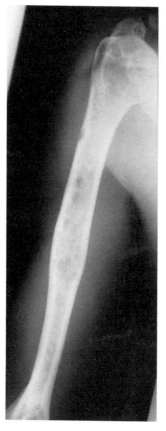

Fig. 26.5 The X-ray of a humerus in an arm with a deep intramuscular and intraosseus venous angioma. The large veins in the bone are visible as multiple X-ray lucent areas.

Investigation

The most useful information is obtained from plain and contrast radiography. A plain film may show the mass and many phleboliths (Fig. 26.4). Nearby bone may show translucent areas if there are dilated veins within it (Fig. 26.5).

A Doppler flow detector is useful when delineating the extent of the lesion and excluding arteriovenous fistulae.

Ascending phlebography usually shows normal axial veins but may fail to fill the haemangioma. It is, however, important to know that the deep axial veins are normal before considering surgical excision (Fig. 26.6a and b).

The extent and the size of the haemangioma are best displayed by a direct injection into one of its veins (Fig. 26.7a and b). This is easy to carry out when the lesion is subcutaneous and visible, but not as easy to perform when it lies deep beneath the muscles; in these circumstances the venous

phase of an arteriogram may reveal the full extent of the lesion more clearly. An arterial phlebogram using digital subtraction angiography is sometimes helpful (Fig. 26.8).

A CT scan after the intravenous injection of a radio-opaque contrast medium will show the relationships between the lesion and nearby muscles, arteries, nerves and joints (Fig. 26.9a and b). Neurovascular bundles are often closely related to deep intermuscular venous haemangiomata.

Arthrography and arthroscopy are important investigations if there are joint symptoms. The filling defects caused by veins bulging into the joint can be enhanced by a tourniquet placed around the limb to produce venous congestion. Joint involvement may also be seen on the venous phase of an arteriogram (Fig. 26.10a and b).

At arthroscopy (through an unaffected part of

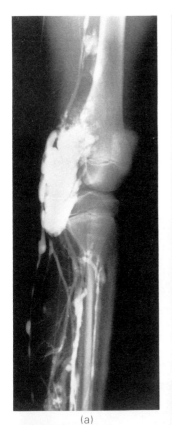
(a)

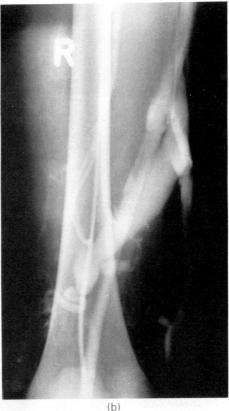
(b)

Fig. 26.6 (a) An ascending phlebogram filling a large venous angioma behind the knee and some abnormal veins in the mid calf.

(b) An ascending phlebogram filling the large draining vessel of a venous angioma in the lower thigh but failing to fill the many veins draining into it.

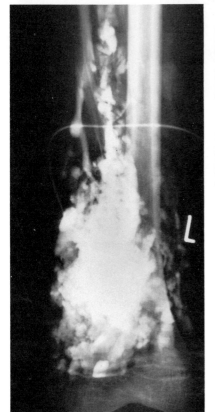
(a)

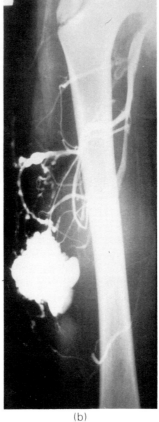
(b)

Fig. 26.7 (a) A direct injection into a venous angioma on the medial side of the lower thigh showing that the lesion extends to the lateral side of the femur and far higher up the thigh than the visible mass had suggested.

(b) A direct injection into a venous angioma on the lateral aspect of the thigh showing that it drains into tributaries of the deep femoral vein.

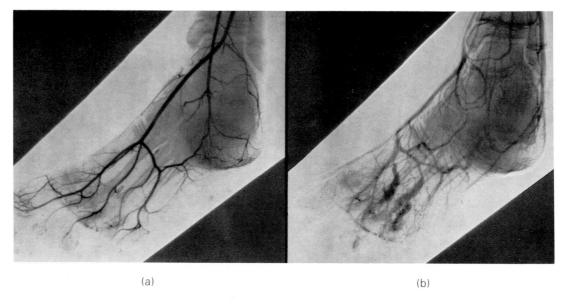

(a)   (b)

Fig. 26.8   (a) The arterial and (b) venous phases of an intra-arterial digital subtraction angiogram. The venous phase reveals the large draining veins of a venous angioma lying deep in the foot between the metatarsal bones.

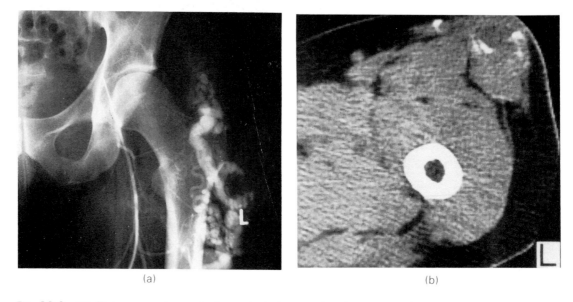

(a)   (b)

Fig. 26.9   (a) The venous phase of a femoral arteriogram showing an extensive venous angioma in the upper thigh.
  (b) The CT scan with vascular enhancement of the same patient showing that the lesion is entirely subcutaneous. Some of the large veins can be seen filled with contrast medium.

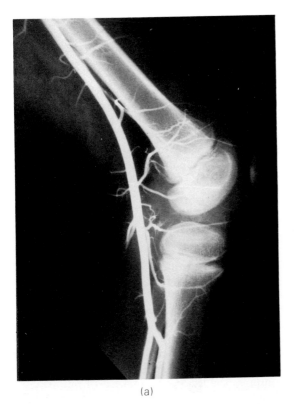
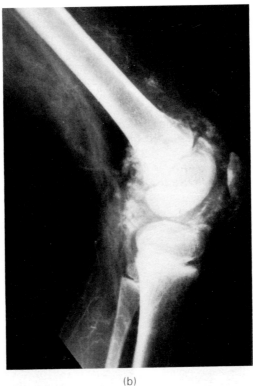

(a)   (b)

Fig. 26.10   (a) The arteriogram of a patient with a large venous angioma around the knee. The arteries are normal; this confirms that no arteriovenous fistulae are present.

(b) The venous phase of the same arteriograph showing an extensive angioma closely related to the synovium of the joint and extending into the quadriceps femoris muscles.

the synovium) the veins can be seen to bulge into the joint making the synovium bosselated and blue.

Arteriography and lymphography are not indicated, unless there is some clinical indication of an arterial or lymphatic abnormality.

Any weakness of the limb should be investigated with a careful neurological examination and, if indicated, electromyography. Clinical examination and phlebography usually exclude the main differential diagnoses (e.g. arteriovenous fistulae, other vascular tumours, lymphangioma circumscriptum and simple varicose veins). When in doubt, all the investigations mentioned above may be necessary, followed on rare occasions, by an incisional biopsy which is a haemorrhagic and difficult procedure.

Treatment

Venous haemangiomata are difficult to excise but complete excision is the best form of treatment. Sclerotherapy with irritant chemicals or boiling water is risky and fails because of the capaciousness of the veins. Venous haemangiomata do not have a large arterial blood supply and therefore embolization is of no help.

Before excision is contemplated, the major axial veins should be shown to be normal and the extent and anatomical relationships of the lesion should be defined as accurately as possible. The patient must be fully appraised of the size of the operation and any likely sequelae (e.g. nerve or joint damage).

Superficial lesions

Superficial lesions are best excised through a longitudinal incision over the mass and through a bloodless field provided by a tourniquet.[30,40] It is important to mark the extent of the lesion before applying the tourniquet, as it may not be visible once the limb is exsanguinated. Involved skin and all the subcutaneous tissue containing the large veins can be excised within the limits imposed by the blood supply of the skin flaps. If it is not possible to remove the whole haemangioma, it can be transected, its cut edge oversewn to prevent bleeding, and the residual abnormality removed through another incision at a second stage operation, 3–6 months later. Subcutaneous nerves are difficult to identify in the middle of a mass of veins and may have to be excised leaving small patches of anaesthetic skin on the limb. This is not a serious complication, provided the nerves at the wrist and ankle which supply the hand and foot are not damaged. The skin must be closed over suction drainage and compressed firmly to reduce the considerable chance of haematoma formation.

Pain in the wound is an indication for early wound inspection. If a large haematoma is found, it should be evacuated as soon as possible. Skin necrosis is an important and undesirable complication. It is usually caused by tension in the skin, secondary to a haematoma or a misguided attempt to achieve a primary closure when too much skin has been excised. Necrotic skin must be excised and the defect covered with a split skin graft after the tendency of the tissues to bleed has stopped and some healthy granulation tissue has formed. Grafting onto any tissue that contains residual haemangioma that might bleed or ooze serum carries a high risk of a further haematoma developing beneath the graft. If a large area of skin has to be excised, the defect can be covered with a rotation or pedicle skin flap or with a vascularized free skin flap.

Deep lesions

Deep venous haemangiomata should also be explored through a bloodless field. A long incision should be made, extending beyond the limits of the lesion, and the deep compartment of the limb should be opened to identify, isolate and protect any major blood vessels or nerves that may be passing through or near to the angioma.

The superficial and lateral surfaces of the angioma are then exposed, until it is possible to see if the angioma can be separated from the surrounding structures, whether any major arteries or nerves pass through it and whether any muscle is extensively involved.

*Inter*muscular angiomata can usually be removed; the last phase is the careful dissection of the mass from any adjacent artery and veins. In the upper limb, deep veins such as the brachial vein can be removed because the superficial veins provide an adequate outflow tract. In the lower limb the main axial veins above the knee must, if possible, be preserved; below the knee one or two pairs of the crural veins can be excised without affecting calf pump function.

*Intra*muscular angiomata are difficult to remove without excising the muscle, and the symptoms rarely justify excising a whole muscle (e.g. the biceps humeris or quadriceps femoris). When a large mass of veins occupies a major part of an important muscle we prefer to obliterate the whole mass with large continuous encircling stitches of a non-absorbable material, for example silk or braided polyethylene. The mass must be dissected clear on three sides, and the deep aspects must not contain a major nerve or artery. A large continuous stitch is then placed around the whole mass. The encircling turns should be approximately 1 cm apart and run the whole length of the mass. The object is to compress the lesion and make it thrombose, yet retain some muscle function and the contours of the limb. When the procedure is completed, the mass looks like a tied up roll of meat. We have found this method to be an effective way of obliterating the mass and stopping the pain, yet preserving function. The same approach can be used on the remnant of a haemangioma when only part of it can be excised.

When the angioma involves a nerve, individual bundles of nerve fibres may be separated by the veins and may be difficult to see. The surgeon must then decide whether to excise the nerve or leave haemangiomatous tissue inside the nerve. The symptoms rarely justify excising a major nerve.

A venous haemangioma which is bulging into a joint should be excised if it is causing recurrent effusions or haemarthroses. It is unusual to be able to excise all the angioma and leave the synovium intact but, fortunately, most of the synovium can be removed from a joint without seriously affecting joint mobility, provided the patient has vigorous postoperative physiotherapy to restore full movement.

In our experience, the joint most often involved is the knee joint, in association with a venous haemangioma in the deep anterior compartment of the thigh. In this situation the abnormal veins in the fat, deep to the rectus femoris muscle, the synovium of the supra-patella pouch, and the synovium on either side of the patella down to the level of the knee joint can be excised with the overlying subcutaneous veins without damaging knee movements. Extensive involvement of the vastus medialis or lateralis is treated by the encircling suture technique. After releasing the tourniquet, it is essential to obtain perfect haemostasis to prevent blood collecting in the joint. Suction drainage and compression are mandatory. Quadriceps exercises must start the day after the operation, but joint movements should not begin for 4–5 days. We have not seen a venous angioma involving the ankle, hip or shoulder joint but have seen two venous angiomata in the back of the arm which impinged upon the elbow joint.

Some young patients who have extensive haemangiomata in and around the knee joint experience severe pain and muscle spasms and develop secondary flexion deformities of the knee joint which cannot be overcome with physiotherapy (see Fig. 26.3). In four patients with this problem we have had to arthrodese the knee joint because the limb shortening resulting from the fixed flexion of the knee was causing a progressing flexion deformity of the hip and ankle and a lumbar scoliosis.

Leiomyoma and leiomyosarcoma of the vein wall

Tumours of smooth muscle are rare; this is surprising in view of the ubiquity of smooth muscle especially in the vascular system. Leiomyosarcomata arising from veins are reported to be more common than those arising from arteries.

The distinction between a benign and low grade malignant smooth muscle tumour is a histological nicety which accounts for the fact that between 1871 and 1984, 93 leiomyosarcomata have been reported[26] whereas only one leiomyoma has been described.[31] For practical purposes, it is wise to assume that all smooth muscle tumours arising in veins are sarcomas with differing degrees of malignancy.

Pathology

The incidence of leiomyosarcomata of the

inferior vena cava found incidentally *post mortem* is probably less than 1 in 25,000;[1,24] the clinical incidence is far less. Most vascular surgeons see only one or two of these tumours in a lifetime. Tumours in the inferior vena cava seem to be more common than tumours in other veins.[25] Tumours in the superior vena cava are very rare.[15] Vena caval tumours are said to occur more often in females than in males but tumours in other veins occur equally in the two sexes.[8,25]

Leiomyosarcomata have a lobulated, grey–pink appearance with a thin fibrous capsule. Histologically, they look like uterine fibroids because they consist of whirls of smooth muscle cells, but they contain a variable number of large, densely-staining nuclei at various stages of mitosis which betray their malignant potential (Fig. 26.11). They tend to grow away from their origin in the wall of a vein, displacing nearby structures rather than infiltrating them, but they can grow along the vein wall and spread within its lumen in a downstream direction. This form of spread blocks the mouths of the tributary veins but the tumour rarely spreads down the lumen of a tributary against the blood flow. Although these tumours are slow growing, they are malignant and ultimately metastasize; only 14 of the 35 patients reviewed by Keiffer were alive 2 years after operation.[26] These tumours must therefore be considered highly malignant, whatever their histological áppearance.

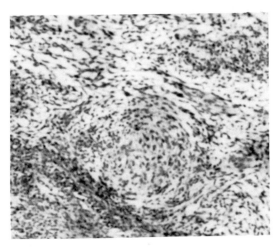

Fig. 26.11 A photomicrograph of a leiomyosarcoma that arose from the wall of the deep femoral vein. It shows the typical whorls of cells with nuclei in different stages of mitosis.

A leiomyosarcoma arising in the wall of the uterus or a uterine myoma occasionally spreads into the lumen of the vena cava and is mistakenly diagnosed as primary vena cava leiomyosarcoma.[7,11]

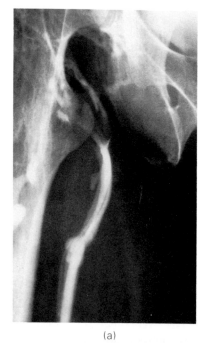

(a)

Clinical presentation

The symptoms and signs depend upon the site of the tumour and its effect on its vein of origin.

Leiomyosarcomata of the inferior vena cava These tumours grow slowly and may not cause symptoms for many years. Abdominal pain is a common feature and is often misinterpreted as indigestion. The pain may radiate to the groin or loin. The patient may complain of swelling of the legs, dilated veins on the abdominal wall and abdominal distention caused by compression or, rarely, by thrombosis of the vena cava.[21]

Examination reveals leg oedema, collateral veins, sometimes an upper abdominal mass slightly to the right-hand side, hepatomegaly and ascites.

When the tumour is below the renal veins the symptoms are mainly of pain and vena caval obstruction. The most common site of origin of

Fig. 26.12 (a) The phlebogram of a patient with a large leiomyosarcoma in the thigh. The deep femoral vein is stretched around the mass, and the upper part of the common femoral vein contains projecting tumour thrombus.

(b) The CT scan of the same patient showing a large homogeneous mass in the upper thigh.

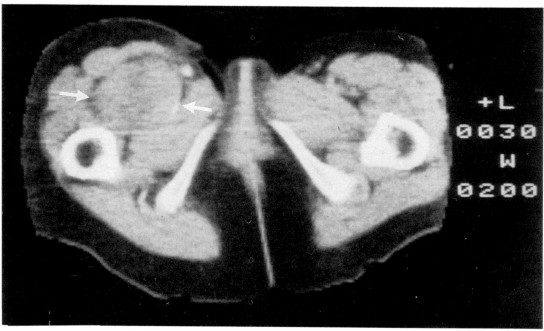

(b)

inferior vena caval tumours is the segment between the renal and hepatic veins. This causes pain and sometimes the symptoms and signs of vena caval obstruction, but it rarely causes uraemia or renal failure, as the slow occlusion of the renal veins allows time for collaterals to develop.

A high tumour at or above the hepatic veins can cause the Budd–Chiari syndrome – ascites, hepatomegaly and jaundice.[10,29,33] Leiomyosarcomata occasionally present with a pyrexia.[16]

Leiomyosarcomata of the iliac and femoral veins These present with pain, a mass, or signs of venous obstruction – oedema and distended veins.[27,39] When a mass is palpable it is usually painful and tender. The patient illustrated in Fig. 26.12 (a and b) had pain in the upper part of the thigh for 10 years, and three surgical explorations of the groin were carried out in different hospitals before a mass appeared and a fourth exploration revealed a leiomyosarcoma arising from a deep tributary of the deep femoral vein. The pain which the patient had experienced for 10 years had been caused by a stretched obturator nerve.

The venous obstruction may cause oedema, but it is often asymptomatic, as it develops slowly and the collaterals are usually good. Venous claudication is rarely seen as a presenting symptom.

It is unusual for patients with leiomyosarcomata to present with debility and weight loss, but these tumours can spread to the lungs and ultimately death is caused by disseminated secondary disease.

Investigations

Phlebography and CT scanning are the most useful investigations (Fig. 26.12a and b). Phlebography defines the venous anatomy, the site of origin of the tumour and the extent of the collateral circulation. CT scanning defines the size of the tumour and its relationship to the surrounding structures.

Gastrointestinal investigations which are ordered because of an incorrect diagnosis of indigestion may reveal a retroperitoneal mass displacing the duodenum, stomach or kidney. Ultrasound can detect a retroperitoneal mass but does not provide the anatomical detail provided by a CT scan.[37,43]

Retrograde catheterization of the vena cava via an arm vein may be needed to obtain a phlebograph that shows the veins above a caval occlusion.

Careful renal and liver function studies must be carried out in patients with vena caval tumours. It may be necessary to measure portal vein pressure and to obtain a liver biopsy.

These tumours are not very vascular and arteriography is therefore not helpful.[14,36] The other causes of similar symptoms (e.g. gastroenterological problems, retroperitoneal tumours and vena caval thrombosis) should be detected by the above investigations.

In spite of the possibility of making a preoperative diagnosis on the basis of all these investigations, the symptoms and signs of vena caval tumours can be so vague that the diagnosis is first made at a laparotomy. When this occurs it is wise to obtain a biopsy and stop the operation so that detailed investigations can be performed and a planned approach to treatment can be formulated.

Treatment

Leiomyosarcomata arising from peripheral limb veins should be treated by wide excision as for any other low grade sarcoma, if possible by compartmentectomy.[27,39] This is often difficult, as these tumours arise from blood vessels which are commonly between, not within, the fascial compartments of the limb. Fortunately, most leiomyosarcomata have a capsule and rarely infiltrate adjacent muscle and bone; they can therefore be dissected free of the surrounding tissues, even though the vessel from which they arise must be excised. This may mean excising the femoral or iliac vein. If the vein is already totally occluded and the symptoms of the venous occlusion are not severe, the excised vein does not need to be replaced provided the collateral veins are not disturbed. If swelling or bursting pain becomes a problem after the operation and all of the tumour has been excised, the excised segment of vein may be replaced with a segment of autogenous vein (e.g. saphenous vein) or a prosthesis (e.g. supported PTFE).

Residual tumour should be irradiated, though these tumours are not very radiosensitive. Leiomyosarcomata are not sensitive to chemotherapy.

Leiomyosarcomata of the inferior vena cava

These tumours have become susceptible to surgical treatment since the advent of venous bypass grafting.

Tumours below the renal veins can be excised with removal of as much of the vena cava as necessary. If a pedunculated tumour is excised with a small piece of vein wall, the vena cava can be sutured or repaired with a patch. The whole infrarenal vena cava can be ligated and excised if necessary.[34] After this operation the patient is likely to develop bilateral leg oedema but this is a relatively small price to pay for complete excision of the tumour. It is better not to replace the vena cava with a prosthesis at the time of the excision to avert the risk of postoperative graft thrombosis and pulmonary embolism. Replacement of the vena cava should be carried out at a later date with a PTFE prosthesis if the patient has symptoms and when it is clear that the patient has no recurrent disease.[25]

By the time they are discovered, tumours between the renal and hepatic veins are usually large and have to be treated by a complete resection of the vena cava from its origin to just below the hepatic veins. The right kidney may have to be removed if its pedicle is involved in the tumour. If the pedicle is not involved, both it and the left renal vein can be tied without causing renal failure because genital, adrenal, and lumbar veins dilate to act as collateral vessels, provided the vein is ligated on the caval side of these vessels.[3,9,13,23,32] Sometimes the left renal vein can be anastomosed to the upper or lower stump of the vena cava. A healthy right kidney that has to have part of its vein excised can be transplanted into the iliac fossa. Reconstruction of the vena cava with a prosthesis and implantation of the renal veins into the prosthesis is rarely indicated.[2]

Tumours at or above the hepatic veins are usually impossible to remove because the tumour has usually spread into the hepatic veins or the liver. Hepatic lobectomy and upper vena caval replacement has been performed when one of the hepatic veins was free of tumour. The success of liver transplantation now presents the possibility of performing a liver and upper vena caval transplant after complete excision of the tumour mass.

When the tumour cannot be excised and the patient has the Budd–Chiari syndrome, some form of portal–systemic shunt should be considered (e.g. a portal or mesenteric–atrial shunt).[12]

References

1. Abell MR. Leiomyosarcoma of the inferior vena cava. *Am J Clin Pathol* 1957; **28**: 272.
2. Adebonojo SA, Atil PC, Christiansen KH, Stainback WC, Williams KR. Acute ligation of inferior vena cava above renal veins. A clinical and experimental appraisal of graft replacement of inferior vena cava above renal veins. *J Cardiovasc Surg* 1973; **14**: 508.
3. Annetts DL, Graham AB. Cystic degeneration of the femoral vein. *Br J Surg* 1980; **67**: 287.
4. Arland R. Venous angiomas. *Phlebologie* 1980; **33**: 547.
5. Atkins HB, Key JA. A case of myxomatous tumour arising in the adventitia of the left external iliac artery. *Br J Surg* 1947; **34**: 426.
6. Baggish MS. Mesenchymal tumours of the uterus. *Clin Obstet Gynaecol* 1947; **17**: 51.
7. Bailey RV, Stribling J, Weitzner S, Hardy JD. Leiomyosarcoma of the inferior vena cava. *Ann Surg* 1976; **184**: 169.
8. Beck AD. Resection of the suprarenal inferior vena cava for retroperitoneal malignant disease. *J Urol* 1979; **121**: 112.
9. Brewster DC, Athanasoulis CA, Darling RC. Leiomyosarcoma of the inferior vena cava. *Arch Surg* 1976; **111**: 1081.
10. Cameron AEP, Graham JC, Cotton LT. Intracaval leiomyomatosis. *Br J Obstet Gynaecol* 1983; **90**: 272.
11. Cameron JL, Herlong HF, Sanfey H, Boitnott J, Kaufman SL, Gott VL, Maddrey WC. The Budd Chiari syndrome: Treatment by mesenteric–systemic venous shunts. *Ann Surg* 1983; **198**: 335.
12. Caplan BB, Halasz NA, Bloomer WE. Resection and ligation of the suprarenal inferior vena cava. *J Urol* 1964; **92**: 25.
13. Chauhan MA, Smith PL, Ferris EJ, Murphy K, Westbrook K, Slayden JE. Leiomyosarcoma of the inferior vena cava: Angiographic and computed tomography findings. *Cardiovasc Intervent Radiol* 1981; **4**: 209.
14. Couinaud C. Tumeurs de la veine cava inferieure. *J Chir (Paris)* 1973; **105**: 411.
15. Flores Torre M, Merino Angulo J, Villaneuva Marcos R, Aguirre Errasti C. Leiomyosarcome de la veine cave inferieure revele par un syndrome febrile. *Nouv Presse Med* 1981; **10**: 3493.
16. Frileux CI, Le Baleur A, Uzan E. Obstruction of the iliac vein by mucoid cyst. *J Cardiovasc Surg* 1979; **20**: 517.
17. Fujiwara Y, Cohn LH, Adams D, Collins JJ. Use of Gore-Tex grafts for replacement of the superior and inferior venae cavae. *J Thorac Cardiovasc Surg* 1974; **67**: 774.

18. Fyfe NCM, Silcocks PB, Browse NL. Cystic mucoid degeneration in the wall of the femoral vein. *J Cardiovasc Surg* 1980; **21**: 703.

19. Ghadially FN, Mehta PN. Multifunctional mesenchymal cells resembling smooth muscle cells in ganglia of the wrist. *Ann Rheum Dis* 1971; **30**: 31.

20. Goerttler U, Noldge G, Baumeister I, Bohn N. Cava Verschluss-Syndrome durch ein Leiomyosarkom der Vena Cava inferior. *Radiologie* 1977; **17**: 350.

21. Gomez-Ferrer F. Cystic degeneration of the wall of the femoral vein. *J Cardiovasc Surg* 1966; 7: 162.

22. Greenfield LJ, Peyton JWR, Crute S. Hemodynamics and renal function following experimental suprarenal vena caval occlusion. *Surg Gynec Obstet* 1982; **155**: 37.

23. Hallock CJ, Watson CJ, Berman L. Primary tumour of the vena cava with clinical features suggestive of Chiari's disease. *Arch Intern Med* 1940; **66**: 50.

24. Kevorkian J, Cento DP. Leiomyosarcoma of large arteries and veins. *Surgery* 1973; **73**: 390.

25. Kieffer E, Berrod JL. Chometter G. Primary tumours of the inferior vena cava. In Bergan JJ, Yao JS (Eds) *Surgery of the Veins*. Orlando. Grune & Stratton 1985; 423.

26. Larmi TKI, Niinimaki T. Leiomyosarcoma of the femoral vein. *J Cardiovasc Surg* 1974; **15**: 602.

27. Lewis GJT, Douglas DM, Reid W, Kennedy Watt J. Cystic adventitial disease of the popliteal artery. *Br Med J* 1967; **2**: 411.

28. Lintner F, Faust U, Nowotny C. Ein malignen entartetes primares Leiomyom der Vena Cava inferior (Leiomyosarkom) unter dem klinishen Bild des Chiari–Buddschen Syndromes. *Wien Klin Wochenschr* 1978; **90**: 485.

29. Lofgren EP, Lofgren KA. Surgical treatment of cavernous haemangiomas. *Surgery* 1985; **97**: 474.

30. Mandelbaum I, Pauletto FJ, Nasser WK. Resection of a leiomyoma of the inferior vena cava that produced tricuspid valvular obstruction. *J Thorac Cardiovasc Surg* 1974; **67**: 561.

31. McCombs PR, Delaurentis DA. Division of the left renal vein: Guidelines and consequences. *Am J Surg* 1979; **138**: 257.

32. McDermott WV, Stone MD, Bothe A Jr, Trey C. Budd Chiari syndrome. *Am J Surg* 1984; **147**: 463.

33. Melchior E. Sarkom der Vena Cava inferior. *Deutsch Z Chir* 1928; **213**: 135.

34. Mentha C. La degenerescence mucoide des veines. *Presse Med* 1963; **71**: 2205.

35. Nyman U, Hellekant C, Jonsson K. Angiography in leiomyosarcoma of the inferior vena cava. *Br J Radiol* 1979; **52**: 273.

36. Picard JD, Denis P, Chambeyron Y, Dufour B, Lubrano JM, Orcel L, Premont M. Leiomyosarcomes de la veine cave inferieure. *Chirurgie* 1983; **109**: 306.

37. Rutner JR. Pathologie Radiologie und Chirugie de zystischen adventitia degeneration peripher blutgefasse. *Vasa* 1977; **6**: 94.

38. Taheri SA, Conner GW. Leiomyosarcoma of the iliac veins. *Surgery* 1983; **94**: 516.

39. Trout HH, McAllister HA, Giordano JM, Rich NM. Vascular malformations. *Surgery* 1985; **97**: 36.

40. Van Der Molen HR. Use of Doppler ultrasound in the examination of the extent of venous angiomas. *Phlebologie* 1976; **29**: 9.

41. Woollard HH. The development of the principal arterial stems in the forelimb of the pig. In *Contribution to Embryology*. Washington DC. Carnegie Institute of Washington 1921; Vol **14** No. 70; 141.

42. Young R, Friedman AC, Hartman DS. Computed tomography of leiomyosarcoma of the inferior vena cava. *Radiology* 1982; **145**: 99.

Index